Pharmacogenetics of Psychotropic Drugs

Pharmacogenetics and pharmacogenomics are areas of rapidly growing importance at the interface of molecular genetics and psychopharmacology, with implications for drug development and clinical practice. This book provides a conceptual framework for understanding and studying the pharmacogenetics of psychotropic drugs; it reviews advances in the field and describes the findings that have already emerged.

Coverage extends to antipsychotics, antidepressants, mood-stabilizing, cognitive-enhancing, and anxiolytic drugs. Chapters also examine the interface of pharmacogenetics with substance dependence and brain imaging, and consider the impact of pharmacogenetics on the biotechnology and pharmaceutical industries.

This book defines the young field of pharmacogenetics as it applies to psychotropic drugs and is, therefore, an essential reference for all clinicians and researchers working in this field.

Bernard Lerer is Professor of Psychiatry and Director of the Biological Psychiatry Laboratory at Hadassah–Hebrew University Medical Center in Jerusalem. He is Director of the National Institute for Psychobiology in Israel, and Editor-in-Chief of the *International Journal of Neuropsychopharmacology*.

Pharmacogenetics of
Psychotropic Drugs

Edited by

Bernard Lerer

Hadassah-Hebrew University Medical Center, Jerusalem, Israel

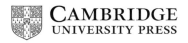
CAMBRIDGE
UNIVERSITY PRESS

PUBLISHED BY THE PRESS SYNDICATE OF THE UNIVERSITY OF CAMBRIDGE
The Pitt Building, Trumpington Street, Cambridge, United Kingdom

CAMBRIDGE UNIVERSITY PRESS
The Edinburgh Building, Cambridge CB2 2RU, UK
40 West 20th Street, New York, NY 10011-4211, USA
477 Williamstown Road, Port Melbourne, VIC 3207, Australia
Ruiz de Alarcón 13, 28014 Madrid, Spain
Dock House, The Waterfront, Cape Town 8001, South Africa

http://www.cambridge.org

© Cambridge University Press 2002

First published 2002

Printed in the United Kingdom at the University Press, Cambridge

Typeface Minion 8.5/12pt   *System* QuarkXPress™   [SE]

A catalogue record for this book is available from the British Library

Library of Congress Cataloguing in Publication data

Pharmacogenetics of psychotropic drugs / edited by Bernard Lerer.
    p.   cm.
  Includes bibliographical references and index.
  ISBN 0 521 80617 8 (hbk.)
    1. Psychotropic drugs.   2. Pharmacogenetics.   I. Lerer, Bernard.
RM315.P446   2002
615′.788–dc21   2001043946

ISBN 0 521 80617 8 hardback

Contents

v

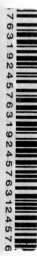

Contributors

Martin Alda
Department of Psychiatry, Dalhousie University, Abbie J. Lane Building, 5909 Jubilee Rd, Halifax, Nova Scotia, B3H 2E2, Canada

Larry Altsteil
Schering-Plough Research Institute, 2015 Galloping Hill Rd, Kenilworth, NJ 07033-1300, USA

Spilios V. Argyropoulos
Psychopharmacology Unit, University of Bristol, University Walk, Bristol BS8 1TD, UK

Maria J. Arranz
Institute of Psychiatry, De Crespigy Park, Denmark Hill, London SE5 8AF, UK

Thomas A. Ban
Vanderbilt University, Nashville, TN, USA

Vincenzo S. Basile
Neurogenetics Section, Centre for Addiction and Mental Health, University of Toronto, Toronto, Canada

Pierre Baumann
Department Universitaire de Psychiatrie Adulte, Adulte Hopital de Cery, CH-1008 Prilly, Switzerland

Jens Benninghoff
Department of Psychiatry, University of Wurzburg, Fuchsleinstr. 15, 97080 Wurzburg, Germany

Marco Catalano
IRCCS H. San Raffaele, Department of Neuropsychiatric Sciences, Milan, Italy

David A. Collier
Institute of Psychiatry, De Crespigy Park, Denmark Hill, London SE5 8AF, UK

Ariel Darvasi
The Life Sciences Institute, The Hebrew University of Jerusalem and IDgene Pharmaceuticals, Jerusalem 91904, Israel

Chin B. Eap
Department Universitaire de Psychiatrie Adulte, Adulte Hopital de Cery, CH-1008 Prilly, Switzerland

Thomas N. Ferraro
Center for Neurobiology and Behavior, Department of Psychiatry, University of Pennsylvania School of Medicine, 415 Curie Blvd, Philadelphia, PA 19104, USA

Joel Gelernter
Department of Psychiatry, Yale University
School of Medicine, New Haven, CT 06516,
USA

Linda K. Hutchinson
Department of Pharmacology, Vanderbilt
University, Nashville, TN 37232, USA

Angela D.M. Kashuba
School of Pharmacy, University of North
Carolina, Chapel Hill, NC, USA

Patrick G. Kehoe
Psychopharmacology Unit, University of
Bristol, University Walk, Bristol, BS8 1TD,
UK

James L. Kennedy
Neurogenetics Section, Centre for Addiction
and Mental Health, University of Toronto,
Toronto, Canada

Robert W. Kerwin
Institute of Psychiatry, De Crespigy Park,
Denmark Hill, London SE5 8AF, UK

Henry Kranzler
Department of Psychiatry, University of
Connecticut, School of Medicine,
Farmington, CT, USA

Bernard Lerer
Biological Psychiatry Laboratory,
Department of Psychiatry, Hadassah-
Hebrew University Medical Center, Ein
Karem, Jerusalem 91120, Israel

K. Peter Lesch
Department of Psychiatry, University of
Wurzburg, Fuchsleinstr. 15, 97080
Wurzburg, Germany

Fabio Macciardi
Unit of Biostatistics and Genetic
Epidemiology, Neurogenetics Section,
Clarke Division, Center for Addiction and
Mental Health, R-32, 250 College Street,
Toronto, Ontario, M5T 1R8, Canada

Anil K. Malhotra
Unit of Molecular Psychiatry, Hillside
Hospital, 75–59 263rd St, Glen Oaks, NY
11004, USA

Dalu Mancama
Institute of Psychiatry, De Crespigy Park,
Denmark Hill, London SE5 8AF, UK

Emanuela Mundo
Department of Psychiatry, University of
Wurzburg, Fuchsleinstr. 15, 97080
Wurzburg, Germany

Janet Munro
Institute of Psychiatry, De Crespigy Park,
Denmark Hill, London SE5 8AF, UK

Colleen M. Niswender
Department of Pharmacology, University of
Washington, Seattle, WA 98195, USA

David J. Nutt
Psychopharmacology Unit, University of
Bristol, University Walk, Bristol, BS8 1TD,
UK

Sarah Osborne
Institute of Psychiatry, De Crespigy Park,
Denmark Hill, London SE5 8AF, UK

Vural Ozdemir
Department of Pharmacogenomics, Drug
Discovery Division, R.W. Johnson
Pharmaceutical Research Institute, Route
202 South, #1000 OMP Building, Raritan,
NJ 08869, USA

Smita A. Pandit
Psychopharmacology Unit, University of
Bristol, University Walk, Bristol, BS8 1TD,
UK

Judes Poirier
Center for Studies in Aging, 6875 Blvd.
Lasalle, Verdun, Quebec, H4H 1R3, Canada

Steven G. Potkin
Brain Imaging Center, University of
California, Irvine Hall, Irvine, CA
92697–3960, USA

William Z. Potter
Lilly Research Laboratory, Lilly Corporate
Center, Drop Code 0532, Indianapolis, IA
46285, USA

Sheldon H. Preskorn
Psychiatric Research Institute, University of
Kansas, 1100 N. St Francis, Wichita, KS
67214, USA

Keith Schappert
Mirador DNA Design, Suite 501, 404 McGill
St, Montreal, Quebec H2Y 2G1, Canada

Angelina Schmitt
Department of Psychiatry, University of
Wurzburg, Fuchsleinstr. 15, 97080
Wurzburg, Germany

Ronnen H. Segman
Biological Psychiatry Laboratory,
Department of Psychiatry, Hadassah-
Hebrew University Medical Center, Ein
Karem, Jerusalem 91120, Israel

Pierre Savigny
Mirador DNA Design, Suite 501, 404 McGill
St, Montreal, Quebec H2Y 2G1, Canada

Anne Shalom
The Life Sciences Institute, The Hebrew
University of Jerusalem, Israel

AnnCatherine Van Lone
Lilly Research Laboratory, Lilly Corporate
Center, Drop Code 0532, Indianapolis, IA
46285, USA

Part I

Introduction

Genes and psychopharmacology: exploring the interface

Bernard Lerer

Biological Psychiatry Laboratory, Department of Psychiatry, Hadassah–Hebrew University Medical Center, Jerusalem, Israel

OVERVIEW

Pharmacogenetics is the study of genetically determined, interindividual differences in therapeutic response to drugs and susceptibility to adverse effects. The principal objective of pharmacogenetics is to identify and categorize the genetic factors that underlie these differences and to apply these observations in the clinic. Individualization of drug treatment to the specific patient is thus a core objective of pharmacogenetics. The goal of this book is to provide a basic conceptual framework for the pharmacogenetics of psychotropic drugs, to address major issues in the design and implementation of studies that seek to advance the field and to provide an overview of findings that have emerged so far. In this introductory chapter, the rationale for psychopharmacogenetics is considered, a brief historical perspective is provided, some of the pivotal concepts and terms are defined, important issues in the design and interpretation of pharmacogenetic studies in psychiatry are considered and optimistic predictions for the future are evaluated. The chapter concludes with a brief overview introducing the reader to the various sections of the book.

Introduction

For as long as medicine has been practiced, physicians have known that patients respond differently to the therapeutic agents that they are administered, even though there are no obvious differences in the nature or severity of their illnesses. Therefore, individual or illness characteristics that might aid the physician in choosing an appropriate treatment have long been sought. The principal objective of pharmacogenetics is to identify and categorize the genetic factors that underlie differences among individuals in their response to drugs and to apply these observations in the clinic.

The pharmacological treatment of psychiatric disorders has made rapid progress since the 1950s. Psychotropic drugs are among the most widely used pharmacological agents worldwide and their number has increased exponentially. These developments have occurred in spite of the highly complex clinical characteristics of psychiatric disorders and the absence of biological anchors for their diagnosis. Both these limitations are a consequence of the fact that the pathophysiological basis of most psychiatric disorders has not yet been defined. A role for genetic factors in the pathogenesis of many of the major psychiatric syndromes is well established. The advent of modern molecular techniques has led to an intensive search for susceptibility genes, efforts that have yielded intriguing leads but no definitive findings.

This book is positioned at the rapidly developing interface between molecular genetics and psychopharmacology. This area is closely related to the search for susceptibility genes but is also separate from it since genes that affect the therapeutic and adverse effects of the drugs used to treat an illness need not be involved in the pathogenesis of the illness. It is an exciting and increasingly productive interface that holds considerable promise. At the same time, the difficulties and complexities are clearly apparent and will grow more evident as optimistic predictions are submitted to empirical testing. The field holds exceptional fascination and it is still a wide-open frontier in that some of the most fundamental studies have yet to be conducted.

The area of basic concepts, experimental approaches and current findings is too large to be comprehensively addressed in a single volume. Nevertheless, there is a very great need to provide the researcher and clinician with an overview of the pivotal topics and to do so in an integrative way. This chapter is intended to serve as a general introduction to psychopharmacogenetics and to the topics covered in this book.

The rationale for psychopharmacogenetics

Whether medicine is an art or a science may seem an outdated, if not naive, debate at the dawn of the twenty-first century. This impression is bolstered by the extensive basis of modern medicine in biomedical science. Powerful diagnostic technology has immeasurably increased the precision of diagnosis, and evidence-based prescription is rapidly becoming a hallowed cornerstone of therapeutics. Yet, one needs to look no further than pharmacotherapy in order to realize how tenuous the scientific roots of our discipline still are. This is particularly true of the pharmacotherapy of psychiatric disorders but is by no means limited to this field. The psychiatrist who initiates drug treatment of a depressed patient is faced with a bewildering set of choices – at least five classes of drug if one applies current definitions, including tricyclic antidepressants, specific serotonin reuptake inhibitors, monoamine oxidase inhibitors and newer agents that specifically inhibit norepinephrine uptake or enhance synaptic availability of both norepinephrine and serotonin (5-hydroxytryptamine (5-HT)) by mechanisms other than reuptake. Within these classes there are subclasses and within each subclass individual drugs that differ from each other in the intensity or specificity of their pharmacological effects. The psychiatrist has no definitive way of knowing which patient will respond to which drug. There is very little hard evidence on which to base a rational choice, certainly not in the area of therapeutic efficacy. Usually the choice is made on the basis of adverse effect profiles or clinical experience.

The situation described is by no means limited to psychopharmacology. The neurologist treating epilepsy and the internist or pediatrician treating asthma (notwithstanding recent advances in the pharmacogenetics of this disorder) are in the similar position of having to make educated guesses regarding the choice of medication on the basis of a far from comprehensive set of evidence-based criteria. This situation is an inevitable consequence of the fact that modern, evidence-based therapeutics is by definition group and not individual oriented. Particularly in psychiatry, large numbers of patients are required to demonstrate unequivocally a significant drug–placebo difference, and drug–placebo differences are the cornerstone of evidence-based medicine. In cases where a drug is effective in two thirds of subjects (versus one third of subjects for placebo), efficacy may be unequivocally demonstrated, but a less appreciated element of the message is that one in three patients will not respond. Moreover, among responders to the active drug, at least one third might be placebo responders.

It is envisaged that pharmacogenetic predictors of response to drugs and of adverse effects will ultimately serve as the basis for simple diagnostic tests that can be applied in the clinic in order to prescribe the appropriate drug to the appropriate patient. In the current era of managed care in medicine and limited resources, this will be a development of major economic importance. As discussed in this chapter, the obstacles on the way to this objective are formidable but not insurmountable. Another very important application of pharmacogenetic screening will be in clinical trials. Knowledge of genetic predictors of response and/or adverse effects, even if this is not at a level of resolution that permits applicability in regular clinical practice, will permit stratification of patients in clinical trials. This will substantially reduce the cost of drug development and shorten the lengthy lag period that currently elapses until a drug is introduced into the clinic.

With the publication of the draft sequence of the human genome, it has become accepted practice to refer to the current era as "postgenomic." In this postgenomic era, pharmacogenetics, a discipline with a long and distinguished "pregenomic" history, has come of age. Powerful tools have been placed at its disposal and optimism abounds as to its anticipated impact on pharmacotherapy.

Historical perspective

Nebert (1997) suggests that Pythagoras was the first to recognize the basic principle of pharmacogenetics when, around 510 BC, he noted the predisposition of some individuals but not others to develop an adverse reaction (hemolytic anemia owing to glucose 6-phosphate dehydrogenase deficiency) after consumption of the fava bean. A century ago, the English physician Archibald Garrod suggested that genetic factors directed chemical transformations in humans. His ideas on the hereditary basis of chemical individuality are extensively discussed in his writings (Garrod, 1902, 1909). A seminal study was that of Snyder (1932), which defined the phenylthiourea nontasting phenomenon as an autosomal recessive trait. According to Propping and Nothen (1995), the relationship between adverse drug reactions and genetically determined variation was first demonstrated by Motulsky (1957). The term "pharmacogenetics" was coined by Vogel in 1959. Another important development was the observation that the antitubercular drug isoniazid could be slowly or rapidly acetylated and that this was under genetic control (Evans et al., 1960). A further milestone was the demonstration by Kalow of an abnormal form of serum cholinesterase that leads to catastrophic adverse reactions to succinylcholine. Kalow also wrote the first systematic account of pharmacogenetics (Kalow, 1962). Polymorphism of the P-450 enzyme now termed CYP2D6 was first observed in the 1970s in healthy volunteers who developed adverse effects when taking the antihypertensive agent debrisoquine. The enzyme was initially named debrisoquine hydroxylase but it was subsequently shown that oxidation of sparteine is by the same enzyme (Mahgoub et al., 1977; Eichelbaum et al., 1979).

For much of its history, the focus of pharmacogenetics has been on drug-metabolizing enzymes. This was because of the availability of techniques to detect phenotypic differences between individuals in the plasma level of drugs and to study their genetic basis. The focus on pharmacodynamic variation is more recent and was given considerable impetus by the advent of techniques to determine the sequence of genes and identify variations.

Definition of terms

Table 1.1 summarizes many of the terms that will be used frequently throughout this book. While *pharmacogenetics* is defined as the study of genetically determined interindividual differences in response to drugs, *pharmacogenomics* refers to the use of genome-based technologies in drug development. The fields are closely related and the terms are often used interchangeably. Nevertheless, it is useful to maintain the distinction because of the different starting points and outcomes. Pharmacogenetics is individual based and its body of information is derived from the relationship between drug effects and genetic predisposition in patients or volunteer subjects. Its outcome is rational drug choice in the treatment of patients, based on the evidence that has accumulated. The starting point of

Table 1.1. A pharmacogenetics glossary

Term	Definition
Pharmacogenetics	The study of genetically determined interindividual differences in response to drugs
Pharmacogenomics	The use of genome-based technologies in drug development
Types of pharmacogenetic effects	
Pharmacokinetic	Genetically based differences that influence bioavailability of a drug
Pharmacodynamic	Genetically based differences in the proteins at which a drug acts
Polymorphism	Genetic variation that occurs with a frequency of 1% or more in the population
Single nucleotide polymorphisms (SNPs)	Differences between individuals in a single base of the genomic sequence; these are the most frequently occurring genetic variation
Coding	Occur in exons (coding regions) of genes
Noncoding	Occur in introns (noncoding regions) of genes
Regulatory	Occur in 3′ or 5′ regulatory regions (promoter)
Synonymous	SNPs in coding regions that do not influence the structure of the protein
Conservative	Alter the structure of the protein but not its function
Functional	Alter the function of the protein
Candidate gene	Chosen for analysis on the basis of an a priori hypothesis regarding the role of the protein coded by the gene in the phenotype under study
Association	Statistical demonstration of a greater than chance occurrence of a polymorphism in a candidate gene in conjunction with the target phenotype
Linkage disequilibrium (LD)	Statistical association of two alleles at a rate greater than would be predicted by chance (owing to the fact that the two alleles are close enough to each other to not undergo recombination)
Polygenic	A trait that is influenced by a number of different genes each of which contributes a portion of the effect
Epistasis	Genetic variance owing to nonadditive effects of alleles at distinct loci
Multifactorial	Both genetic and environmental factors contribute substantially and variably to the phenotype

pharmacogenomics is the human genome sequence and its outcome is the development of new pharmacological agents. The points of interaction between the two approaches are multiple and they complement each other at many levels, so it is inevitable that the distinction is easily blurred.

There are two broad categories within pharmacogenetics, which derive from the fact that differences between individuals can be attributed to two major factors that are under genetic influence. The first set of factors is *pharmacokinetic* and they encompass genetically based differences in processes that influence bioavailability of a drug, i.e., the concentration of the drug and its active metabolites that is available at the site of action). The second major category is *pharmacodynamics* and refers to genetically based differences in the proteins at which the drug acts. Both sets of factors may influence the response of the individual to a given drug and they may interact within the same individual.

Polymorphism is a core term in pharmacogenetics. A polymorphism is a genetic variation that occurs with a frequency of 1% or more in the population. Genetic variations that occur more rarely (mutations) also influence drug response, often dramatically, but these are of less importance on a population-wide basis. *Single nucleotide polymorphisms* (*SNPs*) are differences between individuals in a single base of the genomic sequence and are the most frequently occurring genetic variation. SNPs occur throughout the human genome at a density of approximately 1 per 1000 bases (kilobases, kb) of DNA. It is important to stress that the vast majority of SNPs are unlikely to influence either the structure or function of proteins. SNPs may be classified by their location, occurring in exons (coding regions) or introns (noncoding regions) of genes and in regulatory regions such as the promoter. SNPs in coding regions need not necessarily influence the structure of the protein and are termed synonymous. SNPs that do alter the structure of the proteins need not have functional consequences and are termed conservative or non-functional. SNPs located in intronic regions can have an impact on the coded protein by influencing splicing (Krawezak et al., 1992). SNPs in regulatory regions are a focus of considerable interest and can have major effects on expression of the gene. In fact, it has been suggested that regulatory mutations rather than mutations that affect protein structure may be the prime cause of biological differences in humans (Chakravarti, 1999; Chapter 12). Major efforts are now in progress by public and industry-based consortia to generate SNP databases that will be an invaluable resource for pharmacogenetics in the very near future.

SNPs are not the only type of DNA variation of relevance to pharmacogenetics. Other types of genetic polymorphism result from the insertion or deletion of a few nucleotides (termed *insertion/deletion polymorphisms*) and variation in the number of times a sequence is repeated. *Variable number tandem repeats* (*VNTRs* or *minisatellites*) have several hundred base pairs repeated while *microsatellites* (or *simple tandem repeats, STRs*) have two to four nucleotides repeated a variable number of times. Allelic variations (i.e., variability in the number of repeats) can be considerable and this type of variation is consequently highly polymorphic.

Traditionally, pharmacogenetic studies have sought an association between a specific gene and the response or adverse effect phenotype under study. This is a classical *candidate gene* approach, which is based on an a priori hypothesis regarding the role of the protein coded by the gene in the particular phenotype. However, an SNP or other genetic variation may be statistically associated with a phenotype without having a direct effect. This phenomenon results from *linkage disequilibrium* (LD) and it arises from the fact that the variant examined is close enough to the true predisposing variant that it does not undergo recombination during meiosis and is inherited with it. The marker may be at a different site in the gene itself or may be located outside the gene. Linkage disequilibrium mapping employs dense SNP maps in order to localize genes associated with a phenotype and has been suggested as a powerful approach to identify genes for complex phenotypes (Risch, 2000), although there are dissenting voices that question the feasibility of the strategy (Weiss and Terwilliger, 2000). Linkage disequilibrium approaches are the cornerstone of the large-scale mapping projects in pharmacogenetics that are currently being advocated.

Classical genetics of human disease deals with monogenic disorders in which a single mutation in a single gene is causatively related to the phenotype. This paradigm holds reasonably true in pharmacogenetics for classical "pharmacokinetic" polymorphisms that have a major effect on drug bioavailability (such as the effect of CYP2D6 polymorphism on the metabolism of a variety of psychotropic and other drugs, which is inherited as an autosomal recessive trait). For the most part, however, the accepted view is that pharmacogenetic traits are likely to be *polygenic* and *multifactorial*. A polygenic trait is one that is influenced by a number of different genes each of which contributes a portion of the effect and may do so additively as well as interactively (*epistasis*). The term "multifactorial" indicates that both genetic and environmental factors contribute substantially and variably to the phenotype.

Core issues in pharmacogenetic research design

The classical experimental context for determining pharmacogenetic influences on drug response is a comparison of responders and nonresponders to the drug or of individuals who develop adverse effects and those who do not. This appealingly simple case-control design should be readily applicable in psychopharmacology. Data from such studies are amenable to analysis by two approaches. The first is a categorical approach in which patients are grouped according to the phenotype (responder or nonresponder, develops adverse effect or does not) and the frequency of the genotype of interest in these groups is compared. The second approach utilizes the response variable (or adverse effect measure) in a continuous fashion and compares scores at a single time point or over a period of treatment in patients grouped according to genotype. There are already numerous examples of the application of this approach to psychopharmacology. The paucity of replicable results may be a consequence of a number of relatively elementary factors.

Population effects

It is well known that the frequency of genetic polymorphisms differs markedly among ethnic groups. Therefore, unequal inclusion of individuals of different ethnic backgrounds in groups of subjects being compared can lead to spurious results that reflect ethnic stratification. Methods have been proposed to address these issues (Devlin and Roeder, 1999; Lerer et al., 2001). Nevertheless, it is essential that studies be designed to take them into account prospectively. Another point is that the functional relevance of a particular polymorphism may vary among ethnic groups. Thus, a true finding in a sample from a particular population may not be replicable in a different population.

Demographic variables

Since the basis of interindividual variability in drug response is multifactorial, the impact of demographic variables such as age and gender cannot be ignored. A particular genetic variant may not be functionally relevant without the addition of other factors that also influence the phenotype. An example is the influence of certain 5-HT receptor variants on predisposition to neuroleptic-induced tardive dyskinesia, which was demonstrated in a sample of older patients but was not observed in a sample two decades younger (Segman and Lerer, 2002). It is highly conceivable that gender-specific effects are also operative and that interactions between age and gender will be demonstrated.

Definition and evaluation of the phenotype

Drug response to psychotropic drugs is a phenotype that is very difficult to define for evaluation experimentally. There is an extensive literature that debates how to define a "responder" to an antidepressant drug in the context of a clinical trial. Definitions may be based on percentage improvement on a particular rating scale or by using a specific score on that scale as a threshold. There are conventions that are fairly well accepted for clinical trials of psychopharmacologic agents. It remains to be established whether these conventions can be readily transferred to pharmacogenetic studies (see Rietschel et al., 1999).

Study design

Most recently published studies on the pharmacogenetics of psychotropic drugs are "opportunistic" in that they employ subjects who were previously studied and correlate the phenotypic measures gathered in these studies with genotypic data that are obtained currently. Alternatively, they may be "add-on" in nature. In studies of this type, drawing of blood samples for DNA is included in the protocol of clinical trials for future correlation of genotypes with drug response or adverse effect phenotypes. In both cases, studies are not "purpose designed" to address pharmacogenetic questions. They address the questions that they were designed to answer and do not take into account issues that are pivotal to pharmacogenetics. Since clinical trials demand large sample sizes, there is usually little consideration given to ethnicity of the subjects. The age range may be great and diagnostic boundaries tend to be as wide as possible to insure maximum recruitment. It is likely that even very large samples will not have adequate power to address pharmacogenetic questions when subject groups are stratified in order to control for factors that can spuriously affect the results. A "second generation" of pharmacogenetic studies can be anticipated that are designed to take these issues into account. When this occurs, the issue of placebo control is likely to emerge as a major consideration. On the one hand, it is self-evident that non-placebo-controlled studies greatly impede attempts to differentiate factors associated with "response" from these associated with "response to the active drug." On the other hand, already existing concerns regarding the ethical validity of placebo-controlled trial in disorders such as schizophrenia or depression will be more intense when the aim of the study is refinement of drug prescription rather than demonstration of efficacy. Simulation studies are urgently needed in order to address these issues.

Interaction among multiple loci

Traditionally, pharmacogenetic studies have focused on single genes and on single polymorphisms within these genes. It is becoming clear that this approach is too limited to address the complexity of the situation adequately. Single SNPs may not show an association with treatment effects or with disease susceptibility while combinations do. These may be within a single gene, as demonstrated for the effect of complex haplotypes of SNPs in the coding region and the promoter of the β_2-adrenoreceptor gene on the bronchodilator response to asthma therapy (Drysdale et al., 2000). Interactions (epistasis) may be demonstrated between SNPs in different genes, as recently observed in a study of genetic susceptibility to sporadic breast cancer (Ritchie et al., 2001). In the context of pharmacogenetics, Segman et al. (2002) have observed an interaction between a polymorphism in the gene for cytochrome P17 and the gene for dopamine D_3 receptor that is associated with more neuroleptic-related abnormal involuntary movements in patients who carry both mutant genotypes.

Gene expression

It is not inevitable that the genotype carried by an individual will be expressed functionally as anticipated from the structure of the protein predicted by the DNA sequence. This assumption is inherent in pharmacogenetic studies that seek to correlate DNA variations with a particular phenotype. The reasons for this are numerous and may be found at any point along the long route traversing transcription, translation and post-translational modification between the DNA sequence of a gene and the protein for which it codes. Examples considered in Chapter 7 of this volume are the processes of RNA editing and RNA splicing. Both represent important mechanisms that ultimately contribute to the expression of specific protein isoforms within a given cell. These considerations are of major importance in pharmacogenetics and demand that the functional implications of a specific DNA variant be assessed before it is assumed that association of a trait with the variant can serve as a predictor of response or of adverse effects to a drug.

An age of optimism

In spite of the methodological concerns outlined in the preceding section, there are very substantial reasons for optimism regarding the potential of pharmacogenetics to fulfill some of the expectations that have been assigned to it, although the time frame could well be longer than anticipated.

The identification of DNA variations that serve as a basis for pharmacogenetic studies is proceeding apace. A number of international consortia supported by government, industry, and academic resources are devoting major efforts to identifying and cataloging SNPs throughout the human genome. Much of the information that is being amassed is being placed in the public domain and will thus be available to researchers worldwide. This is an invaluable resource. Once the human genome is covered by a dense SNP map, it will be possible to proceed with large-scale studies that consider thousands of potential markers.

Efforts in the laboratory are being matched by parallel developments in bioinformatics. The enormous body of genetic information that is being created is of little value unless appropriate tools are available for the researcher to access and use this information. Private as well as public efforts are directed at making this possible, and the accessibility of the information can be expected to increase with time. There are also major challenges in data analysis that need to be addressed. Current approaches are inadequate to analyze vast amounts of genotypic information except in the context of sample sizes that are completely unrealistic. Recent reports suggest that novel statistical techniques may allow a number of genetic loci to be considered simultaneously in the context of sample sizes that are within the realm of clinical reality (Ritchie et al., 2001). Another very real problem that has to be adequately addressed is the potential to generate false-positive results from a huge number of repeated tests. Currently applied corrections for this problem run the risk of excluding positive results, while less conservative approaches can lead to the accumulation of nonreplicable chance findings.

To be applicable in the clinic, pharmacogenetic findings will need to cross two thresholds. The first is a replicability threshold that establishes their validity as prognostic markers. The second is that enough of the variance in treatment response must be accounted for by a particular marker (an unlikely scenario) or by a combination of markers to render a test based upon these markers clinically useful. It is clear that this process will take considerably longer than developing the technological means to perform such tests in the clinic. Chip technologies are already available that allow up to several thousand SNPs to be typed at one time. The cost of chips of this type is obviously still very high. It can be anticipated that the costs will drop long before psychopharmacogenetics is able to fill the available slots in a rational way.

In the area of psychopharmacology, there are a few recent pharmacogenetic findings that have been reasonably well replicated, although not by all groups. One example is the association of an insertion–deletion polymorphism in the serotonin transporter promoter and response to antidepressant treatment with serotonin reuptake blockers (see Chapter 12). A second example is the association of a serine to glycine polymorphism in the dopamine D_3 receptor gene with susceptibility to tardive dyskinesia, a serious adverse effect of classical antipsychotic drugs (Chapter 11). Outside of psychopharmacology, asthma therapy has been a very active research focus in pharmacogenetics, with a number of encouraging results reported (Silverman et al., 2001). In patients with coronary atherosclerosis, it was found that a functional polymorphism in the cholesterol ester transfer protein (CETP), which influenced CETP plasma levels, was associated with a stronger ability of the drug pravastatin to lower plasma cholesterol levels (Kuivenhoven et al., 1998).

Pharmacogenetics of psychotropic drugs: an overview

Parts II–IV of the book deal with a selection of important background topics. Chapter 2 discusses the clinical implications of identifying molecular genetic predictors of drug response and basic design issues in studies that are designed to generate data of this type. Chapter 3 reviews the history of psychiatric nosology and its interactions with psychopharmacology and proposes the use of an empirically derived pharmacologically meaningful classification of mental illness in genetic research. Chapter 4 reviews methodological issues facing pharmacogenetic studies in clinical psychopharmacology, considering the drug development process itself, the problems posed by poor signal:noise ratio, and practical problems posed in trying to study whether a genetically defined population is at increased risk for toxicity or other adverse effects at routine drug dosages. Chapter 5 considers optimal approaches to the statistical analysis of pharmacogenetic data with reference to the specific challenges posed and their implications for the design of studies.

Background issues at the molecular level are addressed in Part III. Chapter 6 focuses on serotonergic gene pathways and discusses the potential importance for pharmacogenetics of variation in the structure and expression of genes that play a key role in neurodevelopment of these pathways. Chapter 7 reviews the post-transcriptional processes of RNA editing and alternative splicing and considers how processes such as these, beyond the level of structural DNA variation, can be important in psychopharmacogenetics.

Historically and practically, heritable effects on drug metabolism are of major importance in the pharmacogenetics of psychotropic drugs. Section IV deals with this topic. Chapter 8 reviews and contrasts genetic polymorphisms of the metabolic enzymes CYP2D6 and CYP1A2 and their roles in the pharmacokinetics of psychotropic drugs. This chapter also considers gene–gene and gene–environment interactions. Chapter 9 focuses on the stereoselectivity of cytochrome P-450 isoenzymes towards chiral substrates and its importance in view of the fact that many psychotropic drugs have one or more chiral centers.

Part V of the book focus on specific drug groups and syndromes. Antipsychotic drugs, particularly the atypical drug clozapine, have been fairly extensively studied. In Chapter 10, Collier and colleagues discuss the impact of genetic variation in a number of target receptors on the therapeutic efficacy of clozapine, in the light of their own studies and those other investigators. Chapter 11 covers the genetic predisposition to the movement disorder tardive dyskinesia, the most severe adverse effect of classical antipsychotics, and reviews the possible role of a number of candidate genes.

Chapters 12–14 consider the antidepressants and anxiolytics. Chapter 12 highlights the potentially important role of genetic polymorphisms that are involved in the regulation of gene expression or the activity of key enzymes, as opposed to the structure of receptor sites, in the pharmacogenetics of a variety of antidepressant treatments. In most pharmacogenetic studies of psychotropic drugs, the target phenotype is very simply defined on a response/nonresponse continuum. Mundo and Kennedy in Chapter 15 consider the importance of more homogeneous phenotype definition in studies of antidepressant pharmacogenetics and also discuss and review data concerning the role of novel alternative phenotypes such as antidepressant-induced mania. Chapter 14 focuses on the treatment of anxiety disorders and reviews genetic variations in the gamma-aminobutyric acid (GABA) type A receptor and its subunits and their implications for antianxiety treatments.

Chapter 15 considers the pharmacogenetics of mood-stabilizing drugs such as lithium and anticonvulsants. Alda reviews studies that categorize families segregating bipolar disorder according to the responsiveness of their affected members to lithium treatment. These samples are being used to identify genes associated with treatment response or to map genes for bipolar disorder in families homogeneous for treatment response. Besides lithium, anticonvulsant drugs now have an important place in the treatment of mood disorders. Chapter 16 reviews the pharmacogenetics of anticonvulsants, including extensive work on the polymorphism of cytochrome P-450 isoforms and their influence on the metabolism of these drugs and more limited work on the genes that encode their protein targets.

Chapter 17 focuses on Alzheimer's disease, specifically on the possible role of apolipoprotein E (apoE) genotype as a predictor of response to cholinomimetic treatment. Schappert and colleagues discuss findings in this regard and also a possible role for the butyrylcholinesterase gene in modifying treatment outcome with noncholinergic therapies. Chapter 18 covers the topic of substance abuse and dependence, disorders that involve the ingestion of an exogenous substance that can be expected to interact with pharmacogenetic factors possibly specific for the substance. Examples of such factors are discussed in the broader context of genetic risk factors for substance dependence and the development of pharmacological treatment. Chapter 19 brings brain imaging into the domain of pharmacogenetics. Potkin and colleagues discuss data regarding the regional brain metabolic phenotypic manifestation of specific genotypes (apoE in Alzheimer's disease and the dopamine D_3 receptor gene in tardive dyskinesia) and the possible use of brain imaging in pharmacogenetic evaluation.

The final part of the book (Part VII) provides perspectives from the pharmaceutical and biotechnology industries. Chapter 20 describes the major benefits to be derived from the implementation of pharmacogenetically oriented research protocols in industry-supported studies; the authors discuss the problems and limitations that have prevented such implementation so far and consider how such initiatives may be developed in the context of collaboration between industry and academia. High throughput genotyping is a key element of large-scale pharmacogenetic analysis. Chapter 21 reviews a number of technologies that have been developed, considering both their effectiveness and their cost.

Conclusions

The interface between psychopharmacology and molecular genetics is already a focus of considerable research activity and this is likely to intensify as anticipated technological advances provide the tools for even more sophisticated studies. Pharmacogenetics addresses a core issue in pharmacotherapeutics, the individualization of drug treatment to the specific patient, and promises to provide the tools for making rational clinical decisions that are based on the patient's genetic profile. This will be a major advance in therapeutics and will have enormous impact on patient care and also important pharmacoeconomic implications. Furthermore, the complex and lengthy process of new drug development could be considerably shortened, with cost reductions that would be passed on to the consumer. Translating this optimistic scenario into reality is likely to take substantially longer than anticipated by some and will require considerable investment of resources in the design and execution of appropriate clinical studies as well as the development of novel and considerably more efficient approaches to data analysis. We are positioned at the beginning of a crucial and highly intriguing era; there will undoubtedly be high points, but disappointments and some degree of disillusionment are inevitable given the considerable level of current expectations. It may take longer than originally thought, but ultimately pharmacogenetics and pharmacogenomics will revolutionize the field of clinical psychopharmacology and the development of psychotropic drugs.

REFERENCES

Chakravarti A. (1999). Population genetics – making sense out of sequence. *Nat Genet* 21, 56–60.

Devlin B, Roeder K. (1999). Genomic control for association studies. *Biometrics* 55, 997–1004.

Drysdale CM, McGraw DW, Stack CB et al. (2000). Complex promoter and coding region β_2-adrenergic receptor haplotypes alter receptor expression and predict in vivo responsiveness. *Proc Natl Acad Sci USA* 97: 10483–10488.

Eichelbaum M, Spannbrucher N, Steincke B, Dengler HJ (1979). Defective N-oxidation of sparteine and debrisoquine in man: a new pharmacogenetic defect. *Eur J Clin Pharmacol* 16, 183–187.

Evans DAP, Manley KA, McKusick VA (1960). Genetic control of isoniazid metabolism in man. *Br Med J* 2, 485–491.

Garrod AE (1902). The incidence of alcaptonuria: a study in chemical individuality. *Lancet* ii, 1616–1620.

Garrod AE (1909). *Inborn Errors of Metabolism.* Oxford: Oxford University Press.

Kalow W (1962). *Pharmacogenetics – Heredity and Response to Drugs.* Philadelphia: Saunders.

Krawezak M, Reiss J, Cooper DN (1992). The mutational spectrum of single base-pair substitutions in mRNA splice junctions of human genes: causes and consequences. *Hum Genet* 90, 41–54.

Kuivenhoven JA, Jukema JW, Zwinderman AH et al. (1998). The role of a common variant of the cholesteryl ester transfer protein gene in the progression of coronary atherosclerosis. The Regression Growth Evaluation Statin Study Group. *N Engl J Med* 338, 86–93.

Lerer B, Macciardi F, Segman RH et al. (2001). Variability of 5-HT$_{2C}$ receptor Cys23Ser polymorphism among European populations and vulnerability to affective disorder. *Mol Psychiatry* 6, 579–585.

Mahgoub A, Idle JR, Dring LG, Lancaster R, Smith RL (1977). Polymorphic hydroxylation of debrisoquine in man. *Lancet* ii, 584–586.

Motulsky A (1957). Drug reactions, enzymes and biochemical genetics. *J Am Med Assoc* 165, 835–837.

Nebert DW (1997). Pharmacogenetics: 65 candles on the cake. *Pharmacogenetics* 7, 435–440.

Propping P, Nothen MM (1995) Genetic variation of CNS receptors – a new perspective for pharmacogenetics. *Pharmacogenetics* 5, 318–325.

Rietschel M, Kennedy JL, Macciardi F, Meltzer HY (1999). Application of pharmacogenetics to psychotic disorders: the first consensus conference. The Consensus Group for Outcome Measures in Psychoses for Pharmacological Studies. *Schizophr Res* 37, 191–196.

Risch NJ (2000). Searching for genetic determinants in the new millennium. *Nature* 405, 847–856.

Ritchie MD, Hahn LW, Roodi N et al. (2001). Multifactor-dimensionality reduction reveals high-order interactions among estrogen-metabolism genes in sporadic breast cancer *Am J Hum Genet* 69, 138–147.

Segman RH, Lerer B (2002). Age and the relationship of dopamine, serotonin 2C and serotonin 2A receptor genes to abnormal involuntary movements in chronic schizophrenia. *Mol Psychiatry* 7, 137–139.

Segman RH, Heresco-Levy U, Yakir A et al. (2002). Interactive effect of cytochrome P-450 17α-hydroxylase and dopamine D$_3$ receptor gene polymorphisms on abnormal involuntary movements in chronic schizophrenia. *Biol Psychiatry* 51, 261–263.

Silverman ES, Ligget SB, Gelfand EW et al. (2001). The pharmacogenetics of asthma: a candidate gene approach. *Pharmacogenom J* 1, 27–37.

Snyder LH (1932). Studies in human inheritance 1x. The inheritance of taste deficiency in man. *Ohio J Sci* 32, 436–468.

Vogel F (1959). Moderne probleme der humangenetik. *Ergebn Inn Med Kinderheilk* 12, 52–125.

Weiss KM, Terwilliger JD (2000). How many diseases does it take to map a gene with SNPs? *Nat Genet* 26, 151–157.

Part II

Clinical background and research design

2

From pharmacogenetics to pharmacogenomics of psychotropic drug response

Anil K. Malhotra

Hillside Hospital, Glen Oaks, New York

OVERVIEW

The marked interindividual variation in response to psychotropic drugs creates a clinical dilemma that can only be resolved through often lengthy empirical drug trials. Recent developments in molecular biology have provided an opportunity to identify molecular genetic predictors of drug response, which may have immediate clinical implications as well as provide critical data for future drug development. In this chapter, we will discuss the evidence for a heritable component to psychotropic drug response, review basic methodological issues in pharmacogenetic studies of psychotropic drug response, and then highlight future directions for pharmacogenetics research in psychiatry.

Introduction

Individual differences in clinical response to psychotropic drugs has long been recognized as a fundamental problem in the treatment of the seriously mentally ill patient. This variability in individual response ranges from patients who experience complete symptom remission to a subset of patients often described as "treatment refractory," as well as a marked variability in susceptibility to adverse drug effects. A priori identification of the patients who will respond well to a particular psychotropic drug, or be at a higher risk for development of adverse side effects, has the potential to help clinicians to avoid lengthy ineffective medication trials and to limit a patient's exposure to drug side effects. Moreover, enhanced predictability of treatment response early in the course of a patient's illness may result in enhanced patient compliance and willingness to seek treatment rapidly upon symptom exacerbation or recurrence.

Initial efforts to identify predictors of psychotropic drug response focused on clinical variables such as age at onset of illness, level of premorbid function, and comorbidity (Grebb and Cancro, 1989). Unfortunately, these findings have often been confounded by methodological issues (e.g., selection bias, retrospective assessments of response) and have been limited in their applicability to clinical practice. As the understanding of the biological basis of psychiatric disorders has improved, efforts to identify biological predictors of individual drug response have intensified (Malhotra and Pickar, 1996). Plasma and cerebrospinal fluid levels of neurotransmitter metabolites, neurohormone levels, and brain imaging measures, amongst others, have been hypothesized to provide informative correlates of drug response (Bowers et al., 1984; Pickar et al., 1984; Buchsbaum et al., 1992; Kahn et al., 1993; Szymanski et al., 1995). Despite some initially promising results, consistent data in this regard have remained elusive.

The introduction of molecular genetic techniques into psychiatric research has provided the impetus for renewed investigations into the identification of psychotropic drug response predictors. It is now possible to extract DNA efficiently from blood samples of human subjects, amplify targeted molecular regions for analysis with the polymerase chain reaction, and rapidly genotype individuals at ever increasing numbers of loci in a cost-effective manner. Armed with these techniques, a number of psychiatric research groups, as well as pharmaceutical and biotechnology companies, are currently attempting to determine the genetic basis for the variation in clinical response. This field of inquiry offers the prospect of identification of easily accessible biological predictors of psychotropic drug response and may provide information about the molecular substrates of psychotropic drug efficacy. This chapter reviews the evidence for a heritable component to psychotropic drug response, discusses basic methodological issues in pharmacogenetic studies, and highlights some future directions for pharmacogenetic research in psychiatry.

Heritability of psychotropic drug response

A basic assumption of genetic studies is that the phenotype of interest is significantly heritable. Although data from family, twin and epidemiological studies suggest that the major psychiatric disorders have a significant genetic component (Plomin et al., 1994), this may not be the case for response to the drugs that treat these disorders. Unfortunately, heritability data for psychotropic drug response are extremely limited because of the difficulties in designing and executing appropriately powered heritability studies in this area. For phenotypes such as psychiatric diagnosis, estimates of heritability can be calculated by comparison of concordance rates between monozygotic (MZ) and dizygotic (DZ) twins. The ratio of concordance rates between MZ and DZ twins provides an estimate of the contribution of genes, assuming that the environment is shared equally between twin groups (Gottesman, 1991). Alternatively, evidence for heritability can be provided by the study of twins who are separated at birth (adoption studies) and brought up in distinct environments (Kety et al., 1975). These approaches, however, are difficult to utilize for estimates of the heritability of pharmacogenetic phenotypes. The ascertainment of MZ and DZ twin pairs (or adopted twins) in which one individual is psychiatrically ill is a laborious process in and of itself and the possibility that both members of any one twin pair would first be ill (presumably with the same diagnosis), treated with the same drug, at the same (or similar) dosage, for similar durations of treatment, and that each twin's clinical response would be measured utilizing similarly valid and reliable methods, is extremely unlikely. Moreover, pedigree studies of several generations cannot provide much information in this regard because of the continual development of new psychotropic drugs and subsequent alterations in prescription patterns.

The majority of heritability data on psychotropic drugs is from studies of antidepressant drug response. Angst et al. (1964) examined 41 first-degree relative pairs (parents or siblings of probands) both treated with the tricyclic antidepressant imipramine and reported that 38 pairs were concordant for response. Pare et al. (1962) studied first-degree relatives of 170 depressed patients who had participated in clinical trials of antidepressant drugs to assess concordance rates in the relative pairs with similar treatment trials. In the 12 cases of concordant treatments, both members of the relative pair had similar responses, with an overall response rate of 42%. In a subsequent study (Pare and Mack, 1971), the same group utilized the same approach in a new cohort and found that 10 of 12 cases were concordant for antidepressant response. Moreover, the high level of response concordance between the proband and first-degree relative when treated with an antidepressant of the same class was in contrast to the lack of concordance when drugs of different classes were used. These data are consistent with a retrospective analysis of two generations of a family with multiple ill relatives with major depression in which all four family members (proband, mother, daughter, aunt, and first cousin) who underwent treatment with the monoamine oxidase inhibitor tranylcypromine responded despite being nonresponsive to conventional treatment (O'Reilly et al., 1994).

In these early studies, the actual antidepressant used, the dosage of antidepressant, and duration of treatment were not consistently controlled. In a recent study, however, Franchini et al. (1998) assessed 45 first-degree relative pairs all treated with the same antidepressant, fluvoxamine, at a similar dosage, 200–300 mg per day for at least 6 weeks, and measured response with the structured rating scale, the Hamilton Depression Scale. In this work, 67% of pairs were concordant for response compared with the 50% that would be expected by chance in first-degree relatives. Although these data suggest that heritable factors are involved in antidepressant drug response, none of these studies was designed to examine whether shared environmental effects in antidepressant-treated relative pairs influence response. Therefore, these data can only be viewed as preliminary, and more research in this area is warranted.

Evidence for the heritability of antipsychotic drug response is even more limited. There have been several reports that antipsychotic drug response varies by ethnicity (Frackiewicz et al., 1997), suggesting a genetic component to response; however, it is unclear whether the response variation may simply result from differences in drug metabolism or from other disparities in the clinical treatment of different ethnic groups.

The antipsychotic drug most extensively studied in psychiatric pharmacogenetics is the prototypic atypical agent clozapine. Heritability of clozapine response, however, has not been assessed in a systematic fashion. The only current information is in a single case report (Vojvoda et al., 1996) of a MZ twin pair with schizophrenia concordant for good response to 550 mg per day of clozapine despite prior nonresponse to multiple typical antipsychotic agents. Typical antipsychotics have also received only limited study in psychiatric pharmacogenetics, although DeLisi and Dauphinais (1989) retrospectively assessed 28 schizophrenic sibling pairs and found no more concordance for neuroleptic response than expected by chance. The low overall response rate in this study group (30%) suggests that this was either a particularly nonresponsive group or that the criteria for response were relatively conservative.

Antipsychotic drugs are potent dopamine receptor antagonists. Although heritability data on the behavioral response to these drugs are extremely limited, concordance in twins for behavioral response to a dopamine receptor agonist has been observed. Nurnberger and colleagues (1982) administered 0.3 mg/kg of the dopamine receptor agonist dextroamphetamine (dexamfetamine) to healthy volunteer twin pairs and found that induced alterations in behavioral excitation ($r = 0.70$; $p = 0.003$) as well as changes in plasma growth hormone and prolactin levels that were highly correlated in 12 MZ twins but not in three DZ twin pairs. These results were not accounted for by correlation of plasma amphetamine levels. Although these results may suggest heritability of behavioral response to dopaminergic perturbation, the small sample of DZ twins was not sufficient to conduct accurate heritability estimates. Nevertheless, further research utilizing acute pharmacologic "challenge" paradigms (Malhotra et al., 1998a) may be useful to assess heritability of drug responses if appropriate safeguards are in place.

Methodological issues in the pharmacogenetics of psychotropic drug response

Efforts to find disease-susceptibility genes have utilized two major approaches. The first, whole genome scanning by linkage analysis, is a nonhypothesis-driven approach in which polymorphisms distributed throughout the genome are genotyped in families to identify alleles that are shared by ill relatives more often than predicted by chance. The basic unit of analysis is one family that contains either multiple affected relatives through generations or affected relative pairs. If successful, a chromosomal region is "linked" to a phenotype. Unfortunately, linked regions in genome scans are usually extensive, encompass hundreds of genes, and the ultimate identification of the specific genetic variant that contributes to the linkage result can be laborious and resource intensive (Gusella et al., 1983; Tsui et al., 1985). Moreover, genome scanning is particularly disadvantageous for psychiatric pharmacogenetic studies because of the necessity to specify a genetic model of transmission (for traditional lod score analyses), the low likelihood of ascertainment of families with multiple ill relatives treated with the same medication, and the reduced power of genome scanning to detect genes of small effect.

For these reasons, pharmacogenetic studies in psychiatry have been conducted using a complementary approach to genome scanning – the case-control association design. As the basic unit of analysis in case-control studies is the individual, this approach is particularly well suited for pharmacogenetic studies in which unrelated individuals may be all that are available for study.

There are several basic steps in conducting a pharmacogenetic association study. First, a phenotype of interest is identified and response criteria are established. In psychiatric pharmacogenetics, clinical response to psychotropic drug treatment and adverse effects of drug treatment have been the major focus (Arranz et al., 1995, Masellis et al., 1995, Malhotra et al., 1996, 1998b). Second, a candidate gene is selected for analysis. Candidate genes are identified either by position in a chromosomal region linked to the disorder in a genome scan or upon neurobiological evidence that the gene product influences the phenotype of interest. Third, candidate polymorphisms and candidate alleles (or groups of alleles or haplotypes) are selected within or near the candidate gene. The criteria for candidate polymorphism selection are somewhat arbitrary but potential criteria include allele frequency (polymorphisms with low rare allele frequencies may be minimally informative and, therefore, provide limited power), whether the polymorphism results in an amino acid substitution at the protein level, and the functional consequences of the polymorphism in in vitro systems (Malhotra and Goldman, 1999). Finally, in its most basic form, the frequency of alleles (and/or genotypes) is compared between groups of patients (for instance, between clozapine responders and nonresponders).

The candidate gene pharmacogenetic strategy has been successful in nonpsychiatric diseases such as asthma. Effective pharmacologic treatments for asthma include β_2-adrenoreceptor (B2AR) agonists and 5-lipoxygenase (ALOX5) inhibitors. However, a significant subset of asthma patients fails to respond to treatment and suffer significant morbidity and mortality. Recently, Kotani and colleagues

(1999) conducted a case-control pharmacogenetic association study assessing the role of a *B2AR* polymorphism, Arg16Gly, in the airway responsiveness (as measured by spirometry) of Japanese patients with asthma ($n=92$) treated with the beta-agonist salbutamol. The candidate gene was selected because of the known affinity of salbutamol for the receptor, and the polymorphism was selected because it alters agonist-promoted receptor down regulation. The finding that the patients who were homozygous for Gly16 had significantly lower airway responsiveness suggests that the a priori identification of Gly/Gly homozygotes could increase the overall effectiveness of asthma treatment with beta-agonists. Similarly, Drazen et al. (1999) examined the association between improvements in forced expiratory volume in the first second (FEV_1) in a placebo-controlled trial ($n=221$) of the anti-asthma drug ABT-761 and a promoter region polymorphism in the gene *ALOX5*. In this case, the candidate gene was selected because of the known affinity of ABT-761 for ALOX5 and the polymorphism was chosen based upon in vitro data indicating an effect on *ALOX5* gene transcription. Patient stratification by *ALOX5* genotype did not distinguish between the patients' overall disease severity; however, it did reveal that patients homozygous for the rare allele failed to respond to ABT-761. In fact, the homozygotes' FEV_1 response was no different than the group of patients who received placebo treatment. These data suggest that sequence variation in the genes that code for the targets of a therapeutic agent may influence the clinical variation in drug response and that the case-control methodology can be successfully utilized to identify these relationships.

Limitations of case-control association studies

Although the case-control methodology has several advantages (see below), this approach is subject to distinct limitations. In particular, the selection of candidate genes for case-control psychiatric genetic studies is complicated by the lack of direct biological evidence linking any one protein (and hence, gene) to susceptibility to any psychiatric disorder. Therefore, it has been suggested that association studies of psychiatric phenotypes should be corrected for every gene in the genome that might be expressed in the central nervous system (CNS), thus requiring p values for significance that would range as low as 10^{-7}. This may be an overly conservative threshold for psychiatric pharmacogenetic studies because candidate gene selection in this work can be guided by biological data. For example, the initial targets for many psychotropic drugs and the cascade of molecular events that follow drug binding have been intensively studied (Hyman and Nestler, 1996) and can serve to provide initial candidates for psychotropic drug response. Moreover, phenotypes in psychiatric pharmacogenetics may be more amenable to candidate gene selection than phenotypes based solely upon diagnostic classifications. For

instance, although the list of suitable candidate genes for antipsychotic drug efficacy is relatively broad, the initial candidate genes for a phenotype such as antipsychotic drug-induced extrapyramidal symptoms could be reasonably restricted to
genes within or related to the dopamine system, given the large body of data implicating dopaminergic function in extrapyramidal efffects (Farde et al., 1992).
Moreover, new methods such as differential display should provide new candidates
for psychiatric pharmacogenetics by providing quantitative data on the effects of
psychotropic drug administration on CNS gene expression (Nguyen et al., 1992).
Taken together, these data suggest that rational candidate gene selection for psychiatric pharmacogenetic studies can be accomplished based upon biological data.
Therefore, the establishment of extreme thresholds to achieve significance may
result in inflated type II errors rates and minimize the opportunity to take advantage of the genomic information being generated by the Human Genome Project
and other large-scale sequencing efforts.

A second important consideration in evaluating case-control association studies
is the criteria used to select a candidate polymorphism within the gene of interest.
For genes that have not been scanned for genetic variation, techniques including
single-strand conformational polymorphism analysis (Orita et al., 1989), denaturing gradient gel electrophoresis (Myers et al., 1985) denaturing high performance liquid chromatography (Underhill et al., 1997) and methods using
oligonucleotide-based chip arrays (Chee et al., 1996) can be utilized to detect new
variants. However, since most genes contain a number of sequence variants including single nucleotide polymorphisms (SNPs), the selection of which variant or variants to genotype in a case-control association study may be critical. Several issues
should be considered. First, the frequency of the rare allele of a variant may be
important. Variants with low frequencies of the rare allele may provide little power
to detect significant associations unless the study group size is large or the variant
has a strong influence on the phenotype. Moreover, the number of alleles at a locus
must be considered. Variants with relatively large number of alleles provide a
greater number of potential genotypes, increasing the informativeness of the locus
but complicating the statistical analysis. For instance, the dopamine D_4 receptor
gene (*DRD4*) polymorphism leading to a 16 amino acid repeat may produce more
than 15 different genotypes (Chang et al., 1996), leading to relatively small groups
of subjects with particular genotypes. For this reason, most studies with this *DRD4*
polymorphism have arbitrarily grouped subjects with different genotypes. In
instances where genotypes are to be grouped, this is optimally done on the basis of
similarity of function or evolutionary relationship of alleles in order to maximize
the likelihood of relating a functional variant to phenotype (Templeton et al., 1987).

Perhaps the best criterion for candidate allele selection is functionality. Many
intronic sequence variants do not alter gene splicing or expression and most coding

sequence variants are synonymous substitutions that do not alter the amino acid sequence of the gene product. Association studies utilizing variants with no functional effects, or coding region variants known not to alter protein structure, have a significantly lower prior probability of detecting valid associations than studies using functional variants or "candidate alleles." Positive findings with nonfunctional markers are more likely to be secondary to chance or to inadvertent ethnic stratification of cases and controls. The nonfunctional or silent variant may be in linkage disequilibrium (nonrandom population association) with an as yet undiscovered functional variant. However, a difference in the frequency of a silent variant and the functional variant to which it is linked dilutes the information content of the silent variant. The informativeness of the silent variant is also weakened by population differences in variant frequencies and less than perfect linkage disequilibrium. Moreover, the possibility that a silent variant is in linkage disequilibrium with a functional variant should be viewed with caution if the candidate gene has been rigorously scanned for variation in large, ethnically mixed populations. An illustrative example of this issue is provided by the well-publicized association between the TaqI $A1$ allele near the dopamine D_2 receptor gene ($DRD2$) and risk of alcoholism (Blum et al., 1990). The initial report of this association suggested that variation within $DRD2$ influenced susceptibility to alcoholism. However, the Taq I $A1$ allele is located more than 10 kb downstream from the coding region of $DRD2$ and does not appear to impart any structural or functional effects on the D_2 receptor (Grandy et al., 1989). Gejman and colleagues (1994) scanned the coding sequence of $DRD2$ and were unable to detect additional variants that might account for this association, although a functionally deficient variant giving rise to Ser311Cys, was found but was not linked to alcoholism in a Southwestern American-Indian population (Goldman et al., 1997). Therefore, it is unlikely that the Taq I $A1$ allele is in linkage disequilibrium with a $DRD2$ variant that increases the susceptibility to alcoholism

An alternative approach to single candidate variant selection within a gene is to genotype subjects at several variants within the gene and construct haplotypes. Using haplotype estimation–maximization algorithms (Long et al., 1995), it is possible to assign haplotypes objectively. However, if one is testing the actual variant that produces the phenotype, then haplotype analysis adds to the degrees of freedom but not the information content and increases the possibility of a false-negative result. The power and validity of haplotype-based analysis is dramatically increased by the grouping of haplotypes according to their most likely common origin (Templeton et al., 1987). In this way, a group of haplotypes is most informative for functional genetic variants that first appeared on an ancestral haplotype and tends to be found on the descendants of that haplotype.

Finally, perhaps the most discussed limitation of case-control association studies is the potential for ethnic stratification between subject groups. In the case of psychiatric pharmacogenetic studies, this might arise in a study comparing candidate allele frequencies between drug responders and non responders. If the candidate allele frequency varies between ethnic groups, and responders and nonresponders are not ethnically matched, a significant difference in allele frequencies could be detected that is not associated with drug response. Unfortunately, ethnic variation in allele frequencies is not uncommon. For example, Chang and colleagues (1996) have found that frequencies for the 4-repeat allele of the DRD4 16 amino acid residue repeat varies between 16 and 96% in different populations. The *DRD2* Taq I *A1* allele is twice as frequent in African-Americans and four times as frequent in some American Indians compared with American Caucasians (Goldman et al., 1993).

One method to control for population differences is to analyze ethnically homogeneous samples, or population isolates. Unfortunately, it is difficult to ascertain these samples in Westernized society derived from multiple ethnic groups. Moreover, in pharmacogenetic studies, the phenotypic information is generally collected in the context of a clinical trial in which the objective is to study a wide variety of ethnic groups, and limiting study participation to a sole ethnic group would not be possible. An alternative to seeking ethnically homogeneous data sets is to collect DNA from the parents of probands and analyze data with the transmission disequilibrium test (Spielman and Ewens, 1996). With the family-based association approaches, the frequency of transmission of a candidate allele between parent and child is compared with the frequency of nontransmission. As the nontransmitted alleles represent the control alleles for the transmitted alleles, these tests are not sensitive to ethnic stratification. Although with this approach it is more difficult to collect large samples because of the necessity to ascertain family members, recent modifications of the transmission disequilibrium test involving siblings and the introduction of quantitative data analytic strategies (Allison et al., 1997) suggest that family-based association may represent a useful tool in psychiatric pharmacogenetics.

From pharmacogenetics to pharmacogenomics

The first generation of pharmacogenetic studies have utilized a limited number of polymorphisms in relatively small data sets derived from ethnically heterogenous populations. The next generation of studies, however, may be dramatically different from these early efforts because of impressive advances in genomic information, novel statistical genetic methodologies, and marked improvements in genotyping technologies. The following section briefly discusses some of the recent major advances in these domains.

Table 2.1. The SNP Consortium

Date	SNPs
23 November 1999	2556
23 December 1999	7365
30 March 2000	41209
28 April 2000	102719
21 August 2000	296990
1 November 2000	638372

Notes:
SNP, single nucleotide polymorphism.

Completion of the human genome sequence and identification of single nucleotide polymorphisms

The most important development at the beginning of the twenty-first century was the announcement of the completion of the human genome sequence by the US federally funded Human Genome Project and a private biotechnology firm, Celera Genomics. Although full sequence data are not yet available, the genome sequence that is available is already providing the reference sequence for large-scale efforts aiming to identify the genetic variation among individuals. In particular, there has been a focus on the identification of hundreds of thousands of SNPs within the genome. For example, the SNP Consortium, a group of pharmaceutical companies and academic centers, was formed in 1999 to identify SNPs distributed throughout the genome for use in pharmacogenomic studies. This consortium has, as of this writing, identified over 1000000 SNPs, with the pace of SNP identification continuing to increase rapidly (Table 2.1). In addition, Celera Genomics has recently reported that it has identified more than 2000000 SNPs within the context of its genome sequencing efforts.

Many of the SNPs that are being identified may be useful in pharmacogenetic studies. Cargill et al. (1999) scanned the coding region of 106 genes, many with potential relevance to the CNS, and identified an average of 3.7 coding region SNPs (cSNPs) per gene, of which nearly 50% were nonsynonymous, and 41% of the nonsynonymous cSNPs had a minor allele frequency of greater than 5%. As discussed above, nonsynonymous, coding region SNPs may have a higher a priori probability of altering function and be the most powerful in pharmacogenetic studies. Therefore, the massive SNP identification efforts, coupled with data demonstrating that a significant subset of them may be useful in pharmacogenetic studies, suggest that a large number of novel SNP targets will soon be available for study in the next generation of pharmacogenetic studies.

Developments in statistical genetic methodologies

Previous pharmacogenetic studies have utilized the case-control design. This approach has three major advantages over family-based designs. First, many of the patients participating in clinical trials of psychotropic drugs are already in their mid to late adult years and, therefore, collecting DNA from family members may be difficult because of lack of availability. Second, it has been suggested that probands selected from trios, or other family-based designs, may be subtly different than the general population of cases, thus reducing the generalizability of findings made with the family-based designs (Bruun and Ewald, 1999). Finally, the case-control design has greater statistical power than family-based approaches. Risch and Teng (1998) examined the relative power of the case-control design versus family-based approaches under a number of different genetic models. Under most models, the case-control design was more efficient than family-based designs, with sample sizes of less than 1000 usually sufficient to detect genes of relatively modest effect, even with extremely conservative significance levels (alpha $= 5 \times 10^{-8}$) and minor allele frequencies as low as 5%. These data suggested that the case-control design would be optimal for pharmacogenetic studies; however, as discussed above, the potential for undetected ethnic stratification has tempered enthusiasm for this design (Paterson, 1997).

Fortunately, "genomic control" methods are under development to help to account for ethnic stratification in case-control studies. Genomic control techniques are based upon the idea that study groups (cases versus controls, responders versus nonresponders, etc.) can be assessed for the presence of stratification by assessing the allele frequency of markers, unlinked to the phenotype of interest, in each group. Pritchard and Rosenberg (1999) determined that no more than 40 unlinked markers, and perhaps less, are necessary to achieve 95% probability of detecting stratification in study groups of over 200 subjects. If stratification is detected, subjects can be removed until stratification is not present, or correction factors can be introduced that account for the level of stratification between groups (Devlin and Roeder, 1999). Both approaches reduce study power but minimize the risk that the case-control design results in a false-positive or false-negative result.

Genomic control techniques have not yet been utilized in psychiatric pharmacogenetic studies. However, the considerable advantages of the case-control approach for pharmacogenetic studies, coupled with the genomic control methods, suggest that it should soon be feasible to conduct large-scale pharmacogenetic studies with increased power and with decreased potential for undetected ethnic stratification. Moreover, the extension of genomic control techniques to assess quantitative phenotypes is underway and should provide another compelling reason to consider these approaches in pharmacogenetic studies involving heterogenous populations.

Technology

The availability of over 500 000 SNPs distributed throughout the genome suggests that whole-genome association studies may soon be feasible – provided appropriate high-throughput SNP genotyping technology can be developed. Because SNPs are biallellic, unlike short tandem repeat markers with multiple alleles, they are more amenable to automated genotyping procedures. At the time of this writing, the cost of genotyping a single SNP in a single individual can be a low as 40 cents (US), but even this cost remains prohibitive for studies involving hundreds of patients with tens of thousands of SNPs. For example, to genotype 100 000 SNPs in 1000 individuals at this cost would represent a genotyping expenditure of US$40 million, before including the considerable costs associated with phenotype collection and DNA isolation. New technologies are currently under development within the biotechnology industry that promise to reduce genotyping costs further (with some near-term estimates as low as 3–5 cents per genotype) to a level that makes whole genome analyses more plausible. Moreover, the use of DNA pooling strategies provides an efficient method for generating genotype data on large numbers of subjects in an increasingly efficient manner. These developments suggest that it should soon be feasible to genotype comprehensively large study groups of patients characterized for drug response across thousands of SNPs distributed throughout the genome.

Conclusions

With the developments mentioned above, the next generation of molecular genetic studies of psychotropic drug responses should be markedly different from the first-generation studies. It will soon be possible to collect DNA from patients enrolled in large-scale clinical trials of thousands of patients, select SNPs that occur in each gene expressed in the CNS, and compare and contrast SNP frequencies in responders and nonresponders (or patients who develop side effects and those who do not) in large case-control designs. Moreover, as statistical methods are developed to account for undetected ethnic stratification between groups, the amount of stratification (if any) can be quantified between groups and accounted for in the analyses. Improved bioinformatics tools and statistical methods will be required to deal with the volume of data that will be generated by this approach, but it seems likely that such methods will soon be available given the level of interest in genetic approaches to complex diseases and to phenotypes such as drug response. With these developments in place, the first generation of pharmacogenetic studies that utilized SNPs in relatively limited numbers of candidate genes will be replaced by pharmacogenomic studies in which the complete genome is assessed. Therefore, the prospect for molecular genetic studies of psychotropic drug response seems bright and there is renewed hope that the first genes associated with psychotropic drug response will soon be identified.

REFERENCES

Allison DB (1997). Transmission–disequilibrium tests for quantitative traits. *Am J Hum Genet* 60, 676–690.

Angst J (1964). Antidepressiver effekt und genetische faktoren. *Arzneimittel-Forschung* 14(Suppl), 496–500

Arranz M, Collier D, Sodhi M et al. (1995). Association between clozapine response and allelic variation in 5HT-2A receptor gene. *Lancet* 346, 281–282

Blum K, Noble EP, Sheridan PJ et al. (1990). Allelic association of human dopamine D_2 receptor gene in alcoholism. *J Am Med Assoc* 263, 2055–2060.

Bowers MB, Swigar ME, Jatlow PI, Goicoechea N (1984). Plasma catecholamine metabolites and early response to haloperidol. *J Clin Psychiatry* 45, 248–251.

Bruun TG, Ewald H (1999). Selection bias of susceptibility genes possible when using parent-off-spring trios in genetic association studies. *Mol Psychiatry* 4, 414–416.

Buchsbaum MS, Potkin SG, Marshall JF et al. (1992). Effects of clozapine and thiothixene on glucose metabolic rate in schizophrenia. *Neuropsychopharmacology* 6, 155–163.

Cargill M, Altshuler D, Ireland J et al. (1999). Characterization of single-nucleotide polymorphisms in coding regions of human genes. *Nat Genet* 22, 231–238.

Chang FM, Kidd JR, Livak KJ, Pakstis AJ, Kidd KK (1996). The world-wide distribution of allele frequencies at the human dopamine D4 receptor locus. *Hum Genet* 98, 91–101.

Chee M, Yang R, Hubbell E et al. (1996). Accessing genetic information with high-density DNA arrays. *Science* 274, 610–614.

DeLisi LE, Dauphinais D (1989). Neuroleptic responsiveness in siblings concordant for schizophrenia. *Arch Gen Psychiatry* 46, 477.

Devlin B, Roeder, K (1999). Genomic control for association studies. *Biometrics* 55, 997–1004.

Drazen JM, Yandava CN, Dube L et al. (1999). Pharmacogenetic association between ALOX5 promoter genotype and the response to anti-asthma treatment. *Nat Genet* 22, 168–170.

Farde L, Nordstrom AL, Wiesel FA, Pauli S, Halldin C, Sedvall G (1992). Positron emission tomographic analysis of central D_1 and D_2 dopamine receptor occupancy in patients treated with classical neuroleptics and clozapine. Relation to extrapyramidal side effects. *Arch Gen Psychiatry* 49, 538–544.

Frackiewicz EJ, Sramek JJ, Herrera JM, Kurtz NM, Cutler NR (1997). Ethnicity and antipsychotic response. *Ann Pharmacother* 31, 1360–1369.

Franchini L, Serretti A, Gasperini M, Smeraldi E (1998). Familial concordance of fluvoxamine response as a tool for differentiating mood disorder pedigrees. *J Psychiatric Res* 32, 255–259.

Gejman PV, Ram A, Gelertner et al. (1994). No structural mutation in the dopamine D_2 receptor gene in alcoholism and schizophrenia. *J Am Med Assoc* 271, 204–208.

Goldman D, Brown GL, Albaugh B et al. (1993). *DRD2* dopamine receptor genotype, linkage disequilibrium and alcoholism in American Indians and other populations. *Alcohol Clin Exp Res* 17, 199–204.

Goldman D, Urbanek M, Guenther D, Robin R, Long UC (1997). The dopamine D_2 receptor: Linkage and association of a functional allele [Ser311Cys] and other *D2DR* markers to alcoholism, substance abuse and schizophrenia in Southwestern American Indians. *Neuropsychiat Genet* 74, 386–394.

Gottesman II (1991). *Schizophrenia Genesis: The Origins of Madness.* New York: WH Freeman.

Grandy DK, Litt M, Allen L, Bunzow JR, Marchionni M, Makam H (1989). The human dopamine D_2 receptor gene is located on chromosome 11 at q22–q23 and identifies a TaqI RFLP. *Am J Hum Genet* 45, 889–785.

Grebb JA, Cancro R (1989). Schizophrenia: clinical features. In Kaplan HI, Sadock BJ, eds. *Comprehensive Textbook of Psychiatry.* Baltimore, MD: Williams & Wilkins, pp. 457–486.

Gusella JF, Wezler NS, Conneally PM et al. (1983). A polymorphic DNA marker genetically linked to Huntington's disease. *Nature* 306, 234–238.

Hyman SE, Nestler EJ (1996). Initiation and adaptation: a paradigm for understanding psychotropic drug action. *Am J Psychiatry* 153, 151–162.

Kahn RS, Davidson M, Siever L, Gabriel S, Apter S, Davis KL (1993). Serotonin function and treatment response to clozapine in schizophrenic patients. *Am J Psychiatry* 150, 1337–1342.

Kety SS, Rosenthal D, Wender PH, Schulsinger F, Jacobsen B (1975). Mental illness in the biological and adoptive families of adopted individuals who have become schizophrenic: a preliminary report based on psychiatric interviews. In Fieve RR, Rosenthal D, Brill H (eds) *Genetic Research in Psychiatry.* Baltimore, MD: Johns Hopkins University Press, pp. 147–165.

Kotani Y, Nishimura Y, Maeda H, Yokoyama M (1999). β_2-Adrenergic receptor polymorphisms affect airway responsiveness to salbutamol in asthmatics. *J Asthma* 36, 583–590

Long JC, Williams RC, Urbanek M (1995). An E–M algorithm and testing strategy for multiple-locus haplotypes. *Am J Hum Genet* 56, 799–810.

Malhotra AK, Goldman D (1999). Benefits and pitfalls encountered in psychiatric genetic association studies. *Biol Psychiatry* 45, 544–550

Malhotra AK, Pickar D (1996). Biologic predictors of clozapine response in schizophrenia. *Psychiat Ann* 26, 390–394.

Malhotra AK, Goldman D, Ozaki N, Breier A, Buchanan R, Pickar D (1996). Lack of association between polymorphisms in the 5-HT_{2A} receptor gene and the antipsychotic response to clozapine. *Am J Psychiatry* 153, 1092–1094.

Malhotra AK, Breier A, Goldman D, Picken L, Pickar D (1998a). The apolipoprotein E epsilon 4 allele is associated with blunting of ketamine-induced psychosis in schizophrenia. A preliminary report. *Neuropsychopharmacology* 19, 445–448.

Malhotra AK, Goldman D, Buchanan RW et al. (1998b). The dopamine D_3 receptor (*DRD3*) Ser9Gly polymorphism and schizophrenia: a haplotype relative risk study and association with clozapine response. *Mol Psychiatry* 3, 72–75.

Masellis M, Paterson AD, Badri F et al. (1995). Genetic variation of 5-HT_{2A} receptor and response to clozapine. *Lancet* 346, 1128.

Myers RM, Fischer SG, Lerman LS, Maniatis T (1985). Nearly all single base substitutions in DNA fragments joined to a GC-clamp can be detected by denaturing gradient gel electrophoresis. *Nucl Acids Res* 13, 3131–3145.

Nguyen TV, Kosofsky BE, Birnbaum R, Cohen BM, Hyman SE (1992). Differential expression of c-*fos* and *zip268* in rat striatum after haloperidol, clozapine, and amphetamine. *Proc Natl Acad Sci USA* 89, 4270–4274.

Nurnberger JI Jr., Gershon ES, Simmons S et al. (1982). Behavioral, biochemical and neuroendocrine responses to amphetamine in normal twins and "well-state" bipolar patients. *Psychoneuroendocrinology* 7, 163–176.

O'Reilly RL, Bogue L, Singh SM (1994). Pharmacogenetic response to antidepressants in a multi-case family with affective disorder. *Biol Psychiatry* 36, 467–471.

Orita M, Suzuki Y, Seyiya T, Hayashi K (1989). Rapid and sensitive detection of point mutations and DNA polymorphisms using the polymerase chain reaction. *Genomics* 5, 874–879.

Pare CMB, Mack JW (1971). Differentiation of two genetically specific types of depression by the response to antidepressant drugs. *J Med Genet* 8, 306–309.

Pare CMB, Rees L, Sainsbury MJ (1962). Differentiation of two genetically specific types of depression by the response to anti-depressants. *Lancet* ii, 1340–1343.

Paterson AD (1997). Case-control association studies in complex traits – the end of an era? *Mol Psychiatry* 2, 277–278.

Pickar D, Labaraca R, Linnoila M et al. (1984). Neuroleptic-induced decrease in plasma homovanillic acid and antipsychotic activity in schizophrenic patients. *Science* 225, 954–957.

Plomin R, Owen MJ, McGuffin P (1994). The genetic basis of complex human behaviors. *Science* 264, 1733–1739.

Pritchard JK, Rosenberg NA (1999). Use of unlinked genetic markers to detect population stratification in association studies. *Am J Hum Genet* 65, 220–228.

Risch N, Teng J (1998). The relative power of family-based and case-control designs for linkage disequilibrium studies of complex human diseases I. DNA pooling. *Genome Res* 8, 1273–1288.

Spielman RS, Ewens WJ (1996). The TDT and other family-based tests for linkage disequilibrium and association. *Am J Hum Genet* 59, 983–989.

Szymanski S, Lieberman J, Pollack S et al. (1995). Clozapine effects on neuroendocrine response to apomorhine challenge testing in chronic neuroleptic nonresponsive schizophrenia: preliminary findings. *Biol Psychiatry* 37, 52–55.

Templeton AR, Boerwinkle E, Sing CF (1987). A cladistic analysis of phenotypic associations with haplotypes inferred from restriction endonuclease mapping. I. Basic theory of an analysis of alcohol dehydrogenase activity in *Drosophila*. *Genetics* 117, 343–351.

Tsui LC, Buchwald M, Barker D et al. (1985). Cystic fibrosis locus defined by a genetically linked polymorphic DNA marker. *Science* 230, 1054–1057.

Underhill PA, Jin L, Lin AA et al. (1997). Detection of numerous Y chromosome biallelic polymorphisms be denaturing high-performance liquid chromatography. *Genome Res* 7, 996–1005.

Vojvoda D, Grimmell K, Sernyak M, Mazure CM (1996). Monozygotic twins concordant for response to clozapine. *Lancet* 347, 61

3

Neuropsychopharmacology: the interface between genes and psychiatric nosology

Thomas A. Ban

Vanderbilt University, Nashville TA, USA

OVERVIEW

The observation that mental illness runs in families received substantial support in family, twin and adoption studies. Nonetheless, the heterogeneity within the diagnostic categories of schizophrenia and manic-depressive illness has precluded any meaningful research in the genetics of these disorders. To break the impasse in genetic research of mental illness, consideration was given to split psychiatric disorders into simpler biological or behavioral components. However, all alternative approaches fall short of psychiatric nosology in classifying mental illness in a clinically relevant manner. Neuropsychopharmacology has the unique capability of linking the effect of a psychotropic drug on mental illness with the effect of the substance on brain structures involved in the action mechanism of the drug. Since the primary targets of psychotropic drugs are encoded by genes that have been identified, any form of disease which corresponds with the treatment-responsive population to a psychotropic drug is suitable for the generation and testing of genetic hypotheses relevant to mental illness. To provide orientation points about what nosology could offer genetic research, the history of psychiatric nosology is reviewed and the varying constructs that can be used are illustrated. Kraepelin's (1899) diagnostic concepts of dementia praecox and manic-depressive insanity are artificially derived nosologic constructs, whereas Wernicke's (1899) classification was based on scientific developments that were to become the foundation of neuroscience. Schneider's (1950) rudimentary classification was the first nosology in which it was recognized that mental pathology is expressed in the mode (form) in which the experience appears (processed) and not in the "content" of the experience. Specially devised diagnostic instruments are described that provide more homogeneous populations for genetic research in mental illness. However, the use of nosologic homotypes, derived by the employment of a specially devised nosologic matrix is recommended for obtaining interpretable findings. The data collected by using the nosologic matrix could also serve as the starting point for the development of an empirically derived, pharmacologically meaningful classification of mental illness.

Introduction

The observation that mental illness runs in families has been documented since the mid-18th century (Battie, 1758; Chiarugi, 1793–1794). The first genetic theory of mental illness was formulated in the mid-1850s (Shorter, 1997). Morel's (1857) theory of degeneration is based on the assumption that mental illness is the result of an "innate biological defect" that becomes manifest in increasingly severe mental syndromes in "lineal descents."

Morel's (1857) degeneration theory was replaced by Moebius' (1893) "endogeny theory", which implied a "constitutionally determined predisposition" for developing mental illness. The dichotomy of "endogenous" and "psychogenic" (Wimmer, 1916) psychoses has been lingering on ever since.

Genetics in psychiatry

Epidemiological genetics

The notion that mental illness runs in families was endorsed by Kraepelin (1896) and Magnan (1896). It received substantial support from "family," "twin," and "adoption" studies. The majority of epidemiological genetic studies dealt with Kraepelin's (1899) diagnostic concepts of "manic-depressive insanity" and "dementia praecox." Magnan's (1893) diagnostic concept of "delusional psychoses" received relatively little attention in genetic research.

The risk of developing schizophrenia for relatives of schizophrenics, and manic-depressive (bipolar) illness for relatives of manic depressives, was found to be consistently higher than in the general population. The risk of developing the respective illness in both diagnostic groups was found to be higher for first- than for second-degree relatives (Slater and Cowie, 1971; Kay, 1978).

Concordance rates for schizophrenia and manic-depressive illness were found to be consistently higher in "monozygotic" than in "dizygotic" twins, with concordance rates in monozygotic twins for schizophrenia ranging from 35 to 85.8%, and in manic-depressive illness from 33 to 93%. Concordance rates in "dizygotic" twins in schizophrenia range from 0 to 17%, and in manic-depressive illness from 0 to 8% (Gottesman and Shields, 1966; Tsuang and Vandermey, 1980).

Children of schizophrenic natural (biological) parents adopted into the homes of nonschizophrenic foster parents were found to develop schizophrenia at a much higher rate than "adopted away" children of normal parents (Heston, 1966; Mendlewicz and Rainer, 1977). Mental illness was also encountered at a much higher rate in the biological than in the adoptive families of adopted schizophrenic and manic-depressive children (Kety et al., 1994; Wender et al., 1986).

Mathematical models of inheritance

In spite of findings that genetic factors play an important role in the etiology of schizophrenia and manic-depressive illness, the mode of transmission of these disorders, even with the employment of powerful statistical models, has remained hidden (O'Rourke et al., 1982; Craddock et al., 1995). Based on a comprehensive review of "pedigree and segregation analyses," the Genetics Workgroup of the US National Institute of Mental Health concluded that a "single major locus" cannot account for a large proportion of the "familial aggregation" of either schizophrenia or bipolar illness (a term used for manic-depressive disorder). The group suggested that the mode of inheritance of these disorders is "complex" and very "likely involves multiple interacting genes" (Moldin, 1999).

Molecular genetics: linkage analysis

Findings in "molecular genetic" studies in schizophrenia and manic-depressive illness did not clarify matters further. Employment of "positional cloning" ("backward genetics," "genome scanning") yielded inconsistent, conflicting results.

There are numerous publications reporting susceptibility loci for schizophrenia on chromosomes 1q, 3p, 5q, 6p, 8p, 8q, 9p, 10q, 12q, 13p, 14p, 15q, 20p, or 22q, and for manic-depressive illness on chromosomes 4p, 5p, 6p, 10q, 11p, 12q, 16p, 18p, 18q, 20p, 21q, or 22q. However, the findings in one group of patients could not be replicated in others (Gershon et al., 1998; Moldin, 1999).

Different findings in different samples from the same diagnostic category indicate genetic heterogeneity within the diagnosis (Tsuang and Faraone, 1990, 1995). However, the heterogeneity, which precluded meaningful genetic research, has not interfered with the recognition that "genetic anticipation," the essential feature of the first genetic theory of mental illness, is encountered in some schizophrenic families and also in some families with manic-depressive illness. Genetic anticipation may result from "trinucleotide repeat mutations," an anomaly causally linked with Huntington disease (Petronis and Kennedy, 1995; Faraone et al., 1999).

Molecular genetics: candidate gene approach

Genetic heterogeneity, coupled with heterogeneity in pharmacological responsiveness, has also precluded meaningful research with the employment of "forward genetics" in schizophrenia and manic-depressive illness. Nonetheless, on the basis of the demonstrable therapeutic effectiveness of some psychotropic drugs in schizophrenia and of others in manic-depressive illness, various genes have been implicated in the pathophysiology of these conditions. These genes encode transporters, receptors (e.g., serotonin 5-HT transported and 5-HT type 2A receptor, dopamine transporter 1 and D_2–D_4 receptors), and enzymes (e.g., monoamine oxidase, dopamine-β-hydroxylase, catechol-O-methyltransferase) involved in neuronal transmission. "Association studies," with the employment of the "candidate gene approach," however, have invariably failed to detect significant differences in mutations (polymorphisms) in the implicated genes between normal subjects and schizophrenic or manic-depressive patients (Malhotra and Goldman, 1999; Heiden et al., 2000). If there is a difference in "allelic variations" between the treatment responsive form of illness within these diagnostic categories and normal subjects, it is covered up by the heterogeneity of the patient samples used in the comparisons. An essential prerequisite for the demonstration of a difference in "allelic variations" would be the identification of the treatment-responsive forms of illness within schizophrenia or manic-depressive illness.

Replication studies also failed to support findings that allelic variations in the serotonin 5-HT_{2A} or 5-HT_{2C} receptor genes are responsible for individual differences in the therapeutic response to clozapine (Arranz et al., 1995; Malhotra et al., 1996). If the clozapine-responsive form of illness within schizophrenia could be identified, and the forms of the illness responsive to serotonin 5-HT_{2A} and dopamine D_2 demonstrated, the question whether therapeutic responsiveness to clozapine depends on "allelic variations" in the genes for these proteins would become a testable hypothesis.

Consensus-based diagnostic classifications

The inconsistent and conflicting findings in molecular genetic research in schizophrenia and manic-depressive illness led to a steadily growing dissatisfaction with psychiatric nosology. By the late 1990s, it was recognized that it "would be foolhardy to think" that diagnostic criteria in classifications such as those in the American Psychiatric Association's *Diagnostic and Statistical Manuals of Mental Disorders* (DSM-III, DSM-III-R, and DSM-IV; American Psychiatric Association 1980, 1987, 1994) could "select anything that maps into the genome" (Hyman, 1999). DSM-III and its successors are "consensus-based classifications," i.e., sets of diagnostic formulations agreed upon by a body of well-informed psychiatrists. To accommodate the different orientations in psychiatry, the diagnostic categories in these classifications are broad; because of the inclusion of different forms of disease in the same category of illness, the populations within the diagnostic categories are heterogeneous (Ban, 2000a).

In depressive illness, for example, Kraepelin's (1899) "unitary concept of melancholia" – derived by pooling together six distinct syndromes of "melancholia" (i.e., "simplex," "gravis," "stuporous," "paranoid," "fantastic," and "delirious") – was adopted in DSM-III virtually unchanged. In spite of findings in psychopharmacological, genetic and nosological studies that indicated that depressive illness is heterogeneous (Angst, 1966; Overall et al., 1966), the unitary concept of melancholia has been retained in DSM-III-R and DSM-IV. Depressive disorders in DSM-IV consist of one core syndrome, "major depression," which is so broad that, in a "composite (polydiagnostic) evaluation" in 6 of the 25 diagnostic classifications of the diagnostic instrument, 13.5–35.5% of the patients did not fit any of the depressive diagnoses (Ban, 1992b).

While the diagnosis of "major depression" is eminently suited to reconcile widely different conceptualizations of depressive illness, it is a consensus-based diagnosis that covers up its component diagnoses. Schneider's (1920) concept of "vital depression" – the diagnosis which allowed Roland Kuhn (1957) to recognize imipramine's antidepressant effect – is covered up in DSM-IV to the extent that, even if the patient is so severely ill that he/she displays all the possible symptoms and signs considered for the DSM-IV diagnosis of "major depression," one still would not know whether the patient qualifies for "vital depression." The anti-depressant-responsive forms of depressive illness are also obscured by the DSM-IV. There is no way to predict, within the framework of DSM-IV, which one (or two, including placebo responders) of three patients with the diagnosis of major depression will respond to treatment with an antidepressant drug (Ban, 1987, 1999).

The same defect applies to the DSM-IV diagnostic concept of "schizophrenia" (Ban, 1987, 1999).

Alternative approaches

Discouraged by the limitations of current diagnostic constructs, van Praag (1992, 2000) argues that today's "psychiatric taxonomy" presents diagnostic entities of "dubious validity," and suggests replacing the "nosological disease model" by a "reaction form-based disease model" in which "psychiatric conditions" are classified in eight broad basins: "disturbed reality testing and clear consciousness," "disturbed reality testing and lowered consciousness," "disturbances in affect regulation," "disturbed cognition," "conditions in which social adaptation and affiliative abilities are disturbed," "conditions with disturbed impulse regulation," "syndromes characterized by termination pathology," and "somatic syndromes without manifest somatic pathology." Others propose to break-up psychiatric disorders into "simpler biological or behavioral components" (Lander, 1988; Lander and Schork, 1994). Still others have suggested reconceptualizing mental illness in terms of "discrete neurobiological deficits," i.e., alternative phenotypes. One of the most intensively studied "alternative phenotypes" of schizophrenia is the "abnormality of smooth pursuit eye movement" (Holzman et al., 1988). Another frequently studied "alternative phenotype" is the "P-50 (evoked response) deficit" (Freedman et al., 1999). The former had been linked in genetic studies to a locus on the short arm of chromosome 6 (Arolt et al., 1996), and the latter to the "α_7-nicotinic acid receptor" on the long arm of chromosome 15 (Freedman et al., 1997). Nevertheless, the usefulness of these "alternative phenotypes" in genetic research in schizophrenia is questionable, because both "phenotypes" are encountered several times more frequently in the general population than schizophrenia (Faraone et al., 1999).

It has also been proposed to replace "traditional psychiatric nosology" with a "genetic psychiatric nosology," which would classify patients into categories that "correspond with the genes" (Faraone et al., 1999). While such a nosology could focus attention on overlaps between certain traits (e.g., depression and anxiety), it would group together individuals with genes for a particular disease who fully qualify for the disease and individuals who, despite carrying the genes for the disease, are symptom free.

Neuropsychopharmacology

To-date, there is no alternative methodology to psychiatric nosology for classifying mental pathology in a clinically relevant manner. In the light of the inadequacy of DSM-IV and the failure to replace traditional psychiatric concepts by empirically derived objective measurements, the identification of suitable forms of illness for genetic research in the different nosologies has become of practical importance for progress in the field.

Neuropsychopharmacology, by its unique capability of linking the effect of a psychotropic drug on mental illness with the effect of the substance on brain structures involved in the mechanism of the drug, offers an adequate methodology for the identification of suitable forms of illness for genetic research (Ban, 1999). Since the primary targets of psychotropic drugs in the brain (e.g., G-protein-coupled receptors, nuclear (hormonal) receptors, ion channels, enzymes, etc.) are all encoded by genes that have been identified, any nosologic entity that corresponds with the treatment-responsive population is suitable for the generation and testing of genetic hypotheses relevant to mental illness.

Psychiatric nosology

To provide orientation points about what nosology could offer, and about the nosologies which might be suitable for use in genetic research, the history of psychiatric nosology, with special reference to some of the influential classifications in psychiatry is reviewed. It can be seen that many terms are used to describe the symptoms/syndromes of mental illness, with different classifications implying different groupings.

Boissier de Sauvages

The origin of psychiatric nosology is in the work of Boissier de Sauvages (1768), who classified diseases, including "mania" (insanity), as if they were "specimens of natural history" by dividing them into 244 "species," 295 "genera," and 10 "classes" (Garrison, 1929). His assertion that naturally occurring categories of disease can be identified in a manner which would allow the attribution of each patient to only one class by grouping the symptoms at a particular point (cross-section) in time opened the path for the syndromic classifications of mental illness (Ban, 2000b).

Philippe Pinel

The first clinically employed psychiatric nosology was Pinel's classification (1799, 1801). It was an empirical, "phenetic" classification, based on "meticulous description of the appearance of objects " in which "mental derangements" were "distributed" into five distinct "species" (syndromes): "melancholia (depression) or delirium (delusions) upon one subject exclusively," "mania (insanity) without delirium," "mania with delirium," "dementia or the abolition of the thinking faculty," and "idiotism or obliteration of the intellectual faculties." Pinel's (1801) classification was modified and further elaborated by Esquirol (1838).

Jean-Etienne Dominique Esquirol

Esquirol (1838) divided insanity into five general forms: "lypemany (or melancholy of the ancient)," "monomania," "mania," "dementia," and "imbecility or idiocy." In variance with Pinel (1801), he assigned "melancholia" a distinct status, separated "partial insanity" ("monomania") from "insanity proper" ("mania"), and distinguished within "partial insanity" three distinct forms: "intellectual," "affective," and "instinctive." Esquirol's (1838) distinction between "partial insanity" and "insanity proper" was adopted by Kahlbaum (1863).

Karl Kahlbaum

Kahlbaum (1863) classified mental illness into five categories: (i) "vesanias," corresponding with "insanity proper," in which the syndromic expression of the disease changes through different developmental stages until it reaches dementia; (ii) "vecordias," corresponding with "partial insanity" (e.g., "paranoia", "dysthymia"), in which the syndromic expression remains essentially unchanged and restricted to one mental faculty during lifetime; (iii) "dysphrenias," or symptomatic diseases linked to somatic illness; (iv) "neophrenias," which are inborn or have an onset shortly after birth; and (v) "paraphrenias," with an onset at periods of transition in biological development (e.g., puberty, involution). Kahlbaum's (1874) postulation of a close correspondence between etiology, brain pathology, symptom pattern, and outcome picture had a major impact on nosologic development in psychiatry.

It stimulated Kraepelin (1893) to adopt "Sydenham's disease model" and shift emphasis in his classification of mental illness from cross-sectional syndromes to progression of clinical manifestations (Ban, 2000b).

Emil Kraepelin

Kraepelin's (1883, 1886, 1889) syndromic classification, presented in the first three editions of his textbook, was gradually replaced by his disease-oriented classification. To achieve his objective, Kraepelin (1893), in the fourth edition of his text, brought together three distinct syndromes – "demence precoce" (Morel, 1860), "catatonia" (Kahlbaum, 1874), and "dementia paranoides" (Kraepelin, 1893) under the heading of "psychic degeneration processes". In the fifth edition (1896) he subsumed all psychiatric disorders under two inferential classes: "acquired," and "constitutional." In the sixth edition (Kraepelin, 1899), the unifying diagnostic concept of "dementia praecox," for the three syndromes "hebephrenia (Hecker, 1871), "catatonia," and "dementia paranoides" and the all-embracing diagnostic concept of "manic-depressive insanity," appeared. All the distinct mental syndromes were pooled together and assigned on the basis of their course and outcome to one of these two categories of disease. By the time of the seventh edition (Kraepelin, 1903–1904), the inferential classes of "acquired," and "constitutional" psychiatric disorders were replaced by 15 disease categories, including "manic-depressive insanity" and "dementia praecox." Of the remaining 13 disease categories, seven were based on inferences or guesses about their possible causes ("exhaustion psychoses," "involutional psychoses," "paranoia," "psychogenic neuroses," "constitutional psychopathic states," "psychopathic personalities," and "defective mental development"), and six were attributed to organic, including toxic, etiologies ("infection psychoses," "intoxication psychoses," "thyrogenous psychoses," "dementia paralytica," "organic dementias," and "epileptic insanity"). In the eighth edition (Kraepelin, 1908–1915), the already broad diagnostic concepts were expanded. "Manic-depressive insanity" incorporated "involutional melancholia" (Dreyfus, 1905) and "all cases of affective excess," and "dementia praecox" incorporated Magnan's (1893) diagnostic concept of "delire chronique" (Kraepelin, 1919, 1921; Pichot, 1983). However, in the same edition, Kraepelin (1908–1915) distinguished between the "paranoid form of dementia praecox" and the "paraphrenias." By the time Bleuler (1911) coined the term "schizophrenia" to replace the term "dementia praecox," Kraepelin (1919) recognized 10 different forms of "dementia praecox, i.e., "dementia simplex" (Diem, 1903); "silly deterioration" (replacing the term "hebephrenia"); "depressive deterioration;" "depressive deterioration with delusional formation;" "circular," "agitated," "periodic," "catatonic," and "paranoid" forms; and schizophasia. He also defined nine different end-states of the disease, i.e., "cure"; "cure with defect;" "simple deterioration;" "imbecility with confusion of speech;" "hallucinatory deterioration;" "hallucinatory insanity;" "dementia paranoides;" "flighty, silly deterioration;" and "dull, apathetic dementia" (Fish, 1962; Hamilton, 1976).

Eugen Bleuler

Kraepelin's (1903–1904) classification was adopted by Eugen Bleuler (1916) with some minor modifications. By replacing the term "dementia praecox" with the term "schizophrenia," and redefining schizophrenia as a "group of psychoses" characterized "by a specific type of thinking, feeling and relation to the external world" which "appear in no other disease in this particular fashion," Bleuler (1911) consolidated the diagnostic concept. His "fundamental" or "basic symptoms" remained for well over 50 years the most extensively employed diagnostic criteria of schizophrenia.

Carl Wernicke

Wernicke's (1899) "classification of psychoses" appeared in the same year as the sixth edition of Kraepelin's textbook (1899). It was based on contemporary scientific contributions that were to become the structural foundation of neuroscience, e.g., the description of "multipolar cells" in the cerebral cortex (Golgi, 1883), the recognition that the "neuron" is the morphological and functional unit of the nervous system (Ramon y Cajal, 1897–1904), and the demonstration that the "synapse" is the functional site of transmission from one "neuron" to another (Sherrington, 1896–1897, 1906). By adopting Sechenov's (1866) extension of the concept of the "reflex" as the elementary unit of mental pathology, Wernicke (1900) perceived the different forms of mental illness as "loosening of detachment from the rigid structure of associations," displayed in "hyperfunctioning," "hypofunctioning," or "parafunctioning" in the "psychosensory," "intrapsychic," or "psychomotor" component(s) of the "psychic reflex" (Franzek, 1990). Wernicke (1899) was also first to describe "motility psychosis" and "anxiety-happiness psychosis", to separate memory impairment ("dysmnesia") from personality deterioration ("dementia"), and to divide consciousness into "consciousness of the body" ("somatopsyche"), "consciousness of one's personality" ("autopsyche"), and "consciousness of the external world" ("allopsyche").

Karl Kleist

Wernicke's (1900) contributions were further elaborated by Kleist (1921, 1923), who split the diagnostic concept of "schizophrenia" into two groups of diseases: "typical schizophrenias," which are confined to one neurological system, and "atypical schizophrenias," which affect many different neurological systems in the central nervous system. Kleist (1928) was first to recognize "cycloid psychoses" as a distinct nosological category that include Wernicke's (1900) diagnostic concepts of "anxiety psychosis" and "motility psychosis," and Kleist's own diagnostic concept of "confusion psychosis."

Karl Leonhard

Leonhard (1957) replaced Kleist's dichotomy (1923) of "typical" and "atypical schizophrenias" with the "polarity"-based dichotomy of "systematic" and "unsystematic schizophrenias." He adopted Kleist's (1928) diagnostic concept of "cycloid psychoses" and Neele's (1949) diagnostic concept of "phasic psychoses" and classified "endogenous psychoses" into five classes of illness: "unipolar phasic psychoses," "bipolar manic-depressive disease," "bipolar cycloid psychoses," "bipolar unsystematic schizophrenias," and "unipolar systematic schizophrenias." Furthermore, on the basis of the primarily affected component of the "psychic reflex" – "afferent" (sensory–perceptual–cognitive), "central-intrapsychic" (affective), or "efferent" (motor) – he separated three groups of illnesses within the "systematic schizophrenias" ("paraphrenias," "hebephrenias," and "catatonias), the "unsystematic schizophrenias" ("cataphasia" "affect-laden paraphrenia," and "periodic catatonia"), and the "cycloid psychoses ("confusion psychosis," "anxiety-happiness psychosis," and "motility psychosis"). He also separated "pure mania" and "pure melancholia," diseases in which the "mental pathology" extends to all three components of the "psychic reflex," from the pure "euphorias" and "pure depressions," in which the "mental pathology" is less pervasive. In Leonhard's (1936, 1961, 1986) "differentiated nosology" there are 16 "psychopathology"-based syndromes differentiated within the "systematic schizophrenia" group; five "psychopathology"-based syndromes within each of the "pure euphorias" and the "pure depressions;" and three psychopathology-based syndromes within each of the "unsystematic schizophrenias" and the "cycloid psychoses."

Kurt Schneider

Kurt Schneider's (1959) rudimentary classification was based on Karl Jaspers' (1910, 1913, 1962) recognition that mental illness is expressed in the "form" (i.e., the "mode") in which the experience appears (e.g., "sudden primordial delusional idea put in the mind by hallucinatory voices") and not in the "content" (e.g, "being persecuted") of the experience. About two decades prior to Schneider (1950), a group of German psychiatrists at the "Heidelberg Clinic," began to re-evaluate psychiatric nosology with the employment of Jaspers' (1913) conceptual framework. Their activity ended in 1933 with the removal of Wilmans, the head of the "Clinic" by the Nazi regime. (Gruhle, who was the intellectual leader of the group, left the university and took a position at a provincial psychiatric hospital; Mayer-Gross moved to England, etc.). What was left behind was put together by Schneider

(1959) into a rudimentary classification in which "developmental anomalies" (i.e., "abnormal variations of mental life") are separated from the "effects of illness and defective structure." Included among the "developmental anomalies" are "abnormal intellectual endowment," "abnormal personality," and "abnormal psychic reaction." Included among the "effects of illness" are the "somatically based psychoses," "schizophrenia," and "cyclothymia," the term Schneider (1959) used for "manic-depressive disease." Although Schneider (1950) retained the diagnosis of schizophrenia, he maintained that "there is nothing to which one can point as a common element in all the clinical pictures that are today christened as schizophrenia."

Diagnostic instruments for research

There are two diagnostic instruments specially devised to provide more homogeneous populations for research than the diagnostic categories of consensus-based classifications: these are the Diagnostic Criteria for Research Budapest–Nashville (DCR) and the Composite Diagnostic Evaluation (CODE) system.

DCR Budapest–Nashville

The DCR Budapest-Nashville (Petho et al., 1984, 1988) is an "eclectic classification," devised on the basis of theoretical considerations. It is an integration of nosologic contributions from different schools of psychiatry into a classification in which the original diagnostic concepts are retained.

At the core of the DCR is Leonhard's (1957) classification of "endogenous psychoses." However, the DCR also includes the Scandinavian diagnostic concept of "psychogenic (reactive) psychoses" (Wimmer, 1916; Stromgren, 1974), and a composite of the German diagnostic concept of "delusional development" (Gaupp, 1914; Kretschmer, 1927) and the French diagnostic concept of "delusional psychoses" (Magnan, 1893; Baruk, 1974).

The decision to adopt Leonhard's (1957) classification of "endogenous psychoses" in the DCR was based on findings in epidemiological genetic and psychopharmacological research that were supportive of Leonhard's (1957) diagnostic concepts (Ban, 1990; Ban and Ucha Udabe, 1995). The incidence of "nosologic homotypy" was high, 57–77% in the parents and siblings of patients with "cycloid psychoses" (Perris, 1974a; Ungvari, 1985); the concordance for "polarity" was as high as 80% in twin pairs concordant for "mood disorders" (Zerbin-Rudin, 1967; Tsuang and Vandermey, 1980). Morbidity risk for "endogenous psychoses" was higher in the relatives (parents and siblings) of patients with "bipolar affective psychoses" than in the relatives of patients with "unipolar phasic psychoses" or "cycloid psychoses"; in the relatives of those with "unsystematic schizophrenias" than in the relatives of those with "systematic schizophrenias" or "cycloid psychoses"; and in the relatives of those with "cycloid psychoses" than in the relatives of those with "systematic schizophrenias" (Trostorff, 1968, 1975; Perris, 1974b). Responsiveness to neuroleptic treatment was higher in the "unsystematic schizophrenias" (79%) than in the "systematic schizophrenias" (22%) (Astrup, 1959; Fish, 1964). The different forms (and subforms) of schizophrenia in Leonhard's (1957) classification were to become suitable end-points for molecular genetic research, yielding to the demonstration that "periodic catatonia," one of the three forms of "unsystematic schizophrenia," is associated with a "major disease locus" that "maps" to chromosome 15q15 (Stober et al., 2000).

The diagnostic process in the DCR is based on a decision tree model that consists of 524 variables organized into 179 diagnostic decision clusters, yielding a total of 213 diagnoses (11 undifferentiated; 37 atypical; 21 tentative; 44 provisional; 45 working; and 55 final). An undifferentiated diagnosis in the DCR implies that patient qualifies for "psychosis" but does not fit any of the DCR diagnoses; an atypical diagnosis implies that the patient fulfills only cross-sectional diagnostic criteria of a specific DCR diagnosis.

CODE-system

The CODE system provides a methodology for the detection of the forms of mental illness identified in the different nosologies which are biologically the most homogeneous. It is a set of diagnostic instruments that can assign simultaneously a diagnosis from several diagnostic systems to a patient by specially devised algorithms. Each instrument ("CODE") can provide for a polydiagnostic evaluation in a distinct category of mental illness by employment of an integrated criteria list and standardized data collection. To achieve its purpose, each "CODE" consists of a set of symptoms ("codes"), which yield diagnoses in all the component diagnostic systems; a semistructured interview, suitable for the elicitation of all the symptoms in terms of "present" or "absent"; and diagnostic decision trees, which organize symptoms into distinct psychiatric disorders (Ban, 1991). The CODE system differs from other polydiagnostic systems by the inclusion of all distinct diagnostic formulations relevant to the conceptual development of a diagnostic category, and by its capability to provide readily accessible information relevant to the diagnostic process from the lowest to the highest level of decision making.

The prototype of the CODE System is CODE-DD, the CODE for "unipolar depressive disorders" (Ban, 1989). It consists of a 90-item Rating Scale for Depressive Diagnoses (RSDD) with a 40-item subscale (the Rating Scale for the Assessment of Severity in Depressive Disorders); a Semi-Structured Interview for Depressive Disorders, suitable for the elicitation of the presence or absence of the 90 variables of the RSDD; and decision trees, which provide diagnoses within 25 different classifications of depression. Many of the classifications of depression included in CODE-DD are empirically derived, e.g., those of Kiloh and Garside (1963) and Winokur (1979). Some are based on the conceptual development of depression in Europe, e.g., Schneider (1920), and others on the conceptual development of depression in North America, e.g., Robins and Guze (1972). Included also in CODE-DD are consensus-based classifications, e.g., DSM-III-R of the American Psychiatric Association (1987), and diagnostic criteria for research, e.g., Feighner et al. (1972).

One would expect low inter-rater agreement in such a complex system like CODE-DD. However, in the first reliability study there was an 87.8% inter-rater agreement (regarding the presence or absence of) on the 90 RSDD variables (Morey, 1991). In the second, agreement increased to 100% (Ban et al., 1993). In a validation study that included 230 patients with a clinical diagnosis of major depression, there was a 99.6% correspondence between the clinical DSM-III-R and the CODE-DD diagnosis of major depression. In another validation study, which included 322 patients, the correspondence was 97.2% (Ban, 1992).

Nosologic matrix

Whether DCR, CODE-DD, or any other diagnostic instrument in preparation would provide suitable populations for genetic research is not known. Until the time such an instrument becomes available, the use of "nosologic homotypes" is an essential prerequisite for obtaining interpretable findings in research in the genetics of mental illness. Nosologic homotypes are identical in "elementary units" of mental illness and are assigned the same position in the "nosologic matrix" constructed with consideration for the "nosologic organizing principles" of Esquirol (1838), Kraepelin (1896, 1899), and Leonhard (1957) (Ban, 2000b).

The elementary units of mental illness are psychopathologic symptoms (Jaspers, 1913, 1962). Each psychopathologic symptom represents a distinct pathology in the processing of mental events (Wernicke, 1900), and each distinct "psychopathologic symptom profile" (syndrome) is a potential "phenotype" of mental disorder. The formal characteristics of the "onset" (sudden or insidious), "course" (episodic or continuous), and "outcome" (recovery or defect) of the mental syndrome reflect the pathological process in its "dynamic totality," and the "dynamic totality" of the pathological process, together with the "holistic character" (Petho, 1990) of the clinical picture ("monomorphous," "polymorphous," "amorphous"), provides a "structure" that is " determined by the illness" (Ban, 1987). It is in terms of this structure that each mental illness is defined and assigned a distinct place in the "nosologic matrix," based on the three nosologic organizing principles.

The first organizing principle of psychiatric nosology is the "inclusiveness" of the psychopathological process. Its origin is in Esquirol's (1838) distinction between "insanity proper" and "partial insanity." The prototype of "insanity proper" is Morel's (1860) "demence precoce," and the prototype of "partial insanity" is Lasegue's (1852) "persecutory delusional psychosis." The concept of "partial insanity" (i.e., insanity with preserved personality) was extended to include "abortive insanity." Patients with "abortive insanity" are fully aware (cognizant) that their thinking, feelings, or actions are pathological. The prototype of "abortive insanity" is Westphal's (1878) diagnostic concept of "obsessional neurosis."

The second organizing principle of psychiatric nosology is the "course" and "outcome" of the psychopathological process. Its origin is in Kraepelin's (1899) separation of "manic-depressive insanity" (an episodic and remitting illness) from "dementia praecox" (a continuous and progressing disease). It is within the frame of reference of the second nosologic organizing principle that "attacks" (episodes with brief duration, from minutes to hours, encountered in "panic disorder") are distinguished from "phases" (episodes with long duration, from days to years, encountered in the "phasic psychoses") and from "periods" (phases recurring with regularity, encountered in "seasonal affective disorder"). Similarly, "thrusts" (acute events that yield lasting changes, encountered in the "unsystematic schizophrenias") can be distinguished from "continuous process" (chronic events, that yield highly differentiated end-states, encountered in the "systematic schizophrenias") and from "progressive deterioration" (chronic events that yield increasingly severe "dedifferentiation," encountered in the "organic dementias").

The third organizing principle of psychiatric nosology is "polarity." Its origin is in Leonhard's (1957) distinction between "polymorphous (multiform) bipolar" and "monomorphous (pure) unipolar" psychiatric disorders. "Bipolar illness" swings between two poles of mood (emotions and motility) and displays a continuously changing (variable) clinical picture, whereas "unipolar illness" is restricted to one pole of mood (emotions and motility) and displays the same symptomatology within and across episodes. Each distinct form of "unipolar illness is characterized by a syndrome associated with no other form and not even transitionally related to any other forms."

While "nosologic homotypes," based on a specially devised "nosologic matrix," are biologically more homogeneous populations than any of the diagnostic population identified by the available diagnostic instruments today, the information collected by the use of the "nosologic matrix" would allow completion of the re-evaluation of diagnostic concepts started by the psychiatrists at the "Heidelberg Clinic" in the 1920s. The information collected by the use of the "nosologic matrix" could also serve as the starting point for an empirically derived classification of mental illness.

Considering that "nosologic homotypes" are defined in terms of their effect on "processing of mental events," and psychotropic drugs are defined in terms of their effect on "signal transduction" in the brain (Bloom, 2001), the empirically derived diagnostic categories provide clinical entities which are suitable for testing hypotheses relevant to the relationship between "processing of mental events" and "signal transduction " in the central nervous system. Thus, employment of the "nosologic matrix" could open up a new perspective for the development of a psychiatry in which mental pathology is perceived in terms of pathology in "signal transduction" in the brain, and for the development of a rational pharmacotherapy of mental illness. Within the new frame of reference, genetic research in mental illness would enter a new phase.

Conclusions

The observation that mental illness runs in families received substantial support from findings in epidemiological genetic research. The failure to reveal the mode of inheritance of schizophrenia and manic-depressive disorder with the employment of powerful statistical models led psychiatric geneticists to conclude that the mode of inheritance of these disorders is "complex." However, the inconsistent, conflicting findings in molecular genetic studies of schizophrenia and manic-depressive illness have brought attention to the fact that populations within these diagnostic categories are genetically heterogenous.

Neuropsychopharmacology provides an adequate methodology for the identification of suitable, pharmacologically homogeneous forms of illness for genetic research in the different nosologies. Until this is done, the use of "nosologic homotypes," identified by the employment of a "nosologic matrix," is an essential prerequisite in genetic research for obtaining interpretable findings.

The "nosologic matrix" may also serve as the starting point for the development of an empirically derived pharmacologically meaningful classification of mental illness. A classification in which the relationship between mental pathology and the pathology of "signal transduction" in the brain is recognized would open up a new perspective in genetic research and in the pharmacotherapy of mental illness.

REFERENCES

American Psychiatric Association (1980). *Diagnostic and Statistical Manual of Mental Disorders*, 3rd edn. Washington, DC: American Psychiatric Association.

American Psychiatric Association (1987). *Diagnostic and Statistical Manual of Mental Disorders*, 3rd edn. Revised. Washington, DC: American Psychiatric Association.

American Psychiatric Association (1994). *Diagnostic and Statistical Manual of Mental Disorders*, 4th edn. Washington, DC: American Psychiatric Association.

Angst J (1966). *Zur Aetiologie und Nosologie endogener depressiver Psychosen.* Berlin: Springer.

Arolt V, Lencer R, Nolte A et al. (1996). Eye tracking dysfunction is a putative phenotypic susceptibility marker of schizophrenia and maps to a locus on chromosome 6p in families with multiple occurrence of the disease. *Am J Med Genet* 67, 564–579.

Arranz M, Collier D, Sodhi M et al. (1995). Association between clozapine response and allelic variation in $5HT_{2A}$ receptor gene. *Lancet* 346, 281– 282.

Astrup C (1959). The effects of ataraxic drugs on schizophrenic subgroups related to experimental findings. *Acta Psychiatr Scand* 34(Suppl 136), 388–393.

Ban TA (1987). Prolegomenon to the clinical prerequisite: psychopharmacology and the classification of mental disorders. *Progr Neuropsychopharmacol Biol Psychiatry* 11, 527–580.

Ban TA (1989). *CODE-DD Composite Diagnostic Evaluation of Depressive Disorders.* Nashville, TN: JM Productions.

Ban TA (1990). Clinical pharmacology and Leonhard's classification of endogenous psychoses. *Psychopathology* 23, 331–338.

Ban TA (1991). CODE system: theory and practice. In Aguglia E, Ban TA, eds. *International Symposium on Functional Psychoses Today.* Rome: John Libbey, pp. 279–296.

Ban TA (1992). Composite diagnostic evaluation: methodology and applications. In Ferrero FP, Haynal AE, Sartorius N, eds. *Schizophrenia and Affective Psychoses. Nosology in Contemporary Psychiatry.* Rome: John Libbey, pp. 410–419.

Ban TA (1999). Selective drugs versus heterogenous diagnoses towards a new methodology in psychopharmacologic research. *Psiquiatr Biol* 7, 177–189.

Ban TA (2000a). From DSM-III to DSM-IV: progress or standstill? In Franzek E, Ungvari GS, Ruther E, Beckmann H, eds. *Progress in Differentiated Psychopathology.* Hong Kong: Contemporary Development Company, pp. 1–11.

Ban TA (2000b). Nosology in the teaching of psychiatry. *J Bras Psiquiatr* 49, 39–49.

Ban TA and Ucha Udabe R (1995). *Clasificacion de las Psicosis.* Buenos Aires: Editorial Salerno.

Ban TA, Fjetland OK, Kutcher M, Morey LC (1993). CODE-DD development of a diagnostic scale for depressive disorders. In Hindmarch I, Stonier PD, eds. *Human Psychopharmacology. Measures and Methods,* Vol. 4. Chichester, UK: John Wiley & Sons, pp. 73–85.

Baruk H (1974). Delusions of passion. [Translated by Rohde M.] In Hirsch SR, Shepherd M, eds. *Themes and Variations in European Psychiatry.* Charlottesville, VA: University Press of Virginia, pp. 375–383.

Battie W (1758). *A Treatise of Madness.* London: Whiston.

Bleuler E (1911). *Dementia praecox oder gruppe der Schizophrenien.* Leipzig: Deuticke.

Bleuler E (1916). *Lehrbuch der Psychiatrie.* Berlin: Springer.

Bloom F (2001). Personal perpectives. *Am Coll Neuropsychopharm Bull* 7, 4–8.

Boissier de Sauvages (1768). *Nosologia Methodica.* Amsterdam: Frat de Tournes.

Chiarugi V (1793–1794). *On Insanity and its Classification.* (Republished in English, 1989). Canton, MA: Science History Publishers.

Craddock N, Khodel V, van Eerdewegh P, Reich T (1995). Mathematical limits of multilocus models: the genetic transmission of bipolar disorder. *Am J Hum Genet* 57, 690–702.

Diem O (1903). Die einfach demente Form der Dementia Praecox (Dementia Simplex). *Arch für Psychiatr Nervenkrank* 37, 111–187.

Dreyfus GL (1905). *Die Melancholie ein Zustandsbild des Manisch-Depressiven Irreseins*. Jena: Gustav Fischer.

Esquirol JED (1838). *Des Maladies Mentales Considerees Sous les Raports Medical, Hygienique et Medico-Legal*. Paris: JP. Baillière.

Faraone SV, Tsuang MT, Tsuang DW (1999). *Genetics of Mental Disorders*. New York: Guilford Press.

Feighner JP, Robins E, Guze B, Woodruff JP, Winokur G, Munoz R (1972). Diagnostic criteria for use in psychiatric research. *Arch Gen Psychiatry* 26, 57–63.

Fish F (1962). *Schizophrenia*. Bristol: John Wright.

Fish F (1964). The influence of the tranquilizer on the Leonhard schizophrenic syndromes. *Encephale* 53, 245–249.

Franzek E (1990). Influence of Carl Wernicke on Karl Leonhard's nosology. *Psychopathology* 23, 277–281.

Freedman R, Coon H, Myles-Worsley M et al. (1997). Linkage of a neurophysiological deficit in schizophrenia to a chromosome 15 locus. *Proc Natl Acad Sci, USA* 94, 587–592.

Freedman R, Adler LE, Leonard S (1999). Alternative phenotypes for the complex genetics of schizophrenia. *Biol Psychiatry* 45, 551– 558.

Garrison FH (1929). *An Introduction to the History of Medicine*, 4th edn (reprinted 1960). Philadelphia, PA: Saunders.

Gaupp R (1914). Die Wissenschaftliche Bedeutung des Falles Wagner. *Munch Med Wschr* 61, 633–637.

Gershon ES, Badner J, Goldin LR, Sanders AR, Cravchik A, Detera-Wadleigh SD (1998). Closing in on genes for manic-depressive illness and schizophrenia. *Neuropsychopharmacology* 18, 233–242.

Golgi C (1883). Recherches sur l'histologie des centres nerveux, *Arch Ital Biol Turin* 3, 285–317.

Gottesman II, Shields J (1966). Contributions of twin studies to perspectives on schizophrenia. In Maher BA, ed. *Progress in Experimental Personality Research*. New York: Academic Press, pp. 1–84.

Hamilton M (1976). *Fish's Schizophrenia*, 2nd edn. Bristol: John Wright.

Hecker E (1871). Die Hebephrenie. *Arch Pathol Anat Physiol Klin Med* 52, 394–409.

Heiden A, Schussler P, Itzlinger U et al. (2000). Association studies of candidate genes in bipolar disorder. *Neuropsychobiology* 42(Suppl 1), 18–21.

Heston LL (1966). Psychiatric disorders in foster home reared children of schizophrenic mothers. *Br J Psychiatr* 112, 819– 825.

Holzman PS, Kringlen E, Mathysse S et al. (1988). A single dominant gene can account for eye tracking dysfunctions and schizophrenia in offspring of discordant twins. *Arch Gen Psychiatry* 45, 641–647.

Hyman SE (1999). Introduction to the complex genetics of mental disorders. *Biol Psychiatry* 45, 518–521.

Jaspers K (1910). Eifersuchtswahn: Entwicklung einer Persoenlichkeit oder Prozess. *Z Ges Neurol Psychiatr* 1, 567–637.

Jaspers K (1913). *Allgemeine Psychopathologie*. Springer: Berlin.

Jaspers K (1962). *General Psychopathology*. [Translated from the German 7th edn by Hoenig J, Hamilton MW.] Manchester, UK: Manchester University Press.

Kahlbaum KL (1863). *Die Gruppierung der psychischen Krankheiten und die Enteilung der Seelenstoerungen.* Danzig: AW Kaufman.

Kahlbaum K (1874). *Die Katatonie oder das Spannungsirresein.* Berlin: Hirschwald.

Kay DWK (1978). Assessment of familial risks in the functional psychoses and their application in genetic counselling. *Br J Psychiatr* 133, 385–403.

Kety SS, Wender PH, Jacobsen B et al. (1994) Mental illness in the biological and adoptive relatives of schizophrenic adoptees. Replication of the Copenhagen Study in the rest of Denmark. *Arch Gen Psychiatry* 51, 442–455.

Kiloh LG, Garside RF (1963). The independence of neurotic depression and endogenous depression. *Br J Psychiatry* 109, 451–463.

Kleist K (1921). Autochtone Degenerationspsychosen. *Z Ges Neurol Psychiatr* 69, 1–11.

Kleist K (1923). Die Auffassung der Schizophrenien als Systemkrankheiten. *Klin J Wochenschr* 2, 962–965.

Kleist K (1928). Uber zykloide, paranoide und epileptoide psychosen und uber die Frage der Degenerationspsychosen. *Schweiz Arch Neurol Psychiatr* 23, 1–35.

Kraepelin E (1883). *Compendium der Psychiatrie.* Leipzig: Barth.

Kraepelin E (1886). *Compendium der Psychiatrie,* 2nd edn. Leipzig: Barth.

Kraepelin E (1889). *Compendium der Psychiatrie,* 3rd edn. Leipzig: Barth.

Kraepelin E (1893). *Psychiatrie, Ein Lehrbuch für Studierende und Arzte,* 4th edn. Barth: Leipzig.

Kraepelin E (1896). *Psychiatrie, Ein Lehrbuch für Studierende und Arzte,* 5th edn. Barth: Leipzig.

Kraepelin E (1899). *Psychiatrie, Ein Lehrbuch für Studierende und Arzte,* 6th edn. Barth: Leipzig.

Kraepelin E (1903–1904). *Psychiatrie, Ein Lehrbuch für Studierende und Arzte,* 7th edn. Barth: Leipzig.

Kraepelin E (1908–1915). *Psychiatrie, Ein Lehrbuch für Studierende und Arzte,* 8th edn. Barth: Leipzig.

Kraepelin E (1919). *Dementia Praecox and Paraphrenia.* [Translated by Barclay RM.] Edinburgh: Livingstone.

Kraepelin E (1921). *Manic Depressive Insanity and Paranoia.* [Translated by Barclay RM.] Edinburgh: Livingstone.

Kretschmer E (1927). *Der sensitive Beziehungswahn.* Berlin: Springer.

Kuhn R (1957). Uber die Behandlung depressives Zustande mit einem iminodibenzyl-derivat (G22355). *Schweiz Med Wochenschr* 87, 1135–1140.

Lander ES (1988). Splitting schizophrenia. *Nature* 336, 105–106.

Lander ES, Schork NI (1994). Genetic dissection of complex traits. *Science* 265, 2037–2038.

Lasegue EC (1852). Du delire de persecution. *Arch Gen Med* 28, 129–150.

Leonhard K (1936). *Die Defektschizophrenen Krankheitsbilder.* Leipzig: Thieme.

Leonhard K (1957). *Aufteilung der endogenen Psychosen.* Berlin: Akademie-Verlag.

Leonhard K (1961). Cycloid psychoses – endogenous psychoses which are neither schizophrenic nor manic-depressive. *J Ment Sci* 107, 633–648.

Leonhard K (1986). *Aufteilung der endogenen Psychosen und ihre differenzierte Aetiologie,* 6th edn revised. Berlin: Akademie-Verlag.

Magnan V (1893). *Leconc Cliniques sur les Maladies Mentales,* 2nd edn. Paris: Bataille.

Magnan V (1896). Considerations generales sur la folie (des hereditaires ou degeneres). *Prog Med* 2, 108–110.

Malhotra AK, Goldman D (1999). Benefits and pitfalls encountered in psychiatric genetic association studies. *Biol Psychiatry* 45, 544–550.

Malhotra AK, Goldman D, Mazzani C, Clifton A, Breier A, Pickar D (1996). Lack of association between polymorphism in the *5-HT2A* receptor gene and the antipsychotic response to clozapine. *Am J Psychiatry* 153, 1092–1094.

Mendlewicz J, Rainer JD (1977). Adoption study supporting genetic transmission in manic-depressive illness. *Nature* 268, 326–329.

Moebius JP (1893). *Abriss der Lehre im den Nervenkrankheiten*. Leipzig: Barth.

Moldin S (1999). Report of the National Institute of Mental Health's Genetic Workgroup. Summary of research. *Biol Psychiatry* 45, 573–602.

Morel BA (1857). *Traite de Degenerescences Physiques, Intellectuelles et Morales de l'Espace Humaine*. Paris: Baillière.

Morel BA (1860). *Traite des Maladies Mentales*. Paris: Mason.

Morey LC (1991). Reliability considerations in the development of CODE-DD. In Aguglia E, Ban TA, eds. *International Symposium on Functional Psychoses Today*. Rome: John Libbey, pp. 297–304.

Neele E (1949). *Die Phasischen Psychosen*. Leipzig: JA Barth.

O'Rourke DH, Gottesman II, Suarez BK, Rice JP, Reich T (1982). Refutation of the general single locus model for the etiology of schizophrenia. *Am J Hum Genet* 34, 630–649.

Overall J, Hollister LE, Johnson M, Pennington V (1966). Nosology of depression and differential response to drugs. *J Am Med Assoc* 195, 946–948.

Perris C (1974a). A study of cycloid psychoses. *Acta Psychiatr Scand* 50 (Suppl), 253.

Perris C (1974b). The genetics of affective disorders. In Mendels J, ed. *Biological Psychiatry*. New York: John Wiley, pp. 385–415.

Petho B (1990). Development and structure of the DCR Budapest–Nashville. *Psychopathology* 23, 316–330.

Petho B, Ban TA, Kelemen A et al. (1984). KDK Budapest Kutatasi Diagnosztikai Kriteriumok funkcionalis psychosisok korismezesehez. *Ideggyogyaszati Szemle* 37, 102–131.

Petho B, Ban TA in collaboration with Kelemen A, Ungvari G, Karczag I, Bitter I, Tolna Y (Semmelweis Medical University, Budapest), Jarema M, Ferrero F, Aguglia E, Zurria GL, Fjetland OK (Vanderbilt University, Nashville) (1988). *DCR Budapest–Nashville in the Diagnosis and Classification of Functional Psychoses*. Basel: Karger.

Petronis A, Kennedy JL (1995). Unstable genes – unstable mind. *Am J Psychiatry* 152, 164–172.

Pichot P (1983). *A Century of Psychiatry*. Paris: Editions Roger Dacosta.

Pinel P (1799). *Nosographie Philosophique ou La Methode de l'Analyse Appliquee a la Médicine*. Paris: Brosson.

Pinel P (1801). *Traite Médico-Philosphique sur l'Alienation Mentale ou la Manie*. Paris: Brosson.

Ramon y Cajal S (1897–1904). *Histology of the Nervous System of Man and Vertebrates*. [Original in Spanish; republished 1995 in English.] New York: Oxford University Press.

Robins E, Guze SB (1972). Classification of affective disorders: the primary–secondary, endogenous–reactive and the neurotic–psychotic concepts. In Williams A, Katz MM, Shields JA, eds. *Recent Advances in Psychobiology of the Depressive Illnesses.* Washington, DC: US Government Printing Office, pp. 283–293.

Schneider K (1920). Die Schichtung des emotionalen Lebens und der Aufbau der Depressions zustande. *Z Ges Neurol Psychiatr* 59, 281–285.

Schneider K (1950). *Klinische Psychopathologie,* 3rd edn. Stuttgart: Thieme.

Schneider K (1959). *Clinical Psychopathology.* [Translated by Hamilton MW from the 5th revised edition of the German original.] New York: Grune & Stratton.

Sechenov IM (1866). *Refleksy Golovnogo Mozga.* St Petersburg.

Sherrington CS (1896–1897). On reciprocal innervation of antagonistic muscles. *Proc Roy Soc Lond* 9, 414–417.

Sherrington CS (1906). *The Integrative Action of the Nervous System.* London: Scribner.

Shorter E (1997). *A History of Psychiatry.* New York: John Wiley.

Slater E, Cowie V (1971). *The Genetics of Mental Disorder.* London: Oxford University Press.

Stober G, Saar K, Ruschendorf F et al. (2000). Splitting schizophrenia: periodic catatonia – susceptibility locus on chromosome 15q15. *Am J Hum Genet* 67, 1201–1207.

Stromgren E (1974). Psychogenic psychosis. In Hirsch S, Shepherd M, eds. *Themes an Variations in European Psychiatry.* Charlottesville: University Press of Virginia, pp. 97–117.

Trostorff S (1968). Uber die hereditare Belastung bei den zykloiden Psychosen und den unsystematischen und systematischen Schizophrenien. *Psychiatr Neurol Med Psychol* 20, 98–106.

Trostorff S (1975). Verlauf und psychose in der verwandtshaft beiden systematischen und unsystematischen Schizophrenien und den zykloiden Psychosen. *Psychiatr Neurol Med Psychol (Leipzig)* 27, 80–100.

Tsuang MT, Faraone SV (1990). *The Genetics of Mood Disorders.* Baltimore, MD: Johns Hopkins University Press.

Tsuang T, Faraone SV (1995). The case for heterogeneity in the etiology of schizophrenia. *Schizophr Res* 17, 161–175.

Tsuang MT, Vandermey R (1980). *Genes and the Mind. Inheritance of Mental Illness.* Oxford: Oxford University Press.

Ungvari G (1985). A contribution to the validity of Leonhard's classification of endogenous psychoses. *Acta Psychiatr Scand* 72, 144–149.

van Praag HM (1992). Reconquest of the subjective . Against the waning of psychiatric diagnosing. *Br J Psychiatry* 160, 266–271.

van Praag HM (2000). Nosologomania: a disorder of psychiatry. *World Biol Psychiatry* 1, 151–158.

Wender PH, Kety SS, Rosenthal D, Schulsinger F, Ortman J, Lunde I (1986). Psychiatric disorders in the biological adoptive families of adopted individuals with affective disorders. *Arch Gen Psychiatry* 43, 923–929.

Wernicke C (1899). *Uber die Klassifikation der Psychosen.* Breslau: Schlettersche Buchhandlung.

Wernicke C (1900). *Grundriss der Psychiatrie in Klinischen Vorlesungen.* Leipzig: Thieme.

Westphal C (1878). Ueber Zwangsvorstellungen. *Arch Psychiatr Nervenkrank* 8, 734–750.

Wimmer A (1916). *Psykogene Syndssygdomsformer.* Copenhagen: Lunds.

Winokur G (1979). Unipolar depression. Is it divisible into autonomous subtypes. *Arch Gen Psychiatry* 36, 47–52.

Zerbin-Rudin E (1967). Endogene Psychosen. In Becker PE, ed. *Humangenetik ein Kurzes Handbuch*, Vol. 2. Stuttgart: Thieme, pp. 446–577.

4

Methodological issues in psychopharmacogenetics

Sheldon H. Preskorn

Psychiatric Research Institute, University of Kansas School of Medicine, Wichita, Kansas, USA

OVERVIEW

This chapter will discuss methodological issues relevant to conducting pharmacogenetic studies in clinical psychopharmacology. First, basic pharmacologic principles will be reviewed, followed by a discussion of the drug development process. Last, the research linking cytochrome P-450 CPY2D6 poor metabolizers with increased risk of toxicity on routine doses of tricyclic antidepressants will be reviewed as an example of the methodological issues encountered when conducting such studies.

Introduction

As explained in the introductory chapter, pharmacogenetics is the study of genetically determined interindividual differences in the response to a drug.

This chapter will consider methodological issues that can impinge on the success of pharmacogenetic studies of psychiatric medications. As background for this discussion, a number of elementary pharmacological principles will be reviewed in terms of their importance to both the drug development process and the clinical use of psychiatric medications. For additional information of these topics, the reader is referred to www.preskorn.com.

The effect of any drug is a function of three variables, as illustrated in Equation 4.1:

$$\text{Effect} = \text{Affinity for site of action} \times \text{Drug concentration} \times \text{Biological variance among individuals} \tag{4.1}$$

The potential effect of a drug (i.e., the product of the three variables in Equation 4.1) can be divided into three major categories: toxicity, intolerability, or efficacy. For any investigational drug to reach the market, the manufacturer (i.e., the pharmaceutical company) and the responsible regulatory agency (e.g., the Food and Drug Administration (FDA) in the USA) must decide that the efficacy of the drug outweighs its potential for causing toxicity or tolerability problems. The drug does not have to be absolutely "safe" but simply its efficacy must outweigh its risk for toxicity. Safety considerations weigh against the risk associated with not treating effectively the underlying disease. It is easy to see why there are different safety considerations for a drug that is used to treat a condition that is not life threatening and is self-limited (e.g., seasonal allergies) than for one used in a fulminant and life-threatening condition (e.g., Gram-negative shock or poorly differentiated squamous cell carcinoma of the lung). To be marketed, a drug must be sufficiently safe that its likelihood of causing serious toxicity or tolerability problems is outweighed by its ability to produce efficacy in the population with the target disease.

For any drug to be effective in a given disorder, it must affect a site of action relevant to the pathophysiology underlying the disorder. For the vast majority of drugs (over 95%), their site of action is a regulatory protein such as a receptor, an enzyme, or an uptake pump. Affinity for the site of action in Equation 4.1 is a necessary condition for a drug to be effective in a specific disorder.

However, affinity for site of action is not, in and of itself, a sufficient condition for efficacy; instead an adequate concentration of the drug must reach this target to affect it to a physiologically meaningful degree. That fact is represented by the second variable in Equation 4.1. Of note, the factors that determine drug concentration are summarized in Equation 4.2:

$$\text{Drug concentration (ng/ml)} = \frac{\text{Dosing rate (mg/day)}}{\text{Clearance (ml/min)}} \tag{4.2}$$

Clearance of most drugs is determined by the rate of their oxidative metabolism. That, in turn, is determined by the affinity of the drug for specific drug-metabolizing enzymes, primarily cytochrome P-450 (CYP) enzymes, and the speed and capacity of these enzymes to biotransform the drug into polar metabolites that can be eliminated, usually by the kidneys.

The third variable in Equation 4.1 is the focus of this book. It is the interindividual differences among patients that can shift the dose–response curve for one individual relative to another making them either "sensitive" (i.e., more effect than expected for the dose given) or "resistant" (i.e., less effect than expected for the dose given) to a specific drug. There are a number of factors that account for interindividual variability in response:

• diagnosis
• age
• intercurrent disease
• concomitantly administered drugs or dietary substances
• genetics

The focus of this book is genetic factors only.

Pharmacogenetics and variables affecting drug action

At the beginning of the twenty-first century, conventional clinical trials are primarily focused on variables 1 and 2 in Equation 4.1. Drug discovery is focused on variable 1. The goal in discovery is to develop a new chemical entity that affects the desired site(s) of action in the desired way (i.e., agonism, antagonism, or inverse agonism) (Preskorn, 2000). (See www.preskorn.com for this and related articles.)

The goal of clinical testing is to determine the "usual" dose needed for the "usual" patient in the population enrolled in the study. As illustrated in Equation 4.2, that dose, in turn, determines the "usual" concentration that the "usual" patient enrolled in the trial will achieved. Based on Equation 4.1, that "usual" concentration, in turn, determines the "usual" degree of occupancy or activity of the drug at its site(s) of action. The goal, then, of human testing of an investigational new drug is to determine the "usual" dose in the "usual" patient enrolled in the trial needed to affect the desired site(s) of action to the right degree without encountering tolerability or safety problems, caused either by affecting the desired site of action to an undesired degree or by affecting an undesired site(s) of action to a physiologically meaningful degree. From this perspective, clinical trials are, in essence, population pharmacokinetic studies.

Of relevance to this chapter and book, clinical trials carried out for drug registration have strict inclusion and exclusion criteria. The goal of these criteria is to narrow the population eligible to participate in the study to those who are likely to respond to the treatment and who are not likely to have serious adverse events. From a pharmacogenetic perspective, those criteria are designed to try to make the study population as homogeneous as is possible using clinical assessment and routine laboratory testing. As a result of these inclusion and exclusion criteria, the "usual" patient enrolled in most registration trials of antidepressants can differ appreciably from the "usual" patient in clinical practice, particularly those being referred to a psychiatrist. The major difference is the exclusion of patients with significant comorbidity in terms of both psychiatric and general medical disorders. At least some of those comorbid conditions are likely to be in part genetically determined. That raises the possibility that pharmacogenetic differences exist between the clinical trial population for drug registration and the populations treated by some practitioners.

For most drugs, regulatory proteins are the important mechanisms determining variables 1 and 2 in Equation 4.1. Most drugs have a regulatory protein as their site(s) of action (variable 1). Most drugs require oxidative drug metabolism by an enzyme (i.e., a regulatory protein) as a necessary step in their clearance from the body (variable 2). The expression of these proteins is dependent on the genetic make-up of the individual. Thus, pharmacogenetic differences may either affect the site of action of the drug or the mechanism mediating its clearance from the body.

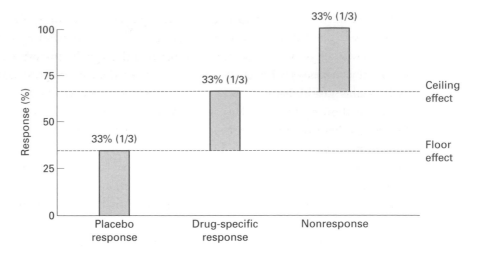

Fig. 4.1.   Rule of thirds in antidepressant clinical trials. Response in such trials is commonly defined as a 50% reduction in symptom severity. A common finding is that one third of patients respond on placebo, two thirds on drug, and one third do not respond because of lack of efficacy, loss to follow-up, or early termination because of intolerable adverse effects. The drug-specific response is therefore one out of three patients (i.e., overall drug response minus placebo response). (Reproduced with permission from www.preskorn.com)

Stated another way, pharmacogenetically determined differences may be either pharmacokinetic or pharmacodynamic. That is fundamental to understanding the role of pharmacogenetics in determining the response of a specific individual to a drug in relationship to the response of the general population.

Efficacy: a poor signal:noise ratio in clinical psychopharmacology

An important methodological issue of relevance to this chapter is the poor signal:noise ratio which plagues most efficacy trials of psychiatric medications. For example, the results of most published antidepressant clinical trials follow the "rule of thirds" (Fig. 4.1): one third of patients enrolled in such studies respond to placebo, one third respond specifically to the antidepressant (i.e., the two third overall response on the drug minus the one third placebo response rate) and one third do not respond regardless of the dose of the antidepressant (Preskorn, 1998a). As a result, the signal:noise ratio in these trials is 1:2: the one third who are responding specifically because of the drug versus the two thirds who are either responding to nondrug factors inherent in the study (e.g., time or supportive psychotherapy (placebo responders)) or who will not respond to the drug. This should be compared with most mature areas of science, where the goal is to have a minimum signal:noise ratio of 10:1.

As discussed below, pharmacogenomic approaches to drug development coupled with parallel pharmacogenetic testing to select specifically responsive populations offers significant promise for improving the signal:noise ratio in clinical psychopharmacology trials in the future. However, the current poor signal:noise ratio means that drugs must have broad effects on brain function to have any chance of showing efficacy relative to placebo. This poor signal:noise ratio is also the reason that two antidepressant clinical trials generally have to be done to get one positive study. Parenthetically, only the positive studies are published; as a result, the existing literature represents a skewed version of the actual data about the efficacy of existing antidepressants. If taken together, a summary of all the clinical trials (published and unpublished) would suggest that current antidepressants produce a specific response in less than one third of patients. As discussed below, this is the reason why studies trying to correlate plasma drug level of antidepressants versus efficacy are virtually guaranteed to fail: there is not sufficient signal:noise power to demonstrate such a relationship even though it obviously must exist based on Equation 4.1 and the basic pharmacological principles underlying that equation.

Given the above background, this chapter will now describe methodological issues that must be addressed to realize the promise that deciphering the human genome has for explaining interindividual differences in drug response and for the optimal practice of clinical psychopharmacology.

Drug development: screening out pharmacogenetic differences

Because of the way in which drug development processes work, pharmacogenetic findings are likely to be limited. First, the goal and intent of the inclusions and exclusion criteria is, in part, to make the study population as homogeneous as possible. Second, the drug would likely fail to receive approval if there were relatively sizable (i.e., $>10\%$) subsets of this presumably homogeneous group with genetically determined differences in their dose–response curves in terms of efficacy or adverse effects.

As alluded to earlier in this chapter, one area that could be fruitful would be the discovery of a pharmacogenetic difference in patients with one of the comorbid conditions (e.g., alcohol abuse) that is generally an exclusion criterion for participation in a clinical trials of psychiatric medications. The discovery of such a pharmacogenetic difference could have significant implications for the use of the drug in that population because that population would have been excluded from the systematic studies that lead to the approval of the drug. Conceivably, this pharmacogenetic difference could mark a population that is more or less responsive to either the beneficial or the adverse effects of the drug.

Theoretically, pharmacogenetic studies of existing drugs could also find subsets in the clinical trial population that have reduced or heightened efficacy on the drug. The identification of a genetically determined subset with reduced efficacy is possible, but, would still be a subset of the one third of the patients enrolled in antidepressant clinical trials who do not respond to current antidepressants. The identification of a subset who are uniquely responsive to the drug is unlikely because of the small fraction of specific drug responders (i.e., one third or less) in the clinical trial population. In fact, drug development as currently practiced is prone to screen out drugs that may be uniquely safe, well tolerated, and/or efficacious in a genetically determined subset of the general (i.e., wild) population with the disease of interest unless that subset is so large that their unique responsiveness is not washed out by nonresponse in the rest of the population. For example, assume that a researcher is following a *"top down"* approach and has discovered a variant regulatory protein that he/she believes is etiopathologically important in a subset (less than 15%) of patients suffering from a psychiatric syndrome such as major depression. It is unlikely that this variant regulatory protein will be the site of action of currently marketed drugs because the signal from such a population would have been too small (15:85) to have been detected in the clinical trials that would have been done to gain registration approval for the drug. Ironically, the researcher might have better success screening investigational antidepressants that failed in earlier development attempts for activity at the new target, because the efficacy signal of those drugs was insufficient to gain registration approval. An even more fruitful approach would be to develop new drugs stereospecifically to affect this new site of action (variable 1 in Equation 4.1) and also to develop a means of screening for the presence of the variant and then requiring that participants must have this variant to be included in the study (see below).

Another possibility is the identification of genetically determined subpopulations less sensitive to the toxicity or tolerability problems caused by the drug. While such a discovery would likely have basic science implications, it is not likely to be clinically useful because this population does not limit the usefulness of the drug or its appropriateness. In other words, the drug is still useful and appropriate for this subpopulation. For that reason, the remainder of this chapter will not consider this scenario but instead will focus on pharmacogenetic studies of existing drugs in which the pharmacogenetic difference causes the drug to be either not useful or not appropriate through heightened risk of toxicity or tolerability problems.

Even in these situations, the results are likely to be limited to a small subset of the clinical trial populations because their heightened sensitivity to tolerability problems and/or toxicity did not prevent the drug from gaining approval. As discussed later in this chapter, the first successful pharmacogenetic finding in psychiatry involved the discovery of just such a subset of the population: individuals who were at increased risk of serious toxicity with tricyclic antidepressants (TCAs) as a result of being genetically deficient in cytochrome P-450 CYP2D6, which preferentially metabolizes these drugs.

Parenthetically, scientists are using this and other related pharmacogenetic discoveries to new chemical entities (NCEs) for subsequent drug development. For example, scientists in drug discovery now use high-throughput screening to determine which CYP enzymes mediate the metabolism of their NCEs. If genetically polymorphic CYP enzymes such as CYP2C19 or CYP2D6 metabolizes the NCE, then that NCE will likely be dropped for future development. The drug discoverers will instead add that finding to their structure–activity relationship paradigm and use it to develop other lead compounds that have desired action on the desired site without being metabolized by that polymorphic CYP enzyme. In essence, drug discoverers are using pharmacogenetic knowledge to screen out drugs that may pose problems in specific pharmacogenetically determined populations.

By using these techniques to refine the structure of the drug, their goal is to take variable 3 (including pharmacogenetic differences) out of Equation 4.1 as a factor determining the effect of the drug in the general human population. The question is whether they may unwittingly also be screening out drugs with unique efficacy or tolerability features. In essence, pharmacogenetics is limiting drug developments by raising the bar of what characteristics a drug must not have to be developed.

Future psychiatric drug development: screening in pharmacogenetic differences

The above situation will further evolve when the knowledge of the human genome uncovers variants (i.e., genetic mutations) in proteins that are etiologically responsible for disease in a sufficiently large number of people in the population to make drug development a commercially viable proposition. Ironically, some subsets of what are now considered to be common diseases (e.g., major depression) may become "orphan" areas for drug development.

To understand the last statement, consider that major depression is likely many different diseases when understood from an etiopathological point of view. Some of those different conditions may be caused by genetic mutations. In this scenario, what is now a common disease affecting a substantial percentage of the general population may become multiple diseases with each subtype affecting only a small portion of the group presently defined as suffering from clinical depression. Some of those genetically determined subsets may be so small as to make it questionable whether drug development for that subset would be commercially viable. From this perspective, pharmacogenetics has the potential to limit the development of psychiatric drugs for some subtypes of what are now considered common diseases.

Nevertheless, subsets will be found that are sufficiently large to support the commercial drug development specifically targeted at that subset. In fact, pharmacogenetics and pharmacogenomics will facilitate and streamline drug development, thus reducing costs and increasing the likelihood of success. As an example, say that a specific form of clinical depression is mediated by a variant of the serotonin uptake pump. That variant now becomes the site of action in Equation 4.1. The site can be expressed and its three-dimensional configuration deciphered. Armed with that knowledge, medicinal chemists can develop more precise structure–activity relationships to design a NCE which stereospecifically interacts with that variant of the wild-type regulatory protein. That is an example of the so-called top-down approach in which a genetic variant is defined and then one works downward to determine whether it mediates a clinically useful difference in outcome.

In addition to aiding in the drug discovery process, such a pharmacogenetic finding would also help with the signal:noise problem discussed earlier as, at the human testing phase of drug development (i.e., phase I through III), scientists can select the specific subset of the population (i.e., those with the genetic variant) likely to respond to the drug. Using this strategy, the inclusion criteria for the clinical trials of this new drug would require that a subject has the genetic variant to be eligible to participate in the study. That would enrich the study sample with individuals likely to be responsive to the drug. That alone could flip the signal:noise ratio around to 2:1, by reducing, if not eliminating altogether, nonresponders. The signal:noise ratio would still be limited by the problem of nonspecific (placebo) response unless this variant population also had a smaller nonspecific response rate. Thus, the discovery of such a pharmacogenetic variant could decrease the cost and speed up the drug development process by focusing the studies and reducing the numbers needed to prove efficacy relative to placebo compared with those needed in current studies with a signal:noise ratio of 1:2.

Pharmacogenetic research in psychiatry could further enhance the signal:noise ratio by finding a genetically determined subset of patients suffering from a psychiatric syndrome who are prone to placebo response. That finding might well have some basic science etiopathological implications. More germane to this chapter, that finding would provide a genetic test to exclude the placebo-responsive patients from enrollment.

Consequently, pharmacogenetic tests could be used to reduce both ends of the current signal:noise ratio problem in clinical psychopharmacology trials. One test could be used as an inclusion criterion, requiring that those who enter the study have the variant that predicts specific responsiveness to the drug. Another test could be done to exclude the subset of the population genetically predisposed to placebo response. That could make drug development less costly, faster, and less of a gamble. At the same time, these tests and population limitations would be reflected in the package insert for the drug and could become part of clinical practice as a condition of prescribing the drug. The question would remain for the developers whether the new product would be commercially viable with these limitations on its potential market size. For example, the development of a test that identifies the one third of the clinical trial population who respond to placebo would provide a test to exclude drug therapy for this segment of the population with the syndrome. If that one third was translated to the general population in clinical practice who take antidepressants, it would have a significant effect on the size of the market.

Pharmacogenetic studies and existing drugs

As mentioned at the beginning of this chapter, there are three main categories of drug outcome (i.e., effect in Equation 4.1). The drug may be toxic, intolerable, or efficacious. The pharmacogenetic problem with the drug may be mediated by its pharmacodynamics (variable 1 in Equation 4.1) or its pharmacokinetics (variable 2 in Equation 4.1). Pharmacogenetic differences mediating variable 2 are much easier to study at the present time than those mediating variable 1.

The reason is twofold. First, the pharmacogenetic differences underlying variable 2 are better understood. The mechanisms accounting for variable 2 (i.e., regulatory proteins such as CYP enzymes) are fewer in number and easier to study than those accounting for variable 1, which for psychiatric medications are a vast number of regulatory proteins in the brain, an organ that is still difficult to study mechanistically.

Variable 2 mechanisms lend themselves to relatively simple in vitro techniques (Beaune and Guengerich, 1988). The results of such in vitro studies are readily extrapolated to in vivo predictions that can then be readily tested in humans (von Moltke et al., 1998; Schmider et al., 1999). For in vitro studies of CYP enzymes, the drug in question can be screened against all known human enzymes by high throughput methods to determine the affinity of the drug for the different enzymes and their speed and capacity for biotransforming the drug. That information can be used to predict which CYP enzyme(s) will likely metabolize it under usual dosing conditions. If the rate-limiting enzyme mediating the oxidative metabolism of the drug is polymorphic, then the drug is likely to have altered clearance in that subset of the population. That can then be tested by measuring the clearance of the drug in a sample of the wild-type population and a sample of the population with the variant enzyme. In this way, the human study becomes a direct extension of the in vitro study. Such screening is now being used to screen out NCEs from further drug development if they may require a change in dosage for the poor metabolizing subpopulation and hence the drug will not meet the desired criteria of having one dose for all patients.

CYP2D6 as an example

CYP2D6 is a polymorphic enzyme that has played a major role in the understanding of the potential impact of pharmacogenetics on the effect of psychiatric medications. This CYP enzyme was a classic example of the *bottom up* approach in which an aberrant response (i.e., increased sensitivity to the dose-dependent adverse effects of a specific drug) was identified, leading to a search for the mechanism that accounted for the increased sensitivity. In the case of CYP2D6, several examples of aberrant responses were observed. One was the increased hypotensive effect of debrisoquine (Maghous et al., 2001). Another was the increased toxicity of TCAs (Sjoqvist and Bertilsson, 1986). In both instances, these increased effects were associated with increased accumulation of the drug (variable 2 in Equation 4.1) on routine doses owing to the slow clearance resulting from the genetically determined deficiency in enzymatic activity.

In this case, the individuals genetically deficient in enzyme activity were analogous to the results of the blank test tube (i.e., no enzyme) in the in vitro studies when the substrate is added (i.e., essentially no metabolism at least via that pathway). This genetic deficiency was easily identified by simple blood sampling and measuring the concentration of the drug. This value could be put into Equation 4.1 and the outcome predicted. In this scenario, the pharmacogenetic difference is like giving a higher dose of the drug to the general population or, in other words, is the same as a left shift in the dose–response curve for toxicity and tolerability problems in the CYP2D6-deficient individuals. Parenthetically, they should for the same reason be more sensitive to the antidepressant effects of TCAs (i.e., responding to lower doses).

However, it is interesting to note that psychiatrists did not readily embrace this idea despite its simplicity. Consider that almost as soon as TCAs were marketed the dose-dependent nature of their propensity to cause serious cardiotoxicity was recognized. After all, the toxicity of these drugs was fulminant following an acute overdose and was a leading cause of drug overdose death in the USA and other countries for over 30 years. Shortly after these drugs were marketed, it was recognized that 5–10% of Caucasians, particularly those of northern European descent, cleared these drugs much slower than the rest of the population and that this phenomenon was genetically determined (Alexanderson et al., 1969). Moreover, it was recognized that these individuals developed blood concentrations many times higher than the general population and could develop toxic levels on routine dosage. Moreover, this phenomenon could be readily detected by monitoring blood levels in these patients.

In essence, therapeutic drug monitoring (TDM) of TCAs was a means of testing for a pharmacogenetically determined difference in oxidative drug metabolism (variable 2) that could seriously shift the dose–response curve in a sizable number, albeit a minority, of patients (5–10%). Despite those simple facts, there was great resistance to the adoption of TDM in clinical practice. Arguments were raised that it was too costly and that physicians could do a better job by simply clinically adjusting the dose. Parenthetically, and somewhat ironically, the same arguments were raised two decades later when it was discovered that some popular drugs (e.g., fluoxetine and paroxetine) could produce phenocopies of genetic deficiency of this enzyme in 50 to 80% of CYP2D6 normal or extensive metabolizers (Preskorn, 1998b). As late as 1984, the task established by the American Psychiatric Association to develop guidelines for the use of laboratory procedures in psychiatry took a "conservative" posture on the use of TDM for TCAs in psychiatry (Task Force on the Use of Laboratory Tests in Psychiatry, 2001).

The reason behind the slow acceptance of TDM for TCAs reveals some of the methodological problems that will likely face future pharmacogenetic discoveries in psychiatry. The first problem was that the focus of the debate was on the wrong aspect of the concentration–response curve: the relationship between concentration and antidepressant efficacy rather than toxicity. The second problem was who was going to do a study to demonstrate that the more relevant problem was increased risk for serious toxicity?

Efficacy as a difficult target for study in psychiatry

At the time the genetic difference in the metabolism of TCAs was being identified, TDM studies were being conducted to examine the potential relationship between drug level and antidepressant efficacy. It should have been recognized then, and certainly now, that such studies are almost certainly doomed to failure. The reason is the poor signal:noise ratio in such studies. The problem is that a typical conventional TDM efficacy study includes all the same patients as a drug registration clinical trial: (a) the one third or less who are drug-specific responders, (b) the one third who are placebo responders, and (c) the one third who are nonresponders. However, the only population who can show a concentration–efficacy relationship is the one third or less who are drug-specific responders. Of course, the placebo responders and drug nonresponders still achieve plasma drug concentrations but their response or lack of response is independent of the drug and hence its concentration. Figure 4.2 illustrates what happens when the concentration–response data from these two groups is superimposed on a clear-cut, plasma concentration–antidepressant response curve from the drug-specific responders: no relationship is found.

The results of such studies lead to the astounding conclusion that drug concentration was meaningless. Ironically, that conclusion was being championed at the

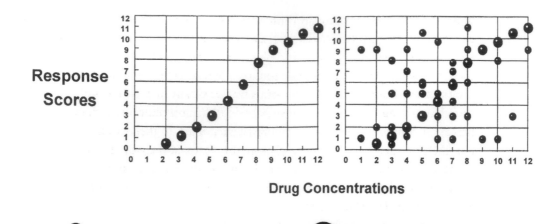

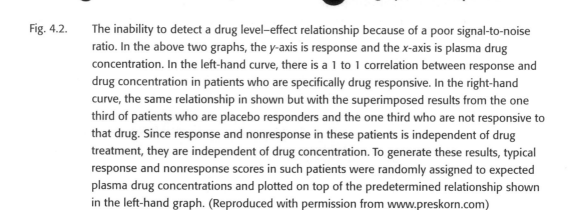

Fig. 4.2.   The inability to detect a drug level–effect relationship because of a poor signal-to-noise ratio. In the above two graphs, the y-axis is response and the x-axis is plasma drug concentration. In the left-hand curve, there is a 1 to 1 correlation between response and drug concentration in patients who are specifically drug responsive. In the right-hand curve, the same relationship in shown but with the superimposed results from the one third of patients who are placebo responders and the one third who are not responsive to that drug. Since response and nonresponse in these patients is independent of drug treatment, they are independent of drug concentration. To generate these results, typical response and nonresponse scores in such patients were randomly assigned to expected plasma drug concentrations and plotted on top of the predetermined relationship shown in the left-hand graph. (Reproduced with permission from www.preskorn.com)

same time that physicians were being berated for using too low a dosage of TCAs as if somehow dose but not concentration mattered.

The fruitful area to study was the relationship between drug concentration and toxicity. Here the signal was clear: seizures, cardiac arrhythmias, and sudden death. However, who would propose doing a study prospectively to define the risk of these serious adverse effects as a function of either dose or interindividual differences in sensitivity (e.g., slow clearance because of CYP2D6 deficiency) – and would any institutional review board let such a study be carried out? Of course, the answer to these two questions are no one and no. Here then is a dilemma in pharmacogenetic studies. A genetically determined population that is likely to be more susceptible to the adverse effects of a drug is defined, but how can it be determined that they are more susceptible if it is unethical to expose to the potential increased risk. One approach would be to use a surrogate marker for the increased risk. That was done with the TCAs. A number of studies were done showing that poor metabolizers developed substantially higher levels of the drugs and asymptomatic prolongation of the QT interval (Preskorn and Fast, 1991). However, drug levels were kept sufficiently low to avoid toxicity and the QT prolongation was asymptomatic. (Additionally, asymptomatic QT prolongation was easier to ignore at that time than it is today.) The absence of clinically obvious toxicity reinforced the idea that drug concentrations could be ignored. A similar situation occurred with studies in the 1990s testing the effects of substantial CYP2D6 inhibitors (e.g., fluoxetine and paroxetine) on CYP2D6 substrates (Preskorn, 1998b). In these studies, the dose of the CYP2D6 substrate was purposely kept low to avoid the risk of serious toxicity. Because no toxicity occurred, some dismissed the finding that fluoxetine and paroxetine could cause 500% increases in the plasma concentrations of drugs such as desipramine (Preskorn, 1999).

While using drug levels as a surrogate for toxicity was met with limited success and skepticism, another approach did prove compelling: naturalistic studies of toxicity under usual dosing conditions (Preskorn and Jerkovich, 1990; Preskorn and Fast, 1991). Here the failure to employ TDM rationally to guide the dose adjustment of the TCAs put a predictable percentage of the vulnerable genetically determined subset of the population at risk for toxicity. When an adverse outcome occurred, plasma drug levels were obtained and found to be unusually high as a result of slowed clearance. Eventually, an upper threshold of 450 ng/ml (450 µg/l) was established beyond which the likelihood of serious toxicity outweighed the likelihood of increase efficacy (Fig. 4.2). Hopefully, future pharmacogenetic findings will be more readily accepted but the history with TCAs and CYP2D6 illustrates that scientific findings are not necessarily rapidly accepted into clinical practice, at least in psychiatry.

Conclusions

This chapter has endeavored to review some of the methodological issues facing those interested in conducting pharmacogenetic studies in clinical psychopharmacology. It began with two equations that illustrate basic pharmacological principles relevant to drug effects in humans and continued to discuss specific methodological issues. First was the drug development process itself, goal of which is to minimize pharmacogenetic differences as a variable affecting the response to a drug. Second was the problems posed by the poor signal:noise ratio, which plagues current efficacy studies in psychiatry. The third issue was the ethical and practical problems posed in trying to study whether a genetically defined population is at increased risk for toxicity or other adverse effects on what is a routine dosage of the drug for the general population. TDM studies with TCAs were used to illustrate this issue.

While the above are all important hurdles in conducting pharmacogenetic studies with existing drugs, this chapter also reviewed the significant potential for advancing psychiatric drug development as a result of improved understanding of the pharmacogenetics and pharmacogenomics relevant to the effects of drugs on the human brain. This includes the discovery of completely novel sites of action and the discovery of pathophysiologically and etiopathologically distinct subsets of what are now likely heterogeneous syndromes such as major depression. These discoveries should have a profound impact on psychiatric drug development in terms of making it more efficient, less costly, and less of a gamble. However, they may also reduce the potential size of the market for any specific agent by better defining what subset actually needs the treatment. In doing so, some subsets of some psychiatric syndromes may be too small to be commercially viable for drug development. Consequently, developments in this area will both promote and restrict psychiatric drug development.

A number of these topics are explored at greater length in other chapters in this book. The interested reader can also find more information at www.preskorn.com.

REFERENCES

Alexanderson B, Evans D, Sjoqvist F (1969). Steady-state plasma levels of nortriptyline in twins: influence of genetic factors and drug therapy. *Br Med J* 4, 764–768.

Beaune PH, Guengerich FP (1988). Human drug metabolism *in vitro*. *Pharmacol Ther* 37, 193–211.

Maghous A, Idle JR, Dring LG, Lancaster R, Smith RL (2001). Polymorphic hydroxylation of debrisoquine in man. *Lancet* ii, 584–586.

Preskorn SH (1998a). Recent dose–effect studies regarding antidepressants. In Balant LP, Benitez J, Dahl SG, Gram LF, Pinder RM, Potter WZ, eds. *European Cooperation in the Field of Scientific and Technical Research*. Belgium: European Commission, pp. 45–61.

Preskorn SH (1998b). Debate resolved: there are differential effects of serotonin selective reuptake inhibitors on cytochrome P-450 enzymes. *J Psychopharmacol* 12, S89–S97.

Preskorn SH (1999). *Outpatient Management of Depression: A Guide for the Primary-Care Practitioner*. Caddo, OK: Professional Communications Inc., pp. 96–97, 256 (this book is also available at www.preskorn.com).

Preskorn SH (2000). The stages of drug development and the human genome project: drug discovery. *J Psychiatr Pract* 6, 341–344. (Also available at www.preskorn.com)

Preskorn SH, Fast GA (1991). Therapeutic drug monitoring for antidepressants: efficacy, safety and cost effectiveness. *J Clin Psychiatry* 52, 23–33.

Preskorn SH, Jerkovich GS (1990). Central nervous system toxicity of tricyclic antidepressants: phenomenology, course, risk factors and role of therapeutic drug monitoring. *J Clin Psychopharmacol* 10, 88–95.

Schmider J, von Moltke LL, Shader RI, Harmatz JS, Greenblatt DJ (1999). Extrapolating in vitro data on drug metabolism to in vivo pharmacokinetics: evaluation of the pharmacokinetic interaction between amitriptyline and fluoxetine. *Drug Metab Rev* 31, 545–560.

Sjoqvist F, Bertilsson L (1986). Slow hydroxylation of tricyclic antidepressants – relationship to polymorphic drug oxidation. In Kalow W, Goedde HW, Agarwal DP, eds. *Ethnic Differences in Reaction to Drugs and Xenobiotics.* New York: Liss, pp. 169–188.

Task Force on the Use of Laboratory Tests in Psychiatry (2001). Tricyclic antidepressants–blood level measurements and clinical outcome. *Am J Psychiatry* 144, 155–162.

von Moltke LL, Greenblatt DJ, Schmider J, Wright CE, Harmatz JS, Shader RI (1998). In vitro approaches to predicting drug interactions in vivo. *Biochem Pharmacol* 55, 113–122.

5

Statistical approaches in psychopharmacogenetics

Fabio Macciardi

Center for Addiction and Mental Health, University of Toronto. Toronto, Canada

OVERVIEW

The statistical analysis of data in psychopharmacogenetics is a key factor in the evaluation of the importance of a gene or of a set of genes in controlling for the response to a given drug or to explain the emergence of a side effect as a consequence of the administered drug. A pharmacogenetic trait is frequently controlled by more than one gene, with different contributions from genes coding for pharmacokinetic traits (absorption, distribution, metabolism, elimination), the ultimate drug target (e.g., receptors, transporters or enzymes), and endogenous ligands. As such, a pharmacogenetic characteristic can be considered a complex trait, with a multifaceted etiology. The best approach to evaluate the genetic bases of a pharmacogenetic trait is the association strategy, where each gene contributing to the expression of the trait conveys only a portion of the overall variability of the characteristic itself. The association strategy conceptually entails the candidate gene paradigm, which is based on a "forward genetics" design. The re-emergence of this analytical approach has become possible as a result of the completion of the sequence for the human genome and the possibility of knowing a priori which genes are involved in the biochemical mechanisms that lead to the drug function. However, several issues must be considered to perform a correct analysis, including a proper definition of the phenotype, a detailed knowledge of the extent and dimension of the genetic variation that is present within and across populations, and the choice of the statistical design.

Introduction

Pharmacogenetics has been defined as the study of variability in drug response owing to heredity, based on the original definition of the term coined by F. Vogel (1959). Indeed, it is a common medical experience to observe that the effect of the same drug, when administered to several patients, can be advantageous in some subjects, deleterious in others and of no consequences in a third group. Understanding the mechanisms responsible for variability in drug response, as well as in the origin of side effects, is the major object of pharmacogenetics, considering how to relate a drug response unequivocally (phenotype) to the genotype (Roses, 2000). To accomplish this task, it is necessary to define a quantifiable clinical response and then to detect the variant(s) of the gene(s) implicated in modulating the response to the drug. Statistics is the tool to prove the relationship between the phenotype and the genotype.

In recent years, the term pharmacogenomics has also been introduced; while the terms pharmacogenetics and pharmacogenomics do not substantially differ from each other in that each recognizes that genes play a substantial role in controlling for the response to the administration of a given drug, there are also conceptual differences. The term pharmacogenomics emphasizes the accepted view that most, if not all, of the "response" traits are potentially controlled by more than a single unique gene and are somewhat influenced by the whole human genome. Under this perspective, several different genetic loci are required to explain the effect, or the lack of effect, of a given drug treatment. This implies that pharmacogenetic traits are not simple Mendelian characteristics and that several genes play a causal role in the genesis of a pharmacogenetic trait. Two nonmutually exclusive alternative possibilities exist: each gene has only a small quantitative effect on the trait ("polygenic" model) or more than one "trait" gene must be simultaneously present in order to produce the phenotypic effect ("epistatic" model). This implicitly means that, taken separately, the individual gene effects are only modest and that the genotype relative risk (i.e., the increased chance that an individual with a particular genotype for a particular allele has the trait) is low. Despite the small effects of these genes, the magnitude of their attributable risk may be large, since they must be quite frequent in the population owing to the high prevalence of the characteristic.

The following sections will show how to analyze the genetic architecture of a pharmacogenetic trait. First, a definition of a pharmacogenetic trait will be presented, with the consequential methods of analysis, followed by some considerations for defining a phenotype suitable for investigation. Then, our present understanding of genetic polymorphisms will be described, with a particular focus on single nucleotide polymorphisms (SNPs). A detailed discussion will follow about ethnic and interindividual differences in the distribution of genetic variants and how they can affect any investigation.

The pharmacogenetic trait: definition and methods of analysis

A pharmacogenetic trait is a complex, multidetermined characteristic, not a disease but rather a "difference" in the expression of a genetically determined mechanism involved in drug metabolism (Nebert, 1999). The distinction is subtle but substantial. At variance with a common/complex disorder, we do not have to detect which genes are relevant for the trait to be manifested, and then to detect their pathological variants. Rather, it should be known, more or less, from our knowledge of biology, pharmacology, or neuroscience, that a given set of "proteins" are implicated and responsible for the drug to function. These proteins comprise drug-metabolizing enzymes, transporters, receptors, drug-binding proteins and other enzymes. The goal is then to detect which specific variant(s) of any one of the genes coding for the specific protein(s) relevant for the drug function may be responsible for the lack of drug efficacy, either acting alone or – more probably – in some kind of combined effect (interaction). The focus of the investigation has, therefore, shifted from the identification of a gene as a causative effect of the trait, as when analyzing the genetic bases of a complex disease, toward the identification of a set of variant(s) that across many genes already known will generate the observed phenotype.

In other words, a pharmacogenetic character is the ultimate effect of an "environmental" stimulus acting on the specific genetic make-up of an individual. The consequence of such a definition of a pharmacogenetic trait is that traditional genetic analytical strategies like linkage or segregation analyses do not apply. Instead, association or linkage disequilibrium (LD) techniques are the methods of choice, privileging an epidemiological biometrical approach over a Mendelian scheme and using a population genetics strategy. Population genetics is a well-developed science that studies how, where, and why the variation in genes is different across different groups or human populations. Population genetics has been active for more than 100 years; however, its methods have only begun to be applied to the variation across different individuals in their response to (or in their susceptibility to develop side effects with) the same medication, i.e., in pharmacogenetics.

Given the number of biochemical mechanisms involved in controlling psychotropic drug actions, the pharmacogenetic "profile" of a given medication can be defined as a "complex trait" that cannot be explained by a simple genetic mechanism like a single major locus. The association strategy has the advantage of being able to detect not only major gene effects but, minor gene effects also; the criteria for a positive association rely on detecting those alleles of the candidate or marker genes under analysis that are preferentially transmitted together with the trait. This provides indirect proof that a still as yet unidentified allele of the locus responsible for the trait cosegregates with the corresponding associated allele of the candidate/marker gene, giving rise to a haplotype (combination of alleles in a chromosome). Under these conditions, association is equivalent to linkage analysis (Baur and Knapp, 1997; Ott, 1999). In extreme favorable circumstances, the marker and the trait locus are identical, and only the individuals with the trait present a given allele at the marker locus.

In recent years there has been a critical debate about the most appropriate design to study genetic associations. Case-control is the simplest method, but it was considered a weak approach because of the difficulty of appropriately selecting a group of controls and because it had the potential for failing to deal adequately with issues of admixture and stratification within the population studied. Consequently, techniques that used "internal" – or family-based – controls were preferred, as in the transmission disequilibrium test (TDT: Spielman et al., 1993). The TDT is based on the detection of unequal transmission of high- versus low-risk alleles from heterozygous parents to affected children. The Mendelian expectation under the null hypothesis of no linkage or association is that either allele carried by a heterozygote has 50:50 odds of being transmitted to an affected child. If the allele is causally related to the disorder, however, then the odds of its being transmitted should exceed 50%. Compared with other within-family association tests (e.g., the affected family based control and haplotype-based haplotype relative risk methods) (Schaid and Sommer, 1993; Spielman and Ewens, 1996), the TDT provides a test of linkage as well as association, robustness against artifacts induced by population stratification, greater statistical power, and the ability to include multiple affected siblings from a family in a test of linkage (but not association) without having to correct for dependence (Spielman et al., 1993; Schaid and Sommer, 1994; Ewens and Spielman, 1995; Spielman and Ewens, 1996, 1998).

Generalizations of the TDT approach are presently available (Monks and Kaplan, 2000) for any kind of family (trios, nuclear, extended, sib-pair, etc.) even when one parent is not available (Spielman and Ewens, 1998). Despite many expectations, however, the TDT has not definitively proven to be superior to other association designs. Moreover, it is also less efficient than the case-control design, being limited to information only from heterozygous parents, and, since the collection of an appropriate sample size is much more time consuming, ultimately leads to a loss of power. Consequently, unrelated case-controls are now re-emerging as a more powerful and efficient approach, in spite of their lack of robustness for possibly inflating type I errors (Risch, 2000). However, it is not possible to avoid false-positive results, and different strategies to deal with this issue are presented in the following paragraphs. In addition to specific strategies, a few simple cautionary approaches, like a priori setting a conservative p value to define a significant finding, help to increase the robustness of the case-control design. The re-emergence of case-control studies in human genetics has also been stimulated by the potential identification of all (or most) of the genes in the human genome, as well as by the identification and cataloguing of the functional variation that occurs naturally within them in human populations. This information will also lead to application of a "forward-genetics" method, rather than a reverse-genetics approach, given the opportunities for studying the impact of those variants on the phenotypic outcome of interest, thus strengthening the candidate gene approach (Risch and Merikangas, 1996; Risch, 2000). However, to avoid the risk of generating biased results, the researcher must adopt a strict methodological strategy that involves a relevant definition of the phenotype and a correct use of the genetic polymorphisms, including the knowledge of their variability within and across populations.

How to define a phenotype in psychopharmacogenetics

The objective of any clinical pharmacogenetic analysis is to consider how to correlate drug response or the emergence of a side effect to the genotype in an unequivocal way. Defining the phenotype of response to a given drug is a critical issue since the expression of the phenotype can be identified only in those subjects who were administered the specific compound. It is obvious that subjects unexposed to a given drug are dormant for the phenotype identification and it will never be known whether those subjects will be responsive or not to the administration of the drug. This makes ascertainment difficult in the general population. Moreover, especially in pharmacogenetics of psychotropic drugs, even the definition of the "response" to a treatment is a challenging task, with serious issues to consider. Apart from some medications and under unusual circumstances, as for example in sophisticated clinical trials, the researcher does not have biological or laboratory indices of response to a given psychotropic drug.

In its simplest form, the classification of responder/nonresponder can be considered a dichotomous trait, with a clear separation between the two classes. In reality, however, the classification is based upon a threshold set up by the researcher. Methods to position the threshold are largely drawn from classical pharmacology guidelines as derived from clinical trials or from epidemiological investigations. Despite the apparent simplicity of the concept and the appeal of getting a simple yes/no answer, the nominal definition of responder entails a large set of information that need to be critically evaluated before being synthesized into the proposed classification.

Alternatively, the responder/nonresponder phenotype can be measured as a quantitative variable. This allows a more flexible definition of response without the need to impose a rigid bipartition of the phenotype. In this case the degree of responsiveness is measured along a continuous scale, which may be arbitrary or more probably represents a summary measure of various clinical domains. The correspondence between the degree of responsiveness and the genetic make-up can be evaluated using the full range of responsiveness in a straightforward way, but alternatives are possible. One option is to use only the extremes of the scale, that is subjects lying in the areas that contain the "best" and the "worst" responders, usually constituting the upper and lower 5% of a continuous Gaussian distribution (Nebert, 1999). Comparison between extreme discordant subjects in looking for the role of a significant effect of a genetic component is a powerful technique that has already been proven successful (Lifton, 1996; Halushka et al., 1999).

Ultimately, the classification of patients into responder/nonresponder mostly relies on the clinical judgement of the physician who evaluates the improvement of the patient following the administration of the therapeutic compound. Criteria about the reliable definition of responder and nonresponder must, therefore, be agreed among investigators and must reasonably guarantee against the risk of statistical errors in future genetic studies for an associated genetic polymorphism. For example, if responders are defined as those patients who show a 20% improvement over the baseline of their psychopathological symptoms, measured with a certain scale, this will eventually give rise to a sample size of patients where the proportion of responders will be much bigger than if the trait definition had to have a 30% improvement threshold. The consequence of this is that, when studying a possible association with a polymorphic variant with high frequency (e.g., $> 10–20\%$) in the general population, the possibility of a positive finding are a priori larger in the "20% improvement" phenotype, irrespective of the real meaning of the association, unless stringent significance levels are used to define a positive association. In fact, relaxing the criteria for the identification of the phenotype increases the risk of including false-positive responders and leads to an unknown corresponding increment of type I error. Unfortunately, in the absence of objective criteria, the phenotypic definition of responder is frequently based upon loose clinical criteria, and researchers are naturally inclined to prefer phenotype definitions that maximize the efficiency of the analysis. In this case, a "broad" formal definition of the phenotype allows a relatively small sample of patients to be recruited. Even though this small sample size can be justified by a power analysis showing that there is enough power to detect an association, the risk of drawing erroneous conclusions is high. The error results from incorrect premises rather than incorrect procedures. To avoid these kinds of error and since the definition of the phenotype is entirely arbitrary, it is best that one group (responder) be unequivocally separated from the other group (nonresponder). It must be also pointed out that virtually all the "common" traits – either diseases or pharmacogenetic characters – represent multiplex phenotypes in the sense that they are polygenic (derived from the contribution of two or more genes). Therefore, the best possible approach in humans is to quantify the pharmacogenetic phenotype in much the same way as geneticists have done in studying hypertension: instead of looking at subjects as hypertensive/not hypertensive, the identification of relevant genes was possible when researchers looked at the quantitative phenotype "blood pressure" (Jacob et al., 1991; Schork et al., 1995; Brown et al., 1996; Halushka et al., 1999). Various examples of alternative phenotypic definitions useful for psychopharmacogenetic analyses can be found in other chapters (e.g., Chs. 10–13) and the interested reader can find more specific details there.

In principle, the definition of a "side effect" phenotype is not as difficult as the responder/nonresponder phenotype. Many side effects present with objective clinical signs, as in tardive dyskinesia during long-term administration of antipsy-chotic medications, or are measurable with laboratory tests, as in the decrease in white blood cells count in patients treated with clozapine or thioridazine. In these and other similar cases, the recognition of the phenotype is relatively easy, not pre-senting the same difficulties as the clinical-response phenotype. However, here too the possibility exists to define the phenotype as a qualitative or a quantitative char-acteristic. In some cases, the selection of one or the other method might induce a difference in the way the phenotype is considered, and the researcher should clearly establish the focus of the analysis at the beginning. For example, if the phenotype is defined as present/absent, an established correlation with a given gene points to this gene as one of the "causes" of the phenotype. The same conclusion does not necessarily apply if the phenotype is defined quantitatively, since – depending upon the quantitative dimension of the phenotype that is being considered – the meaning of the "phenotype" in this case might be different from the simple concept of presence/absence and could be related to other characteristics of the phenotype itself, like the degree of severity. Consequently, given that the trait has a multigene mechanism, a qualitative or a quantitative definition of the phenotype could, in principle, pinpoint different genetic components.

Association and linkage disequilibrium methods

To understand the genetic architecture of complex traits and to dissect the genetic component of the trait into its basic elements is a considerable challenge, despite the remarkable advances in knowledge and the sophistication of contemporary technology. A general view of complex genetic traits is that the contributing genes are genes of small or minor effect, as opposed to major genes characteristic of simple Mendelian traits (Ott and Hoh, 2000); however, opinions differ as to the best way to describe the contribution that each small gene exerts on the trait.

The assumption that complex traits follow a similar genetic model to that seen, for example, in late-onset Alzheimer's disease, which is associated with the *apoE4* allele (Corder et al., 1993), or in type I diabetes mellitus, which is associated with class I alleles of the insulin gene minisatellite (Bennet et al., 1995), has not yet been demonstrated, suggesting that not all predisposing alleles to complex traits are common. In Alzheimer's disease and diabetes, common alleles/variants of genes implicated in the etiology of the diseases can be found with medium to high fre-quencies in all populations. Under this scenario, the common trait–common variant hypothesis (Risch and Merikangas, 1996; Collins et al., 1997; Chakravarty, 1999), the allele variants are not pathological per se and represent a risk factor for a given disease only when they are present in a particular multigene combination. In other words it is only when they appear concurrent with other "risk" variants at other loci that the combination produces the ultimate genetic risk. An alternative theory suggests that a large pool of alleles with low population frequency and varying effects on risk (the common trait–rare variant hypothesis) could explain the genetic component of common traits (Terwilliger and Weiss, 1998; Wright et al., 1999; Weiss and Terwilliger, 2000; Pritchard, 2001).

It is probable that a more realistic model lies between these two extreme hypotheses, where predisposing alleles of varying population frequencies may represent a true allelic heterogeneity in some cases or a locus heterogeneity in other circumstances, and alleles would act either independently or epistatically to influence trait outcome (van Hauwe et al., 1999; Johnson and Todd, 2000). It is clear that if we are going to maximize the chances of success in complex trait mapping, we must design our analytical strategies so that we can detect subtle genetic effects under a variety of genetic models.

Polymorphic variants in the human genome

The sequence of human DNA is characterized by a high number of variants (polymorphisms) that are widely distributed across the various chromosomes and are generally termed markers. A detailed description of the various types of polymorphism is beyond the scope of this chapter, but it is nonetheless important to introduce some definitions and describe in simple details the most widespread form of genetic variants: the SNPs. By polymorphisms, geneticists mean any variant of the sequence of a locus that is represented in the general population with a frequency $>1\%$, while the most represented form of a gene is called the wild type. Another usual term to define the different form that a gene can take is allele: a gene can be present with any number of alleles, from 1, when the gene is not polymorphic, to several hundreds, like in the loci controlling for the HLA complex. It is common for genes to be polymorphic, and this simple fact does not mean that a given variant is pathological. On the contrary, mutations are generally rare variants of a gene, usually $<1\%$, and the present use of the term mutation indicates a pathological form of a gene, generally leading to a disorder.

Among the many variants present in DNA, the most common is the result of a variation in a single base pair or a simple insertion/deletion of a small number of base pairs; these polymorphisms are defined as single nucleotide polymorphisms (SNPs) (Collins et al., 1999). At present there are already more than 2.5 million SNPs mapped into the human DNA, by the same group of investigators that have sequenced the human genome (International SNP Map Working Group, 2001) and by a consortium of private and public researchers (Venter et al., 2001). A rough estimate of the frequency of SNPs is that there could be a variant of the sequence every 500/1000 base pairs (Cargill et al., 1999; Kruglyak, 1999), generating a potential number of at least 3 to 6 million SNPs. SNPs are further subdivided according to their "location" with respect to the coding sequence of a gene. SNPs within the coding region of a gene can lead to nonconservative alterations (type I), conservative amino acid substitutions (type II) or synonymous substitutions (type III). Noncoding SNPs have been classified into 5′ untranslated (UTR) region (type IV), 3′ UTR (type V), and other noncoding regions (type VI). There is already the proposal that type VI SNPs be divided into further subtypes, depending whether they are found at exon/intron boundaries, in putative intronic AP1 sites, etc., while type IV SNPs might comprise also putative promoter regions. Therefore, it appears very likely that multiple SNPs will be found in and around each and every gene in the human genome, and each locus would be potentially highly polymorphic and consequently amenable to a detailed investigation. It is also important to note that changes in the coding sequence (SNP type I to III) are not the only candidates for functional variation, and that SNPs in perigenic regulatory regions can also have a large phenotypic impact (Halushka et al., 1999), as well as having a role in evolution (Beaumont, 1999; Chakravarty, 1999).

SNPs are less frequent in coding regions than in noncoding regions, particularly those that lead to amino acid substitutions (type I) and, therefore, have functional (phenotypic) implications; also SNPs lying in noncoding regions but having relevant functional effect, like those SNPs in the putative promoter regions of genes (type IV), are infrequent. The majority of these SNPs (type I and IV) usually have a low allelic frequency for the less-represented allele, usually $<15\%$ and frequently $<5\%$, with obvious consequences in sampling and for the statistical analyses.

Sample size required for candidate gene studies

The number of patients required to find a statistically significant association between a SNP and a trait depends on a number of factors, including the frequency of the drug response, the proportion of patients having the SNP allele, the minimum detectable effect, the level of statistical significance (p value) and the power. The "effect size" of the association is the likelihood of response to a drug in individuals with the susceptibility allele (O_1) compared with those without the allele (O_0). The magnitude of the effect in a typical case-control study is measured by the odds ratio (OR $= O_1/ O_0$), which is expected to be low, 1.5–4.0, given the multigene characteristic of pharmacogenetic traits. If some of the factors that affect the possibility of finding a significant association are known or can be guessed, then we can also calculate the sample size needed to perform a meaningful study.

For example, if it is known, or can be postulated, that (i) the proportion of response to a drug for patients having a given allele is 41% (O_1), (ii) the magnitude of the effect that is attributed to the gene is around 2 (OR), and (iii) the frequency of the allele of interest is 0.46, we can calculate the required sample size (N) using traditional formulae such as those in Fliess (1981) or Agresti (1966). A simple way to calculate the number of cases and controls is (Agresti, 1966):

$$N_{cases} = N_{controls} = (z_{\alpha/2} + z_\beta)^2 [O_1(1 - O_1) + O_0(1 - O_0)]/(O_1 - O_0)^2$$

where $z_{\alpha/2}$ is the statistics corresponding to the p value (if $p=0.05$, then $z_{\alpha/2}=1.96$) and z_β is the statistical value corresponding to the type II error, equivalent to $1-\beta$ (i.e., power: 0.84 for power 80%). In this example, $O_0=22\%$ ($O_1/1.95$, if $O_1=41\%$) and $N=91$. If the frequency of drug response is assumed to be 30% in the general population, approximately 300 subjects must be screened to reach N. It is evident that this scenario can widely vary, depending upon the various assumptions. If the response to the drug is as low as 10% of all the treated subjects, then approximately 900 patients must be screened. Other than the rate of drug response, another critical factor in determining the sample size is the relative frequency of the allele of interest. As already noted, the occurrence of the less frequent alleles for type I and type IV SNPs may be much lower than for noncoding SNPs: less than 10–15%. In this case, the sample size required to detect a difference between responders and nonresponders in relation with the given polymorphism may become very high, beyond the range attainable by a single independent investigator. Table 5.1 shows an example of this range of computations. For a quantitative phenotype, the "effect size" of the association is relative to the percentage difference of the response measure for the drug treatment in subjects with or without the susceptibility allele. Specific formulae for continuous measures, under determined type I and II errors, give the required sample size to detect what fraction of the variability can be attributed to the allelic effect, in a similar way to the case for qualitative outcomes.

A potential alternative to improve the low "power" of coding SNPs is to use them together with other noncoding SNPs that are present within the same gene. Instead of using a single polymorphism, an array of SNPs are used that are linearly arranged within a short chromosomal area, usually within 1–2 cM, and that are close enough to each other to be not randomly associated, constituting a haplotype. This specific combination of alleles (SNPs) at different loci that are physically close to, or within, a particular gene variant is more likely to be inherited together with that gene variant than alleles that are further apart and are said to be in LD. LD is dependent on the actual physical distance between the polymorphisms and the evolutionary time when the polymorphisms originated (Chakravarty, 1999). LD decays over time as a function of the recombination fraction between loci, but for very close loci, equivalent to very high LD, the decay is negligible. Haplotypes can mark the chromosomal position where the variant of interest is located more efficiently than individual SNPs and haplotype/LD mapping has been already proved to be a useful technique to map genes for several complex traits (Hästbacka et al., 1994;

Table 5.1. Determination of sample size for the association of a single nucleotide polymorphism (SNP) with a drug response in six different scenarios[a]

Study population characteristics with varying general population response rates	Freq of A1=0.46; OR=1.85		Freq of A1=0.23; OR=1.30		Freq of A1=0.10; OR=1.11	
	1	2	3	4	5	6
General response 40%						
Responder with A1 (%)	41	30	41	30	41	30
Responders without A1 (%)	22	16	32	23	37	27
N cases required[b]	91	142	404	638	2214	3546
N cases to be screened[c]	228	356	1009	1596	5535	8866
General response 30%						
Responder with A1 (%)	41	30	41	30	41	30
Responders without A1 (%)	22	16	32	23	37	27
N cases required[b]	91	142	404	638	2214	3546
N cases to be screened[c]	304	474	1346	2128	7380	11821
General response 20%						
Responder with A1 (%)	41	30	41	30	41	30
Responders without A1 (%)	22	16	32	23	37	27
N cases required[b]	91	142	404	638	2214	3546
N cases to be screened[c]	457	712	2019	3192	11071	17731
General response 10%						
Responder with A1 (%)	41	30	41	30	41	30
Responders without A1 (%)	22	16	32	23	37	27
N cases required[b]	91	142	404	638	2214	3546
N cases to be screened[c]	913	1423	4037	6383	22141	35463

Notes:

OR, odds ratio.

[a] The scenarios cover three different frequencies for the SNP allele A1 (1,2; 3,4; and 5,6); each frequency is considered with two different percentage responses for those with and without the allele of interest (1,3,5 and 2,4,6). Details of the calculations needed to compute the sample size are reported in the text.

[b] The p value (α) is set at 0.05 and the power ($1-\beta$) at 80% for all scenarios.

[c] Number that must be screened to find N responders.

Nickerson et al., 1998; McPeek and Strahs, 1999; Rieder et al., 1999; Jorde, 2000; Martin et al., 2000). Association studies with SNPs are not heavily conditioned by allelic heterogeneity, as may be the case for microsatellite polymorphisms, given the biallelic nature of SNPs, but the finding of the association can be affected by locus heterogeneity or by the presence of a yet undetected genetic interaction. However, it is very difficult to address these issues, and thus avoid speculating with theoretical hypotheses, until a first initial result makes it easier to understand the specific genetic architecture of the trait.

Methods of analysis: study design

The analysis of a case-control genetic association is straightforward using traditional statistical techniques, like the chi-square and associated measures for qualitative data (e.g., log-linear or logistic modeling) or the t-test and ANOVA (analysis of variance)/regression for quantitative phenotype definitions (Agresti, 1966; Sokal and Rohlf, 1995). A review of association methods in statistical genetics can be found in Sham (1998). Methods have been developed to account for the lack of robustness in case-control association studies, either by using extensions of the specific techniques, like the Mantel–Haenszel test (1958), for qualitative data or the use of covariates for continuous measure. Moreover, simply defining a conservative p value (i.e., $p \ll 0.05$) to conclude a significant positive finding may help to avoid spurious associations (Risch, 2000).

Other methods that correct for the risk of confounding, mostly from the chance of population admixture in case-control studies, make use of alternative strategies. One example is the method of genomic control (Devlin and Roeder, 1999), which uses the genome itself to determine appropriate corrections for population-based association tests. The test accounts for nonindependence caused by population stratification and cryptic relatedness by genotyping multiple loci unlikely to affect liability. These are called null loci because they are assumed to have no effect on the disease under study. For a case-control analysis of candidate genes, genomic control computes chi-square test statistics for independence for both null and candidate loci. By means of the variability and magnitude of the test statistics observed at the null loci, which are inflated by the impact of population stratification and cryptic relatedness, a multiplier is derived to adjust the critical value for significance tests for candidate loci. In this way, genomic control permits analysis of stratified case-control data without an increased rate of false positives. If population stratification and cryptic relatedness are not detected from null loci, then genomic control is identical to a standard test of independence for a case-control design (Bacanu et al., 2000). Other similar methods have been proposed to test for stratification (Pritchard and Rosenberg, 1999) and these methods are now being successfully applied to genetic association studies.

A statistical design, however, tests whether the observed distribution of a given allele/genotype in responders and nonresponders deviates from the statistical expectation. The test does not consider any population genetic information from the population-specific background, nor can it usually handle more complicated patterns such as those represented by the analysis of haplotypes. In these cases, a LD strategy is the design of choice. LD is based on the principle that most individuals with a specific phenotype in a population carry a polymorphic variant (or a set of variants/alleles) responsible for that phenotype and that such an allele is derived from a single ancestor. For LD to exist, we assume that a given locus A is a disease gene with two alleles A_j and A_i where the allele A_i is the "affected" variant; another locus B is close to A and is polymorphic, with two variants i and j. The B_i variant originated at some point in evolution and on the same chromosome where the A_i variant was already present. Given the close proximity of loci A and B, the two alleles A_i and B_i tend to be transmitted together across many generations, creating an A_iB_i haplotype. Only in very rare cases a crossover occurs between loci A and B, exchanging B_i with B_j and leading to an A_iB_j haplotype. Therefore, the majority of affected individuals in the population present with the $(A_i)B_i$ haplotype. Since we can genotype the B locus in real subjects, finding a disproportionate higher rate of B_i alleles in "affected" subjects implies that the yet unobserved A_i allele responsible for the trait is located in the molecular vicinity of locus B. The measure of LD is a complex topic, but in its simplest formulation LD can be measured by D (Lewontin, 1964), which represents the difference from the product of allelic frequencies at two loci with the actual frequency observed in the data:

$$D = p(A_iB_i) - p(A_i)p(B_i)$$

LD can vary from 0, equivalent to no LD, to 1, when the alleles at the two loci are in complete LD and are always simultaneously co-occurring. A positive value for D less than 1 is indicative of a certain degree of LD. The magnitude of the observed disequilibrium is dependent upon a number of different factors, most notably the distance between loci A and B. Despite the fact that the recombination events that lead to this condition are not observable – differing from linkage observed in families – they can nonetheless be inferred by analyzing the degree of DNA shared segments on the actual chromosomes. Compared with recombination, LD is a property of populations and depends extensively on their demographic and social histories, in short, on the evolutionary history of the populations (Chakravarty, 1999; Wright et al., 1999). Isolated populations like Finns and Ashkenazi Jews show extensive LD around rare disease mutations. The degree to which the same will be true for higher-frequency variants is uncertain, although as a general rule the disequilibrium is likely to decline with increasing allele frequency owing to an older coalescence time (Kingman, 2000). Consequently, the advantage of using such populations depends not only on the prevalence of the trait in the population but also on unknown factors, such as the age and frequency of the trait allele(s). For example, the frequency of the *NAT2* rapid acetylator trait is more than 90% in Japanese, but only about 8% in Middle-Eastern Arabs, owing to striking allelic differences in the gene polymorphisms (Kalow and Bertilsson, 1994). It is speculated that the age of origin of the allelic variant is different between the two populations.

Other than theoretical studies (Lio and Goldman, 1998), practical approaches have been developed to infer the age of a given allele at least at a marker locus, i.e., at a SNP (Bertorelle and Rannala, 1998), thus leading to the possibility of studying LD via evolutionary trees (Lam et al., 2000; Seltman et al., 2001). However, because LD reflects the history of recombinations, populations with different demographic histories will often display different LD patterns (Goddard et al., 2000; Pritchard and Przeworki, 2001). In particular, most studies demonstrate higher levels of LD in recently founded populations than in "older" populations such as those in Africa (e.g., Kidd et al., 1998; Tishkoff et al., 1998). In recent founded groups, such as the Finns, LD may be seen for loci separated by several centimorgans or more, suggesting that younger populations may be most useful for the initial detection of a trait locus via LD at large distances. Subsequently, older populations, in which more recombinants have accumulated, may be more useful for the fine-scale LD mapping of the trait locus, assuming that the ages of trait-causing alleles are correlated with the age of a population. In addition, for complex traits, it assumes that the relative effect of each susceptibility locus will be roughly similar in diverse populations (Ott, 2000).

LD can be computed using different mathematical methods (e.g., Devlin and Risch, 1995; Terwilliger, 1995; Devlin et al., 1996; Xiong and Guo, 1997; Lazzeroni, 1998) for single and multilocus models. The incorporation of information from multiple loci – haplotype – can enhance the power and accuracy of LD mapping, mostly if there is the possibility to accommodate for multiple founder mutations and locus heterogeneity, as in Lazzeroni (1998). The multilocus LD mapping involves the analysis of haplotype regions shared in affected cases, taking into account the relationships among groups of markers (Service et al., 1999; Mander and Clayton, 2000). LD can be measured both in large and small (triad) families and in unrelated individuals with numerous ad hoc programs, thus making an LD analysis feasible under many different sampling designs (e.g., Kerem et al., 1989). For unrelated individuals, the reconstruction of the haplotype is based upon probabilistic models, since the "phase" of the linked alleles at their sites is usually unknown.

The growing relevance of this approach, and of its associated issues, is highlighted by the recent finding of a positive association between the response to salbutamol and the interaction of multiple SNPs within a haplotype (Drysdale et al., 2000) and between a haplotype at the μ-opiod receptor gene (*OPRM1*) and heroin addiction (Hoehe et al., 2000). In these cases, only the LD-haplotype analyses supported these findings. Other researchers have already questioned the relevance of the findings, considering that only individual SNP variants, and not a haplotype, are important and can be considered the "real" causative factors (Davidson, 2000).

Gene interactions

In complex trait genetics, a large majority of investigators are beginning to think that almost every trait is determined by the joint and synergistic effect of more than one gene. However, as yet a complete theory of gene–gene interaction has not been developed, as indicated by the imprecision of the terminology used to describe these phenomena (Phillips, 1998). The analysis of a gene interaction is theoretically clear and simple for any biallelic system and mostly depends on whether the outcome phenotype is represented by a quantitative or by a qualitative variable. For a single gene controlling for a quantitative variable, the additive genotypic value is defined as half the difference between the genotypic values for the two homozygotes [$a = (G_{22} - G_{11})/2$], while the dominance genotypic value is given by the deviation of the heterozygote from the point midway between the two homozygotes [$d = G_{12} - (G_{11} + G_{22})/2$]. Using a regression approach, it is possible to estimate values for a and d, using $G_{11} = -1.0$, $G_{12} = 0$ and $G_{22} = +1.0$. Extending this notation to multiple loci, the estimate of an epistatic effect is straightforward: for two interacting loci A and B, there are nine genotypic values (for example, $Ga_{11}b_{11}$) and by simply adding an additional locus values for a and d can be calculated for the two-locus model. Here, there will be four epistatic genotypic values, referred to as additive-by-additive (aa), additive-by-dominant (ad), dominant-by-additive (da) and dominant-by-dominant (dd). Again, a regression approach allows for the estimation of these four parameters (Cheverud, 2000).

For a qualitative phenotype, the case-control association or the TDT must be represented in the form of a logistic regression (Sham, 1998) to allow for the interaction to be evaluated. The simple coding of genotypes at both loci A and B as dominant (e.g., $G_{11} = G_{12} = 1.0$, $G_{22} = 0.0$), codominant ($G_{11} = 1.0$, $G_{12} = 0.5$, $G_{22} = 0.0$) or recessive ($G_{11} = 1.0$, $G_{12} = G_{22} = 0.0$) and the consequent test of the nine possible models (e.g., dominant-by-dominant, dominant-by-codominant, dominant-by-recessive, etc.) allows the estimation of the presence of a specific form of epistatic interaction (Phillips, 1998; Goodnight, 2000).

Conclusions

The present brief review of the methods existing and under development for statistical analysis in pharmacogenetics should emphasize the great efforts that geneticists and statisticians are making to improve the ability to detect the complex genetic architecture of pharmacogenetic traits. Indeed, there are already the theoretical backgrounds and the practical techniques to detect the relevance of a given gene for the expression of a complex trait. The methodological approaches must take into account a large set of issues, ranging from the proper estimation of the required sample size to the extent of LD in the particular population under analysis, but, in principle, a positive significant result is predictable in many cases. At present, there are still major limitations when there are not obvious candidate genes or candidate regions to explore in order to relate the pharmacogenetic trait to its genetic determinants. In this case, the researcher is faced with the enormous task of performing a LD mapping across the human genome. In fact, to detect a gene with a LD approach without any a priori assumption requires genotyping each person in the study for every one of 60 000 to 500 000 SNPs. These are the figures estimated to cover a map of the human genome with a SNP every 100 to 10 kb: such a number of polymorphisms allows the detection of LD in most regions but still may be insufficient to detect genes in regions where LD is less extensive. Although the existing genotyping technologies are powerful, the current average cost of approximately US$1 per genotype could make a large-scale SNP genotyping study prohibitively expensive. It is possible to predict different scenarios with a dramatic reduction of costs achieved through new technologies, such as DNA microchips, but even at 1 cent per genotype, a large-scale LD mapping for a single patient would cost about $5000. If the number of subjects required to detect a gene in a complex pharmacogenetic trait is considered, it becomes obvious that even in favorable circumstances a pharmacogenetic study represents a notable economic challenge. Among the solutions proposed to deal with the cost of these studies, the proposal to pool patient DNA samples (e.g., Barcellos et al., 1997) has gained favor. However, pooling methods rule out the possibilities of subgrouping and performing haplotype analyses, in addition to presenting technical difficulties. In these cases we are still awaiting the significant advances that will make extensive genotyping a standard component of the investigations of complex traits.

Acknowledgement

The work described in this chapter has been partially supported by a NARSAD Investigator Initiated 2000 Award.

REFERENCES

Agresti A (1966). *Introduction to Categorical Data Analysis*. New York: John Wiley.

Bacanu SA, Devlin B, Roeder K (2000). The power of genomic control. *Am J Hum Genet* 66, 1933–1944.

Barcellos LF, Klitz W, Field LL et al. (1997). Association mapping of disease loci by use of a pooled DNA genomic screen. *Am J Hum Genet* 61, 876–884.

Baur M, Knapp M (1997). Association studies in genetic epidemiology. In Pawlowitzki IH, Edwards JH, Thompson EA, eds. *Genetic Mapping of Disease Genes*. San Diego: Academic Press, pp. 159–172.

Beaumont M (1999). Detecting population expansion and decline using microsatellites. *Genetics* 153, 2013–2029.

Bennett ST, Lucassen AM, Gough SCL et al. (1995). Susceptibility to human type 1 diabetes at IDDM2 is determined by tandem repeat variation at the insulin gene minisatellite locus. *Nat Genet* 9, 284–292.

Bertorelle G, Rannala B (1998). Using rare mutations to estimate population divergence times: a maximum likelihood approach *Proc Natl Acad Sci USA* 95, 15452–15457.

Brown DM, Provoost AP, Daly MJ, Lander ES, Jacob HJ (1996). Renal disease susceptibility and hypertension are under independent genetic control in the fawn-hooded rat. *Nat Genet* 12, 44–51.

Cargill M, Altschuler D, Ireland J et al. (1999). Characterization of single-nucleotide polymorphisms in coding regions of human genes. *Nat Genet* 22, 231–248.

Chakravarty A (1999). Population genetics – making sense out of sequence. *Nat Genet* 21, 56–60.

Cheverud JM (2000). Detecting epistasis in quantitative trait loci. In: Wolf JB, Brodie ED III, Wade MJ, eds. *Epistasis and the Evolutionary Process.* New York: Oxford University Press, pp. 58–81.

Collins A, Longjou C, Morton NE (1999) Genetic epidemiology of single-nucleotide polymorphisms. *Proc Natl Acad Sci USA* 96, 15173–15177.

Collins FS, Guyer MS, Chakravarty A (1997). Variation on a theme: cataloguing human DNA sequence variation. *Science* 278, 1580–1581.

Corder EH, Saunders AM, Strittmatter WJ et al. (1993). Gene dose of apolipoprotein E type 4 allele and the risk of Alzheimer's disease in late onset families. *Science* 261, 921–923.

Davidson S (2000). Research suggests importance of haploytpes over SNPs. *Nat Biotech* 18, 1134–1135.

Devlin B, Risch N (1995). A comparison of linkage-disequilibrium measures for fine-scale mapping. *Genomics* 29, 311–322.

Devlin B, Roeder K (1999). Genomic control for association studies. *Biometrics* 55, 997–1004.

Devlin B, Risch N, Roeder K (1996). Disequilibrium mapping: composite likelihood for pairwise disequilibirum. *Genomics* 36, 1–16.

Drysdale CM, McGraw DW, Stack CB et al. (2000). Complex promoter and coding region β_2-adrenergic receptor haplotypes alter receptor expression and predict in vivo responsiveness. *Proc Natl Acad Sci USA* 97, 10483–10488.

Ewens WJ, Spielman RS (1995). The transmission/disequillibrium test: history, subdivision and admixture. *Am J Hum Genet* 57, 455–464.

Fliess JL (1981). *Statistical Methods for Rates and Proportions.* New York: John Wiley.

Goodnight CJ (2000). Modeling gene interaction in structure populations. In Wolf JB, Brodie ED III, Wade MJ, eds. *Epistasis and the Evolutionary Process.* New York: Oxford University Press, pp. 129–145.

Halushka MK, Fan JB, Bentley K et al. (1999). Patterns of single-nucleotide polymorphisms in candidate genes for blood-pressure homeostasis. *Nat Genet* 22, 239–247.

Hästbacka J, de la Chapelle A, Mahtani MM et al. (1994). The diastrophic dysplasia gene encodes a novel sulfate transporter: positional cloning by fine-structure linkage disequilibrium mapping. *Cell* 78, 1073–1087.

Hoehe MR, Köple K, Wendel B et al. (2000). Sequence variability and candidate gene analysis in complex disease: association of μ opioid receptor gene variation with substance dependence. *Hum Mol Genet* 19, 2895–2908.

International SNP Map Working Group (2001). A map of human genome sequence variation containing 1.42 million single nucleotide polymorphisms *Nature* 409, 928–923.

Jacob HJ, Lindpaintner K, Lincoln SE et al. (1991). Genetic mapping of a gene causing hypertension in the stroke-prone spontaneously hypertensive rat. *Cell* 67, 213–224.

Johnson GCL, Todd JA (2000). Strategies in complex disease mapping. *Curr Opin Genet Dev* 10, 330–334.

Jorde LB (2000). Linkage disequilibrium and the search for complex disease genes. *Genome Res* 10, 1035–1044.

Goddard KAB, Hopkins PJ, Hall JM, Witte JS (2000). Linkage disequilibrium and allele-frequency distributions for 114 single-nucleotide polymorphisms in five populations. *Am J Hum Genet* 66, 216–234.

Kalow W, Bertilsson L (1994). Interethnic factors affecting drug response. *Adverse Drug Res* 23, 1–53.

Kerem B, Rommens JM, Buchanan JA et al. (1989). Identification of the cystic fibrosis gene: genetic analysis. *Science* 245, 1073–1080.

Kidd KK, Morar B, Castiglione CM et al. (1998). A global survey of haplotype frequencies and linkage disequilibrium at the *DRD2* locus. *Hum Genet* 103, 211–227.

Kingman JFC (2000). Origin of the colascent: 1974–1982. *Genetics* 156, 1461–1463.

Kruglyak L (1999). Prospects for whole-genome linkage disequilibrium mapping of common disease genes. *Nat Genet* 22, 139–144.

Lam JC, Roeder K, Devlin B (2000). Haplotype fine mapping by evolutionary trees. *Am J Hum Genet* 66, 659–673.

Lazzeroni LC (1998). Linkage disequilibrium and gene mapping: an empirical least-squares approach. *Am J Hum Genet* 62, 159–170.

Lewontin RC (1964). The interaction of selection and linkage. 1. General considerations; heterotic models. *Genetics* 49, 49–67.

Lifton RP (1996). Molecular genetics of human blood pressure variation. *Science* 272, 676–680.

Lio' P, Goldman N (1998). Models of molecular evolution and phylogeny. *Genome Res* 8, 1233–1244.

Mander A, Clayton D (2000). Haplotype frequency estimation using an EM algorithm and log-linear modeling. *Stat Tech Bull* 57, 5–7.

Mantel N, Haenszel W (1958). Statistical aspects of the analysis of data from retrospective studies of disease. *J Nat Cancer Inst* 4, 719–748.

Martin ER, Gilbert JR, Lai EH et al. (2000). Analysis of association at single nucleotide polymorphisms in the APOE region. *Genomics* 63, 7–12.

McPeek MS, Strahs A (1999). Assessment of linkage disequilibrium by the decay of haplotype sharing, with application to fine-scale genetic mapping. *Am J Hum Genet* 65, 858–875.

Monks SA, Kaplan NL (2000). Removing the sampling restrictions from family-based tests of association for a quantitative-trait locus. *Am J Hum Genet* 66, 576–592.

Nebert DW (1999). Pharmacogenetics and pharmacogenomics: why is this relevant to the clinical geneticist? *Clin Genet* 56, 247–258.

Nickerson DA, Taylor SL, Weiis KM et al. (1998). DNA sequence diversity in a 9.7-kb region of the human lipoprotein lipase gene. *Nat Genet* 19, 233–240.

Ott J (1999). *Analysis of Human Genetic Linkage*, 3rd edn. Baltimore: Johns Hopkins University Press.

Ott J (2000). Predicting the range of linkage disequilibrium. *Proc Natl Acad Sci, USA* 97, 2–3.

Ott J, Hoh J (2000). Statistical approaches to gene mapping. *Am J Hum Genet* 67, 289–294.

Phillips PC (1998). The language of gene interaction. *Genetics* 149, 1167–1171.

Pritchard JK (2001). Are rare variants responsible for susceptibility to complex diseases? *Am J Hum Genet* 69, 124–137.

Pritchard JK, Przeworki M (2001). Linkage disequilibrium in humans: models and data. *Am J Hum Genet* 69, 1–14.

Pritchard JK, Rosenberg NA (1999). Use of unlinked genetic markers to detect population stratification in association studies. *Am J Hum Genet* 65, 220–228.

Rieder MJ, Taylor SL, Clark AG, Nickerson DA (1999). Sequence variation in the human angiotensin converting enzyme. *Nat Genet* 22, 59–62.

Risch N (2000). Searching for genetic determinants in the new millennium. *Nature* 405, 847–856.

Risch N, Merikangas K (1996). The future of genetic studies of complex human diseases. *Science* 273, 1561–1517.

Roses AD (2000). Pharmacogenetics and the practice of medicine. *Nature* 405, 857–865.

Schaid DJ, Sommer SS (1994). Comparison of statistics for candidate-gene association studies using cases and parents. *Am J Hum Genet* 55, 402–409.

Schaid DJ, Sommer SS (1993). Genotype relative risks: methods for design and analysis of candidate-gene association studies. *Am J Hum Genet* 53, 1115–1126.

Schork NJ, Krieger JE, Trolliet MR et al. (1995). A biometrical genome search in rats reveals the multigenic basis of blood pressure variation. *Genome Res* 5, 164–172.

Seltman H, Roeder K, Devlin B (2001). Transmission/disequilibrium test meets measured haplotype analysis: family-based association analysis guided by evolution of haplotypes. *Am J Hum Genet* 68, 1250–1263.

Service SK, Lang DW, Freimer NB, Sandkuijl LA (1999). Linkage-disequilibrium mapping of disease genes by reconstruction of ancestral haplotypes in founder populations. *Am J Hum Genet* 64, 1728–1738.

Sham PC (1998). Statistical methods in psychiatric genetics. *Stat Meth Med Res* 7, 279–300.

Sokal RR, Rohlf FJ (1995). *Biometry*, 3rd edn. San Francisco: Freeman.

Spielman RS, Ewens WJ (1996). Invited editorial: the TDT and other family-based tests for linkage test for linkage disequilibrium and association. *Am J Hum Genet* 59, 983–989.

Spielman RS, Ewens WJ (1998). A sibship test for linkage in the presence of association: the sib transmission/disequilibrium test. *Am J Hum Genet* 62, 450–458.

Spielman RS, McGinnis RE, Ewens WJ (1993). Transmission test for linkage disequilibrium: the insulin gene region and insulin-dependent diabetes mellitus (IDDM). *Am J Hum Genet* 56, 777–787.

Terwilliger JD (1995). A powerful likelihood method for the analysis of linkage-disequilibrium between trait loci and one or more polymorphic markers. *Am J Hum Genet* 56, 777–787.

Terwilliger JD, Weiss KM (1998). Linkage disequilibrium mapping of complex disease: fantasy or reality? *Curr Opin Biotechnol* 9, 578–594.

Tishkoff SA, Goldman A, Calafell F et al. (1998). A global haplotype analysis of the myotonic dystrophy locus: implications for the evolution of modern humans and for the origin of myotonic dystrophy mutations. *Am J Hum Genet* 62, 1389–1402.

van Hauwe P, Coucke PJ, Declau F et al. (1999). Deafness linked to *DFNA2*: one locus but how many genes? *Nat Genet* 21, 363.

Venter J et al. (2001). The sequence of human genome. *Science* 291, 1304–1351.

Vogel F (1959). Moderne probleme der Humangenetik. *Ergebn Inn Med Kinderheilk* 12, 52–125.

Weiss KM, Terwilliger JD (2000). How many diseases does it take to map a gene with SNPs? *Nat Genet* 26, 151–157.

Wright AF, Carothers AD, Pirastu M (1999). Population choice in mapping genes for complex diseases. *Nat Genet* 23, 397–404.

Xiong M, Guo SW (1997). Fine-scale genetic mapping based on linkage disequilibrium: theory and application. *Am J Hum Genet* 60, 629–640.

Part III

Molecular background

6

The psychopharmacogenetic–neurodevelopmental interface in serotonergic gene pathways

K. Peter Lesch, Jens Benninghoff and Angelika Schmitt

Department of Psychiatry and Psychotherapy, University of Wuerzburg, Wuerzburg, Germany

OVERVIEW

Individual differences in drug effects and treatment response are relatively enduring, continuously distributed, and substantially heritable; they are, therefore, likely to result from an interplay of multiple genomic variations with environmental influences. As the etiology and pathogenesis of behavioral and psychiatric disorders are genetically complex, so is the response to drug treatment. Psychopharmacological drug response depends on the structure and functional expression of gene products, which may be direct drug targets or may indirectly modify the development and synaptic plasticity of neural networks critically involved in drug response. While formation and integration of these neural networks is dependent on the action of manifold proteins, converging lines of evidence indicate that genetically controlled variability in the expression of genes critical to the development and plasticity of distinct neurocircuits influences a wide spectrum of quantitative traits including treatment response. During brain development, neurotransmitter systems (e.g., the serotonergic system), which are frequently targeted by psychotropic drugs, control neuronal specification, differentiation, and phenotype maintenance. The formation and maturation of these neurotransmitter systems, in turn, is directed by an intrinsic genetic program. Based on the notion that complex gene–gene and gene–environment interactions in the regulation of brain plasticity contribute to interindividual differences in drug response, the concept of developmental psychopharmacogenetics is emerging. This chapter appraises prototypical genomic variation with impact on gene expression, and complementary studies of gene *and* environmental effects on brain development and synaptic plasticity in the mouse model. Although special emphasis is given to molecular mechanisms of neurodevelopmental genetics, relevant conceptual and methodological issues pertinent to the dissection of the psychopharmacogenetic–neurodevelopmental interface are also considered.

Introduction

Psychopharmacogenetics is an emerging scientific discipline examining the genetic basis for individual variations in response to psychotherapeutic drugs (Catalano,

1999). While pharmacogenetics cannot improve the efficacy of a given drug, it may help in selecting patients who are likely to respond well. Psychopharmacological drug response depends on the structure and functional expression of a large number of gene products representing either pharmacokinetic or pharmacodynamic determinants. For most drugs, variations in drug response have, until recently, been considered a result of pharmacokinetic rather than pharmacodynamic differences. However, it now seems that pharmacodynamic variability in humans is large, reproducible, and usually more pronounced than pharmacokinetic variability. Many drug targets (e.g., receptors, transporters, enzymes) that contribute to the pharmacodynamics of drug response are not only key players in the regulation of neurotransmitter systems but also directly or indirectly modify the development and plasticity of neural networks involved in drug effects. Both variation of structure (which is rare) and variation of expression (which is common) influence gene product availability and function.

Gene expression involves many facets of regulation ranging from transcription, transcript processing, translation, post-translational modification and intracellular trafficking. It is controlled by multiple regulatory proteins (Lesch and Heils, 2000). These regulatory proteins represent gene products themselves and have been expressed sequentially following an intrinsic genetic program. This developmental blueprint controls the hierarchical cascade of gene expression whose different stages subject to similar regulatory principles. There is now considerable evidence that variability of expression of genes critical to neurocircuit development and function influences drug responses. This chapter describes fundamental aspects of the genetics of complex traits including drug response, provides an appraisal of quantitative genetic research, and reviews genomic variations with impact on gene expression.

Psychopharmacological drug response as a complex trait

Considerable evidence has been assembled that treatment response is influenced by genetic factors and that the genetic component is highly complex, polygenic, and epistatic. Moreover, treatment response is believed to involve both genetic and environmental factors. Most likely, the contribution of single genes to drug response is modest, if not minimal. However, interactions between different genes could result in a dramatic modification of drug response (additive, nonadditive or synergistic gene effects). The challenge is to identify genes of relative small effect against a background of substantial genetic and environmental variation.

Many genes that influence complex traits and psychopharmacological drug responses are likely to be distributed continuously. Such genes are, therefore, referred to as quantitative trait loci (QTLs). In contrast to the focus of quantitative genetics on phenotypes of interest and on naturally occurring genetic variation responsible for phenotypic differences, molecular genetics focused on genes and techniques to create new mutations in model organisms such as the worm (*Caenorhabditis elegans*), fruit fly (*Drosophila melanogaster*), or mouse in order to investigate how genes work. The pace of integration of quantitative and molecular genetics has been accelerated remarkably as a result of the *Drosophila*, Mouse, and Human Genome Projects, which have opened the postgenomic era in which the genome of humans and other species is known. While several million DNA variations (polymorphisms) have been identified in the genomic sequence, approximately 30 000–60 000 common polymorphisms are located in coding and regulatory regions of genes that are the ultimate causes of the heritability of complex traits (McPherson et al., 2001; Sachidanandam et al., 2001). New technologies, such as DNA microarrays, have made it possible to investigate the role of thousands of DNA variants in complex traits. Because behavioral traits are the most complex traits of all, response to psychopharmacological drugs, which modify behavior, is likely to profit from this integration. Moreover, behavioral pharmacogenetics will make a major contribution to functional genomics. Although functional genomics has been equated with a bottom-up approach that begins with genes and their protein products in cells – and the importance of this level of analysis is not doubted – the phenotypical level of analysis is also crucial and should provide benefits in terms of diagnosing, treating, and preventing behavioral and psychiatric disorders. The term pharmacogenomics emphasizes the importance of the behavioral level of analysis in understanding how genes work at the developmental interface between the organism and its environment. Bottom-up molecular approaches will eventually meet top-down behavioral research in the brain, the ultimate target for functional genomic analysis of behavior and treatment response.

Several genes related to monoaminergic neurotransmission are currently under investigation, including the dopaminergic, noradrenergic, and serotonergic systems, which may contribute to the genetic variance of response to antidepressant, anxiolytic, and antipsychotic treatment. However, molecular genetics has so far failed to identify a genomic variation that can consistently contribute to psychopharmacological drug responses (Stoltenberg and Burmeister, 2000). Since components of the monoaminergic neurotransmitter system not only participate in the function and plasticity of the adult brain but also represent key players in the development of the brain, genetic variation in neurodevelopment further complicates assessment of the interplay of genotype and drug efficacy. Emerging genetic and genomic techniques now offer the prospect of identifying functionally relevant gene variants that participate in the development and adult plasticity of the brain relating to psychopharmacological drug responses.

Variation of structure and expression of pharmacodynamic factors

The pace of discovery of genes associated with complex traits, such as drug response, is currently increasing as systematic QTL scans can be conducted using functional DNA variants in the brain that affect coding regions or gene regulation. Of a total approximately 40 000 genes, approximately 50% are expressed in the brain. However, a substantial proportion of these are housekeeping genes, which provide structure or maintain basic physiological functions of cells. Consequently, fewer than 15 000 tissue-specific genes may be expressed in the brain. Identifying the estimated 8000–16 000 functional DNA variants in coding regions of these genes and the DNA variants that regulate the expression of these genes is a high priority for pharmacogenetic research because these genes are likely to be the source of the heritable influence on psychopharmacological drug response. Several classes of genomic variation in coding and regulatory regions of genes are of particular interest. These range from single nucleotide polymorphisms (SNPs) to microdeletions (or insertions), and polymorphic simple sequence repeats (SSRs) of 2 to 50+ nucleotides in length (Fig. 6.1).

Although many features of drug targets, their protein components or subunits, and their spliced or edited isotypes have been revealed, less is known about the genetic elements and transcription factors involved in the regulation of gene expression. Even less still is known about the impact of genomic variation within regulatory regions and elements on gene expression. Nevertheless, there is consensus that the basal promoter and associated regulatory elements are located upstream of a transcribed gene, although adjunct regulatory units may be located across the entire region of a gene. In contrast to constitutively active core promoters, which effectively drive expression in a large variety of tissues, tissue-selective regulatory elements, which are frequently located upstream of the core promoter unit, confer cell-restricted activity such that the gene is transcribed only in distinct cell types, such as neurons or glial cells (Fig. 6.1).

DNA variants in coding and regulatory regions of genes will be both useful for systematic genome scans, for identifying genes associated with drug response, and for examining integrated systems of gene pathways as an important step on the route to functional genomics. Initiatives focused on genes expressed in the brain and the creation of a brain "transcriptome" map in which gene expression is mapped throughout the brain in mice would greatly facilitate postgenomic research on the links between genes, brain, behavior, and treatment response. Connecting drug response with relevant functional DNA variants in the brain and with differences in gene expression in brain regions represents the ultimate goal for pharmacogenetic research. The serotonergic gene pathways may be a rewarding area of investigation because of the numerous and essential functions of the central

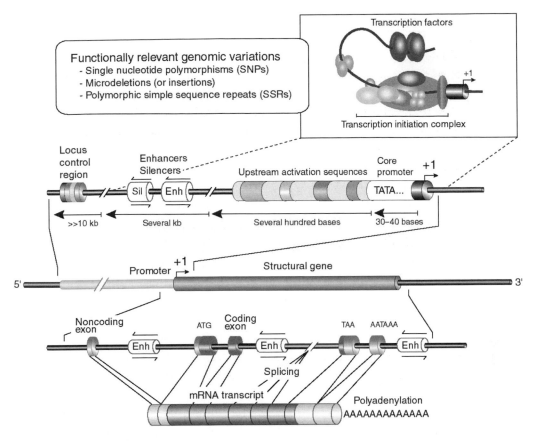

Fig. 6.1.   Gene organization, transcriptional control region, and common functionally relevant genomic variations. Frequency of initiation of mRNA synthesis depends on transcription factors that interact with specific elements in the gene promoter, other regulatory sites, and optional locus control regions. The transcription initiation complex comprises multiple factors, including the TATA box-binding protein (TBP) with TBP-associated factors, coactivators, and basal factors. These components associate to a complex with RNA polymerase that are bound to the TATA and enhancer (Enh) motifs. Several structures and motifs characteristic for binding of activators are indicated. Activators bind to enhancer motifs and transduce their signals to coactivators; they control gene activation by increasing transcription rate. Repressors bind to silencer elements (Sil), inhibit activator function and slow down transcription. Coactivators are adapter molecules that integrate signals of activators/repressors and transfer the information on basal factors. Basal factors facilitate binding and activation of RNA polymerase at the transcription start site.

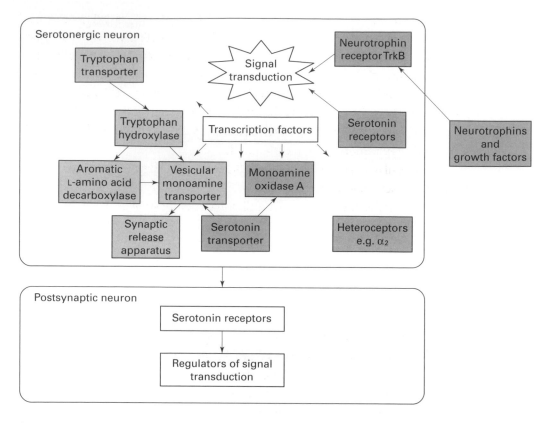

Fig. 6.2.   Serotonergic gene pathways and different components of serotonergic system development, plasticity, and function currently under psychopharmacogenetic investigation.

serotonin (5-HT) system, the striking wealth of drug targets within this system, and the impressive range of serotonergic compounds available in the clinical setting (Fig. 6.2).

Representative genomic variants in serotonergic gene pathways

Serotonin receptors

Ligand-binding experiments and the study of functional responses to agonists/antagonists initially defined four 5-HT receptor subfamilies, 5-HT_{1-4}. Molecular biology has subsequently both confirmed this classification and also revealed the existence of novel 5-HT receptor subtypes for which few pharmacological or functional data exist ($5\text{-HT}_{1E/F}$, $5\text{-HT}_{3A/B}$, $5\text{-HT}_{5A/B}$, 5-HT_{6}, and 5-HT_{7}) (Hoyer and Martin, 1997; Barnes and Sharp, 1999). In the genes for 5-HT_{2-7} receptors, the coding region is interupted by introns, whereas the genes for $5\text{-HT}_{1A\text{-}F}$

receptors contain no introns. The genes for 5-HT$_{2B}$, 5-HT$_4$, 5-HT$_6$, and 5-HT$_7$ receptors are alternatively spliced, and RNA editing of 5-HT$_{2C}$ receptor subtype in the second intracellular loop confers differential receptor functionality, thus increasing the complexity of the 5-HT receptor superfamily (Gerald, 1995; Canton et al., 1996; Heidmann, 1997; Olsen et al., 1999). The present challenge is to determine the physiological relevance of these gene products, establish their functionality as endogenous receptors, find selective ligands, and determine potential therapeutic application of these compounds.

The molecular characterization of different 5-HT receptor families has simplified the elucidation of gene transcription, mRNA processing and translation, intracellular trafficking, and post-translational modification relevant to synaptic and postreceptor signaling (for review see Lesch and Heils (2000)). Transcriptional control regions have been cloned for several 5-HT receptor subtypes, and functional promoter mapping data are available for the genes for 5-HT$_{1A}$, 5-HT$_{2A}$, 5-HT$_{2C}$, and 5-HT$_3$ receptors. The analysis of genomic regulatory regions of 5-HT receptor genes and modeling variable 5-HT receptor gene function in genetically engineered mice (constitutive and conditional knockout) provides critical knowledge regarding the respective role of these receptors in neurodevelopment, synaptic plasticity, and behavior (Bonasera and Tecott, 2000). For example, behavioral evaluation of 5-HT$_{1B}$ knockout mice has implicated this 5-HT autoreceptor in alcohol-seeking and aggressive behavior (Brunner et al., 1999). Mice with targeted disruption of the 5-HT$_{2C}$ gene display anxiety-related behavior, hyperphagia-evoked weight gain, and deficits in spatial learning (Tecott and Barondes, 1996).

Several potentially functional variations in genes of 5-HT receptors have recently been associated with behavioral traits, psychopathological conditions, and psychopharmacological drug response. Since this area has recently been reviewed comprehensively (for example, in Cichon et al. (2000) and Veenstra-VanderWeele et al. (2000)), only a few prototypical polymorphisms with evidence for functional impact on gene expression and function will be discussed here. Studies in a Finnish population and a southwestern American Indian tribe revealed that the silent Gly861Cys (G861C) polymorphism in the 5-HT$_{1B}$ receptor is associated with antisocial alcoholism. In a family-based study, a polymorphism in the 5′-regulatory region of the gene for the 5-HT$_{2A}$ (Ala1438Gly (A1438G)) was associated with schizophrenia (Spurlock et al., 1997). Analysis of the A1438G polymorphism revealed no effect of genotype on basal or cyclic adenosine monophosphate (cAMP) and protein kinase C-induced gene transcription in a cell model and no difference in lymphocyte 5-HTR$_{2A}$ mRNA expression between 1438G/G and A/A homozygotes. However, a preliminary autopsy study demonstrated higher prefrontal 5-HT$_{2A}$ binding in subjects with the 1438A allele (Turecki et al., 1999). The common polymorphism Cys23Ser (C23S) in the coding region of the 5-HT$_{2C}$

receptor gene shows only weak associations with schizophrenic psychosis but influences psychotic symptoms, clinical course (including duration of hospitalization) and drug response (Cichon et al., 2000). A recently identified polymorphic compound dinucleotide repeat in the 5′-regulatory region of the $5-HT_{2C}$ gene (J. Meyer and K.P. Lesch, unpublished data), which is unique to humans and nonhuman primates, contributes to the predictive power of several variants in serotonergic gene pathways (i.e., $5-HT_{2A}$, $5-HT_{2C}$, 5-HT transporter (5-HTT)) for clozapine response in schizophrenia (Arranz et al., 2000), whereas no association with panic disorder was detected (Deckert et al., 2000).

Serotonin transporter

In humans, transcriptional activity of the gene for the transporter 5-HTT is modulated by a polymorphic repetitive element (5-HTT gene-linked polymorphic region, 5-HTTLPR) located upstream of the transcription start site. Additional variations have been described in the 5′ untranslated region (5′-UTR) through alternative splicing of exon 1B (Bradley and Blakely, 1997), in intron 2 (a 16/17 variable number tandem repeat, VNTR-17) (Lesch et al., 1994), and in the 3′ UTR (Battersby et al., 1999). Comparison of different mammalian species confirmed the presence of the 5-HTTLPR in simian primates but not in prosimian primates and other mammals (Lesch et al., 1997). The majority of alleles are composed of either 14- or 16-repeat elements in humans (short (*s*) and long (*l*) allele, respectively), while alleles with 15, 18, 19, 20, or 22 repeat elements and variants with single-base insertions/deletions or substitutions within individual repeat elements are rare. A predominantly Caucasian population displayed allele frequencies of 57% for the *l* allele and 43% for the *s* allele, with a 5-HTTLPR genotype distribution of 32% *l/l*, 49% *l/s*, and 19% *s/s* (Lesch et al., 1996). Different allele and genotype distributions were found in other populations (Gelernter et al., 1997; Ishiguro et al., 1997; Kunugi et al., 1997).

The unique structure of the 5-HTTLPR gives rise to the formation of DNA secondary structure that has the potential to regulate the transcriptional activity of the associated 5-HTT gene promoter. When fused to a luciferase reporter gene and transfected into human 5-HTT-expressing cell lines, the *s* and *l* 5-HTTLPR variants differentially modulate transcriptional activity of the 5-HTT gene promoter (Lesch et al., 1996). The effect of 5-HTTLPR length variability on 5-HTT function was determined by studying the relationship between 5-HTTLPR genotype, 5-HTT gene transcription, and 5-HT uptake activity in human lymphoblastoid cell lines. Cells homozygous for the *l* variant of 5-HTTLPR produced higher concentrations of 5-HTT mRNA than cells containing one or two copies of the *s* form. Membrane preparations from *l/l* lymphoblasts showed higher inhibitor binding than did *s/s* cells. Furthermore, the rate of specific 5-HT uptake was more than twofold higher in cells homozygous for the *l* form of the 5-HTTLPR than in cells carrying one or two copies of the *s* variant of the promoter. The association of the *s* form with lower 5-HTT expression and function is supported by studies of 5-HTT promoter activity in other cell lines (Mortensen et al., 1999), mRNA concentrations in the raphe complex of human postmortem brain (Little et al., 1998), platelet 5-HT uptake and content (Hanna et al., 1998; Greenberg et al., 1999; Nobile et al., 1999) and in vivo SPECT (single photon emission computed tomography) imaging of human brain 5-HTT (Heinz et al., 1999).

The secondary structure of the 5-HTTLPR is also likely to precipitate a 381 bp somatic deletion in the promoter region (del(17)(q11.2)) of the 5-HTT gene, observed in 20–60% of genomic DNA isolated from human brain and mononuclear cells (Lesch and Mössner, 1999). The localization of the deletion breakpoints adjacent to identical putative signal sequences suggests a recombinase-like rearrangement event. This suggests that mosaicism of the 5-HTT gene promoter-associated deletion is likely to be regulated by brain region-selective and possibly 5-HTTLPR-dependent mechanisms. This extraordinary feature provides further evidence for complex 5-HTT gene organization and regulation.

A growing body of evidence suggests a role of 5-HTTLPR-dependent allelic variation in 5-HTT expression and function in anxiety-, depression-, and aggression-related personality traits and syndromal dimensions of various psychiatric disorders (for review see Lesch, 2001a). The finding that individuals with reduced 5-HTT function are at risk to develop affective illness would seem at odds with the fact that 5-HT reuptake inhibitors (SRIs), which competitively block 5-HT uptake, are effective in anxiety disorders and depression. The regional variation of 5-HTT expression and the complex autoregulatory processes of 5-HT function that are operational in different brain areas may lead to a plausible hypothesis to explain this apparent contradiction (Routledge and Middlemiss, 1996). The impaired ability for rapid 5-HT clearance associated with the *s*-allele of 5-HTTLPR following 5-HT release into the synaptic cleft, may elicit acute increases of 5-HT in the vicinity of serotonergic cell bodies and dendrites in the raphe complex and may exert a somatodendritic 5-HT$_{1A}$ receptor-mediated negative feedback that leads to an overall decrease of 5-HT neurotransmission. By comparison, chronic SRI treatment induces adaptive changes in the 5-HTT/5-HT$_{1A}$ receptor-modulated negative feedback regulation that eventually leads to an overall enhancement of terminal 5-HT. In this regard it has been proposed that concurrent antagonism of this autoreceptor during 5-HT reuptake blockade may have the potential to accelerate the antidepressant effect of 5-HTT inhibition, which could be particularly advantageous in 5-HTTLPR genotype-related SRI nonresponders (Blier and de Montigny, 1997; Smeraldi et al., 1998).

Based on theoretical consideration, a complex interaction between genotype, behavioral or syndromal dimensions, and drug response has been predicted (Catalano, 1999). A given genetic predisposition, such as allelic variation in 5-HTT function, may lead to increased susceptibility to anxious or depressive features and to less favorable antidepressant responses in patients affected by mood disorders. Impaired 5-HTT function apparently confers only a very modest susceptibility, if any, to depressed states, because adaptive mechanisms are likely to compensate for the deficiency, while more robust alterations of 5-HT turnover observed during antidepressant treatment may reveal 5-HTTLPR genotype effects that lead to variable SRI efficacy. Smeraldi and associates (1998) investigated whether the 5-HTTLPR genotype is related to the antidepressant response to the SRI fluvoxamine and/or to augmentation with the 5-HT_{1A} receptor antagonist pindolol. Their study included patients with major depression with psychotic features (n = 102) who had been randomly assigned to treatment with a fixed dose of fluvoxamine and either placebo or pindolol for 6 weeks. Both *l/l* homozygotes and *l/s* heterozygotes showed a better response to fluvoxamine than for 5-HTTLPR *s/s* homozygotes. In the group treated with fluvoxamine plus pindolol, all the genotypes acted like *l/l* homozygotes treated with fluvoxamine alone. Thus, SRI efficacy in delusional depression seems to be related, in part, to allelic variation within the promoter of the 5-HTT gene. This 5-HTTLPR genotype effect on antidepressant response has recently been replicated in an independent sample of depressed patients treated with the SRI paroxetine (Zanardi et al., 2000). Furthermore, an interaction between 5-HTTLPR genotype and therapeutic efficacy of the antimanic/antibipolar agent lithium, which is assumed to act via serotonergic mechanisms, was demonstrated (Del Zompo et al., 1999). Finally, drug-free patients with bipolar depression who were *l/l* homozygotes for 5-HTTLPR showed better mood improvement after total sleep deprivation than those with the *s/l* and *s/s* genotypes (Benedetti et al., 1998). These findings support the notion that 5-HTTLPR genotyping may represent a useful pharmacogenetic tool to individualize treatment of depression and that 5-HTT function is critical for the antidepressant mechanism of action of sleep deprivation.

Monoamine oxidase

Monoamine oxidase A (MAO-A) oxidizes 5-HT, norepinephrine, and dopamine. It is expressed in a cell type-specific manner. Abnormalities in MAO-A activity have been implicated in a wide range of behavioral and psychiatric disorders (for review see Lesch and Merschdorf (2000)). Interestingly, deficiency in MAO-A owing to a hemizygous chain termination mutation in its gene has been shown to be associated with impulsive aggression and hypersexual behavior in affected males from a single large family. Transgenic mice lacking the gene for MAO-A exhibit aggressive behavior in adult males.

While there is considerable controversy regarding the site where MAO-A mRNA synthesis is initiated, tissue-specific length variability of the 5′-UTR has been reported, with multiple transcription start sites clustered primarily around an initiator element, which may also act as a negative *cis* element (Denney et al., 1994; Zhu et al., 1994; Zhu and Shih, 1997). The core promoter region contains two 90 bp repeat sequences, which are further divided into four imperfect tandem repeats, each containing an Sp1 binding site in reversed orientation. A polymorphic 30 bp repeat was recently identified in the promoter region of the *MAO-A* that differentially modulated gene transcription (Sabol et al., 1998; Deckert et al., 1999). Variation in the number of repeats (3 to 5) of this *MAO-A* gene-linked polymorphic region (*MAO-A-LPR*) resulted in different transcriptional efficiencies when the gene was fused to a luciferase reporter gene and transfected into cell lines. The transcriptional efficiency of the 3-repeat allele was twofold lower than those with longer repeats (3a, 4, and 5). Interestingly, there was an up to eightfold higher MAO-A activity in human male skin fibroblasts associated with the 4-repeat MAO-A-LPR genotype ((Denney et al., 1999)). Jonsson and associates (2000)) found increased cerebrospinal fluid (CSF) levels of hydroxyindoleacetic acid (5-HIAA) and homovanillic acid in women with at least one copy of the 3.5- or 4-repeat promoter allele, but not in men. This finding further supports the gender-specific effect of the MAO-A-LPR previously reported in panic disorder (Deckert et al., 1999).

The MAO-A-LPR is, therefore, an attractive genomic variation to investigate behavioral disorders that are associated with abnormalities in monoaminergic transmission as well as response to psychopharmacological drugs affecting these neurotransmitter systems. Recent studies showed associations of MAO-A-LPR length variation in alcoholics with dissocial behavior and in female patients with panic anxiety (Deckert et al., 1999; Samochowiec et al., 1999). The findings suggest that the 3-repeat allele of the MAO-A-LPR confers vulnerability to dissocial behavior rather than alcohol-seeking behavior in alcohol-dependent males. Among females with panic disorder, the longer alleles (3a, 4, and 5) were more frequent than in the corresponding control populations. Together with the observation that inhibition of MAO-A is clinically effective in the treatment of panic disorder, particularly in women, these results suggest that increased MAO-A activity is a risk factor for panic disorder in females.

Brain development and serotonin

While being important pharmacodynamic factors themselves, components of monoaminergic neurotransmitter systems such as receptors, transporters, and modifying enzymes also participate in brain development and thus set the stage for brain (dys)function and influence presence as well as function of drug targets and many other pharmacodynamically important factors.

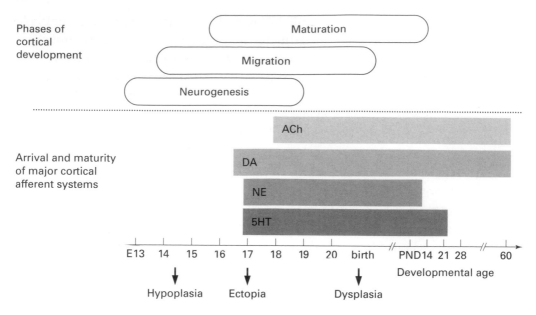

Fig.6.3.   Neurotransmitters in brain development and plasticity. Timeline for different phases of cortical development and for the arrival and maturity of major cortical afferents. ACh, acetylcholine; DA, dopamine; NE, norepinephrine; 5HT, 5-hydroxytryptamine (serotonin); PND, postnatal day. (Modified from Berger-Sweeney and Hohmann, 1997.)

Development of the brain, including the neocortex, involves a complex series of rigorously timed stages that are subdivided into generation, migration, and differentiation of neurons and glia (Berger-Sweeney and Hohmann, 1997) (Fig. 6.3). These events occur during distinct time windows that span the perinatal period and create intricate neural circuits and networks critical in the integration of sensory and cognitive functions and aspects of behavioral responses. Evidence indicates that variation in gene function as well as environmental factors at certain stages of neurodevelopment may lead to circumscribed alterations including hypoplasia (reduced cell number), ectopia (abnormality in migration), and dysplasia (alteration in number and structure). Harmonizing these sequential stages and reaching developmental milestones is critical to guide assembly of neuronal cells from different regions of the brain at the appropriate times and locations to form functional circuits. Several models of manipulations that affect different stages of cortical development, particularly those that compromise ontogeny of neurotransmitter-defined afferent systems, have implicated acetylcholine, norepinephrine, dopamine, and 5-HT (Fig. 6.3). Given the complexity of the processes that will eventually be regulated by these circuits, it is conceivable that neurodevelopment is exquisitely prone to allelic variation in functional gene expression.

There are several lines of evidence that 5-HT system homeostasis is critical to the genesis, differentiation, and maturation of neuronal cells and networks in brain regions controlling sensory inputs, stimulus processing, and motor output. 5-HT is a mitogenic and morphogenetic factor as well as a differentiation signal in cortical development. For instance, 5-HT modulates neurite outgrowth of thalamocortical glutamatergic neurons in culture, which involves both 5-HT$_{1A}$ and 5-HT$_{1B}$ receptors (Lavdas et al., 1997). Furthermore, it promotes differentiation of cortical glutamatergic neurons via 5-HT$_{1B}$ (Lieske et al., 1999), increases the probability of long-term potentiation in the visual cortex by activation of 5-HT$_{2C}$ (Kojic et al., 2000), and stimulates hippocampal neurogenesis resulting in antidepressant effects, which is likely to be mediated by 5-HT$_{1A}$ (Gould, 1999; Malberg et al., 2000).

Serotonergic projections to cortical regions including sensory areas come almost exclusively from the dorsal and median raphe nuclei of the brainstem. Raphe neurons are generated in mice at embryonic days (E) 11–15 and arrive at cortical areas at about E17. At birth, serotonergic fibers infiltrate all cortical layers and display a transient profuse distribution pattern; this is pruned considerably to the pattern of the mature brain around postnatal week 3. Subtle alterations in cortical morphogenesis have been reported following perinatal pharmacologically induced 5-HT depletion. In the rat, emergence of the thalamocortical innervation pattern is delayed and whisker representation in the somatosensory cortex is reduced, although maturation (i.e., overall somatotropic organization of thalamocortical afferents) is eventually achieved. Other indirect evidence further supports a role for 5-HT in cortical development and behavior. Treatment of neonatal rats with MAO inhibitors reduces serotonergic projections to the cortex and impairs passive avoidance in juvenile rats. In mice, prenatal hypoxia delays serotonergic and other fiber ingrowth into the parietal cortex and induces hyperactivity and impairment in attention and spatial memory in adult mice. In general, mouse models have become essential as behavioral pharmacogenetics enters the postgenomics era and as the field moves beyond identifying genes associated with drug response toward understanding how they accomplish their effect.

Mouse models and the emerging concept of developmental pharmacogenetics

Mouse models increasingly contribute to pharmacogenomic research, especially in terms of brain mechanisms and circuits that mediate genetic effects. In addition to the ability to manipulate the genome through transgenic and knockout mice, the models also make it possible to control and to manipulate the environment, which will facilitate elucidation of gene–gene and gene–environment interactions. Although mouse models already play an important role in behavioral pharmacogenetics, there is consensus that these models are quite limited behaviorally (Lesch,

2001b). In other areas such as emotionality and psychopathology, few mouse models are available. What is especially needed are batteries of multiple tasks that can be used to assess a latent construct relatively free of test-specific factors (Crawley and Paylor, 1997; Crawley, 1999). Nonetheless, mice provide a practical model to study the impact of gene knockouts on development and the plasticity of the brain, including regionalization and connectivity of the cerebral cortex and subcortical structures. Obviously, mouse models are essential in the dissection of the psychopharmacogenetic–neurodevelopmental interface.

It has been suggested that the differentiation of cortical areas is controlled by an interplay of intrinsic genetic programs (sequential activation of transcription factors and expression of cell adhesion molecules, such as cadherins) and extrinsic mechanisms including those mediated by thalamocortical afferents (Nakagawa et al., 1999). Both transcription factors and cell adhesion molecules display graded and areal expression patterns. Experimental embryological and developmental genetics has made considerable progress in the elucidation of the molecular events regulating the generation of distinct neuronal cell types at precise locations and in appropriate numbers in the neural tube, which is separated into transverse and longitudinal domains at early embryonic stages. The forebrain neuroepithelium is subdivided into six so-called prosomeric units, which prevent progenitor cell mixing across their boundaries (Puelles and Rubenstein, 1993). The six transverse domains of the prosomeres can be further subdivided longitudinally by the restricted pattern of a wide spectrum of regulatory proteins. In the embryonic telencephalon, which constitutes cortical areas dorsally and the ventral basal ganglia, homeobox genes *Emx* and *Lhx*, and paired homeobox *Pax* genes, are expressed exclusively in dorsal progenitor cells, whereas ventral progenitors express homeobox genes of the *Nkx*, *Otx*, *Gbx*, and *Dlx* families (Rubenstein et al., 1998; Cecchi et al., 2000; Simeone, 2000). Knockout studies have demonstrated that thalamocortical connections also require several transcription factors (e.g., Tbr1, Gbx1, Pax6) as well as secreted molecules and cell surface axon guidance proteins (Rubenstein et al., 1999).

Morphological analyses revealed a crucial role of 5-HT in the formation and plasticity of neocortical and subcortical structures, suggesting that it acts as a differentiation signal in brain development. Moreover, the timing of serotonergic innervation coincides with pronounced growth and synaptogenesis in the cortex, and perinatal manipulations of 5-HT affect cortical 5-HT receptors (Fig. 6.3). The period for 5-HT action corresponds to the period when incoming axons begin to establish synaptic interactions with target neurons and to elaborate a profuse branching pattern (Cases et al., 1996). Investigations of 5-HT participation in neocortical development and plasticity have concentrated on the rodent somatosensory cortex (SSC), because of its one-to-one correspondence between each whisker and its cortical barrel-like projection area (Killackey et al., 1995) (Fig. 6.4*a*). The

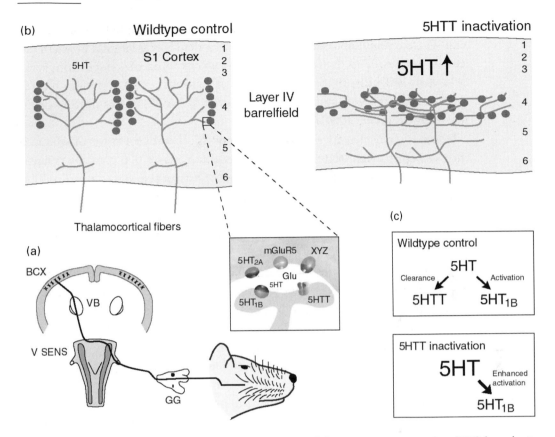

Fig. 6.4.   Serotonin in the development and plasticity of the somatosensory cortex (SSC) in rodents. (*a*) One-to-one correspondence between each whisker and its cortical barrel-like projection area. (*b*) SSC in wild-type mice and in knockout mice for the serotonin transporter. (*c*) The deleterious effects of excess serotonin are mediated by the serotonin transporter and by the serotonin receptor subtype 1B (see text for details). GG, ganglion gasseri; V SENS, sensory nerve V; VB, ventrobasal thalamus; BCX, barrelfield cortex; 5HT, serotonin; $5HT_{1B/2A}$ serotonin receptor subtypes; Glu, glutamate; mGluR5, metabotropic glutamate receptor 5; XYZ, unknown receptors.

processes underlying patterning of projections in the SSC have been intensively studied, with a widely held view that the formation of somatotropic maps does not depend on neural activity (Katz and Shatz, 1996). While pharmacologically induced 5-HT depletion at birth yields smaller barrels but does not prevent the formation of the barrel pattern itself (Bennett-Clarke et al., 1994; Osterheld-Haas et al., 1994) excess of extracellular 5-HT (present for example in mice with an inactivation of the gene for MAO-A) results in the complete absence of cortical barrel patterns (Cases et al., 1996). Additional evidence for a role of 5-HT in the development of neonatal rodent SSC derives from the transient barrel-like distribution of

5-HT, 5-HT_{1B} and 5-HT_{2A} receptors, and of the 5-HTT (Fuchs, 1995; Lebrand et al., 1996; Mansour-Robaey et al., 1998). The transient barrel-like 5-HT pattern visualized in layer IV of the SSC of neonatal rodents apparently stems from 5-HT uptake and vesicular storage in thalamocortical neurons, which express both the 5-HTT and the vesicular monoamine transporter (VMAT2) at this developmental stage (Lebrand et al., 1996).

Inactivation of the gene for 5-HTT profoundly disturbs formation of the SSC, with altered cytoarchitecture of cortical layer IV, the layer that contains synapses between thalamocortical terminals and their postsynaptic target neurons (Fig. 6.2). Brains of 5-HTT knockout mice display no or only very few barrels (Bengel et al., 1998; Persico et al., 1999). Cell bodies as well as terminals, typically more dense in barrel septa, appear homogeneously distributed in layer IV of adult 5-HTT knockout brains. Injections of a 5-HT synthesis inhibitor within a narrow time window of 2 days postnatally completely rescued formation of SSC barrel fields. Of note, heterozygous knockout mice develop all SSC barrel fields but frequently present irregularly shaped barrels and less-defined cell gradients between septa and barrel hollows. These findings demonstrate that excessive concentrations of extracellular 5-HT are deleterious to SSC development and suggest that transient 5-HTT expression in thalamocortical neurons is responsible for barrel patterns in neonatal rodents; its permissive action is required for normal barrel pattern formation, presumably by maintaining extracellular 5-HT concentrations below a critical threshold. Because there is normal synaptic density in SSC layer IV of 5-HTT knockout mice, it is more likely that 5-HT affects SSC cytoarchitecture by promoting dendritic growth toward the barrel hollows and by modulating cytokinetic movements of cortical granule cells, similar to concentration-dependent 5-HT modulation of cell migration described in other tissues (Moiseiwitch and Lauder, 1995; Choi et al., 1997; Tamura et al., 1997). Since the reduction in 5-HTT availability in heterozygous knockout mice, which leads to a modest delay in 5-HT uptake but distinctive irregularities in barrel and septum shape, is similar to that reported in humans carrying the low-activity allele of 5-HTTLPR, it may be speculated that allelic variation in 5-HTT function also affects the human brain during development, with due consequences for disease liability and therapeutic response.

Two key players of serotonergic neurotransmission appear to mediate the deleterious effects of excess 5-HT: the 5-HTT and the 5-HT_{1B} receptor (Fig. 6.4c). Both molecules are expressed in primary sensory thalamic nuclei during the period when the segregation of thalamocortical projections occurs (Bennett-Clarke et al., 1996; Lebrand et al., 1996; Hansson et al., 1998). 5-HT is internalized via 5-HTT in thalamic neurons and is stored in axon terminals (Lebrand et al., 1996; Cases et al., 1998). The presence of VMAT2 within the same neurons allows internalized 5-

HT to be stored in vesicles and used as a cotransmitter of glutamate. Lack of 5-HT degradation in MAO-A knockout mice as well as severe impairment of 5-HT clearance in mice with an inactivation of the 5-HTT results in an accumulation of 5-HT and overstimulation of 5-HT receptors all along thalamic neurons (Cases et al., 1998). Since 5-HT$_{1B}$ receptors are known to inhibit the release of glutamate in the thalamocortical somatosensory pathway (Rhoades et al., 1994), excessive activation of 5-HT$_{1B}$ receptors could prevent activity-dependent processes involved in the patterning of afferents and barrel structures (Fig. 6.4c). This hypothesis is supported by a recent study using a strategy of combined knockout of MAO-A, 5-HTT, and 5-HT$_{1B}$ receptor genes (Salichon et al., 2001). While only partial disruption of the patterning of somatosensory thalamocortical projections was observed in 5-HTT knockout, MAO-A/5-HTT double knockout mice showed that 5-HT accumulation in the extracellular space causes total disruption of the patterning of these projections. Moreover, the removal of 5-HT$_{1B}$ receptors in MAO-A and 5-HTT knockout as well as in MAO-A/5-HTT double knockout mice allowed a normal segregation of the somatosensory projections. These findings point to an essential role of the 5-HT$_{1B}$ receptor in mediating the deleterious effects of excess 5-HT in the somatosensory system. If 5-HT and serotonergic gene expression is involved in a myriad of processes during brain development as well as in synaptic plasticity in adulthood, thus setting the stage for brain (dys)function, complex behavior and psychopharmacological drug response are likely to be influenced by genomic variations within the serotonergic gene pathway.

Regulatory genes of neurodevelopment

Developmental neurogenetics has generally taken a reductionist approach to elucidate how the brain is built and functions, focusing on neurite outgrowth and axonal pathfinding as well as synaptogenesis and synapse function. Although these studies have not been carried out in ways that would likely identify genes that specify neural networks, investigations aimed at dissecting various sensory modalities, such as the somatosensory systems, have unquestionably advanced the understanding of the basic workings of neurocircuits. A complementary approach to studies of expression and function of proteins that regulate the function of brain neurotransmitter systems encompasses investigation of genes and their protein products implicated in the specification of monoaminergic neurocircuits. Regulatory genes, such as transcription factors, neurotrophins, and other growth or axon guidance factors, functioning in hierarchies across time and space are required for particular aspects of development to occur (Ragsdale and Grove, 2001; Rhinn and Brand, 2001). Analogous to, and frequently in concert with, other morphogenetic factors, neurotrophins act via specific receptors at the cell membrane, and their intracellular signal tranduction pathways converge at the level of gene expression by activation of transcription factors.

The development of distinct neurons is defined by the unique profiles of genes that these neurons express. Transcriptional control regions and their associated *cis* and *trans* regulatory elements are targets for modulation of gene expression (Fig. 6.1). It is widely accepted that neuronal genes are initially regulated at the point of transcription initiation, although other mechanisms of gene regulation including alternative splicing, mRNA editing, and mRNA elongation may also be crucial. A large variety of transcription factors has been identified and characterized that activate or repress the transcription of specific genes in the brain, resulting in changes of the neuronal phenotype.

Transcription factors bind to specific motifs in the regulatory sequence of a target gene, resulting in spatio-temporal alterations in promoter-driven gene transcription. Furthermore, they have the potential to be highly specific in their target recognition, and transcription factors from different families may interact with each other when bound to DNA at composite response elements. This has two striking consequences: ubiquitous factors can affect cell specificity, and closely related factors from a given family can produce very different regulatory patterns. Therefore, transcription factors play a key role in the control of development and differentiation.

Different stimuli lead to the activation or repression of different transcription factors, and circumstantial evidence indicates that transcription factors may be targeted by psychoactive drugs such as 5-HT_{2A} and 5-HT_{2C} receptor agonists and antagonists or lithium (for review see Lesch and Heils (2000)). The mechanisms by which they exert therapeutic effects still require to be studied in detail, but inducible transcription factors such as Fos and Zif268 are believed to mediate between receptor-activated second messenger systems and the transcriptional apparatus of genes involved in the complex functions of neuronal cells (Herdegen and Leah, 1998). Taken together, a large number of genes coding for transcriptional regulators, which are either indirect drug targets or pharmacodynamically important factors, play a key role in the control of neuronal development, differentiation, and phenotype maintenance.

Developmental specification and differentiation of serotonergic neurons

Despite the widespread importance of the central serotonergic neurotransmitter system, little is known about the molecular mechanisms controlling the development of 5-HT neurons. Several regulatory genes (including those for transcription factors, other morphogenetically relevant regulators of gene expression, neurotrophins, and growth factors as well as 5-HT itself) contribute to the specification, differentiation, and phenotype maintenance of the raphe serotonergic system.

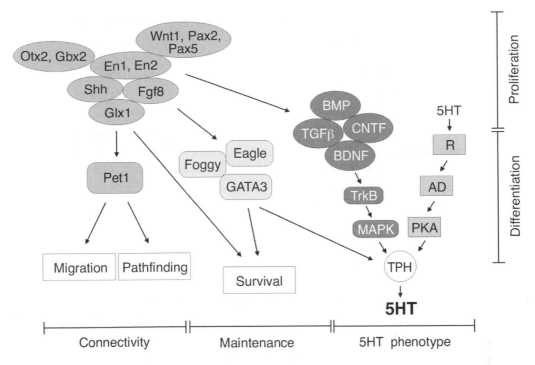

Fig. 6.5.   Genetic pathways in the development of the raphe serotonin (5HT) system. Wnt1, Pax2, Pax5, Otx2, Glx2, En1, En2, Shh, Fgf8, Glx1, Pet1, Foggy, Eagle, and GATA3 are transcription factors. BMP (bone morphogenetic protein), TGFβ (transforming growth factor β), CNTF (ciliary neurotrophic factor), and BDNF (brain-derived neurotrophic factor) are neurotrophins and other growth factors. TrkB, neurotrophin receptor; MAPK, MAP kinase; AD, adenylyl cyclase; PKA, protein kinase A; TPH, tryptophan hydroxylase; R, receptor. (Modified for 5HT from Burbach, 2000.)

Induction of the floor plate at the ventral midline of the neural tube is one of the earliest events in the establishment of dorsoventral polarity in the vertebrate brain. Fibroblast growth factors (FGF8) and "Sonic hedgehog" (Shh) signals control serotonergic and dopaminergic cell fate in the anterior neural plate (Ye et al., 1998; Hynes et al., 2000). While the transcription factor Gli2 is also required for induction of floor plate and adjacent cells, including serotonergic (and dopaminergic) neurons throughout the midbrain, hindbrain and spinal cord (van Doorninck et al., 1999), expression of Pet1, a ETS (electrical transcranial stimulation) domain transcription factor, is restricted to the hindbrain and closely associated with developing serotonergic neurons in the raphe nuclei (Hendricks et al., 1999) (Fig. 6.5). Moreover, consensus Pet1-binding motifs are present in the 5′-regulatory regions of genes for both the human and murine 5-HT$_{1A}$ receptor, 5-HTT, tryptophan hydroxylase, and aromatic L-amino acid decarboxylase genes; this expression profile is characteristic of the serotonergic neuron phenotype, i.e., 5-HT synthesis, release, uptake, and metabolism. These findings identify Pet1 as a critical regulator of serotonergic system specification. Even within the relatively circumscribed serotonergic raphe complex, gene expression in discrete subsystem appears to be differentially controlled by transcriptional regulators. The transcription factor GATA3 plays a critical role in the development of the serotonergic neurons of the caudal raphe nuclei and thus in locomotor performance (Matise et al., 1998). Beyond the point of transcription initiation, the role of mRNA elongation and other mechanisms of neural gene regulation are increasingly attracting systematic scrutiny. Foggy, a phosphorylation-dependent, dual regulator of transcript elongation, affects development of 5-HT (and dopamine)-containing neurons in the zebrafish (Guo et al., 2000). In the fruit fly, Eagle, a zinc finger transcription factor with homology to the steroid receptor family, is required for the specification of 5-HT neurons (Lundell and Hirsh, 1998).

Finally, several neurotrophins and growth factors also modulate the phenotype of serotonergic neurons (Fig. 6.2). These include family members of the neuro-trophins, such as FGF, transforming growth factor-β, bone morphogenetic protein, and neurokines (e.g., ciliary neurotrophic factor) (Galter and Unsicker, 2000a, b). 5-HT itself regulates the serotonergic phenotype of neurons by sequential activation of the 5-HT$_{1A}$ receptor, brain-derived neurotrophic factor and its receptor TrkB, as well as a wide spectrum of signal transduction pathways. In particular, transcriptional regulation appears to be dependent on stimulation of the adenylyl cyclase/protein kinase A signaling pathway mediated by a family of cAMP-responsive nuclear factors (including cAMP response element B, cAMP response element modulator, and activating transcription factor 1) (Herdegen and Leah, 1998). These factors contain the basic domain/leucine zipper motifs and bind as dimers to cAMP-responsive elements (CREs). Galter and Unsicker (2000a, b) have, therefore, proposed the neurotrophin receptor TrkB as the master control protein that integrates a diverse array of signals which elicit and maintain serotonergic differentiation. Interestingly, heterozygous mice deficient in brain-derived neuro-trophic factor develop intermale aggressiveness and hyperphagia in conjunction with decreased forebrain 5-HT concentrations and fiber densities (Lyons et al., 1999). Based on the increasing body of evidence that genetically driven variability of transcriptional regulators, neurotrophins, and growth factors is associated with complex behavioral traits (Okladnova et al., 1998; Stoeber et al., 1998; Krebs et al., 2000; Kunugi et al., 2001), investigations are increasingly examining the molecular basis of gene regulation in psychopharmacological drug response. Although the remarkable impact of serotonergic neurons on brain development and behavioral functions is clear, the mechanisms underlying their developmental genetics are only beginning to emerge. Unraveling the interactions of these determinants of development remains a daunting task but it may eventually lead to the discovery of novel drug targets or factors relevant to the genetics of psychotherapeutic drug response.

Are epistatic interactions relevant to brain development?

Although still in its infancy, investigation of gene–gene and gene–environment interactions support the view that both genetic and environmental factors influence brain development, neuroplasticity, and drug response. Despite evidence for a substantial contribution of genetic and environmental factors to the formation of synaptic connections in the brain during development, adult life, and old age, detailed knowledge of the molecular mechanisms is only beginning to accumulate. The resolution of epistatic interactions that are operative in this fine-tuning process is indeed among the last frontiers of genetic research.

Ebstein and coworkers (1998) investigated the behavioral effects of VNTR polymorphism in exon 3 of the dopamine D_4 receptor (DRD4), which had previously been linked to the personality trait of novelty seeking, and the 5-HTTLPR, which seems to influence neuroticism and harm avoidance, in two week-old neonates. Neonate temperament and behavior were assessed using a neonatal assessment scale. In addition to a significant association of the DRD4 polymorphism across four behavioral clusters relevant to temperament, including orientation, motor organization, range of state and regulation of state, an interaction was also observed between the DRD4 polymorphism and 5-HTTLPR. The presence of the 5-HTTLPR *s/s* genotype decreased the orientation score for the group of neonates carrying the long (*l*) allelic variant of DRD4. The DRD4 polymorphism–5-HTT-LPR interaction was also assessed in a sample of adult subjects. Interestingly, there was no significant effect of *l* DRD4 genotype in those homozygotes with 5-HTTLPR when they were grouped by the 5-HTTLPR, whereas in the group without the homozygous genotype the effect of *l* DRD4 was significant and represented 13% of the variance in novelty-seeking scores between groups. Temperament and behavior of these infants were psychometrically re-examined at 2 months (Auerbach et al., 1999). There were significant negative correlations between neonatal orientation and motor organization at 2 weeks and negative emotionality, especially distress in daily situations, at 2 months of age. Furthermore, grouping of the infants by DRD4 polymorphism and 5-HTTLPR revealed significant main effects for negative emotionality and distress. Infants with *l* DRD4 alleles had lower scores on negative emotionality and distress than infants with DRD4 *s* alleles. In contrast, infants homozygous for the 5-HTTLPR s allele had higher scores on negative emotionality and distress than infants with the *l/s* or *l/l* genotypes. Infants with the *s/s* genotype who also were lacking the novelty seeking-associated DRD4 *l* alleles showed most negative emotionality and distress, traits that possibly contribute to the predisposition for emotional instability. These findings represent a benchmark example for future research on gene–gene interaction in behavioral development.

Following up on the landmark studies concerning early environmental regulation of spatial learning and memory, hippocampal synaptogenesis, and stress reactivity by Meaney and associates (Meaney et al., 1996, 2000; Francis et al., 1999; Liu et al., 2000), evidence for a role of gene–environment interactions in brain development also comes from studies of rhesus macaques, a nonhuman primate species that, like humans, carries the 5-HTT gene-associated polymorphism (rh5-HTTLPR). Previous work in rhesus monkeys has shown that early adverse experiences have long-term consequences for the functioning of the central 5-HT system, as indicated by robustly altered CSF 5HIAA levels, in monkeys deprived of their parents at birth and raised only with peers (Higley et al., 1991, 1992). Association between central 5-HT turnover and rh5-HTTLPR genotype was recently tested in rhesus monkeys with well-characterized environmental histories (Bennett et al., 2001). The monkeys' rearing fell into one of the following four categories: mother-reared, either with the biological mother or cross-fostered, or peer-reared, either with a peer group of three or four monkeys or with an inanimate surrogate and daily contact with a playgroup of peers. Peer-reared monkeys were separated from their mothers, placed in the nursery at birth, and given access to peers at 30 days of age either continuously or during daily play sessions. Mother-reared and cross-fostered monkeys remained with the mother, typically within a social group. At roughly 7 months of age, mother-reared monkeys were weaned and placed together with their peer-reared cohort in large, mixed-gender social groups.

Since the monkey population comprised two groups that received dramatically different social and rearing experience early in life, the interactive effects of environmental experience and the rh5-HTTLPR on cisternal CSF 5HIAA levels and 5-HT-related behavior was assessed. CSF 5HIAA concentrations were significantly influenced by genotype for peer-reared but not for mother-reared subjects. Peer-reared rhesus monkeys with the low-activity rh5-HTTLPR *s* allele had significantly lower concentrations of CSF 5HIAA than their homozygous *l/l* counterparts. Low 5-HT turnover in monkeys with the *s* allele is congruent with in vitro studies that show reduced binding and transcriptional efficiency of the 5-HTT gene associated with the 5-HTTLPR *s* allele (Lesch et al., 1996). This suggests that the rh5-HTTLPR genotype is predictive of CSF 5HIAA concentrations, but that early experiences make unique contributions to variation in later 5-HT functioning. This finding provides evidence of an environment-dependent association between a polymorphism in the 5'-regulatory region of the 5-HTT gene and a direct measure of 5-HT functioning, cisternal CSF 5HIAA concentration, thus revealing an interaction between rearing environment and rh5-HTTLPR genotype.

Similar approaches have also been applied to the neonatal period to facilitate investigation of the contribution of genotype *and* rearing environment to the development of behavioral traits. Rhesus macaque infants heterozygous for the *s* and *l* variants of the rh5-HTTLPR displayed higher behavioral stress reactivity compared with infants homozygous for the long variant of the allele (*l/l*) (Champoux et al., 1999). Mother-reared and peer-reared monkeys were assessed on a standardized primate neurobehavioral test designed to measure orienting, motor maturity, reflex functioning, and temperament. Main effects of genotype and, in some cases, interactions between rearing condition and genotype were demonstrated for items indicative of orienting, attention, and temperament. In general, heterozygotes demonstrated diminished orientation, lower attentional capabilities, and increased affective responding relative to *l/l* homozygotes. However, the genotype effects were more pronounced for monkeys raised in the neonatal nursery than for those reared by their mothers.

Taken together, these findings provide evidence of an association between allelic variation of 5-HTT expression and central 5-HT function. In addition, they demonstrate the contributions of rearing environment and genetic background, and their interaction, in a nonhuman primate model of neural and behavioral development. The developmental and behavioral results of deleterious early experiences of social separation are consistent with the notion that the 5-HTTLPR may influence the risk for affective spectrum disorders and the response to treatment. Nonhuman primate studies are, therefore, useful to help to identify environmental factors that either compound the vulnerability conferred by a particular genetic makeup or, conversely, act to influence the therapeutic outcome associated with that genotype.

Conclusions

Pharmacogenomics, in general, will not improve the efficacy of a given drug, but pharmacogenetic profiling may assist the selection of patients who are likely to respond favorably. Thus, pharmacogenomics provides a view of drug behavior and sensitivity useful for improving the efficacy of drug development and utilization. Progress in developmental psychopharmacogenetics is currently accelerated by closer integration of behavioral, developmental, and genetic approaches. Integration of emerging tools and technologies for genetic analysis will provide the groundwork for an advanced stage of gene identification and functional studies in pharmacogenetics. The documented heterogeneity of both genetic and environmental constituents of brain development and function suggests the futility of searching for unitary determinants of psychopharmalogic drug response. This vista should, therefore, encourage the pursuit of quantitative approaches to pharmacogenetics.

Several refined concepts should be adopted regarding future behavioral pharmacogenetic research. First, pharmacogenetic studies require to employ randomized, double-blind clinical trial methodology, and, in order to detect a small gene effects, a dimensional, quantitative approach to behavioral phenotypes and treatment effects arising from standardized psychometric trait and response assessment is needed. Given the limitation of the diagnostic and psychometric approach, future studies will require extended, homogeneous, and ethnically matched samples. In order to control for nonindependence within case-controlled samples, and thus to minimize the risk of population stratification bias, rigorous methods of "genomic control" have been designed. These statistical strategies are based on the assessment of 60 SNPs or genotypes of 100 unlinked microsatellite markers spread throughout the genome to adjust the significance level of a candidate gene polymorphism (Bacanu et al., 2000; Pritchard et al., 2000). With recent advances in molecular genetics, the rate-limiting step in identifying candidate genes has become definition of phenotype and therapeutic outcome.

Second, more functionally relevant polymorphisms in genes within a single neurotransmitter system, or in genes that constitute a developmental and functional unit in their concerted actions, need to be identified and assessed in large association studies to avoid stratification artifacts and to elucidate complex epigenetic interactions of multiple loci. Although great strides have been made in understanding the diversity of the human genome, such as the frequency, distribution, and type of genetic variation that exists, the feasibility of applying this information to uncover useful pharmacogenomic markers remains uncertain. Based on the first draft sequence of the human genome, more than 1.4 million SNPs in the human genome have been identified (Consortium, 2001; Sachidanandam et al., 2001). The health care industry is heavily relying on the commercialized access to SNP databases for use in research in the hope of revolutionizing the drug development process. However, the reality of using SNPs to uncover drug response markers is rarely addressed; this requires considerations such as patient sample size, SNP density and genome coverage, SNP functionality, and data interpretation, which will be important for determining the suitability of pharmacogenomic information. Success will depend on the availability of SNPs in the coding or regulatory regions of a large number of candidate genes as well as knowledge of the average extent of linkage disequilibrium between SNPs, the development of high-throughput technologies for genotyping SNPs, identification of protein-altering SNPs by DNA and protein microarray-assisted expression analysis, and collection of DNA from well-assessed patients. As more and more appreciation of the potential for polymorphisms in gene regulatory regions to impact gene expression is gained, knowledge of novel functional variants is likely to emerge.

Third, genetic influences are not the only pathway that lead to individual differences in personality dimensions, behavior, psychopathology, and drug response. Complex traits are most likely to be generated by a complex interaction of environmental and experiential factors with a number of genes and their products. Even pivotal regulatory proteins of cellular pathways and neurocircuits will have only a very modest impact, while noise from nongenetic mechanisms may obstruct identification of relevant gene variants. Although current methods for the detection of gene–gene and gene–environment interaction in behavioral genetics are largely indirect, the most relevant consequence of gene identification for behavioral traits and psychopharmacological drug response may be that it will provide the tools required to clarify systematically the effects of gene–environment interaction on brain development and plasticity.

Finally, future benefits will stem from the development of techniques involving molecular cell biology, transgenics, and gene transfer technology, which could facilitate novel drug design. In a postgenomics world, behavioral pharmacogenetics research will require integration of research on genomics, DNA variants, gene expression, proteomics, brain development, structure and function, and behavior in a wide spectrum of species. Although bioinformatic resources are evolving in most of these areas, integration of these resources from the perspective of psychopharmacogenomics will greatly facilitate research.

REFERENCES

Arranz M, Nunro J, Birkett J et al. (2000). Pharmacogenetic prediction of clozapine response. *Lancet* 355, 1615–1616.

Auerbach J, Geller V, Lezer S et al. (1999). Dopamine D_4 receptor (DRD4) and serotonin transporter promoter (5-HTTLPR) polymorphisms in the determination of temperament in 2-month-old infants. *Mol Psychiatry* 4, 369–373.

Bacanu SA, Devlin B, Roeder K (2000). The power of genomic control. *Am J Hum Genet* 66, 1933–1944.

Barnes NM, Sharp T (1999). A review of central 5-HT receptors and their function. *Neuropharmacology* 38, 1083–1152.

Battersby S, Ogilvie AD, Blackwood DH et al. (1999). Presence of multiple functional polyadenylation signals and a single nucleotide polymorphism in the 3′ untranslated region of the human serotonin transporter gene. *J Neurochem* 72, 1384–1388.

Benedetti F, Serretti A, Colombo C et al. (1998). Influence of a functional polymorphism within the promoter of the serotonin transporter gene on the effects of total sleep deprivation in bipolar depression. *Am J Psychiatry* 156, 1450–1452.

Bengel D, Murphy DL, Andrews AM et al. (1998). Altered brain serotonin homeostasis and locomotor insensitivity to 3, 4-methylenedioxymethamphetamine ("Ecstasy") in serotonin transporter-deficient mice. *Mol Pharmacol* 53, 649–655.

Bennett AJ, Lesch KP, Heils A et al. (2002). Early experience and serotonin transporter gene variation interact to influence primate CNS function. *Mol Psychiatry*, 7, 118–122.

Bennett-Clarke CA, Leslie MJ, Lane RD, Rhoades RW (1994). Effect of serotonin depletion on vibrissa-related patterns of thalamic afferents in the rat's somatosensory cortex. *J Neurosci* 14, 7594–7607.

Bennett-Clarke CA, Chiaia NL, Rhoades RW (1996). Thalamocortical afferents in rat transiently express high-affinity serotonin uptake sites. *Brain Res* 733, 301–306.

Berger-Sweeney J, Hohmann CF (1997). Behavioral consequences of abnormal cortical development: insights into developmental disabilities. *Behav Brain Res* 86, 121–142.

Blier P, de Montigny C (1997). Current psychiatric uses of drugs acting on the serotonin system. In Baumgarten HG, Göthert M, eds. *Serotonergic Neurons and 5-HT Receptors in the CNS.* Berlin: Springer, pp. 727–751.

Bonasera SJ, Tecott LH (2000). Mouse models of serotonin receptor function: toward a genetic dissection of serotonin systems. *Pharmacol Ther* 88, 133–142.

Bradley CC, Blakely RD (1997). Alternative splicing of the human serotonin transporter gene. *J Neurochem* 69, 1356–1367.

Brunner D, Buhot MC, Hen R, Hofer M (1999). Anxiety, motor activation, and maternal–infant interactions in 5-HT$_{1B}$ knockout mice. *Behav Neurosci* 113, 587–601.

Burbach JP (2000). Genetic pathways in the developmental specification of hypothalamic neuropeptide and midbrain catecholamine systems. *Eur J Pharmacol* 405, 55–62.

Canton H, Emeson RB, Barker EL et al. (1996). Identification, molecular cloning, and distribution of a short variant of the 5-hydroxytryptamine 2C receptor produced by alternative splicing. *Mol Pharmacol* 50, 799–807.

Cases O, Vitalis T, Seif I, De Maeyer E, Sotelo C, Gaspar P (1996). Lack of barrels in the somatosensory cortex of monoamine oxidase A-deficient mice: role of a serotonin excess during the critical period. *Neuron* 16, 297–307.

Cases O, Lebrand C, Giros B et al. (1998). Plasma membrane transporters of serotonin, dopamine, and norepinephrine mediate serotonin accumulation in atypical locations in the developing brain of monoamine oxidase A knock-outs. *J Neurosci* 18, 6914–6927.

Catalano M (1999). The challenges of psychopharmacogenetics. *Am J Hum Genet* 65, 606–610.

Cecchi C, Mallamaci A, Boncinelli E (2000). *otx* and *emx* homeobox genes in brain development. *Int J Dev Biol* 44, 663–778.

Champoux M, Bennett A, Lesch KP et al. (1999). Serotonin transporter gene polymorphism and neurobehavioral development in rhesus monkey neonates. *Soc Neurosci Abstr* 25, 69.

Choi D, Ward S, Messaddeq N, Launay J, Maroteaux L (1997). 5-HT2B receptor-mediated serotonin morphogenetic functions in mouse cranial neural crest and myocardial cells. *Development* 124, 1745–1755.

Cichon S, Nothen MM, Rietschel M, Propping P (2000). Pharmacogenetics of schizophrenia. *Am J Med Genet* 97, 98–106.

Consortium IHGS (2001). Initial sequencing and analysis of the human genome. *Nature* 409, 860–921.

Crawley JN (1999). Behavioral phenotyping of transgenic and knockout mice: experimental design and evaluation of general health, sensory functions, motor abilities, and specific behavioral tests. *Brain Res* 835, 18–26.

Crawley JN, Paylor R (1997). A proposed test battery and constellations of specific behavioral paradigms to investigate the behavioral phenotypes of transgenic and knockout mice. *Horm Behav* 31, 197–211.

Deckert J Catalano M, Syagailo YV et al. (1999). Excess of high activity monoamine oxidase A gene promoter alleles in female patients with panic disorder. *Hum Mol Genet* 8, 621–624.

Deckert J, Meyer J, Catalano M et al. (2000). Novel 5′-regulatory region polymorphisms of the 5-HT$_{2C}$ receptor gene: association study with panic disorder. *Int J Neuropsychopharmacol* 3, 321–325.

Del Zompo M, Ardau R, Palmas M, Bocchetta A, Reina A, Piccardi M (1999). Lithium response: association study with two candidate genes. *Mol Psychiatry* 4(Suppl), 66–67.

Denney RM, Sharma A, Dave SK, Waguespack A (1994). A new look at the promoter of the human monoamine oxidase A gene: mapping transcription initiation sites and capacity to drive luciferase expression. *J Neurochem* 63, 843–856.

Denney RM, Koch H, Craig IW (1999). Association between monoamine oxidase A activity in human male skin fibroblasts and genotype of the MAO-A promoter-associated variable number tandem repeat. *Hum Genet* 105, 542–551.

Ebstein RP, Levine J, Geller V, Auerbach J, Gritsenko I, Belmaker RH (1998). Dopamine D$_4$ receptor and serotonin transporter promoter in the determination of neonatal temperament. *Mol Psychiatry* 3, 238–46.

Francis D, Diorio J, Liu D, Meaney MJ (1999). Nongenomic transmission across generations of maternal behavior and stress responses in the rat. *Science* 286, 1155–1158.

Fuchs JL (1995). Neurotransmitter receptors in developing barrel cortex. In Jones EG, Diamond IT, ed. *Cerebral Cortex*. New York: Plenum Press, pp. 375–409.

Galter D, Unsicker K (2000a). Brain-derived neurotrophic factor and TrkB are essential for cAMP-mediated induction of the serotonergic neuronal phenotype. *J Neurosci Res* 61, 295–301.

Galter D, Unsicker K (2000b). Sequential activation of the 5-HT1A serotonin receptor and TrkB induces the serotonergic neuronal phenotype. *Mol Cell Neurosci* 15, 446–455.

Gelernter J, Kranzler H, Cubells JF (1997). Serotonin transporter protein (SLC6A4) allele and haplotype frequencies and linkage disequilibria in African- and European-American and Japanese populations and in alcohol-dependent subjects. *Hum Genet* 101, 243–246.

Gerald C (1995). The 5-HT$_4$ receptor: molecular cloning and pharmacological characterization of two splice variants. *EMBO J* 14, 2806–2815.

Gould E (1999). Serotonin hippocampal neurogenesis. *Neuropsychopharmacology* 21, 46S-51S.

Greenberg BD, Tolliver TJ, Huang SJ, Li Q, Bengel D, Murphy DL (1999). Genetic variation in the serotonin transporter promoter region affects serotonin uptake in human blood platelets. *Am J Med Genet* 88, 83–87.

Guo S, Yamaguchi Y, Schilbach S et al. (2000). A regulator of transcriptional elongation controls vertebrate neuronal development. *Nature* 408, 366–369.

Hanna GL, Himle JA, Curtis GC et al. (1998). Serotonin transporter and seasonal variation in blood serotonin in families with obsessive-compulsive disorder. *Neuropsychopharmacology* 18, 102–111.

Hansson SR, Mezey E, Hoffman BJ (1998). Serotonin transporter messenger RNA in the developing rat brain: early expression in serotonergic neurons and transient expression in non-serotonergic neurons. *Neuroscience* 83, 1185–1201.

Heidmann DE (1997). Four 5-hydroxytryptamine 7 (5-HT$_7$) receptor isoforms in human and rat produced by alternative splicing: species differences due to altered intron–exon organization. *J Neurochem* 68, 1372–1381.

Heinz A, Jones DW, Mazzanti C et al. (1999). A relationship between serotonin transporter genotype and in vivo protein expression and alcohol neurotoxicity. *Biol Psychiatry* 47, 643–649.

Hendricks T, Francis N, Fyodorov D, Deneris ES (1999). The ETS domain factor Pet-1 is an early and precise marker of central serotonin neurons and interacts with a conserved element in serotonergic genes. *J Neurosci* 19, 10348–10356.

Herdegen T, Leah JD (1998). Inducible and constitutive transcription factors in the mammalian nervous system: control of gene expression by Jun, Fos and Krox, and CREB/ATF proteins. *Brain Res Rev* 28, 370–490.

Higley JD, Suomi SJ, Linnoila M (1991). CSF monoamine metabolite concentrations vary according to age, rearing, and sex, and are influenced by the stressor of social separation in rhesus monkeys. *Psychopharmacology* 103, 551–556.

Higley JD, Suomi SJ, Linnoila M (1992). A longitudinal assessment of CSF monoamine metabolite and plasma cortisol concentrations in young rhesus monkeys. *Biol Psychiatry* 32, 127–145.

Hoyer D, Martin G (1997). 5-HT receptor classification and nomenclature: towards a harmonization with the human genome. *Neuropharmacology* 36, 419–428.

Hynes M, Ye W, Wang K et al. (2000). The seven-transmembrane receptor smoothened cell-autonomously induces multiple ventral cell types. *Nat Neurosci* 3, 41–46.

Ishiguro H, Arinami T, Yamada K, Otsuka Y, Toru M, Shibuya H (1997). An association study between a transcriptional polymorphism in the serotonin transporter gene and panic disorder in a Japanese population. *Psychiatr Clin Neurosci* 51, 333–335.

Jonsson EG, Norton N, Gustavsson JP, Oreland L, Owen MJ, Sedvall GC (2000). A promoter polymorphism in the monoamine oxidase A gene and its relationships to monoamine metabolite concentrations in CSF of healthy volunteers. *J Psychiatr Res* 34, 239–244.

Katz LC, Shatz CJ (1996). Synaptic activity and the construction of cortical circuits. *Science* 274, 1133–1138.

Killackey HP, Rhoades RW, Bennett-Clarke CA (1995). The formation of a cortical somatotopic map. *Trends Neurosci* 18, 402–407.

Kojic L, Dyck RH, Gu Q, Douglas RM, Matsubara J, Cynader MS (2000). Columnar distribution of serotonin-dependent plasticity within kitten striate cortex. *Proc Natl Acad Sci USA* 97, 1841–1844.

Krebs MO, Guillin O, Bourdell MC et al. (2000). Brain derived neurotrophic factor (BDNF) gene variants association with age at onset and therapeutic response in schizophrenia. *Mol Psychiatry* 5, 558–562.

Kunugi H, Hattori M, Kato T et al. (1997). Serotonin transporter gene polymorphisms: ethnic difference and possible association with bipolar affective disorder. *Mol Psychiatry* 2, 457–462.

Kunugi H, Ueki A, Otsuka M et al. (2001). A novel polymorphism of the brain-derived neurotrophic factor (BDNF) gene associated with late-onset Alzheimer's disease. *Mol Psychiatry* 6, 83–86.

Lavdas AA, Blue ME, Lincoln J, Parnavelas JG (1997). Serotonin promotes the differentiation of glutamate neurons in organotypic slice cultures of the developing cerebral cortex. *J Neurosci* 17, 7872–80.

Lebrand C, Cases O, Ådelbrecht C et al. (1996). Transient uptake and storage of serotonin in developing thalamic neurons. *Neuron* 17, 823–835.

Lesch KP (2001a). Molecular foundation of anxiety disorders. *J Neural Transm* 108, 717–746.

Lesch KP (2001b). Serotonin transporter: from genomics and knockouts to behavioral traits and psychiatric disorders. In Briley M, Sulser F, eds. *Molecular Genetics of Mental Disorders*. London: Martin Dunitz, pp. 221–267.

Lesch KP, Heils A (2000). Serotonergic gene transcriptional control regions: targets for antidepressant drug development? *Int J Neuropsychopharmacol* 3, 67–79.

Lesch KP, Merschdorf U (2000). Impulsivity, aggression, and serotonin: a molecular psychobiological perspective. *Behav Sci Law* 18, 581–604.

Lesch KP, Mössner R (1999). 5-HT$_{1A}$ receptor inactivation: anxiety or depression as a murine experience. *Int J Neuropsychopharmacol* 2, 327–331.

Lesch KP, Balling U, Gross J et al. (1994). Organization of the human serotonin transporter gene. *J Neural Transm Gen Sect* 95, 157–162.

Lesch KP, Bengel D, Heils A et al. (1996). Association of anxiety-related traits with a polymorphism in the serotonin transporter gene regulatory region. *Science* 274, 1527–1531.

Lesch KP, Meyer J, Glatz K et al. (1997). The 5-HT transporter gene-linked polymorphic region (5-HTTLPR) in evolutionary perspective: alternative biallelic variation in rhesus monkeys. *J Neural Transm* 104, 1259–1266.

Lieske V, Bennett-Clarke CA, Rhoades RW (1999). Effects of serotonin on neurite outgrowth from thalamic neurons in vitro. *Neuroscience* 90, 967–974.

Little KY, McLaughlin DP, Zhang L et al. (1998). Cocaine, ethanol, and genotype effects on human midbrain serotonin transporter binding sites and mRNA levels. *Am J Psychiatry* 155, 207–213.

Liu D, Diorio J, Day JC, Francis DD, Meaney MJ (2000). Maternal care, hippocampal synaptogenesis and cognitive development in rats. *Nat Neurosci* 3, 799–806.

Lundell MJ, Hirsh J (1998). *Eagle* is required for the specification of serotonin neurons and other neuroblast 7–3 progeny in the *Drosophila* CNS. *Development* 125, 463–472.

Lyons WE, Mamounas LA, Ricaurte GA et al. (1999). Brain-derived neurotrophic factor-deficient mice develop aggressiveness and hyperphagia in conjunction with brain serotonergic abnormalities. *Proc Natl Acad Sci USA* 96, 15239–15244.

Malberg JE, Eisch AJ, Nestler EJ, Duman RS (2000). Chronic antidepressant treatment increases neurogenesis in adult rat hippocampus. *J Neurosci* 20, 9104–9110.

Mansour-Robaey S, Mechawar N, Radja F, Beaulieu C, Descarries L (1998). Quantified distribution of serotonin transporter and receptors during the postnatal development of the rat barrel field cortex. *Dev Brain Res* 107, 159–163.

Matise MP, Epstein DJ, Park HL, Platt KA, Joyner AL (1998). Gli2 is required for induction of floor plate and adjacent cells, but not most ventral neurons in the mouse central nervous system. *Development* 125, 2759–2770.

Meaney MJ, Diorio J, Francis D et al. (1996). Early environmental regulation of forebrain gluco-corticoid receptor gene expression: implications for adrenocortical responses to stress. *Dev Neurosci* 18, 49–72.

Meaney MJ, Diorio J, Francis D et al. (2000). Postnatal handling increases the expression of cAMP-inducible transcription factors in the rat hippocampus: the effects of thyroid hormones and serotonin. *J Neurosci* 20, 3926–3935.

McPherson JD, Marra M, Hillier L et al. (2001). A physical map of the human genome. *Nature* 409, 934–941.

Moiseiwitch JRD, Lauder JM (1995). Serotonin regulates mouse cranial neural crest migration. *Proc Natl Acad Sci USA* 92, 7182–7186.

Mortensen OV, Thomassen M, Larsen MB, Whittemore SR, Wiborg O (1999). Functional anal-ysis of a novel human serotonin transporter gene promoter in immortalized raphe cells. *Brain Res Mol Brain Res* 68, 141–148.

Nakagawa Y, Johnson JE, O'Leary DD (1999). Graded and areal expression patterns of regulatory genes and cadherins in embryonic neocortex independent of thalamocortical input. *J Neurosci* 19, 10877–10885.

Nobile M, Begni B, Giorda R et al. (1999). Effects of serotonin transporter promoter genotype on platelet serotonin transporter functionality in depressed children and adolescents. *J Am Acad Child Adolesc Psychiatry* 38, 1396–1402.

Okladnova O, Syagailo YV, Tranitz M et al. (1998). A promoter-associated polymorphic repeat modulates Pax-6 expression in human brain. *Biochem Biophys Res Commun* 248, 402–405.

Olsen MA, Nawoschik SP, Schurman BR et al. (1999). Identification of a human 5-HT$_6$ receptor variant produced by alternative splicing. *Brain Res Mol Brain Res* 64, 255–263.

Osterheld-Haas MC, van der Loos H, Hornung JP (1994). Monoaminergic afferents to cortex modulate structural plasticity in the barrelfield of the mouse. *Dev Brain Res* 77, 189–202.

Persico AM, Revay RS, Mössner R et al. (1999). Barrel pattern formation in somatosensory cor-tical layer IV requires serotonin uptake by thalamocortical endings, while vesicular mono-amine release is necessary for development of supragranular layers. *J Neurosci* 21, 6862–6873.

Pritchard JK, Stephens M, Rosenberg NA, Donnelly P (2000). Association mapping in structured populations. *Am J Hum Genet* 67, 170–181.

Puelles L, Rubenstein JL (1993). Expression patterns of homeobox and other putative regulatory genes in the embryonic mouse forebrain suggest a neuromeric organization. *Trends Neurosci* 16, 472–479.

Ragsdale CW, Grove EA (2001). Patterning the mammalian cerebral cortex. *Curr Opin Neurobiol* 11, 50–58.

Rhinn M, Brand M (2001). The midbrain–hindbrain boundary organizer. *Curr Opin Neurobiol* 11, 34–42.

Rhoades RW, Bennett-Clarke CA, Shi MY, Mooney RD (1994). Effects of 5-HT on thalamocor-tical synaptic transmission in the developing rat. *J Neurophysiol* 72, 2438–2450.

Routledge C, Middlemiss DN (1996). The 5HT hypothesis of depression revisited. *Mol Psychiatry* 1, 437.

Rubenstein JL, Shimamura K, Martinez S, Puelles L (1998). Regionalization of the prosencephalic neural plate. *Annu Rev Neurosci* 21, 445–477.

Rubenstein JL, Anderson S, Shi L, Miyashita-Lin E, Bulfone A, Hevner R (1999). Genetic control of cortical regionalization and connectivity. *Cereb Cortex* 9, 524–532.

Sabol SZ, Hu S, Hamer D (1998). A functional polymorphism in the monoamine oxidase A gene promoter. *Hum Genet* 103, 273–279.

Sachidanandam R, Weissman D, Schmidt SC et al. (2001). A map of human genome sequence variation containing 1.42 million single nucleotide polymorphisms. *Nature* 409, 928–933.

Salichon N, Gaspar P, Upton AL et al. (2001). Excessive activation of serotonin (5-HT) 1B receptors disrupts the formation of sensory maps in monoamine oxidase A and 5-HT transporter knock-out mice. *J Neurosci* 21, 884–896.

Samochowiec J, Lesch KP, Rottmann M et al. (1999). Association of a regulatory polymorphism in the promoter region of the monoamine oxidase A gene with antisocial alcoholism. *Psychiatry Res* 86, 67–72.

Simeone A (2000). Positioning the isthmic organizer where *Otx2* and *Gbx2* meet. *Trends Genet* 16, 237–240.

Smeraldi E, Zanardi R, Benedetti F, Di Bella D, Perez J, Catalano M (1998). Polymorphism within the promoter of the serotonin transporter gene and antidepressant efficacy of fluvoxamine [see comments]. *Mol Psychiatry* 3, 508–511.

Spurlock G, Heils A, Holmans P et al. (1997). A family based association study of the T102C polymorphism in 5HT$_{2A}$ and schizophrenia plus identification of new polymorphisms in the promoter. *Mol Psychiatry* 3, 42–49.

Stoeber G, Jatzke S, Meyer J et al. (1998). Short CAG repeats within the *hSKCa3* gene associated with schizophrenia: results of a family-based study. *Neuroreport* 9, 3595–3599.

Stoltenberg SF, Burmeister M (2000). Recent progress in psychiatric genetics – some hope but no hype. *Hum Mol Genet* 9, 927–935.

Tamura K, Kanzaki T, Saito Y, Otabe M, Saito Y, Morisaki N (1997). Serotonin (5-hydroxytryptamine, 5-HT) enhances migration of rat aortic smooth muscle cells through 5-HT$_2$ receptors. *Atherosclerosis* 132, 139–143.

Tecott LH, Barondes SH (1996). Genes and aggressiveness. *Behav Genet Curr Biol* 6, 238–240.

Turecki G, Briere R, Dewar K et al. (1999). Prediction of level of serotonin 2A receptor binding by serotonin receptor 2A genetic variation in postmortem brain samples from subjects who did or did not commit suicide. *Am J Psychiatry* 156, 1456–1458.

van Doorninck JH, van der Wees J, Karis A et al. (1999). GATA-3 is involved in the development of serotonergic neurons in the caudal raphe nuclei. *J Neurosci* 19, RC12.

Veenstra-VanderWeele J, Anderson GM, Cook EH Jr. (2000). Pharmacogenetics and the serotonin system: initial studies and future directions. *Eur J Pharmacol* 410, 165–181.

Ye W, Shimamura K, Rubenstein JL, Hynes MA, Rosenthal A (1998). FGF and Shh signals control dopaminergic and serotonergic cell fate in the anterior neural plate. *Cell* 93, 755–766.

Zanardi R, Benedetti F, Di Bella D, Catalano M, Smeraldi E (2000). Efficacy of paroxetine in depression is influenced by a functional polymorphism within the promoter of the serotonin transporter gene. *J Clin Psychopharmacol* 20, 105–107.

Zhu Q, Shih JC (1997). An extensive repeat structure down-regulates human monoamine oxidase A promoter activity independent of an initiator-like sequence. *J Neurochem* 69, 1368–1373.

Zhu QS, Chen K, Shih JC (1994). Bidirectional promoter of human monoamine oxidase A (MAO A) controlled by transcription factor Sp1. *J Neurosci* 14, 7393–7403.

7

RNA processing regulation and interindividual variation

Colleen M. Niswender[1] and Linda K. Hutchinson[2]

[1] The Department of Pharmacology, University of Washington, Seattle, USA
[2] The Department of Pharmacology, Vanderbilt University, Nashville, USA

OVERVIEW

In the search for causes of human disease and variability of drug response, the study of inter-individual differences in RNA processing has lagged substantially behind analyses at the DNA level. The processes of RNA editing and RNA splicing represent important mechanisms that ultimately contribute to the expression of specific protein isoforms within a given cell. Moreover, these events are subject to complex regulation that differs with each cell's make-up, permitting intricate regulation of the cellular protein repertoire. This review will focus upon the post-transcriptional processes of RNA editing and alternative splicing and consider the contribution of aberrations within these events to the efficacy of pharmacotherapy for psychiatric diseases. Specific examples of RNA processing defects within receptors for various neurotransmitters such as dopamine, glutamate, and serotonin will be presented. In addition, mechanisms involved in the regulation of RNA editing and splicing will be addressed as contributors to disease etiology and treatment. It is anticipated that studies of RNA processing regulation will enhance our understanding of disease pathology and eventually improve the rational design of therapeutic compounds.

Introduction

The sequencing of the human genome will almost certainly unlock the secrets of a multitude of human diseases. For the first time, both exonic and intronic regions of the genetic code will be available for analyses of potential disease-causing mutations. For disorders such as depression and schizophrenia, the identification of individual genetic variability will almost certainly provide information as to their etiology and treatment. Despite the answers that the human genome may provide, the possibility remains that dysregulation of post-transcriptional processing events could contribute to the cause or the response to treatment of different diseases. In this review, defects in the RNA processing steps of splicing and editing will be considered as potential causes of disease and as mechanisms complicating the efficacy of pharmacotherapy.

Overview of post-transcriptional RNA processing

Messenger RNA (mRNA) transcripts are generated by the transcriptional activity of RNA polymerase II (Pol II). Increasing evidence suggests that processing and transcription of RNA transcripts are closely coupled. Indeed, many of the factors necessary for RNA processing have been shown to bind to, or be closely associated with, the highly phosphorylated C-terminal domain of Pol II. Transcript RNAs may undergo several processing events prior to translation, including 5′-end capping, RNA editing, constitutive and alternative splicing, and polyadenylation.

Capping is the earliest processing event to take place on the nascent RNA transcript. Three enzymes, a phosphatase, a guanyl transferase, and a methylase, add 7-methyl guanine to the trisphosphate end of the transcript (Proudfoot, 2000). This modification occurs before the transcript is ~30 nucleotides in length and may mark the switch from transcription initiation to elongation. Transcripts without the 5′-end protective cap are sensitive to exonuclease attack and subsequent degradation.

Chronologically, RNA editing is probably the next processing event to occur. RNA editing is defined as an RNA processing event (excluding splicing) that generates a transcript with a primary nucleotide sequence that differs from its gene (Simpson and Emeson, 1996; Smith et al., 1997). RNA editing events can be divided into two major categories: base modification and insertion/deletion. In mammals, cytidine-to-uridine (C-to-U) and adenosine-to-inosine (A-to-I) base modifications are the predominant forms of editing that have been identified. This review will focus on A-to-I editing and its role in the processing of several RNA transcripts in the central nervous system, including glutamate receptor subunits, the serotonin (5-HT) 2C receptor (5-HT$_{2C}$R), and one of the enzymes catalyzing A-to-I modifications, adenosine deaminase (ADA), which acts on RNA 2 (or ADAR2).

In an A-to-I RNA editing event, adenosine is converted to inosine by hydrolytic deamination at the C-6 position of the purine ring and this is accomplished by the coordinate action of enzymes of the ADAR family (Rueter and Emeson, 1998). ADAR1 and ADAR2, the best-characterized members of this enzyme family, contain a catalytic deaminase domain and three or two double-stranded (ds) RNA-binding domains, respectively. Their activity is dependent on the presence of an RNA duplex structure in the substrate RNA (Rueter and Emeson, 1998). In all of the A-to-I editing events characterized to-date, this duplex is formed between inverted repeat sequences by base pairing of exonic and intronic regions of the transcript.

Because the double-stranded RNA structures necessary for editing depend on the coordinate interaction of exonic and intronic sequences, editing must precede splicing in the processing of the RNA transcript. The spliceosome, a dynamic macromolecular complex of small nuclear ribonucleoprotein particles (snRNPs) and extrinsic (non-snRNP) proteins that assemble on the 5′- and 3′-splice sites, is responsible for pre-mRNA splicing. Introns are excised in two transesterification reactions in which the upstream exon is cleaved from the intron and ligated to the downstream exon (Fig. 7.1).

Assembly of the spliceosome begins with recruitment of U1 snRNP to the 5′ splice donor site and U2 snRNP to the branchpoint of the 3′ acceptor site (Fig. 7.1). The consensus sequence for the 5′ donor site is GURAGU, in which the initial GU dinucleotide is almost invariant, and the consensus sequence for the 3′ acceptor site is $(Y)_n$XCAG (Mount, 1982; Jackson, 1991). Three other snRNPs, U4, U5, and U6, as well as up to 50 other proteins, are involved in the splicing reaction (Murray and Jarrell, 1999). These additional proteins include splicing regulatory (SR) proteins, CTD (C-terminal domain)-associated SR-like protein (CASP), and an SR-like CTD-associated factor (SCAF) (Proudfoot, 2000). The SR proteins typically contain one or two RNA recognition motifs (RRM) that bind RNA as well as an arginine-and-serine-rich domain (RS domain). The RS domain appears to serve as a molecular "glue", allowing RS–RS interactions that promote spliceosome assembly and targeting to regulatory sequences. The assembly of all of these proteins with the target RNA transcript is critical for the proper splicing events to occur in the maturation process.

Polyadenylation and 3′-cleavage are likely the final events of transcript maturation. At least six factors are required for polyadenylation and 3′-cleavage of mammalian transcripts, ensuring the correct length of the poly-A tail and cleavage at the appropriate sites (Minvielle-Sebastia and Keller, 1999). Following complete transcript maturation, the mRNA is released from the Pol II complex and exported to the cytoplasm.

RNA processing defects in psychiatric disorders

While the examination of genomic DNA can identify disease-segregating mutations in regulatory elements necessary for post-transcriptional processing (such as mutations within splice sites), the generation of the expressed protein often involves events "hidden" from genomic DNA. These may include alternative splice site selection or the occurrence of editing within an RNA transcript. The discovery that a growing number of transcripts expressed in the brain undergo alternative splicing and RNA editing events that alter protein function suggest that interindividual variation in RNA processing may play a critical role in the response to drugs. A few candidate substrates have been examined directly for aberrant processing in psychiatric disorders; these will be reviewed as examples of the types of event that may affect drug function.

(a)

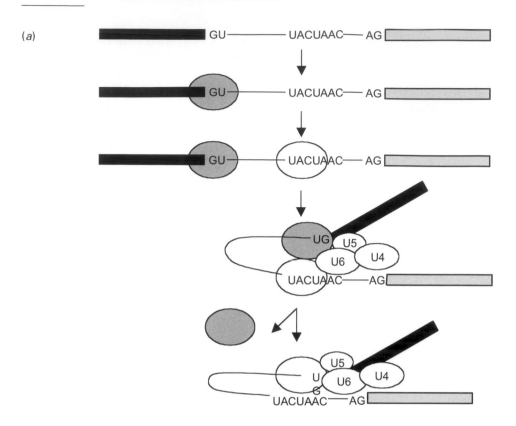

(b)

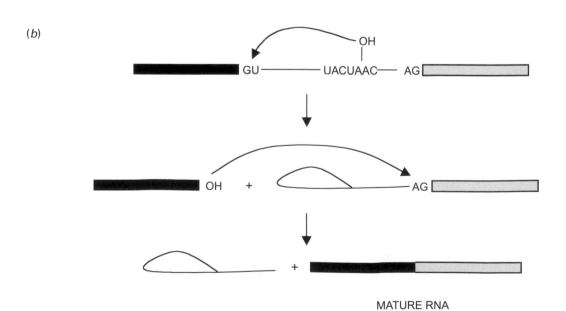

MATURE RNA

Aberrant alternative splicing of RNA transcripts in psychiatric disorders

RNA transcripts

A small number of RNA transcripts have been reported to exhibit alterations in RNA splicing patterns in various psychiatric populations. Included among these are RNAs encoding several receptors for neurotransmitters such as glutamic acid, γ-aminobutyric acid (GABA), and dopamine. Because of the ability of antipsychotic and antidepressant drugs to modulate neurotransmitter receptor function, defects within the splicing of these RNAs may affect the efficacy of drug treatment as well as the manifestation of the disease.

The NMDA R1 subunit of ionotropic glutamate receptor

The *N*-methyl-D-aspartate (NMDA) receptor is a multisubunit ion channel that gates sodium, potassium, and calcium ions. Two subunits, arising from five distinct genes, form the basis of the NMDA receptor channel. The NR1 subunit is common to all functional NMDA receptors and is encoded by a single gene (Moriyoshi et al., 1991). The NR2 subunits (NR2A, NR2B, NR2C, NR2D) are generated from different genes (Ikeda et al., 1992; Kutsuwada et al., 1992; Meguro et al., 1992; Monyer et al., 1992; Ishii et al., 1993) and can substitute for each other within the channel. Receptors are only active in the presence of NR1 (Monyer et al., 1994). Mice that are homozygous null for the NR1 gene die at postnatal day 0, presumably from respiratory arrest (Forrest et al., 1994). Interestingly, mice expressing a hypomorphic allele of NR1 that results in 5–10% of normal protein levels exhibit behaviors that resemble aspects of human schizophrenia, such as stereotypy and inappropriate social behaviors (Mohn et al., 1999).

The involvement of NMDA receptors in schizophrenia has been based largely

Fig. 7.1.   Mechanisms of RNA splicing. This diagram represents a simplistic model of RNA splicing. Many other proteins, not depicted, are involved in the reaction. (*a*) In the first step of RNA splicing, U1 snRNP (small nuclear ribonucleoprotein; shown as a gray oval) is recruited to the 5′ donor site of an upstream exon (black). U2 snRNP (white oval) is then recruited to the branchpoint (UACUAAC) of the 3′ acceptor site of the downstream exon (gray box). A U4/U5/U6 trimer binds with U1, recognizing the 5′ site of the upstream exon and U6 binds to U2. U1 is then released and U5 shifts from the exon to the intron. (*b*) The removal of the intron occurs by two transesterification reactions. The first step, catalyzed by U6 snRNP, occurs when the branchpoint adenosine "attacks" the 5′ donor, resulting in the formation of an intronic "lariat" structure. The second reaction occurs when the 3′ end of the upstream exon attacks the acceptor site of the downstream exon. Subsequent cleavage at the 3′ site results in final ligation of the exons and release of the matured RNA transcript.

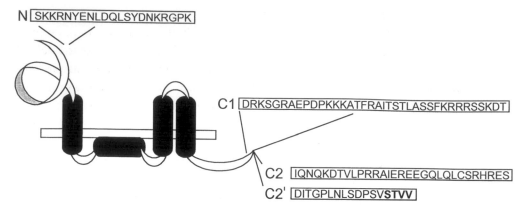

Fig. 7.2.   Alternative splice variants of the NR1 subunit of *N*-methyl-D-aspartate (NMDA receptor). The topology of the rat NR1 subunit is shown with three putative transmembrane domains and one membrane-associated domain. The amino acid sequences of the alternatively spliced regions are shown. The N-terminal cassette represents an inclusion or exclusion of exon 3 (Hollmann et al., 1993). C1 is encoded by exon 21 (Hollmann et al., 1993). Cassettes C2 and C2′ reside within the same exon (exon 22; Hollmann et al., 1993) and encode alternative splice acceptor sequences; if C2 is skipped, the normally 3′ untranslated C2′ region is converted into 22 translated amino acid residues. The postsynaptic density protein 95 interaction sequence (STVV) within the C2′ cassette is indicated in bold.

upon the observations that noncompetitive receptor antagonists, such as phency-clidine (PCP) and ketamine, can induce psychotic symptoms. It has been proposed that excess glutamatergic signaling, induced by hypofunction of the NMDA receptor and a subsequent disinhibition of normal NDMA receptor-mediated negative feedback, can produce psychotic symptoms (Olney et al., 1999). Studies examining the RNA expression levels of various NMDA subunits have shown alterations in the brains of schizophrenics (Akbarian et al., 1996; Humphries et al., 1996; Sokolov, 1998; Grimwood et al., 1999; Le Corre et al., 2000). In the case of NR1, mRNA levels have been observed to be substantially decreased in the superior temporal gyrus of patients with cognitive impairment (Humphries et al., 1996) and in the frontal cortex of an elderly subset of schizophrenic individuals (Sokolov, 1998). These results have suggested that defects in NR1 mRNA expression or regulation might underlie or result from disease pathology in certain subjects.

NR1 RNA can give rise to at least eight distinct protein isoforms, which are generated by alternative splicing at the N- and C-terminal ends of the protein (Hollmann et al., 1993) (Fig. 7.2). Several splicing events generate alternative C-terminal tails of NR1; these isoforms have been shown to exhibit differences in surface expression and calcium influx in a tissue culture system (Okabe et al.,

1999). Le Corre and colleagues (2000) found that the splice variant of NR1 that lacks both the C1 and C2 terminal cassettes (Fig. 7.2) was elevated in the superior temporal gyrus of schizophrenics by 22%, resulting in a 15% increase in total NR1 mRNA levels. These data conflict with reports of a downregulation of total NR1 mRNA expression in selected subjects (Humphries et al., 1996; Sokolov, 1998). They substantiate other studies, however, showing an increase in NR1 ligand binding in the superior temporal gyrus of middle-aged schizophrenics (Grimwood et al., 1999).

Le Corre and coworkers (2000) suggest that these discrepancies may represent distinct phases of the disease, with increased NR1 levels early and decreased amounts as the disease progresses. It is interesting to note that the isoform found to be upregulated in this study is one that, in contrast to several of the other splice variants, targets efficiently to the cell surface in vitro (Okabe et al., 1999). This NR1 variant also contains a motif necessary for interacting with postsynaptic density protein 95 (PSD-95) (Kornau et al., 1995), a clustering molecule important for the integration of cellular signaling (Fig. 7.2). Based on these observations, it is possible that the amount of signaling-competent receptor expressed at the cell surface is changed in susceptible patients, altering glutamatergic activity in selected brain regions. In regard to the NDMA receptor "hypofunction" model (Olney et al., 1999), the increase in surface expression of this NR1 variant may reflect an attempt at compensation for altered NMDA receptor signaling, perhaps transiently during an affected individual's lifetime. It may also reveal a time period in which NMDA receptor-based therapeutics may be most effective during the course of illness.

The GABA-A receptor

GABA is the major inhibitory neurotransmitter in the mammalian central nervous system. Pharmacological agents that target the GABAergic system have therapeutic roles in anxiety, depression, and schizophrenia. Previous studies have suggested that GABAergic dysfunction occurs in various schizophrenic populations, either at the level of the transmitter (Simpson et al., 1989; Reynolds et al., 1990; Sherman et al., 1991; Akbarian et al., 1995a; Ohnuma et al., 1999) or the receptor (Squires et al., 1993). These observations have prompted further examination of GABA-mediated neurotransmission in psychiatric disorders.

GABA-A receptors are composed of subunits termed α, β, and γ. The γ_2 subunit is responsible for high-affinity benzodiazepine binding (Pritchett et al., 1989; von Blankenfeld et al., 1990; Wafford et al., 1991) and is regulated by alternative splicing to produce a long and short form ($\gamma_2 L$ and $\gamma_2 S$, respectively) that differ in length by eight amino acid residues (Whiting et al., 1990; Kofuji et al., 1991) (Fig. 7.3). The long form, $\gamma_2 L$, contains an additional phosphorylation site for protein kinase C (PKC). While both the $\gamma_2 L$ and $\gamma_2 S$ subunits are negatively regulated by PKC

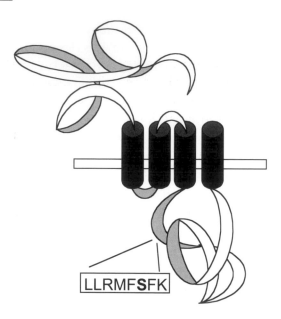

Fig. 7.3.   Alternative splice variants of the γ-aminobutyric acid (GABA) γ_2 subunit. The predicted topology of a GABA γ_2 subunit protein is shown. Alternative splicing within γ_2 RNA results in the production of two variants, the γ_2S and the γ_2L receptors. The γ_2L isoform is produced by the inclusion of 24 additional nucleotides, leading to the inclusion of eight additional amino acid residues. The additional protein kinase C phosphorylation site within the γ_2L receptor is indicated in bold.

phosphorylation, the additional site within the γ_2L protein renders channels containing this subunit particularly susceptible to PKC inhibition (Krishek et al., 1994). It would be predicted that a biased inclusion of the γ_2L protein into functional GABA-A receptors would further reduce channel ion conductance. Individual differences in PKC phosphorylation might also affect the activity of these receptors, possibly enhancing or blunting the effect of γ_2L-containing receptors.

Studies by Akbarian et al. (1995b) and Huntsman et al. (1998) demonstrated a selective 50% reduction in γ_2S mRNA expression in the prefrontal cortex of a subset of five schizophrenic individuals compared with control subjects, resulting in an increased ratio of γ_2L:γ_2S RNA. Further knowledge of the expression patterns of these isoforms in patient populations might enable more effective drug treatment. For example, the predicted dampened activity of γ_2L-containing receptors may prevent GABAergic agonists from functioning as effectively at these receptors, implying that subjects with high γ_2L receptor levels may respond better to alternative drug treatments rather than therapeutics targeting the GABA system.

The dopamine D_2 and D_3 receptors

Dopamine receptors belong to the G-protein coupled receptor superfamily; D_2 and D_3 receptors are targets for many clinically active antipsychotics. Both D_2 and D_3 receptor RNAs undergo alternative splicing in regions of the receptor that are important for interaction with cellular signaling machinery. D_2 receptor RNA has previously been shown to undergo alternative splicing to produce two major RNA isoforms, termed D_{2long} and D_{2short}, that differ by 29 amino acid residues within the third intracellular loop of the receptor protein (Fig. 7.4a) and show distinct expression patterns (Giros et al., 1989; Monsma et al., 1989). It has been reported that the short form of the receptor exhibits increased sensitivity to certain classes of antipsychotic agent (Castro and Strange, 1993; Malmberg et al., 1993). In these studies, benzamide-substituted antipsychotics such as raclopride and remoxipride, as well as the atypical antipsychotic clozapine, exhibited higher affinity for the D_{2short} form of the receptor. In contrast, Leysen and colleagues (1993) found equivalent affinities for a large number of antipsychotics at these receptor variants. The differences in expression systems and the radioligands chosen for competition assays may have contributed to the observed discrepancies. These studies are suggestive, however, of potential differences in the antipsychotic response of these alternatively spliced D_2 receptor isoforms. Recently, mice have been generated that express only the D_{2short} form of the receptor (Usiello et al., 2000; Wang et al., 2000b). While these investigators report discrepancies in the locomotor behaviors observed in these animals, both studies agree that the D_{2short} mice show a blunted response to the catalepsy induced by haloperidol administration. These results suggest that the D_{2long} form of the receptor may mediate important aspects of the extrapyramidal side effects of haloperidol-like antipsychotics as well as define the presynaptic versus postsynaptic locations of these two receptor populations (Usiello et al., 2000).

D_3 receptor RNA undergoes a number of alternative splicing events. One event results in the deletion of 98 nucleotide bases within the third cytoplasmic loop of the receptor, causing a frameshift and predicted truncation of the D_3 receptor protein (Schmauss et al., 1993; Liu et al., 1994). Previous studies (Schmauss et al., 1993) had shown that this alternatively spliced RNA transcript, termed D_{3nf}, was expressed in the prefrontal cortex of schizophrenics, whereas full-length D_3 RNA was lost. In an expansion of these findings, D_{3nf} RNA was found to be produced by an unusual splicing event in which the deleted 98 nucleotide bases were recognized as an atypical intron (Schmauss, 1996) (Fig. 7.4b,c). Determination of the relative levels of D_3 RNA to D_{3nf} RNA revealed a loss of full-length D_3 RNA with a concomitant increase in D_{3nf} message in the anterior cingulate cortex of an examined schizophrenic population (Schmauss, 1996). These results suggest that, in chronic schizophrenia, there may be aberrant RNA processing events that change the

(*a*)

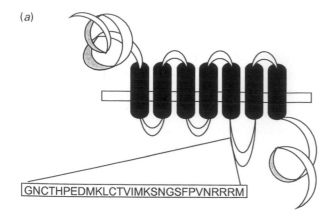

GNCTHPEDMKLCTVIMKSNGSFPVNRRRM

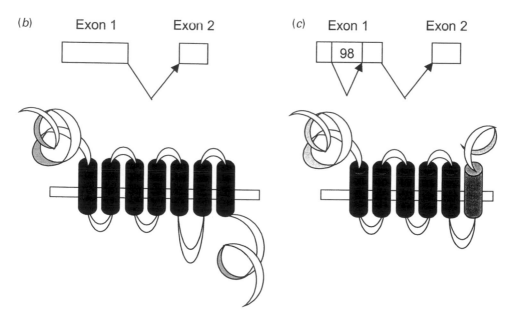

Fig. 7.4.   Alternative splice variants of the D_2 and D_3 dopamine receptors. (*a*) Topology of the D_2 receptor with the position of insertion of the 29 amino acid residues specific to the D_{2Long} receptor indicated. (*b*) Splicing of exon 1 to exon 2 results in the formation of full-length D_3 receptor RNA, encoding the complete seven-transmembrane spanning receptor. (*c*) Use of an alternative splice acceptor within exon 1 promotes the removal of a 98 nucleotide base minor class intron and results in the formation of D_{3nf} RNA. Translation of this alternative splice product results in a receptor variant with a frameshift mutation; it has been hypothesized that this variant may contain a unique C-terminal transmembrane-spanning region (gray) (Elmhurst et al., 2000).

splicing of the primary D_3 transcript, ultimately reducing the level of message that is competent for normal protein generation. D_{3nf} RNA is translated into protein (Liu et al., 1994) and it has been shown that D_3 and D_{3nf} receptors can heterodimerize (Liu et al., 1994). This interaction has been shown to decrease the dopamine-binding ability of the D_3 receptor (Elmhurst et al., 2000), suggesting that an enhanced expression of D_{3nf} protein may exert a dominant negative effect and "antagonize" D_3 receptor signaling.

Potential mechanisms for splicing alterations

Protein isoforms expressed from alternatively spliced RNA may affect drug responsiveness in a number of ways. For example, alterations that affect the production of a functional receptor, or the manner in which that receptor binds ligand and transmits a signal, are ways in which appropriate RNA processing contributes to an effective response of agonists or antagonists. There are several means by which genetic differences among individuals may affect alternative splicing. These mechanisms fall into two broad categories: differences that occur within *cis*-acting elements and those within *trans*-acting factors. *Cis*-acting elements are defined as the nucleotide sequences and structures of the RNA molecule itself, whereas *trans*-acting factors are the numerous proteins and other RNA components that assemble and form the cellular splicing machinery.

Many genomic changes that affect RNA splicing occur within the splice donor and acceptor sequences, causing or contributing to disease (Krawczak et al., 1992). Often, however, a mutation may be linked to disease manifestation but not occur within known splicing elements (Krawczak et al., 1992; Cooper and Mattox, 1997; Valentine, 1998). Novel *cis*-active splicing elements, termed exonic splicing enhancers (ESEs) and exonic splicing suppressors (ESSs), are gaining recognition for their potential role in aberrant splicing (Cooper and Mattox, 1997; Blencowe, 2000; Philips and Cooper, 2000). ESE sequences are interaction sites for SR proteins involved in modulating splicing specificity and efficacy (Blencowe, 2000). Point mutations within ESEs, therefore, could alter SR protein binding and affect selection and efficiency of splicing from a given site. RNAs involved in several disorders, such as Becker muscular dystrophy (Shiga et al., 1997) and spinal muscular atrophy (Lorson et al., 1999), have recently been shown to undergo inappropriate exon skipping or exon inclusion as a result of ESE or ESS mutations. Importantly, these mutations may occur within coding regions of the gene and result in relatively minor changes at the amino acid level (for example, silent mutations at wobble positions). A sequence that has been considered a "silent" polymorphism may actually affect splice site choice, possibly contributing to disease or the effectiveness of drugs that interact with the protein product.

Individual differences in *cis*-active elements within one gene might be predicted to limit altered processing to that particular transcript. Mutations affecting the *trans*-acting factors of the splicing machinery, however, would be predicted to produce more global effects (Philips and Cooper, 2000). While mutation of a ubiquitous splicing factor might prove lethal, alteration of an alternative splicing protein might affect only a subset of RNAs and only in cells where the factor is expressed. In addition, some alternatively spliced sites are regulated by the competition of splicing proteins for specific sites on the RNA; relatively small changes in the level of one protein may disrupt this delicate balance. All of these factors contribute to the final repertoire of spliced proteins and the effects those proteins have on cellular function.

Editing of RNA transcripts implicated in psychiatric disorders

RNA transcripts

Glutamate receptors

The AMPA (α-amino-3-hydroxy-5-methyl-4-isoxazolepropionic acid) and kainate subtypes of glutamate receptors are multisubunit ion channels permeable to sodium and potassium (Bettler et al., 1990; Boulter et al., 1990; Keinanen et al., 1990; Nakanishi et al., 1990; Sakimura et al., 1990; Hollmann et al., 1991; Dingledine et al., 1999). Certain subunit combinations of AMPA and kainate receptors have also been shown to conduct calcium, a property previously attributed solely to the NMDA subtype of glutamate receptors (Mayer and Westbrook, 1987; Mayer et al., 1987; Collingridge and Lester, 1989). Calcium influx into the postsynaptic neuron is critical for normal neurophysiological processes and may underlie activity-dependent changes necessary for the initiation and maintenance of memory (Collingridge and Singer, 1990). Glutamate receptors may also be involved in chronic and acute neurodegenerative disorders, including epilepsy, amyotrophic lateral sclerosis, Parkinson's disease and stroke (Choi and Rothman, 1990; Olney, 1990). The observation that AMPA and kainate receptors may contribute to neuronal calcium influx has led to further examination of their biological roles and regulation of subunit composition.

Four subunits, GluR1, GluR2, GluR3, and GluR4, in homomeric or heteromeric combinations, make up the AMPA subtype of glutamate receptor (Boulter et al., 1990; Keinanen et al., 1990; Nakanishi et al., 1990; Hollmann et al., 1991; Sakimura et al., 1990). Channels containing the GluR2 subunit display negligible permeability to calcium, a phenotype dependent on a specific arginine residue located in second hydrophobic domain of the GluR2 protein (Hume et al., 1991; Mishina et al., 1991; Verdoorn et al., 1991). Greater than 99% of GluR2 transcripts contain an arginine (CGG) codon at this position although the genomic sequence encodes a glutamine residue (CAG). It has subsequently been shown that RNA editing generates the altered base at this position (the Q/R site) through an A-to-I conversion in these transcripts (Sommer et al., 1991; Burnashev et al., 1992) (Fig. 7.5). This RNA editing event is unique to the GluR2 subunit.

While Q/R site editing does not occur in the other subunits of the AMPA receptor, another RNA editing event occurs within the GluR2, GluR3, and GluR4 subunits (Lomeli et al., 1994). Conversion of A to I at this site alters an arginine (AGA) codon to a glycine (GGA) codon. This site is referred to as the R/G site and is immediately upstream of an alternative splice site preceding the fourth hydrophobic domain (TM4) (Fig. 7.5). The alteration of this single amino acid increases the rate of recovery from receptor desensitization, presumably enhancing receptor activity (Lomeli et al., 1994).

The kainate receptor family consists of five subunits, KA1, KA2, GluR5, GluR6, and GluR7 (Dingledine et al., 1999). GluR5 and GluR6 are edited at a site analogous to the GluR2 Q/R site in 40 and 80% of transcripts in adult rat brain, respectively (Sommer et al., 1991) (Fig. 7.5). The GluR6 subunit RNA can undergo two additional editing events in the first predicted transmembrane domain (TM1), resulting in the conversion of an isoleucine codon to a valine codon (I/V site) and a tyrosine codon to a codon for cysteine (Y/C site) (Egebjerg and Heinemann, 1993; Kohler et al., 1993) (Fig. 7.5). Calcium permeability of GluR6-containing kainate receptors is dependent on the pattern of editing at all three sites, indicating that both TM1 and TM2 are involved in the ion permeation and electrophysiological properties of the kainate receptors.

Mice have been generated with a deletion of essential intronic sequences forming the RNA duplex region required for editing of the Q/R site of GluR2 (Brusa et al., 1995; Sprengel et al., 1999). Heterozygous mice carrying this editing-incompetent allele develop epileptic seizures and die by 3 weeks of age. It is interesting to note the distinct phenotype of these animals compared with mice that lack the GluR2 protein completely (Jia et al., 1996). GluR2-null animals, while exhibiting increased calcium permeability in principal neurons and defects in long-term potentiation similar to GluR2 editing-incompetent mice, do not exhibit seizures and death at postnatal day 21. These results indicate that the presence of nonedited GluR2 within an AMPA receptor is distinguishable from a receptor assembled from combinations of the other three subunits, even though both of these scenarios generate calcium-permeable receptors.

The above mouse model suggests that GluR2 Q/R site editing may be involved in the disease pathology of epilepsy and other disorders in humans (Sprengel et al., 1999). A recent study of the surgically excised hippocampi of patients with refractory epilepsy showed that some of these patients had decreased editing at the Q/R site of GluR2 RNA (Grigorenko et al., 1998). Other studies have revealed a

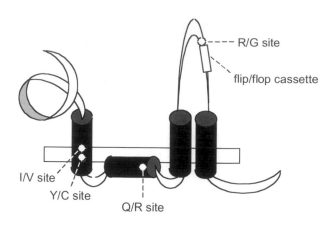

	I/V	Y/C	Q/R	R/G
GluR2			F M Q Q	S S L R
genomic			TTT ATG CAG CAA	TCC TCA TTA AGA
cDNA			TTT ATG CGG CAA	TCC TCA TTA GGA
			F M R Q	S S L G
GluR3				S S L R
genomic				TCC GCA TTA AGA
cDNA				TCC GCA TTA GGA
				S S L G
GluR4				S S L R
genomic				TCC TCA TTA AGA
cDNA				TCC TCA TTA GGA
				S S L G
GluR5			L M Q Q	
genomic			CTC ATG CAG CAA	
cDNA			CTC ATG CGG CAA	
			L M R Q	
GluR6	Y I L L A Y L		L M Q Q	
genomic	TAT ATT CTG CTG GTC TAC TTG		CTC ATG CAG CAA	
cDNA	TAT GTT CTG CTG GTC TGC TTG		CTC ATG CGG CAA	
	Y V L L A C L		L M R Q	

Fig. 7.5.   RNA editing events within glutamate receptor (GluR) subunits. The predicted topology of GluR subunits is shown with three putative transmembrane domains and one membrane-associated domain. The location of the editing sites is indicated by the white circles. The I/V and Y/C sites of GluR5 and GluR6 are located within the first transmembrane domain. The Q/R site lies near the end of the membrane-associated domain, and the R/G site is located "near" the third transmembrane domain. Below the structure, genomic DNA and cDNA sequences are aligned to show the consequences of RNA editing at these positions within the GluR1–GluR6 subunits. Adenosine-to-inosine editing results in adenosine to guanosine discrepancies between genomic DNA and cDNA sequences and changes the coding potential of the edited region of the receptor. I, isoleucine; V, valine; Y, tyrosine; C, cysteine.

significant elevation in the ratio of unedited to edited GluR2 in the prefrontal cortex of individuals with Alzheimer's disease or schizophrenia and in the striatum of subjects with Huntington's disease when compared with age-matched controls (Akbarian et al., 1995b). The increase in unedited (Q) GluR2 subunits in these diseases may have neurotoxic consequences, causing increased levels of intracellular calcium, which in turn trigger events that lead to structural damage and potential cell death. Whether the decrease in Q/R editing leads to these disorders or is a consequence of the disease in these patients remains to be explored.

The serotonin 2C receptor

The serotonin 2C receptor (5-HT$_{2C}$ receptor or 5-HT$_{2C}$R) is a G-protein-coupled receptor that is linked to activation of phospholipase C and the production of inositol phosphates. A-to-I editing within human 5-HT$_{2C}$R RNA occurs at five major positions, termed the A, B, C, D, and E sites (Niswender et al., 1998, 1999; Fitzgerald et al., 1999), resulting in the alteration of amino acids within the second intracellular loop of the receptor (Fig. 7.6). Different combinations of adenosine and inosine at these five positions are predicted to generate as many as 32 distinct RNA species encoding 24 different protein isoforms. Editing levels vary among brain areas (Burns et al., 1997; Fitzgerald et al., 1999; Wang et al., 2000b; Niswender et al., 2001), resulting in tissue-specific isoform expression. It has been reported that the human receptor variant that is edited at all five positions, termed the 5-HT$_{2C-VGV}$R, undergoes a unique splicing event in the amygdala to produce a frameshifted and inactive protein (Wang et al., 2000b). This observation places into question the expression of this isoform as a full-length receptor in certain regions of the brain.

The amino acid alterations that occur as a result of editing within 5-HT$_{2C}$R RNA result in differential G-protein coupling profiles of the receptors (Burns et al., 1997; Fitzgerald et al., 1999; Herrick-Davis et al., 1999; Niswender et al., 1999; Wang et al., 2000a). It has been proposed that these distinct coupling profiles result from differential ability of the receptors to isomerize spontaneously into a constitutively active conformation, giving each receptor isoform a unique "signal to noise" ratio (Herrick-Davis et al., 1999; Niswender et al., 1999). As a result of the alterations in G-protein coupling exhibited by the edited isoforms, agonists show unique potencies when interacting with distinct receptor variants. For example, the hallucinogens ($\pm$)-1-(4-iodo-2,5-dimethoxyphenyl)-2-aminopropane (DOI) and N,N-dimethyltryptamine (DMT) stimulate phosphoinositide turnover when interacting with the completely nonedited form of the receptor (termed the 5-HT$_{2C-INI}$R). When interacting with the fully edited receptor, or 5-HT$_{2C-VGV}$R, these drugs showed an approximately 50- to 100-fold reduction in potency, relative to the potency at the 5-HT$_{2C-INI}$R (Niswender et al., 1999). Unique among agonists examined thus far, (+)-lysergic acid diethylamide (LSD) stimulates phosphoinositide

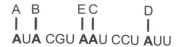

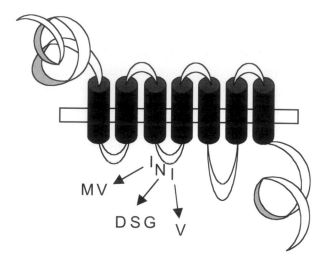

Fig. 7.6.   RNA editing events within the serotonin 2C receptor (5-HT$_{2C}$R). The nonedited RNA sequence of the 5-HT$_{2C}$R is shown at the top with the position of the five editing sites indicated in bold. Below is shown the predicted topology of the 5-HT$_{2C}$R protein with the amino acid changes introduced by adenosine-to-inosine editing. Specific combinations of editing can induce distinct amino acid changes at certain sites; for example, editing at the A position alone or the A and B positions concurrently introduces a valine at position 156 of the human receptor. Editing at the B site alone, however, results in the inclusion of a methionine at this site, leading to three amino acids that may be encoded at this position (isoleucine, valine, or methionine) depending upon editing status. I, isoleucine; N, asparagine; M, methionine; V, valine; D, aspartic acid; S, serine; G, glycine.

production when interacting with the 5-HT$_{2C\text{-INI}}$R but appears completely inactive at the 5-HT$_{2C\text{-VGV}}$R (Backstrom et al., 1999; Fitzgerald et al., 1999; Niswender et al., 2001). In addition, pretreatment of 5-HT$_{2C\text{-VGV}}$R-expressing cells with LSD results in a blockade of subsequent activation by 5-HT, suggesting that LSD may function as an antagonist at certain 5-HT$_{2C}$R isoforms (Niswender et al., 2001). These results indicate that some hallucinogenics may interact efficiently only with distinct 5-HT$_{2C}$R edited isoforms and also suggests that individual responses to hallucinogens may be determined by the isoforms expressed.

Many drugs used in the treatment of schizophrenia and depression interact with high affinity at the 5-HT$_{2C}$R. Several of these agents act as simple antagonists of the system, blocking the activity of agonists. Other drugs, such as clozapine, also inhibit the basal, or constitutive, activity of the 5-HT$_{2C}$R (Barker et al., 1994;

Westphal and Sanders-Bush, 1994); these drugs are termed inverse agonists. The affinity of agonists and inverse agonists for a G-protein-coupled receptor is regulated by G-protein interaction. Agonists exhibit higher affinity for the G-protein-coupled form of the receptor, and inverse agonists preferentially interact with the uncoupled form. Recently, several inverse agonists have been shown to exhibit higher affinity at the $5\text{-HT}_{2C\text{-INI}}$ isoform compared with the $5\text{-HT}_{2C\text{-VGV}}R$ (Niswender et al., 2001). These results again suggest that the isoforms have differential abilities to "precouple" to G-proteins, with the $5\text{-HT}_{2C\text{-INI}}R$ residing predominantly in the precoupled state and the $5\text{-HT}_{2C\text{-VGV}}R$ existing preferentially in an uncoupled form. Several groups have now assessed the ability of a large number of antipsychotics and antidepressants to block constitutive activity of $5\text{-HT}_{2C}Rs$, finding that some agents are effective inverse agonists while others behave as neutral antagonists (Herrick-Davis et al., 2000; Rauser et al., 2001; Weiner et al., 2001). The inverse agonist or neutral antagonist profile of a drug also depends upon the edited receptor examined because of the distinctions in basal activity between variants (Niswender et al., 2001; Rauser et al., 2001). It is intriguing to speculate that the clinical efficacy of certain agents may be related to their ability to block constitutive receptor activation and that failure rates for certain antipsychotics may involve interindividual differences in the edited receptor repertoire.

Because of the observed differences in interaction of both hallucinogenic drugs and antipsychotic medications with various $5\text{-HT}_{2C}Rs$, it is possible that changes in editing status may be involved in psychiatric diseases. Examination of $5\text{-HT}_{2C}R$ RNA editing levels from the prefrontal cortex of 13 normal individuals, 13 subjects with major depression, and 13 individuals with schizophrenia revealed a small but significant increase in the level of editing at the A position in patients who had committed suicide (Niswender et al., 2001). Recently, Sodhi et al. (2001) also performed a detailed sequencing analysis on RNA samples derived from control and schizophrenic cortex, finding a significant increase in the expression of the $5\text{-HT}_{2C\text{-INI}}R$ and a decreased expression of the $5\text{-HT}_{2C\text{-VNV}}R$ and $5\text{-HT}_{2C\text{-VSV}}R$ isoforms. These results suggest that these patients express unique repertoires of edited receptors, possibly resulting in changes in 5-HT-mediated signaling through the involvement of this area of the receptor in coupling efficiency (Wong et al., 1990; Moro et al., 1993; Pin et al., 1994; Arora et al., 1995, 1997; Blin et al., 1995; Verrall et al., 1997; Ballesteros et al., 1998). These results, coupled with the potential differences in interaction of psychiatric medications with various $5\text{-HT}_{2C}Rs$, suggest that detailed analyses from large numbers of affected and control individuals are warranted.

Potential mechanisms for editing alterations

As is the case for splicing, both *cis*- and *trans*-active elements are critical for the maintenance of efficient editing. A-to-I RNA editing relies upon the presence of a dsRNA structure formed by base pairing between inverted repeat sequences within the RNA (Rueter and Emeson, 1998). In the examples of A-to-I editing identified so far, one half of the repeat resides within the intron immediately downstream of the editing sites. The folding pattern of this RNA template helps to direct editing target choice; only a few adenosines are edited within a large sequence of RNA. Interindividual polymorphisms or mutations may affect folding of this RNA structure, altering editing choice or efficiency.

The *trans*-acting factors responsible for A-to-I editing are a family of dsRNA-specific ADARs. Both ADAR1 and ADAR2 appear to be expressed in most tissues and tissue culture cell lines (Wagner et al., 1990) but exhibit differing substrate specificity. *In vitro*, ADAR1 can efficiently edit the R/G site of GluR subunits, the Q/R site of GluR5 RNA (Herb et al., 1996; Maas et al., 1996) and the A and B sites of the 5-HT$_{2C}$R transcripts (Burns et al., 1997). ADAR2 can also edit the R/G site of GluR subunits but, unlike ADAR1, is able efficiently to edit the Q/R site of GluR2 RNA (Melcher et al., 1996) and the C and D sites of 5-HT$_{2C}$R transcripts (Burns et al., 1997).

These enzymes undergo alternative splicing events that may control the level of editing activity in the cell. Two isoforms of ADAR1 have been described (Patterson and Samuel, 1995). One is a 150 kDa interferon (IFN)-inducible variant expressed in both the cytoplasm and nucleus of human amnion and neuroblastoma cell lines. The other, a 110 kDa isoform, is constitutively expressed exclusively in the nucleus. Two promoters, one IFN inducible and the other not, initiate transcription of the gene *ADAR1* (George and Samuel, 1999). Alternative splicing of unique exon 1 structures to a common exon 2 junction results in expression of either the 110 kDa ADAR1 protein or the IFN-induced 150 kDa ADAR1 protein (George and Samuel, 1999). Three variants of the IFN-inducible human ADAR1 have been described, termed ADAR1a, ADAR1b, and ADAR1c (Liu et al., 1997) (Fig. 7.7*a*). All three isoforms exhibit similar dsRNA ADAR activities for a synthetic RNA duplex, although mutagenic analyses of the three dsRNA-binding domains suggest that the role of each in the activity or specificity of spliced ADAR1 isoforms may not be identical (Liu et al., 1997).

ADAR2 may also undergo several alternative splicing events (Fig. 7.7*b*). Compared with ADAR2a, ADAR2b contains an insertion of 120 nucleotide bases within the deaminase domain (Gerber et al., 1997; Lai et al., 1997). Comparison of the activities of recombinant ADAR2a and ADAR2b reveal that ADAR2a is approximately twice as active as ADAR2b for all RNA substrates (Gerber et al., 1997). Further ADAR2 diversity is generated by alternative splicing at the 3′ end of the coding region, generating four isoforms. ADAR2c and ADAR2d, which have a truncated C-terminus, exhibit negligible editing activity for the Q/R and R/G sites of GluR2 pre-mRNA (Lai et al., 1997). It has been suggested that these protein isoforms may serve as competitive inhibitors of the other editing-competent isoforms or that the altered C-terminal structure allows them to modify adenosine residues within currently unidentified RNA targets (Lai et al., 1997).

ADAR2 expression is further regulated by "autoediting", which directs the production of two additional isoforms (2e and 2f) (Rueter et al., 1999). In this case, ADAR2 edits its own RNA to generate a new splice acceptor site, resulting in the inclusion of an inactivating 47 nucleotide base cassette (Fig. 7.7c). Inclusion of this alternatively spliced region only occurs after the sequence AA has been modified to AI, effectively mimicking a functional AG splice acceptor. Addition of these 47 nucleotide bases alters the reading frame and results in truncation of the protein. It has been hypothesized that "autoediting" may serve as a mechanism to regulate the levels of functional ADAR2 protein. For example, transgenic mice designed to overexpress a cytidine deaminase (APOBEC-1) involved in the C-to-U editing of apolipoprotein B transcripts have been shown to develop liver tumors as a result of editing of substrates that are not normal targets in control animals (Yamanaka et al., 1995). Extrapolation of these findings to the ADAR enzymes suggests that cellular expression may be tightly regulated to ensure editing of the correct nucleotides.

Mice were recently generated that are homozygous for a targeted null allele of ADAR2 (Higuchi et al., 2000). Editing in these mice is reduced at many of the described editing positions in several transcripts. The mutant mice die between postnatal days 0 and 20, becoming progressively seizure prone after postnatal day 12. Interestingly, this phenotype can be rescued by replacing both GluR2 alleles with alleles encoding the edited (R) version of GluR2. While these studies indicate that ADAR2 expression and GluR2 Q/R site editing is critical for viability, the consequences of reduced editing at other sites has not been addressed. It is anticipated that differences in ADAR splice variant production, as well as potential polymorphisms/mutations with *cis*-active editing elements, will determine the amounts and patterns of edited proteins expressed by a given individual.

Conclusions

Understanding the regulation of RNA processing is certain to enhance our ability to treat disease. The capacity of drugs to interact uniquely with certain splice variants or edited proteins represents an opportunity to tailor pharmacotherapy to a given individual. Knowledge that patients with a specific disease express an altered subset of edited 5-HT$_{2C}$Rs, for example, may allow the rational design or use of drugs that target these receptor variants. It is also important to consider that changes in alternative splicing/editing events may represent a cellular compensatory mechanism; using drugs that antagonize a cell's attempts to compensate for (*a*) Adenosine deaminase that acts on RNA 1

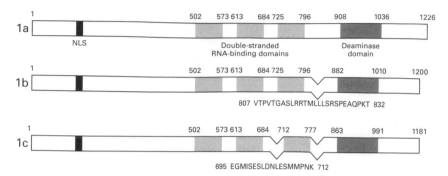

(*b*) Adenosine deaminase that acts on RNA 2

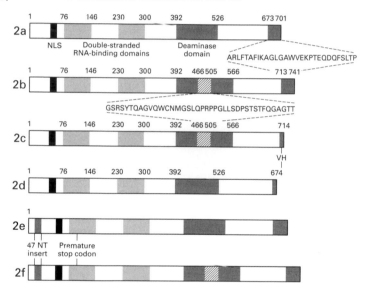

(*c*)

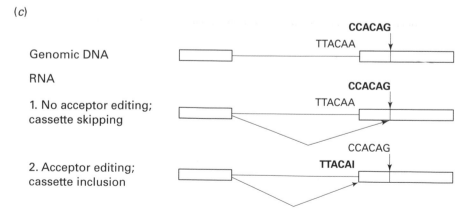

disease-induced alterations may prove ineffective. In addition, changes in RNA processing may *result* from drug treatment. For example, drugs that affect IFN production may influence the activity of ADAR1, possibly changing editing efficiency. The identification of RNA processing events that affect psychotropic drug activity will continue to be challenging. Understanding these processes, however, will certainly contribute to effective disease treatment.

Acknowledgements

The authors would like to thank Dr Ron Emeson, Dr Elaine Sanders-Bush, Ray Price, and T. Renee Dawson for critical reading of the manuscript. This work was supported by an NRSA fellowship (CMN).

REFERENCES

Akbarian S, Huntsman MM, Kim JJ et al. (1995a). GABAA receptor subunit gene expression in human prefrontal cortex: comparison of schizophrenics and controls. *Cereb Cortex* 5, 550–560.

Akbarian S, Smith MA, Jones EG (1995b). Editing for an AMPA receptor subunit RNA in prefrontal cortex and striatum in Alzheimer's disease, Huntington's disease and schizophrenia. *Brain Res* 699, 297–304.

Akbarian S, Sucher NJ, Bradley D et al. (1996). Selective alterations in gene expression for NMDA receptor subunits in prefrontal cortex of schizophrenics. *J Neurosci* 16, 19–30.

Arora KK, Sakai A, Catt KJ (1995). Effects of second intracellular loop mutations on signal transduction and internalization of the gonadotropin-releasing hormone receptor. *J Biol Chem* 270, 22820–22826.

Fig. 7.7.   RNA processing events within human RNA-specific adenosine deaminases (ADAR) 1 and 2. Schematic representations of ADAR1 (*a*) and ADAR2 (*b*) protein isoforms are shown, with the locations of the nuclear localization signal (NLS) (black boxes), double-stranded RNA-binding domains (light gray boxes) and the adenosine deaminase domain (dark gray boxes) indicated. The amino acid residues deleted in the ADAR1b and ADAR1c isoforms are indicated with the one-letter amino acid code. Also indicated are the amino acids inserted in the deaminase domain of ADAR2b and ADAR2c as well as at the C-termini of the ADAR2 isoforms. The location of the 47 nucleotide insertion in ADAR2e and ADAR2f is also indicated. (*c*) The genomic sequence and the sequence of nonedited and edited ADAR2 RNA are shown. If editing at the upstream splice acceptor does not occur, splicing to the downstream acceptor is preferred and results in the formation of RNA encoding full-length ADAR2. Adenosine-to-inosine editing of the upstream acceptor results in the inclusion of the 47 nucleotide base inactivating cassette, causing a frameshift and truncation of the protein.

Arora KK, Cheng Z, Catt KJ (1997). Mutations of the conserved DRS motif in the second intracellular loop of the gonadotropin-releasing hormone receptor affect expression, activation, and internalization. *Mol Endocrinol* 11, 1203–1212.

Backstrom JR, Chang MS, Chu H, Niswender CM, Sanders-Bush E (1999). Agonist-directed signaling of serotonin 5-HT$_{2C}$ receptors: differences between serotonin and lysergic acid diethylamide (LSD). *Neuropsychopharmacology* 21, 77S–81S.

Ballesteros J, Kitanovic S, Guarnieri F et al. (1998). Functional microdomains in G-protein-coupled receptors. The conserved arginine-cage motif in the gonadotropin-releasing hormone receptor. *J Biol Chem* 273, 10445–10453.

Barker EL, Westphal RS, Schmidt D, Sanders-Bush E (1994). Constitutively active 5-hydroxytryptamine 2C receptors reveal novel inverse agonist activity of receptor ligands. *J Biol Chem* 269, 11687–11690.

Bettler B, Boulter J, Hermans-Borgmeyer I et al. (1990). Cloning of a novel glutamate receptor subunit, GluR5: expression in the nervous system during development. *Neuron* 5, 583–595.

Blencowe BJ (2000). Exonic splicing enhancers: mechanism of action, diversity and role in human genetic diseases. *Trends Biochem Sci* 25, 106–110.

Blin N, Yun J, Wess J (1995). Mapping of single amino acid residues required for selective activation of Gq/11 by the M$_3$ muscarinic acetylcholine receptor. *J Biol Chem* 270, 17741–17748.

Boulter J, Hollmann M, O'Shea-Greenfield A et al. (1990). Molecular cloning and functional expression of glutamate receptor subunit genes. *Science* 249, 1033–1037.

Brusa R, Zimmermann F, Koh DS et al. (1995). Early-onset epilepsy and postnatal lethality associated with an editing-deficient *GluR-B* allele in mice. *Science* 270, 1677–1680.

Burnashev N, Monyer H, Seeburg PH, Sakmann B (1992). Divalent ion permeability of AMPA receptor channels is dominated by the edited form of a single subunit. *Neuron* 8, 189–198.

Burns CM, Chu H, Rueter SM et al. (1997). Regulation of serotonin-2C receptor G-protein coupling by RNA editing. *Nature* 387, 303–308.

Castro SW, Strange PG (1993). Differences in the ligand binding properties of the short and long versions of the D$_2$ dopamine receptor. *J Neurochem* 60, 372–375.

Choi DW, Rothman SM (1990). The role of glutamate neurotoxicity in hypoxic-ischemic neuronal death. *Annu Rev Neurosci* 13, 171–182.

Collingridge GL, Lester RA (1989). Excitatory amino acid receptors in the vertebrate central nervous system. *Pharmacol Rev* 41, 143–210.

Collingridge GL, Singer W (1990). Excitatory amino acid receptors and synaptic plasticity. *Trends Pharmacol Sci* 11, 290–296.

Cooper TA, Mattox W (1997). The regulation of splice-site selection, and its role in human disease. *Am J Hum Genet* 61, 259–266.

Dingledine R, Borges K, Bowie D, Traynelis SF (1999). The glutamate receptor ion channels. *Pharmacol Rev* 51, 7–61.

Egebjerg J, Heinemann SF (1993). Ca^{2+} permeability of unedited and edited versions of the kainate selective glutamate receptor GluR6. *Proc Natl Acad Sci, USA* 90, 755–759.

Elmhurst JL, Xie Z, BF OD, George SR (2000). The splice variant D$_{3nf}$ reduces ligand binding to the D$_3$ dopamine receptor: evidence for heterooligomerization. *Res Mol Brain Res* 80, 63–74.

Fitzgerald LW, Lyer G, Conklin DS et al. (1999). Messenger RNA editing of the human serotonin 5-HT$_{2C}$ receptor. *Neuropsychopharmacology* 21, 82S–90S.

Forrest D, Yuzaki M, Soares HD et al. (1994). Targeted disruption of NMDA receptor 1 gene abolishes NMDA response and results in neonatal death. *Neuron* 13, 325–338.

George CX, Samuel CE (1999). Human RNA-specific adenosine deaminase ADAR1 transcripts possess alternative exon 1 structures that initiate from different promoters, one constitutively active and the other interferon inducible. *Proc Natl Acad Sci, USA* 96, 4621–4626.

Gerber A, O'Connell MA, Keller W (1997). Two forms of human double-stranded RNA-specific editase 1 (hRED1) generated by the insertion of an Alu cassette. *RNA* 3, 453–463.

Giros B, Sokoloff P, Martres MP, Riou JF, Emorine LJ, Schwartz JC (1989). Alternative splicing directs the expression of two D$_2$ dopamine receptor isoforms. *Nature* 342, 923–926.

Grigorenko EV, Bell WL, Glazier S, Pons T, Deadwyler S (1998). Editing status at the Q/R site of the GluR2 and GluR6 glutamate receptor subunits in the surgically excised hippocampus of patients with refractory epilepsy. *Neuroreport* 9, 2219–2224.

Grimwood S, Slater P, Deakin JF, Hutson PH (1999). NR2B-containing NMDA receptors are upregulated in temporal cortex in schizophrenia. *Neuroreport* 10, 461–465.

Herb A, Higuchi M, Sprengel R, Seeburg PH (1996). Q/R site editing in kainate receptor GluR5 and GluR6 pre-mRNAs requires distant intronic sequences. *Proc Natl Acad Sci, USA* 93, 1875–1880.

Herrick-Davis K, Grinde E, Niswender CM (1999). Serotonin 5-HT$_{2C}$ receptor RNA editing alters receptor basal activity: implications for serotonergic signal transduction. *J Neurochem* 73, 1711–1717.

Herrick-Davis K, Grinde E, Teitler M (2000). Inverse agonist activity of atypical antipsychotic drugs at human 5-hydroxytryptamine 2C receptors. *Pharmacol Exp Ther* 295, 226–232.

Higuchi M, Maas S, Single FN et al. (2000). Point mutation in an AMPA receptor gene rescues lethality in mice deficient in the RNA-editing enzyme ADAR2. *Nature* 406, 78–81.

Hollmann M, Hartley M, Heinemann S (1991). Ca^{2+} permeability of KA-AMPA-gated glutamate receptor channels depends on subunit composition. *Science* 252, 851–853.

Hollmann M, Boulter J, Maron C et al. (1993). Zinc potentiates agonist-induced currents at certain splice variants of the NMDA receptor. *Neuron* 10, 943–954.

Hume RI, Dingledine R, Heinemann SF (1991). Identification of a site in glutamate receptor subunits that controls calcium permeability. *Science* 253, 1028–1031.

Humphries C, Mortimer A, Hirsch S, de Belleroche J (1996). NMDA receptor mRNA correlation with antemortem cognitive impairment in schizophrenia. *Neuroreport* 7, 2051–2055.

Huntsman MM, Tran BV, Potkin SG, Bunney WE Jr., Jones EG (1998). Altered ratios of alternatively spliced long and short gamma2 subunit mRNAs of the gamma-aminobutyrate type A receptor in prefronal cortex of schizophrenics. *Proc Natl Acad Sci, USA* 8, 15066–10571.

Ikeda K, Nagasawa M, Mori H et al. (1992). Cloning and expression of the epsilon 4 subunit of the NMDA receptor channel. *FEBS Lett* 313, 34–38.

Ishii T, Moriyoshi K, Sugihara H et al. (1993). Molecular characterization of the family of the N-methyl-D-aspartate receptor subunits. *J Biol Chem* 268, 2836–2843.

Jackson IJ (1991). A reappraisal of non-consensus mRNA splice sites. *Nucl Acids Res* 19, 3795–3798.

Jia Z, Agopyan N, Miu P et al. (1996). Enhanced LTP in mice deficient in the AMPA receptor GluR2. *Neuron* 17, 945–956.

Keinanen K, Wisden W, Sommer B et al. (1990). A family of AMPA-selective glutamate receptors. *Science* 249, 556–560.

Kofuji P, Wang JB, Moss SJ, Huganir RL, Burt DR (1991). Generation of two forms of the gamma-aminobutyric acid A receptor gamma 2-subunit in mice by alternative splicing. *J Neurochem* 56, 713–715.

Kohler M, Burnashev N, Sakmann B, Seeburg PH (1993). Determinants of Ca^{2+} permeability in both TM1 and TM2 of high affinity kainate receptor channels: diversity by RNA editing. *Neuron* 10, 491–500.

Kornau HC, Schenker LT, Kennedy MB, Seeburg PH (1995). Domain interaction between NMDA receptor subunits and the postsynaptic density protein PSD-95. *Science* 269, 1737–1740.

Krawczak M, Reiss J, Cooper DN (1992). The mutational spectrum of single base-pair substitutions in mRNA splice junctions of human genes: causes and consequences. *Hum Genet* 90, 41–54.

Krishek BJ, Xie X, Blackstone C, Huganir RL, Moss SJ, Smart TG (1994). Regulation of GABAA receptor function by protein kinase C phosphorylation. *Neuron* 12, 1081–1095.

Kutsuwada T, Kashiwabuchi N, Mori H et al. (1992). Molecular diversity of the NMDA receptor channel. *Nature* 358, 36–41.

Lai F, Chen CX, Carter KC, Nishikura K (1997). Editing of glutamate receptor B subunit ion channel RNAs by four alternatively spliced DRADA2 double-stranded RNA adenosine deaminases. *Mol Cell Biol* 17, 2413–2424.

Le Corre S, Harper CG, Lopez P, Ward P, Catts S (2000). Increased levels of expression of an NMDARI splice variant in the superior temporal gyrus in schizophrenia. *Neuroreport* 11, 983–986.

Leysen JE, Gommeren W, Mertens J et al. (1993). Comparison of in vitro binding properties of a series of dopamine antagonists and agonists for cloned human dopamine D_2S and D_2L receptors and for D_2 receptors in rat striatal and mesolimbic tissues, using [^{125}I] 2′-iodospiperone. *Psychopharmacology (Berl)* 110, 27–36.

Liu K, Bergson C, Levenson R, Schmauss C (1994). On the origin of mRNA encoding the truncated dopamine D_3-type receptor D_{3nf} and detection of D_{3nf}-like immunoreactivity in human brain. *J Biol Chem* 269, 29220–29226.

Liu Y, George CX, Patterson JB, Samuel CE (1997). Functionally distinct double-stranded RNA-binding domains associated with alternative splice site variants of the interferon-inducible double-stranded RNA-specific adenosine deaminase. *J Biol Chem* 272, 4419–4428.

Lomeli H, Mosbacher J, Melcher T et al. (1994). Control of kinetic properties of AMPA receptor channels by nuclear RNA editing. *Science* 266, 1709–1713.

Lorson CL, Hahnen E, Androphy EJ, Wirth B (1999). A single nucleotide in the *SMN* gene regulates splicing and is responsible for spinal muscular atrophy. *Proc Natl Acad Sci, USA* 96, 6307–6311.

Maas S, Melcher T, Herb A et al. (1996). Structural requirements for RNA editing in glutamate receptor pre-mRNAs by recombinant double-stranded RNA adenosine deaminase. *J Biol Chem* 271, 12221–12226.

Malmberg A, Jackson DM, Eriksson A, Mohell N (1993). Unique binding characteristics of antipsychotic agents interacting with human dopamine D_2A, D_2B, and D_3 receptors. *Mol Pharmacol* 43, 749–754.

Mayer ML, Westbrook GL (1987). Permeation and block of *N*-methyl-D-aspartic acid receptor channels by divalent cations in mouse cultured central neurones. *J Physiol* 394, 501–527.

Mayer ML, MacDermott AB, Westbrook GL, Smith SJ, Barker JL (1987). Agonist- and voltage-gated calcium entry in cultured mouse spinal cord neurons under voltage clamp measured using arsenazo III. *J Neurosci* 7, 3230–3244.

Meguro H, Mori H, Araki K et al. (1992). Functional characterization of a heteromeric NMDA receptor channel expressed from cloned cDNAs. *Nature* 357, 70–74.

Melcher T, Maas S, Herb A, Sprengel R, Seeburg PH, Higuchi M (1996). A mammalian RNA editing enzyme. *Nature* 379, 460–464.

Minvielle-Sebastia L, Keller W (1999). mRNA polyadenylation and its coupling to other RNA processing reactions and to transcription. *Curr Opin Cell Biol* 11, 352–357.

Mishina M, Sakimura K, Mori H et al. (1991). A single amino acid residue determines the Ca^{2+} permeability of AMPA-selective glutamate receptor channels. *Biochem Biophys Res Commun* 180, 813–821.

Mohn AR, Gainetdinov RR, Caron MG, Koller BH (1999). Mice with reduced NMDA receptor expression display behaviors related to schizophrenia. *Cell* 98, 427–436.

Monsma FJ Jr., McVittie LD, Gerfen CR, Mahan LC, Sibley DR (1989). Multiple D_2 dopamine receptors produced by alternative RNA splicing. *Nature* 342, 926–929.

Monyer H, Sprengel R, Schoepfer R et al. (1992). Heteromeric NMDA receptors: molecular and functional distinction of subtypes. *Science* 256, 1217–1221.

Monyer H, Burnashev N, Laurie DJ, Sakmann B, Seeburg PH (1994). Developmental and regional expression in the rat brain and functional properties of four NMDA receptors. *Neuron* 12, 529–540.

Moriyoshi K, Masu M, Ishii T, Shigemoto R, Mizuno N, Nakanishi S (1991). Molecular cloning and characterization of the rat NMDA receptor. *Nature* 354, 31–37.

Moro O, Lameh J, Hogger P, Sadee W (1993). Hydrophobic amino acid in the i2 loop plays a key role in receptor–G protein coupling. *J Biol Chem* 268, 22273–22276.

Mount SM (1982). A catalogue of splice junction sequences. *Nucl Acids Res* 10, 459–72.

Murray HL, Jarrell KA (1999). Flipping the switch to an active spliceosome. *Cell* 96, 599–602.

Nakanishi N, Shneider NA, Axel R (1990). A family of glutamate receptor genes: evidence for the formation of heteromultimeric receptors with distinct channel properties. *Neuron* 5, 569–581.

Niswender CM, Sanders-Bush E, Emeson RB (1998). Identification and characterization of RNA editing events within the 5-HT_{2C} receptor. *Ann NY Acad Sci* 861, 38–48.

Niswender CM, Copeland SC, Herrick-Davis K, Emeson RB, Sanders-Bush E (1999). RNA editing of the human serotonin 5-hydroxytryptamine 2C receptor silences constitutive activity. *J Biol Chem* 274, 9472–9478.

Niswender CM, Herrick-Davis K, Gilley GE et al. (2001). RNA editing of the human serotonin 5-HT_{2C} receptor: alterations in suicide and implications for serotonergic pharmacotherapy. *Neuropsychopharm* 24, 478–491.

Ohnuma T, Augood SJ, Arai H, McKenna PJ, Emson PC (1999). Measurement of GABAergic parameters in the prefrontal cortex in schizophrenia: focus on GABA content, GABA(A) receptor alpha-1 subunit messenger RNA and human GABA transporter-1 (HGAT-1) messenger RNA expression. *Neuroscience* 93, 441–448.

Okabe S, Miwa A, Okado H (1999). Alternative splicing of the C-terminal domain regulates cell surface expression of the NMDA receptor NR1 subunit. *J Neurosci* 19, 7781–7792.

Olney JW (1990). Excitotoxic amino acids and neuropsychiatric disorders. *Annu Rev Pharmacol Toxicol* 30, 47–71.

Olney JW, Newcomer JW, Farber NB (1999). NMDA receptor hypofunction model of schizophrenia. *J Psychiatr Res* 33, 523–533.

Patterson JB, Samuel CE (1995). Expression and regulation by interferon of a double-stranded-RNA-specific adenosine deaminase from human cells: evidence for two forms of the deaminase. *Mol Cell Biol* 15, 5376–5388.

Philips AV, Cooper TA (2000). RNA processing and human disease. *Cell Mol Life Sci* 57, 235–49.

Pin JP, Joly C, Heinemann SF, Bockaert J (1994). Domains involved in the specificity of G protein activation in phospholipase C-coupled metabotropic glutamate receptors. *EMBO J* 13, 342–348.

Pritchett DB, Sontheimer H, Shivers BD et al. (1989). Importance of a novel GABAA receptor subunit for benzodiazepine pharmacology. *Nature* 338, 582–585.

Proudfoot N (2000). Connecting transcription to messenger RNA processing. *Trends Biochem Sci* 25, 290–293.

Rauser L, Savage JE, Meltzer HY, Roth BL (2001). Inverse agonist actions of typical and atypical antipsychotic drugs at the human 5-hydroxytryptamine 2C receptor. *J Pharmacol Exp Ther* 299, 83–89.

Reynolds GP, Czudek C, Andrews HB (1990). Deficit and hemispheric asymmetry of GABA uptake sites in the hippocampus in schizophrenia. *Biol Psychiatry* 27, 1038–1044.

Rueter SM, Emeson RB (1998). Adenosine-to-inosine conversion in mRNA. In Grosjean H, Benne R, eds. *Modification and Editing of RNA*. Washington, DC: ASM Press, pp. 343–361.

Rueter SM, Dawson TR, Emeson RB (1999). Regulation of alternative splicing by RNA editing. *Nature* 399, 75–80.

Sakimura K, Bujo H, Kushiya E et al. (1990). Functional expression from cloned cDNAs of glutamate receptor species responsive to kainate and quisqualate. *FEBS Lett* 272, 73–80.

Schmauss C (1996). Enhanced cleavage of an atypical intron of dopamine D_3-receptor pre-mRNA in chronic schizophrenia. *J Neurosci* 16, 7902–9790.

Schmauss C, Haroutunian V, Davis KL, Davidson M (1993). Selective loss of dopamine D_3-type receptor mRNA expression in parietal and motor cortices of patients with chronic schizophrenia. *Proc Natl Acad Sci, USA* 90, 8942–8946.

Sherman AD, Hegwood TS, Baruah S, Waziri R (1991). Deficient NMDA-mediated glutamate release from synaptosomes of schizophrenics. *Biol Psychiatry* 30, 1191–1198.

Shiga N, Takeshima Y, Sakamoto H et al. (1997). Disruption of the splicing enhancer sequence within exon 27 of the *dystrophin* gene by a nonsense mutation induces partial skipping of the exon and is responsible for Becker muscular dystrophy. *J Clin Invest* 100, 2204–2210.

Simpson L, Emeson RB (1996). RNA editing. *Annu Rev Neurosci* 19, 27–52.

Simpson MD, Slater P, Deakin JF, Royston MC, Skan WJ (1989). Reduced GABA uptake sites in the temporal lobe in schizophrenia. *Neurosci Lett* 107, 211–215.

Smith HC, Gott JM, Hanson MR (1997). A guide to RNA editing. *RNA* 3, 1105–1123.

Sodhi MS, Burnet PW, Makoff AJ, Kerwin RW, Harrison PJ (2001). RNA editing of the 5-HT(2C) receptor is reduced in schizophrenia. *Mol Psychiatry* 6, 373–379.

Sokolov BP (1998). Expression of NMDAR1, GluR1, GluR7, and KA1 glutamate receptor mRNAs is decreased in frontal cortex of "neuroleptic-free" schizophrenics: evidence on reversible up-regulation by typical neuroleptics. *J Neurochem* 71, 2454–2464.

Sommer B, Kohler M, Sprengel R, Seeburg PH (1991). RNA editing in brain controls a determinant of ion flow in glutamate-gated channels. *Cell* 67, 11–19.

Sprengel R, Higuchi M, Monyer H, Seeburg PH (1999). Glutamate receptor channels: a possible link between RNA editing in the brain and epilepsy. *Adv Neurol* 79, 525–534.

Squires RF, Lajtha A, Saederup E, Palkovits M (1993). Reduced [^{3}H]flunitrazepam binding in cingulate cortex and hippocampus of postmortem schizophrenic brains: is selective loss of glutamatergic neurons associated with major psychoses? *Neurochem Res* 18, 219–223.

Usiello A, Baik J-H, Rouge-Pont F et al. (2000). Distinct functions of the two isoforms of dopamine D$_2$ receptors. *Nature* 408, 199–203.

Valentine CR (1998). The association of nonsense codons with exon skipping. *Mutat Res* 411, 87–117.

Verdoorn TA, Burnashev N, Monyer H, Seeburg PH, Sakmann B (1991). Structural determinants of ion flow through recombinant glutamate receptor channels. *Science* 252, 1715–1718.

Verrall S, Ishii M, Chen M, Wang L, Tram T, Coughlin SR (1997). The thrombin receptor second cytoplasmic loop confers coupling to G$_q$-like G proteins in chimeric receptors. Additional evidence for a common transmembrane signaling and G protein coupling mechanism in G protein-coupled receptors. *J Biol Chem* 272, 6898–6902.

von Blankenfeld G, Ymer S, Pritchett DB et al. (1990). Differential benzodiazepine pharmacology of mammalian recombinant GABAA receptors. *Neurosci Lett* 115, 269–273.

Wafford KA, Burnett DM, Leidenheimer NJ et al. (1991). Ethanol sensitivity of the GABAA receptor expressed in *Xenopus* oocytes requires 8 amino acids contained in the gamma 2L subunit. *Neuron* 7, 27–33.

Wagner RW, Yoo C, Wrabetz L et al. (1990). Double-stranded RNA unwinding and modifying activity is detected ubiquitously in primary tissues and cell lines. *Mol Cell Biol* 10, 5586–5590.

Wang Q, O'Brian PJ, Chen CX, Cho DS, Murray JM, Nishikura K (2000a). Altered G protein-coupling functions of RNA editing isoform and splicing variant serotonin 2C receptors. *J Neurochem* 74, 1290–1300.

Wang Y, Xu R, Sasaoka T, Tonegawa S, Kung M-P, Sankoorikal EB (2000b). Dopamine D$_2$ long receptor-deficient mice display alterations in striatum-dependent function. *J Neurosci* 20, 8305–8314.

Weiner DM, Burstein ES, Nash N et al. (2001). 5-Hydroxytryptamine 2A receptor inverse agonists as antipsychotics. *J Pharmacol Exp Ther* 299, 268–276.

Westphal RS, Sanders-Bush E (1994). Reciprocal binding properties of 5-hydroxytryptamine type 2C receptor agonists and inverse agonists. *Mol Pharmacol* 46, 937–942.

Whiting P, McKernan RM, Iversen LL (1990). Another mechanism for creating diversity in gamma-aminobutyrate type A receptors: RNA splicing directs expression of two forms of gamma 2 phosphorylation site. *Proc Natl Acad Sci, USA* 87, 9966–9970.

Wong SK, Parker EM, Ross EM (1990). Chimeric muscarinic cholinergic: beta-adrenergic receptors that activate Gs in response to muscarinic agonists. *J Biol Chem* 265, 6219–6224.

Yamanaka S, Balestra ME, Ferrell LD et al. (1995). Apolipoprotein B mRNA-editing protein induces hepatocellular carcinoma and dysplasia in transgenic animals. *Proc Natl Acad Sci, USA* 92, 8483–8487.

Part IV

Pharmacokinetics

8

Pharmacogenetics of psychotropic drug metabolism

Vural Ozdemir[1, 2], Angela D.M. Kashuba[3], Vincenzo S. Basile[1], and James L. Kennedy[1]

[1] Centre for Addiction and Mental Health, University of Toronto, Canada
[2] Department of Pharmacology, University of Toronto, Canada
[3] School of Pharmacy, University of North Carolina, Chapel Hill, USA

OVERVIEW

Drug metabolism is a critical determinant of therapeutic and adverse effects of many psychotropic drugs. Research since the 1960s has firmly established that genetic factors play a prominent role in marked person-to-person variability in drug metabolism. Pharmacogenetics is the study of the hereditary basis of individual differences in drug response. The present chapter reviews the basic concepts and definitions pertinent to pharmacogenetics of psychotropic drug metabolism from a clinical psychiatry perspective. The focus of pharmacogenetic investigations has traditionally been unusual and extreme drug metabolism phenotypes resulting from a single gene effect. To this end, we discuss the *CYP2D6* genetic polymorphism as a classic example of a monogenic variation in drug metabolism and as a high-affinity and low-capacity elimination route. This is contrasted with *CYP1A2*, a nonpolymorphic variation in drug metabolism under polygenic control. In addition to genetic contribution to interindividual differences in drug metabolism, we review various sources of intraindividual variations and gene–environment interactions of relevance for psychopharmacology. For example, we describe the extent and mechanistic basis of drug and nutraceutical (e.g., St. John's wort) interactions and disease influences (e.g., human immunodeficiency virus (HIV) infection) on drug metabolism. Lastly, we highlight some of the future research directions in psychotropic drug metabolism. In particular, we emphasize the need to evaluate genetic variability in drug metabolism in conjunction with other genes encoding drug transporters, receptors and ion channels, which can all influence an individual's risk for adverse drug reactions or therapeutic failure. It is anticipated that these pharmacogenetic inquiries in the first decade of the twenty-first century will provide a framework for the rational choice and dosage of psychotropic drugs.

Introduction

Rational drug treatment in psychiatry has a relatively brief history. The introduction of lithium in 1949 and chlorpromazine in the 1950s represents the first examples where pharmacological adjuncts were used to alleviate mental health disorders. At that time, it also became evident that therapeutic doses of psychotropic medications vary markedly from person to person, with some patients failing to respond despite treatment with high dosages. Early on, it was proposed that genetic factors were likely to explain differences between individuals and populations in response to drugs and other foreign chemicals (Motulsky, 1957; Kalow, 1962). The term pharmacogenetics was coined to establish a new medical subspecialty devoted to study of the hereditary basis of variability in drug effects (Vogel, 1959; Kalow, 1962). Subsequently, a series of seminal twin studies in the 1970s firmly established that heredity is indeed a key determinant of a drug's pharmacological effects (Endrenyi et al., 1976; Vesell, 1978). More recently, advances in molecular genetics put on record numerous examples of genetic polymorphisms in drug-metabolizing enzymes (DMEs), with important therapeutic and toxicological ramifications (Ingelman-Sundberg et al., 1999; Kalow, 1999).

Among many factors that may influence drug response, hepatic function and drug metabolism are of great importance for nearly all medications used in psychiatry (Bertilsson and Dahl, 1996; Brøsen, 1996; Cohen and DeVane, 1996). After more than four decades of research, it is interesting to point out that relatively little effort has been made to translate the established knowledge-base in pharmacogenetics to discrete treatment guidelines for rational choice of drugs and dose-titration regimens. The lack of recognition of functional variability in DMEs and the "one-dose-fits-all" approach to pharmacotherapy are important shortcomings of the current patient care in psychiatry (Chou et al., 2000). For example, the incidence of serious and fatal adverse drug reactions caused by such nonoptimal treatment regimens in North America ranks between the fourth to sixth leading cause of death, ahead of pneumonia and diabetes (Lazarou et al., 1998).

The purpose of this chapter is to provide an overview of the basic concepts pertinent to pharmacogenetics of psychotropic drug metabolism, with an emphasis on clinical applications and future research directions. In addition to differences between individuals, we also discuss intraindividual (within person) variations in drug metabolism capacity and gene–environment interactions. An adequate knowledge of these factors is important for a balanced interpretation of findings from pharmacogenetic studies and individualized therapeutics in psychiatry.

Phase I and phase II drug metabolism

Many of the psychotropic drugs are lipophilic in nature. Hence, they usually undergo oxidative biotransformation to form more water-soluble metabolites to facilitate their disposition from the body. Drug metabolism is generally divided into two phases. Phase I reactions involve oxidative, reductive, and hydrolytic reactions that unmask or introduce a functional group (e.g., a hydroxyl moiety) in the parent compound. This results in an increase in polarity of medications. Phase II reactions involve conjugation (e.g., with glucuronic acid, glutathione, or acetate) of the metabolite produced in phase I reactions, or the parent compound, to more hydrophilic and usually less-toxic metabolites. Phase I reactions are mediated principally by the cytochrome P-450 (CYP) enzymes, which are mostly found attached to the smooth endoplasmic reticulum of hepatocytes. By contrast, most phase II metabolism takes place in the cytosol (e.g., by glutathione S-transferases) with certain exceptions, such as glucuronidation by membrane-bound microsomal UDP-glucuronosyl transferases (Eaton and Bammler, 1999). Ideally, phase I and phase II biotransformation should be evaluated in concert for a thorough understanding of drug disposition and its clinical significance. Notably, however, the majority of studies on psychotropic drug metabolism have been conducted with a focus on CYP enzymes.

Physicochemical properties and nomenclature for cytochrome P-450s

CYP enzymes are heme-containing membrane-bound proteins (Omura and Sato, 1964a). The heme moiety consists of a protoporphyrin IX molecule and an iron atom and serves as the prosthetic group for the CYP apoprotein. An important characteristic of the CYP enzymes is that they exhibit a unique spectral feature: when the heme iron is in its reduced ferrous form (Fe^{2+}) and bound to carbon monoxide, a maximum absorption is observed at a wavelength of 450 nm. This spectral feature is the basis for the CYP name and is also used to measure the total CYP content of a given tissue in solution (Omura and Sato, 1964a, b).

The current nomenclature for CYPs is based on the differences in amino acid sequence homology (Nelson et al., 1996). A CYP gene is named starting with the italicized *CYP*, followed by an Arabic number signifying the gene family, an upper case letter signifying the gene subfamily, and another Arabic number for the individual gene (e.g., *CYP2D6*). The same letters and numbering in nonitalicized form are used to name the corresponding gene products (i.e., mRNA, cDNA and protein). A CYP enzyme from one gene family has ≤40% homology with the amino acid sequence of a CYP enzyme from any other family. In other words, in a given family, there is >40% homology in amino acid sequences of its members. However, a point to keep in mind is that belonging to the same family or subfamily does not necessarily imply similarities in substrate preference, catalytic functions, or regulation of gene expression. Further information on CYP nomenclature and new CYP alleles can be obtained from the worldwide web (http://www.imm.ki.se/CYPalleles/).

The extent of metabolism of a drug by a given CYP isoform is determined by both the affinity of the substrate–enzyme complex and the relative abundance of the particular CYP protein in relation to the total CYP content (Eaton, 2000).

Table 8.1. Relative content of individual CYP isoforms determined immunochemically in relation to total CYP content in the human liver[a]

CYP isoform	Percentage of total P-450 content	Coefficient of variation (%)[b]
CYP1A2	12.7	49
CYP2A6	4.0	80
CYP2B6	0.2	150
CYP2C	18.2	37
CYP2D6	1.5	87
CYP2E1	6.6	44
CYP3A	28.8	36

Notes:
[a]Data are presented as mean values from 60 samples.
[b]The coefficient of variation [(SD/mean) $\times$ 100] is a measure of intcrindividual variability in CYP content.
Source: Shimada et al., 1994.

Approximately 72% of the total CYP content in the human liver can be attributed to seven subfamilies (Table 8.1). Although the CYP3A and CYP2C subfamilies appear to account for almost half of the total CYP content, it is notable that a significant portion of the total CYP content (i.e., 28%) is attributable to other unidentified enzymes in the CYP superfamily (Shimada et al., 1994). Since these data reflect the CYP content, that is the amount of enzyme protein, caution is needed when evaluating their functional (catalytic) and clinical importance.

Genetic variability in drug metabolism

CYP2D6 polymorphism: a classical example of monogenic control in drug metabolism

The *CYP2D6* genetic polymorphism (debrisoquine/sparteine) was discovered in late 1970s and represents one of the most intensively studied monogenic variations in drug metabolism (Nebert, 1999; Sjöqvist, 1999). Approximately 7% of Caucasians are poor metabolizers (PMs) of CYP2D6 substrates while the rest are considered as extensive metabolizers (EMs) (Bertilsson et al., 1992). CYP2D6 enzyme has particular significance for clinical psychiatry as it is involved in clearance of many psychotropic medications such as tricyclic antidepressants (e.g., desipramine), selective serotonin reuptake inhibitors (SSRIs, e.g., paroxetine), classical antipsychotics (e.g., perphenazine), some of the atypical antipsychotic agents (e.g., risperidone), drugs of abuse, and codeine (Bertilsson and Dahl, 1996; Brøsen, 1996).

In vivo, CYP2D6 activity can vary up to 1000-fold in the population (Bertilsson

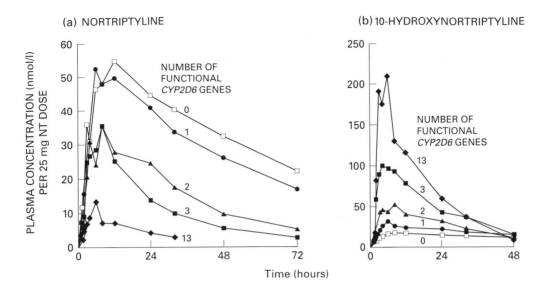

Fig. 8.1.   Average plasma concentrations of nortriptyline (*a*) and 10-hydroxynortriptyline (*b*) after a
25 mg single oral dose in Caucasian healthy volunteers with 0, 1, 2, 3, and 13 functional
copies of *CYP2D6*. Note that the concentration of nortriptyline and its metabolite 10-
hydroxynortriptyline are inversely affected by the number of functional *CYP2D6* copies.
(Reprinted with permission from Dalén et al., 1998.)

et al., 1992; Meyer and Zanger, 1997). This is a consequence of the presence of more
than 50 *CYP2D6* alleles which encode enzymes with inactive, decreased, increased
or normal catalytic function. Genotype–phenotype correlation studies indicate
that the number of functional *CYP2D6* predicts drug and metabolite concentrations in the plasma (Fig. 8.1) (Dalén et al., 1998). From a clinical perspective, as a
general rule, PMs are at risk for drug toxicity during treatment with standard doses
(Pollock et al., 1995). Hence, PMs may present with poor compliance early in the
course of drug treatment. For prodrugs that require activation (e.g., codeine), PM
phenotype may lead to treatment resistance (Sindrup and Brøsen, 1995). At the
other extreme of CYP2D6 activity, in ultrarapid metabolizers with multiple copies
of *CYP2D6*, conventional dose titration regimens may cause delays in therapeutic
response and lead to prolonged inpatient hospital stay and institutionalization.
CYP2D6 genotyping may be clinically invaluable to differentiate ultrarapid
metabolizers with unusually low plasma drug concentrations from patients who do
not comply with drug treatment (Bertilsson et al., 1985; Dalén et al., 1998).
Interestingly, approximately 29% of Ethiopians carry duplicated or multiduplicated functional *CYP2D6* alleles (Aklillu et al., 1996). Identification of such populations with ultrarapid drug metabolism is important as it may provide a
mechanistic basis for treatment resistance to some psychotropic drugs.

A notable and well-established interethnic difference in *CYP2D6* expression occurs between Caucasians and Asians (Bertilsson et al., 1992; Lin et al., 1996). The prevalence of PM phenotype is only 1% in Asians. Another frequently overlooked difference is that the distribution of CYP2D6 activity is significantly shifted towards lower values in Asian EMs. The molecular genetic basis of a slower CYP2D6 activity in Asian EMs was shown to be the result of a cytosine-to-thymine change at position 188 (C188T) in exon 1, leading to Pro34Ser amino acid substitution in a highly conserved region (Pro-Pro-Gly-Pro) of the CYP2D6 enzyme (Johansson et al., 1994; Bertilsson, 1995). Importantly, this allele (*CYP2D6*10*) has a high frequency in Asians (51% in Chinese) and causes a 10-fold decrease in catalytic activity in vivo (Johansson et al., 1994). Therefore, interindividual differences in therapeutic/adverse effects of psychotropics in Asian populations may be explained in part by the presence of *CYP2D6*10* allele. Further information on interethnic differences in CYP2D6 expression is available elsewhere (Bertilsson, 1995).

CYP2D6 with identical pharmacological and molecular properties was also identified in the brain (Britto and Wedlund, 1992). Hence, it is conceivable that CYP2D6 may contribute to local clearance of psychotropics at the site of action. CYP2D6 in the brain is functionally associated with the dopamine transporter and shares similarities in substrates and inhibitors (e.g., *d*-amphetamine), suggesting a role in dopaminergic neurotransmission (Niznik et al., 1990). Differences in personality traits between EMs and PMs were noted in both Swedish and Spanish healthy Caucasian subjects, further suggesting that there may be an endogenous substrate for CYP2D6 (Llerena et al., 1993). At present, little is known on the biological significance and regulation of drug metabolism in the brain, but this is a topic of considerable relevance for personalized therapeutics in psychiatry (Miksys et al., 2000).

Although the *CYP2D6* polymorphism has been known since the 1980s, routine application of this information in clinical practice was hampered, in part, by the lack of cost-effectiveness analyses for pharmacogenetic testing. Recently, Chou et al. (2000) estimated that the annual cost of treating patients at extremes for CYP2D6 activity (PMs and ultrarapid metabolizers) is on average US$4000–$6000 greater than for the rest of the population. Moreover, the total duration of hospital stay appears to be more pronounced in PMs, presumably because of a higher incidence of adverse drug events (Chou et al., 2000). In the near future, further pharmacoeconomic evaluations of genetic variability in drug metabolism and its impact on health outcomes may convince the insurers and other third-party payers to incorporate pharmacogenetic testing into the list of routinely available diagnostic tests. Examples of genetic polymorphisms in other DMEs and their major variant alleles are presented in Table 8.2.

Table 8.2. Human polymorphic cytochrome P-450 enzymes and the global distribution of their major variant alleles

Enzyme	Major variant alleles	Mutation	Consequences for enzyme function	Allele frequencies (%)			
				Caucasians	Asians	Black Africans	Ethiopians and Saudi Arabians
CYP2A6	CYP2A6*2	Leu160His	Inactive enzyme	1–3	0	ND	ND
	CYP2A6*del	Gene deletion	No enzyme	1	15	ND	ND
CYP2C9	CYP2C9*2	Arg144Cys	Reduced affinity for P-450 oxidoreductase	8–13	0	ND	ND
	CYP2C9*3	Ile359Leu	Altered substrate specificity	6–9	2–3	ND	ND
CYP2C19	CYP2C19*2	Aberrant splice site	Inactive enzyme	13	23–32	13	14–15
	CYP2C19*3	Premature stop codon	Inactive enzyme	0	6–10	ND	0–2
CYP2D6	CYP2D6*2xN	Gene duplication or multiduplication	Increased enzyme activity	1–5	0–2	2	10–16
	CYP2D6*4	Defective splicing	Inactive enzyme	12–21	1	2	1–4
	CYP2D6*5	Gene deletion	No enzyme	2–7	6	4	1–3
	CYP2D6*10	Pro34Ser, Ser486Thr	Unstable enzyme	1–2	51	6	3–9
	CYP2D6*17	Thr107Ile, Arg296Cys, Ser486Thr	Reduced affinity for substrates	0	ND	34	3–9

Notes:

ND, not determined.

Source: Reprinted with permission from Ingelman-Sundberg et al., 1999.

Nonpolymorphic drug metabolism with polygenic control: an example with CYP1A2

Historically, CYP2D6 and other genetically polymorphic DMEs have received much research attention in psychopharmacology. Although CYP2D6 is clearly important for the metabolism of many psychotropic drugs, it accounts for only 2% of the total CYP content in the human liver. Consequently, CYP2D6 is considered a "high affinity–low capacity" metabolic clearance pathway (Murphy et al., 2000). Consistent with this, the contribution of CYP2D6 to disposition of substrates is comparatively reduced during multiple- versus single-dose drug administration (Sindrup et al., 1992). Therefore, it is likely that metabolism by pathways other than CYP2D6 may also contribute to disposition of psychotropic drugs, especially under steady-state conditions during multiple-dose treatment. A related point to keep in mind is that CYP2D6 is practically *not* inducible by environmental factors such as smoking and cruciferous vegetable consumption, while such factors may upregulate the expression of certain nonpolymorphic forms of CYPs (e.g., CYP1A2) and thereby increase their contribution to drug clearance.

There is a growing recognition that metabolic routes without a clear-cut polymorphic pattern in distribution of their activity may be subject to "polygenic" regulation (Casley et al., 1999; Kurth, 2000). For example, CYP1A2 enzyme is constitutively expressed in human liver and accounts, on average, for 13% of the total CYP content (Shimada et al., 1994). CYP1A2 activity varies greatly (up to 130-fold) among individuals in many populations and contributes to disposition of several important psychotropic medications, including clozapine, olanzapine and tacrine (Bertilsson et al., 1994; Eaton et al., 1995; Ring et al., 1996; Fontana et al., 1998). Studies in monozygotic and dizygotic twins indicate that genetic factors play a prominent role in regulation of CYP1A2 activity ($h_1 = 0.83$, with 3-methylxanthine formation from theophylline) (Miller et al., 1984). Using a genome-wide interval mapping approach in a mouse model, Casley et al. (1999) recently provided intriguing data that three independent loci on chromosomes 1, 4, and 9 (the last colocalizes with the murine *CYP1A2* locus) explain 63.2% of variability in caffeine N-3 demethylation (an index of CYP1A2 activity). This is a notable landmark study because it is the first application of a genome-wide interval mapping approach to characterize polygenic variation in drug metabolism (Casley et al., 1999). In the near future, it is likely that similar genome-wide searches will provide further insights into polygenic control of drug metabolism.

Genetic contribution to interindividual variability in drug metabolism

Relevance for the design and interpretation of genetic studies of complex diseases

An important corollary of genetic variability in DMEs is that it may potentially lead to a selection bias in candidate gene studies of complex diseases such as schizophrenia. For example, patients who are at risk for drug toxicity (e.g., PMs of CYP2D6) may use inpatient services more commonly and, thus, may have a greater chance of being included in research studies (see discussion by Steen et al. (1997)). In other words, some of the false-positive as well as false-negative genetic studies on complex diseases may be attributed to such population stratification secondary to pharmacogenetic reasons – and not a real disease-causing genetic factor. In future pharmacogenetic investigations, it is advisable, therefore, to stratify and match control and patient populations not only with respect to known confounders such as gender and ethnicity, but also for inpatient and outpatient status. Alternatively, the robustness of conclusions concerning the genetic basis of psychiatric diseases may be ascertained with use of "inpatient status" as another potentially relevant covariate during data analysis.

Intraindividual variations in drug metabolism and gene–environment interactions

Traditionally, genetic factors have mainly been evaluated in relation to interindividual (between person) variations in psychotropic drug metabolism and its clinical significance. Relatively less attention has been given to intraindividual (within person) differences in DME activity, but this variability is also important to consider, particularly for medications that have narrow therapeutic ranges (a high risk of toxicity or therapeutic failure after slight changes in plasma concentrations) and when using compounds for chronic conditions, or for extended periods of time. In these situations, it is important to recognize whether the required dose of a medication administered today will be the same required by the patient 6 months, 1 year, or 5 years from now (e.g., consider the treatment of patients for chronic major depression or schizophrenia). Moreover, intraindividual variability may potentially mimic some of the hereditary drug metabolism phenotypes (Preskorn, 1997; Alfaro et al., 1999). For example, during the course of treatment with potent CYP2D6 inhibitors (e.g., paroxetine, quinidine), EMs may clinically appear as PMs (Alfaro et al., 2000). Thus, drug-induced or physiological variations in drug metabolism may confound the interpretation and conclusions of pharmacogenetic studies (Meyer et al., 1996).

Intraindividual variability in DME activity can be quantified with phenotyping. Although more cumbersome than determining genotype, phenotyping may be clinically more useful as it describes an individual's enzyme activity at any one point in time and accounts for the combined inductive or inhibitory effects of genetic, environmental, and physiological influences. This method involves the oral or intravenous administration of a carefully selected "biomarker compound," and subsequently examining urine, plasma, or saliva concentrations of parent drug and/or metabolites (Carrillo et al., 2000; Streetman et al., 2000a).

Short-term (2 to 6 months) intraindividual variability data in healthy volunteers exist for a number of DMEs (Kashuba et al., 1998a–c; Labbe et al., 2000). When repeated phenotyping measures are performed in healthy volunteers, and coefficients of variation are calculated, intraindividual variability in CYP1A2 phenotype ranges from approximately 5 to 50%, CYP2D6 phenotype varies from 12 to 140%, CYP3A4 phenotype varies from 5 to 21%, N-acetyltransferase 2 (NAT2) phenotype varies from 2 to 27%, and xanthine oxidase phenotype varies from 2 to 13%. A proportion of this intraindividual variability may be ascribed to experimental variation in sample collection and assay techniques, and the variability in other DMEs that may contribute to the biomarker compounds' metabolism. In general, short-term temporal variability in DME activity in diet-restricted, drug-free healthy volunteers appears to be relatively stable. However, environmental and physiological influences on drug–drug interactions in patient populations can all significantly affect intraindividual variability in DME activity.

The following is a synopsis of the frequently encountered environmental and physiological influences that may modify genetically determined variations in drug metabolism. Further information on gene–environment interactions of relevance for drug metabolism are available elsewhere (Eaton and Klaassen, 1996; Costa, 2000).

Dietary influence on intraindividual variability

Certain dietary and environmental factors can significantly alter intestinal and hepatic cytochrome P-450 activity (Walter-Sack and Klotz, 1996). Studies clearly demonstrate that consumption of charcoal-broiled and smoked foods (containing polycyclic aromatic hydrocarbons) can increase the activity of the CYP1A subfamily of isozymes in the intestinal epithelium and hepatocytes (Conney et al., 1976; Kappas et al., 1978; Kall and Clausen, 1995). Cruciferous vegetables such as brussels sprouts, cabbage, broccoli, cauliflower, kale, spinach, and watercress can also alter the activity of selected CYP isozymes: indole-containing vegetables (cabbage, cauliflower) upregulate CYP1A (Pantuck et al., 1989), and isothiocyanate-containing vegetables (watercress) can inhibit CYP2E1 (Kim and Wilkinson, 1996). Organosulfur compounds in garlic, like diallylsulfide, have been found to be inhibitors of CYP2E1 and inducers of the CYP1A, CYP3A, and phase II biotransformation enzymes (Wilkinson, 1997).

Several components of grapefruit juice acting on enterocytes can increase the bioavailability of CYP3A (and in some cases, CYP1A) substrates by four- to five-fold (Bailey et al., 1994; Dresser et al., 2000). A number of phytochemicals found in grapefruit juice that may be responsible for CYP3A (and possibly CYP1A) inhibition and degradation have been investigated. Although the exact compound or compounds is/are currently unknown, ingestion of grapefruit juice can lead to large apparent intraindividual variability, primarily in the pharmacokinetics of

CYP3A compounds. Additionally, certain vitamins and spices have been implicated in altering DME activity (Wilkinson, 1997).

Although the diet contains many more potentially active compounds than have been formally investigated, it is important to recognize that the body is exposed to a constantly changing variety of chemicals that are capable of modulating DMEs in both the intestine and the liver. Many of these may have opposing effects, resulting in complex and often unpredictable interactions, which can contribute to intraindividual variability in drug metabolism and response.

Drug–drug interactions and nutraceutical influences on drug metabolism

Large intraindividual variability in drug metabolism can also be caused by concomitant medication therapy. A wide variety of medications are known to induce or inhibit DME activity profoundly, such as the rifamycins, anticonvulsants, macrolide antibiotics, azole antifungal agents, nefazodone, and certain selective serotonin reuptake inhibitors (SSRIs). The effects of medications on DME activities have been extensively reviewed elsewhere (Lin and Lu, 1998; Fang and Gorrow, 1999; Tanaka and Hisawa, 1999; Flockhart and Oesterheld, 2000). Patients initiating or terminating a medication or compound that can profoundly influence DME activity may experience altered responses to concomitant medications.

For centuries, herbs and other dietary compounds have played a significant role in the treatment of disease in many traditional cultures. In developed countries, there is now increasing interest in the use of the active constituents of these products for medical benefit. Along with this increased use has come the knowledge that these are not innocuous compounds. The detrimental effects of extracts of St. John's wort (*Hypericum perforatum*), used for mild to moderate states of depression, on drug availability have recently been described. Kerb et al. (1997) first demonstrated that taking 300 mg of St. John's wort three times a day for 14 days significantly enhanced urinary 6β-hydroxycortisol excretion, a marker of CYP3A activity. After 14 days of therapy with St. John's wort, the protease inhibitor indinavir had a mean 60% decrease in exposure (area under the concentration-versus-time curve: AUC) and an 80% decrease in trough concentrations (C_{min}) (Piscitelli et al., 2000), indicative of large CYP3A induction effects on hepatic and intestinal activity. In women taking St. John's wort and oral contraceptives, breakthrough bleeding with potential loss of contraceptive efficacy has also been reported (Ernst, 1999). Another recent report demonstrated that ciclosporin (cyclosporine) concentrations decreased in one kidney transplant recipient sporadically taking St. John's wort, necessitating a 46% increase in dose (Mai et al., 2000).

Mechanisms of these nutraceutical effects are under investigation. Wentworth et al. (2000) found that St. John's wort enhanced the transcriptional activity of the steroid X receptor, a member of the nuclear receptor superfamily that is activated by drugs such as rifampin, which are potent inducers of hepatic cytochrome P-450 CYP3A enzyme activity. St. John's wort also appears to alter P-glycoprotein (P-gp) activity. P-gp is a transmembrane efflux pump that removes drugs from the cell and deposits them into the extracellular space (Kashuba and Bertino, 2000; von Moltke and Greenblatt, 2000). It has been suggested that CYP3A and P-gp might play complementary roles in drug disposition by biotransformation and antitransport. This is especially pertinent in enterocytes, where CYP3A and P-gp can act synergistically to decrease drug bioavailability (Wacher et al., 1995). Currently, little is known about the significance of P-gp-mediated transport of psychotropics during distribution. Johne et al. (1999) administered 300 mg dried *Hypericum* extract three times per day, along with digoxin (a P-gp substrate) 0.25 mg once per day in five healthy volunteers. After 10 days of treatment with St. John's wort, digoxin exposure (AUC) decreased 25% and trough concentrations decreased 20–30%. The authors postulated that P-gp activity, transporting digoxin from enterocytes into the intestinal tract, might be activated upon exposure to St. John's wort.

The effects of St. John's wort on both CYP3A and P-gp activity are not completely unexpected. It has been determined that most, but not all (e.g., midazolam), compounds that are metabolized by CYP3A are substrates for P-gp. Most recently, Piscitelli et al. (2001) have demonstrated that, in the presence of garlic supplementation taken twice daily for 3 weeks, steady-state AUC and trough concentrations of saquinavir (a CYP3A and P-gp substrate) both decrease approximately by 50%. This effect appears to be exceedingly prolonged, as these parameters returned to only 60–70% of baseline values 10 days after stopping the garlic supplementation. Much work is still needed to examine the effects of nutraceuticals on psychotropic drug disposition, and how significantly they contribute to intraindividual variability in DME activity and therapeutic response.

Influence of aging on drug metabolism

Beginning in the third decade of life, both liver blood flow and liver volume decline linearly over time. By the time an individual reaches 80–90 years of age, these values are approximately 20–40% less (Durnas et al., 1990). In rodents and other animal models, aging is often associated with impaired drug metabolism; however, extrapolation of these findings to humans is difficult (Schmucker, 1989). In addition, problems such as large interindividual variability and small sample sizes hinder the extrapolation of in vitro human data to the clinical situation (Wilkinson, 1997).

Nonetheless, the available in vitro data suggest that age-related effects on DME activity are modest. Generally, it appears that CYP1A2, CYP2C9/10, CYP2C18/19, and CYP3A4/5 are moderately reduced in the elderly. There are no data on intestinal CYP activity changes in the elderly (Kinirons and Crome, 1997). Although the extent of change is unpredictable with respect to specific drug and particular individual, it appears to be greatest with drugs exhibiting significant (>80%) first-pass effects in young subjects. Fortunately, very few currently marketed drugs possess this characteristic.

Influence of disease on variability in drug metabolism

In addition to genetics, diet, concomitant medications/nutraceuticals and physiologic effects such as aging, the presence of physical diseases can also be a major determinant of variability in drug disposition and clinical response. However, non-psychiatric disease states are frequently overlooked in patients with mental health problems and during their treatment with psychotropic drugs.

As early as the 1960s, acute inflammation and infection were demonstrated to affect the metabolism of drugs and toxins in animals, thereby modulating pharmacological and toxicological effects (Wooles and Borzelleca, 1966; Renton and Mannering, 1976). The earliest report of infection altering human DME activity occurred a decade later, with quinine concentrations consistently elevated in subjects experimentally infected with *Plasmodium falciparum* malaria (Trenholme et al., 1976). Since that time, numerous reports have described alterations in drug metabolism with viral and bacterial infections (Brockmeyer et al., 1998; Shedlofsky et al., 1994), and with traumatic events such as surgery and bone marrow transplantation (Gidal et al., 1996). The effects of inflammation and infection on P-450 activity are ascribed to stimulation of the cellular immune response (Renton, 2000). Although many different mediators may be involved, there has been particular focus on the major proinflammatory cytokines interleukins 1 and 6 and tumor necrosis factor (Watkins et al., 1995; Haas, 2000).

Very little information exists concerning the influence of chronic infection on DME activity. Recently, the effects of HIV infection on drug metabolism have been investigated (Lee et al., 1993; Gotzkowsky et al., 2000; O'Neil et al., 2000). The most comprehensive data were reported by Gotzkowsky et al. (2000), who examined 17 HIV-infected individuals (with disease stage 1A of the Centers for Disease Control and Prevention classification) taking no medications known to alter DME activity. Most notably it was demonstrated that, compared with age- and sex-matched healthy volunteers, CYP3A and CYP2D6 activities were significantly decreased by 30–90%, and 25% of HIV-infected individuals exhibited genotype–phenotype discordance for CYP2D6 (all were EMs by genotype, but PMs by phenotype). These findings indicate that the concurrent presence of HIV infection may limit the utility of genotype-based approaches for the assessment of DME activity in patients who use psychotropic mediations.

Liver disease can also modify blood flow and reduce the activity of DMEs. In acute disease, the major alteration is in hepatocellular function, but in chronic liver disease (cirrhosis), the major abnormality lies with liver blood flow and possibly alteration in liver function. The effects of liver disease appear to be highly variable and difficult to predict (Morgan and McLean, 1995). Several studies with liver biopsy samples have found reduced protein concentrations and/or catalytic activity associated with CYP1A (Bechtel et al., 2000), CYP2D6, CYP2E1, and CYP3A (George et al., 1995; Wilkinson, 1997), although the results were not uniformly consistent in other investigations (Adedoyin et al., 1998). Generally, hepatic impairment appears to be greater in cirrhotic livers than in patients with less severe forms of hepatic dysfunction, including chronic active hepatitis and cholestasis (Vesell, 1984; Wilkinson, 1997).

Genetic variability in drug metabolism and therapeutic drug monitoring

While there is considerable interest in identification of patients with unusual drug metabolism traits through genetic testing, this also raises an important question. Should metabolism by a genetically polymorphic pathway be a sufficient reason to restrict prescription of drugs in certain subpopulations?

The answer is intimately related to how we view the variability in drug response. A contribution from a polymorphic metabolic pathway implies considerable uncertainty in clearance and pharmacological effects of a drug. This uncertainty can take the form of drug toxicity but also can involve lack of efficacy owing to sub-therapeutic concentrations in association with ultrarapid metabolism. On the basis of such therapeutic uncertainties, the initial temptation is to avoid this variability by limiting the prescription of compounds that undergo genetically polymorphic metabolism. By contrast, this strategy may prevent the development of newer and efficacious drugs. This has particular significance for therapeutic fields where there are no well-established efficacious medicines (e.g., Alzheimer's disease and other neurodegenerative disorders). If a new compound demonstrates therapeutic efficacy either alone or in combination, and prolongs the lives of patients, then variability in its metabolism should not be a constraint for clinical development. For example, some of the classical antipsychotics (e.g., perphenazine) developed more than two decades ago are still widely used in many countries and demonstrate efficacy in approximately 70% of patients with major psychosis. Yet many of them are eliminated by CYP2D6-mediated oxidative metabolism. Such compounds can be used safely, provided adequate dose adjustments are made before drug administration. Moreover, as discussed previously, the implicit assumption that nonpolymorphic drug metabolism is associated with less variability is not always valid (e.g., consider the case with CYP1A2). In short, variability in drug metabolism is the rule, rather than the exception (Okey, 1990).

An alternative to avoidance of variability in drug metabolism would be to characterize medications early in the course of their development with respect to primary phase I and phase II biotransformation enzymes responsible for their disposition. Since the DMEs will continue to exist and play an important role in clearance of drugs and other xenobiotics, this approach needs to be complemented by advances in our understanding of the regulation of expression of DMEs. It is a common clinical practice to adjust the doses of medications eliminated predominantly by the kidney in patients with acute or chronic renal failure. Interestingly, marked interindividual differences in drug metabolism typically receive much less attention in routine clinical practice. This *dual* metabolic profiling strategy, that is of medications as well as patients, should allow a more optimal use of psychotropic drugs that are metabolized by a genetically polymorphic pathway. There is evidence that drug metabolism is already beginning to play a significant role in psychotropic drug development. For example, a recent survey conducted by the US Food and Drug Administration found that nearly 70% of the drugs approved by the Division of Neuropharmacological Products contained in vitro drug interaction and metabolism studies (Yuan et al., 1999).

Therapeutic drug monitoring through genotyping and/or phenotyping of DMEs offer several advantages over the traditional approach based on measurement of plasma drug concentrations (Freeman and Oyewumi, 1997). The knowledge of major DMEs that contribute to clearance of a drug is useful to forecast its pharmacokinetic variability in the general population, since the distribution of catalytic activity of most DMEs is established in different populations. Further, this information may provide mechanistic insights to predict inhibitory or inductive drug–drug interactions. In patient populations with known compliance problems or in those exposed to inducers of DMEs (e.g., tobacco smoke), information on individual drug metabolism capacity may help to establish a *quantitative* index of compliance to drug treatment at any given dosage. Lastly, certain DMEs are expressed both in the liver and the brain (e.g., CYP2D6 and CYP1A2) (Farin and Omiecinski, 1993). Therefore, genetic profiling of DMEs may provide an estimate of not only plasma drug concentrations but also psychotropic drug disposition at the site of action.

Conclusions

The theoretical foundations of genetic variability in drug metabolism have been firmly established since the 1960s (Kalow, 1997; Weber, 1997; Grant, 1999). The earlier pioneering pharmacogenetic studies on drug metabolism were conducted mainly in healthy volunteers or in small numbers of selected patients who present with unusual adverse drug reactions (Pfost et al., 2000). Recent advances in molecular biology, along with the declining costs and increased throughput of genetic analyses, now make prospective validation of pharmacogenetic hypotheses entirely feasible in most clinical settings. Notably, pharmacogenetic inquiries are no longer solely dependent on observations of unusual drug metabolism phenotypes and can be initiated directly at the molecular genetic level (Nebert, 1999). The next few years will likely witness a proliferation in the number and scope of correlative "genotype versus clinical outcome" studies in psychopharmacology.

In the midst of this exciting molecular genetic revolution, some cautionary restraint and reflection over past accomplishments as well as methodological short-comings are needed to gain a balanced context for the future. Until recently, much emphasis was placed on monogenic control in drug metabolism (e.g., CYP2D6 genetic polymorphism), with little attention to multigenic regulation of gene expression (Cichon et al., 2000; Nebert, 2000). A case in point is the CYP3A4 enzyme, the most abundant CYP in the human liver. Twin and repeated drug administration studies indicate that heredity plays a prominent role in regulation of *CYP3A4* expression (Penno et al., 1981; Ozdemir et al., 2000). Yet, despite inten-sive research efforts, few polymorphisms could be found within the coding or the immediate promotor regions of *CYP3A4*. It is likely that the marked interindivid-ual variability in CYP3A4 activity is attributable to multigenic control, but little is known on the identity and precise physical location of such putative regulatory loci in the genome. With the completion of the Human Genome Project in 2001, vir-tually all genes in the human genome will be available to examine novel gene–gene interactions and molecular genetic mechanisms for regulation of *CYP3A4* and other DMEs. Assumption-free genome-wide association studies and linkage anal-yses may prove to be very useful tools to discover unprecedented regulatory genetic loci of relevance for drug metabolism that may not be readily predicted by the exist-ing list of plausible candidate genes (Casley et al., 1999; Goodman, 1999; Malhotra and Goldman, 1999).

It is estimated that the human genome contains more than 1 000 000 single nucleotide polymorphisms (SNPs) and these may explain differences in drug metabolism between individuals and populations. However, a point to keep in mind is that not all SNPs will influence the function of the encoded proteins, even though they may alter the amino acid sequences. Hence, it is conceivable that one of the critical determinants of success in pharmacogenetic research in the postge-nomic period will be the ability to perform gene expression and functional genomic studies. These investigations will provide the much needed mechanistic rationale to choose the battery of most relevant candidate genes and SNPs in subsequent clinical pharmacogenetic "validation" studies in humans (Evans and Relling, 1999).

The final pharmacological effects of medications are determined by a complex interplay of numerous genes and environmental factors (Masellis et al., 2000). Dietary factors, smoking, physiological and disease states, drug interactions, and nutraceutical interactions may all modify or cause phenocopying of drug metabolism. Hence, these factors can mimic some of the hereditary drug metabolism traits (e.g., PM versus EM). An adequate knowledge of gene–environment interactions is central to proper interpretation of pharmacogenetic studies in psychiatry.

The contribution of genetic factors to drug metabolism has been mainly sought in the context of *constitutive* person-to-person variability, in the absence of inhibitors or inducers of DMEs. Recently, some progress has been made in understanding the genetic basis of individual differences in DME induction. For example, smoking has been known for a long time as a potent inducer of CYP1A2 activity. Although the extent of exposure to tobacco smoke may explain part of the variability in *CYP1A2* induction, our knowledge of the putative genetic factors that may influence *CYP1A2* induction has been limited. A recent study in a sample of Caucasian volunteers identified a single nucleotide polymorphism (cytosine to adenosine) in intron 1 of *CYP1A2* (*CYP1A2*1F*) at position 734 downstream from the transcription initiation site (Sachse et al., 1999). The *CYP1A2*1F* allele reportedly accounts for 18% of variability in CYP1A2 activity in Caucasian smokers and appears to influence caffeine disposition and the risk for tardive dyskinesia (Sachse et al., 1999; Basile et al., 2000). Clearly, the design of future pharmacogenetic studies may benefit from further explorations of similar gene–environment interactions.

Although genotyping is central to any psychiatric pharmacogenetic study, phenotyping of DMEs with biomarker compounds (e.g., caffeine) will continue to play a significant role in validation of observations on associations between a particular DME genotype and clinical end-points. Progress has also been made in the development of rapid phenotyping procedures or "probe cocktails" for convenient measurement of multiple DME activities in tandem (Svensson and Bertilsson, 1999; Carrillo et al., 2000; Streetman et al., 2000b).

Pharmacogenetics provides a rational framework for evaluation of genetic variation in DMEs as well as in genes encoding drug transporters, receptors, and ion channels, which can all influence an individual's risk for adverse drug reactions or therapeutic failure (Arranz and Kerwin, 2000; Meyer, 2000; Sjöqvist, 2000). It can be anticipated that psychiatric pharmacogenetics will reduce the uncertainty and trial-and-error in choice and dosing of medications in the near future, thereby importantly contributing to development of personalized treatment guidelines in clinical psychiatry.

Acknowledgements

The authors thank Drs Werner Kalow, Laszlo Endrenyi, and Allan B. Okey for many insightful discussions and support.

REFERENCES

Adedoyin A, Arns PA, Richards WO, Wilkinson GR, Branch RA (1998). Selective effect of liver disease on the activities of specific metabolizing enzymes; investigation of cytochromes P-450 2C19 and 2D6. *Clin Pharmacol Ther* 64, 8–17.

Aklillu E, Persson I, Bertilsson L, Johansson I, Rodrigues F, Ingelman-Sundberg M (1996). Frequent distribution of ultrarapid metabolizers of debrisoquine in an Ethiopian population carrying duplicated and multiduplicated functional CYP2D6 alleles. *J Pharmacol Exp Ther* 278, 441–446.

Alfaro CL, Lam YW, Simpson J, Ereshefsky L (1999). CYP2D6 status of extensive metabolizers after multiple-dose fluoxetine, fluvoxamine, paroxetine, or sertraline. *J Clin Psychopharmacol* 19, 155–163.

Alfaro CL, Lam YW, Simpson J, Ereshefsky L (2000). CYP2D6 inhibition by fluoxetine, paroxetine, sertraline, and venlafaxine in a crossover study: intraindividual variability and plasma concentration correlations. *J Clin Pharmacol* 40, 58–66.

Arranz MJ, Kerwin RW (2000). Neurotransmitter-related genes and antipsychotic response: pharmacogenetics meets psychiatric treatment. *Ann Med* 32, 128–133.

Bailey DG, Arnold JMO, Spence JD (1994). Grapefruit juice and drugs – how significant is the interaction? *Clin Pharmacokinet* 26, 91–98.

Basile VS, Ozdemir V, Masellis M et al. (2000). A functional polymorphism of the cytochrome P-450 1A2 (CYP1A2) gene: association with tardive dyskinesia in schizophrenia. *Mol Psychiatry* 5, 410–417.

Bechtel YC, Haffen E, Lelouet H et al. (2000). Relationship between the severity of alcoholic liver cirrhosis and the metabolism of caffeine in 226 patients. *Int J Clin Pharmacol Ther* 38, 467–475.

Bertilsson L (1995). Geographical/interracial differences in polymorphic drug oxidation. Current state of knowledge of cytochromes P-450 (CYP) 2D6 and 2C19. *Clin Pharmacokinet* 29, 192–209.

Bertilsson L, Dahl ML (1996). Polymorphic drug oxidation. Relevance to the treatment of psychiatric disorders. *CNS Drugs* 5, 200–223.

Bertilsson L, Aberg-Wistedt A, Gustafsson LL, Nordin C (1985). Extremely rapid hydroxylation of debrisoquine: a case report with implication for treatment with nortriptyline and other tricyclic antidepressants. *Ther Drug Monit* 7, 478–480.

Bertilsson L, Lou YQ, Du YL et al. (1992). Pronounced differences between native Chinese and Swedish populations in the polymorphic hydroxylations of debrisoquin and S-mephenytoin. *Clin Pharmacol Ther* 51, 388–397.

Bertilsson L, Carrillo JA, Dahl ML et al. (1994). Clozapine disposition covaries with CYP1A2 activity determined by a caffeine test. *Br J Clin Pharmacol* 38, 471–473.

Britto MR, Wedlund PJ (1992). Cytochrome P-450 in the brain. Potential evolutionary and therapeutic relevance of localization of drug-metabolizing enzymes. *Drug Metab Dispos* 20, 446–450.

Brockmeyer NH, Barthel B, Mertins L, Goos M (1998). Changes of antipyrine pharmacokinetics during influenza and after administration of interferon-alpha and -beta. *Int J Clin Pharmacol Ther* 36, 309–311.

Brøsen K (1996). Drug-metabolizing enzymes and therapeutic drug monitoring in psychiatry. *Ther Drug Monit* 18, 393–396.

Carrillo JA, Christensen M, Ramos SI et al. (2000). Evaluation of caffeine as an in vivo probe for CYP1A2 using measurements in plasma, saliva, and urine. *Ther Drug Monit* 22, 409–417.

Casley WL, Menzies JA, Whitehouse LW, Moon TW (1999). Detection of quantitative trait loci affecting caffeine metabolism by interval mapping in a genome-wide scan of C3H/HEJ × APN F_2 mice. *Drug Metab Dispos* 27, 1375–1380.

Cohen LJ, DeVane CL (1996). Clinical implications of antidepressant pharmacokinetics and pharmacogenetics. *Ann Pharmacother* 3, 1471–1480.

Chou WH, Yan FX, de Leon J et al. (2000). Extension of a pilot study: impact from the cytochrome P-450 2D6 polymorphism on outcome and costs associated with severe mental illness. *J Clin Psychopharmacol* 20, 246–251.

Cichon S, Nöthen MM, Rietschel M, Propping P (2000). Pharmacogenetics of schizophrenia. *Am J Med Genet* 97, 98–106.

Conney AH, Pantuck EJ, Hsiao KC et al. (1976). Enhanced phenacetin metabolism in human subjects fed charcoal broiled beef. *Clin Pharmacol Ther* 20, 633–642.

Costa LG (2000). The emerging field of ecogenetics. *Neurotoxicology* 21, 85–90.

Dalén P, Dahl ML, Ruiz ML, Nordin J, Bertilsson L (1998). 10-Hydroxylation of nortriptyline in white persons with 0, 1, 2, 3, and 13 functional CYP2D6 genes. *Clin Pharmacol Ther* 63, 444–452.

Dresser GK, Spence JD, Bailey DG (2000). Pharmacokinetic–pharmacodynamic consequences and clinical relevance of cytochrome P-450 3A4 inhibition. *Clin Pharmacokinet* 38, 41–57.

Durnas C, Loi CM, Cusack BJ (1990). Hepatic drug metabolism and aging. *Clin Pharmacokinet* 19, 359–389.

Eaton DL (2000). Biotransformation enzyme polymorphism and pesticide susceptibility. *Neurotoxicology* 21, 101–111.

Eaton DL, Bammler TK (1999). Concise review of the glutathione *S*-transferases and their significance to toxicology. *Toxicol Sci* 49, 156–164.

Eaton DL, Klaassen CD (1996). Principles of toxicology. In Klaassen CD, ed. *Casarett and Doull's Toxicology: The Basic Science of Poisons*, 5th edn. New York: McGraw-Hill, pp. 13–33.

Eaton DL, Gallagher EP, Bammler TK, Kunze KL (1995). Role of cytochrome P-4501A2 in chemical carcinogenesis: implications for human variability in expression and enzyme activity. *Pharmacogenetics* 5, 259–274.

Endrenyi L, Inaba T, Kalow W (1976). Genetic studies of amobarbital elimination based on its kinetics in twins. *Clin Pharmacol Ther* 20, 701–714.

Ernst E (1999). Second thoughts about safety of St. John's wort. *Lancet* 254, 2014–2016.

Evans WE, Relling MV (1999). Pharmacogenomics: translating functional genomics into rational therapeutics. *Science* 286, 487–491.

Fang J, Gorrow JW (1999). Metabolism, pharmacogenetics, and metabolic drug–drug interactions of antipsychotic drugs. *Cell Mol Neurobiol* 19, 491–510.

Farin FM, Omiecinski CJ (1993). Regiospecific expression of cytochrome P-450s and microsomal epoxide hydrolase in human brain tissue. *J Toxicol Environ Health* 40, 317–335.

Flockhart DA, Oesterheld JR (2000). Cytochrome P-450-mediated drug interactions. *Child Adolesc Psychiatr Clin N Am* 9, 43–76.

Fontana RJ, deVries TM, Woolf TF et al. (1998). Caffeine based measures of CYP1A2 activity correlate with oral clearance of tacrine in patients with Alzheimer's disease. *Br J Clin Pharmacol* 46, 221–228.

Freeman DJ, Oyewumi LK (1997). Will routine therapeutic drug monitoring have a place in clozapine therapy? *Clin Pharmacokinet* 32, 93–100.

George J, Murray M, Byth K, Farrell GC (1995). Differential alterations of cytochrome P-450 proteins in livers from patients with severe chronic liver disease. *Hepatology* 21, 120–128.

Gidal BE, Reiss WG, Liao JS, Pitterle ME (1996). Changes in interleukin-6 concentrations following epilepsy surgery: potential influence on carbamazepine pharmacokinetics. *Ann Pharmacother* 30, 545–546.

Goodman L (1999). Hypothesis-limited research. *Genome Res* 9, 673–674.

Gotzkowsky SK, Kim J, Tonkin J et al. (2000). Altered drug metabolizing enzyme activity and genotype-phenotype discordance in HIV-infected subjects. *40th Interscience Conference on Antimicrobial Agents and Chemotherapy*, Toronto, Canada, abstract 1169:301.

Grant DM (1999). Pharmacogenomics and the changing face of clinical pharmacology. *Can J Clin Pharmacol* 6, 131–132.

Haas CE (2000). Drug–cytokine interactions. In Piscitelli SC, Rodvold KA, eds. *Drug Interactions in Infectious Diseases*. Totowa NJ: Humana Press, pp. 287–310.

Ingelman-Sundberg M, Oscarson M, McLellan RA (1999). Polymorphic human cytochrome P-450 enzymes: an opportunity for individualized drug treatment. *Trends Pharmacol Sci* 20, 342–349.

Johansson I, Oscarson M, Yue QY, Bertilsson L, Sjöqvist F, Ingelman-Sundberg M (1994). Genetic analysis of the Chinese cytochrome P-4502D locus: characterization of variant CYP2D6 genes present in subjects with diminished capacity for debrisoquine hydroxylation. *Mol Pharmacol* 46, 452–459.

Johne A, Brockmoller J, Bauer S, Maurer A, Langheinrich M, Roots I (1999). Pharmacokinetic interaction of digoxin with an herbal extract from St Johns wort (*Hypericum perforatum*). *Clin Pharmacol Ther* 66, 338–345.

Kall MS, Clausen J (1995). Dietary effect on mixed function P-450 1A2 activity assayed by estimation of caffeine metabolism in man. *Hum Exp Toxicol* 14, 801–807.

Kalow W (1962). *Pharmacogenetics: Heredity and the Response to Drugs*. Philadelphia, PA: Saunders, pp. 1–231.

Kalow W (1997). Pharmacogenetics in biological perspective. *Pharmacol Rev* 49, 369–379.

Kalow W (1999). Pharmacogenetic research: a revolutionary science. *J Psychiatr Neurosci* 24, 139–140.

Kappas A, Alvares AP, Anderson KE et al. (1978). Effects of charcoal-broiled beef on antipyrine and theophylline metabolism. *Clin Pharmacol Ther* 23, 445–450.

Kashuba ADM, Bertino JS Jr. (2000). Mechanisms of drug interactions. In Piscitelli SC, Rodvold KA, eds. *Drug Interactions in Infectious Diseases*. Totowa, NJ: Humana Press, pp. 13–38.

Kashuba AD, Bertino JS Jr., Kearns GL et al. (1998a). Quantitation of three-month intra-individual variability and influence of sex and menstrual. cycle phase on CYP1A2,

N-acetyltransferase-2, and xanthine oxidase activity determined. with caffeine phenotyping. *Clin Pharmacol Ther* 63, 540–551.

Kashuba AD, Bertino JS Jr., Rocci ML Jr., Kulawy RW, Beck DJ, Nafziger AN (1998b). Quantification of 3-month intraindividual variability and the influence of sex and menstrual cycle phase on CYP3A activity as measured by phenotyping with intravenous midazolam. *Clin Pharmacol Ther* 64, 269–277.

Kashuba AD, Nafziger AN, Kearns GL, et al. (1998c). Quantification of intraindividual variability and the influence of menstrual cycle phase on CYP2D6 activity as measured by dextro-methorphan phenotyping. *Pharmacogenetics* 8, 403–410.

Kerb R, Bauer S, Brockoller J, Roots I (1997). Urinary 6β-hydroxycortisol excretion rate is affected by treatment with hypericum extract [abstract]. *Eur J Clin Pharmacol* 52(Suppl), A186.

Kim RB, Wilkinson GR (1996). Watercress inhibits human CYP2E1 activity in vivo as measured by chlorzoxazone 6-hydroxylation. *Clin Pharmacol Ther* 59, 170.

Kinirons MT, Crome P (1997). Clinical pharmacokinetic considerations in the elderly: an update. *Clin Pharmacokinet* 33, 302–312.

Kurth JH (2000). Pharmacogenomics: future promise of a tool for identifying patients at risk. *Drug Info J* 34, 223–227.

Labbe L, Sirois C, Pilote S, et al. (2000). Effect of gender, sex hormones, time variables and physiological urinary pH on apparent CYP2D6 activity as assessed by metabolic ratios of marker substrates. *Pharmacogenetics* 10, 425–438.

Lazarou J, Pomeranz BH, Corey PN (1998). Incidence of adverse drug reactions in hospitalized patients: meta-analysis of prospective studies. *J Am Med Assoc* 279, 1200–1205.

Lee BI., Wong D, Benowitz NL, Sullam PM (1993). Altered patterns of drug metabolism in patients with acquired immunodeficiency syndrome. *Clin Pharmacol Ther* 53, 529–535.

Lin JH, Lu AY (1998). Inhibition and induction of cytochrome P-450 and the clinical implications. *Clin Pharmacokinet* 35, 361–90.

Lin KM, Poland RE, Wan Y-JY, Smith MW, Lesser IM (1996). The evolving science of pharmacogenetics: clinical and ethnic perspectives. *Psychopharmacol Bull* 32, 205–217.

Llerena A, Edman G, Cobaleda J, Benitez J, Schalling D, Bertilsson L (1993). Relationship between personality and debrisoquine hydroxylation capacity. Suggestion of an endogenous neuroactive substrate or product of the cytochrome P-4502D6. *Acta Psychiatr Scand* 87, 23–28.

Mai I, Kruger H, Budde K et al. (2000). Hazardous pharmacokinetic interaction of Saint John's wort (*Hypericum perforatum*) with the immunosuppressant cyclosporin. *Int J Clin Pharmacol Therap* 38, 500–502.

Malhotra AK, Goldman D (1999). Benefits and pitfalls encountered in psychiatric genetic association studies. *Biol Psychiatry* 45, 544–550.

Masellis M, Basile VS, Ozdemir V, Meltzer HY, Macciardi FM, Kennedy JL (2000). Pharmacogenetics of antipsychotic treatment: lessons learned from clozapine. *Biol Psychiatry* 47, 252–266.

Meyer UA (2000). Pharmacogenetics and adverse drug reactions. *Lancet* 356, 1667–1671.

Meyer UA, Zanger UM (1997). Molecular mechanisms of genetic polymorphisms of drug metabolism. *Annu Rev Pharmacol Toxicol* 37, 269–296.

Meyer UA, Amrein R, Balant LP et al. (1996). Antidepressants and drug-metabolizing enzymes – expert group report. *Acta Psychiatr Scand* 93, 71–79.

Miksys S, Rao Y, Sellers EM, Kwan M, Mendis D, Tyndale RF (2000). Regional and cellular distribution of CYP2D subfamily members in rat brain. *Xenobiotica* 30, 547–564.

Miller M, Opheim KE, Raisys VA, Motulsky AG (1984). Theophylline metabolism: variation and genetics. *Clin Pharmacol Ther* 35, 170–182.

Morgan DJ, McLean AJ (1995). Clinical pharmacokinetic and pharmacodynamic considerations in patients with liver disease: an update. *Clin Pharmacokinet* 29, 370–391.

Motulsky AG (1957). Drug reactions, enzymes and biochemical genetics. *J Am Med Assoc* 165, 835–837.

Murphy MP, Beaman ME, Clark LS et al. (2000). *Pharmacogenetics* 10, 583–590.

Nebert DW (1999). Pharmacogenetics and pharmacogenomics: why is this relevant to the clinical geneticist? *Clin Genet* 56, 247–258.

Nebert DW (2000). Suggestions for the nomenclature of human alleles: relevance to ecogenetics, pharmacogenetics and molecular epidemiology. *Pharmacogenetics* 10, 279–290.

Nelson DR, Koymans L, Kamataki T et al. (1996). P-450 superfamily: update on new sequences, gene mapping, accession numbers and nomenclature. *Pharmacogenetics* 6, 1–42.

Niznik HB, Tyndale RF, Sallee FR et al. (1990). The dopamine transporter and cytochrome P450IID1 (debrisoquine 4-hydroxylase) in brain: resolution and identification of two distinct [^{3}H]GBR-12935 binding proteins. *Arch Biochem Biophys* 276, 424–432.

Okey AB (1990). Enzyme induction in the cytochrome P-450 system. *Pharmacol Ther* 45, 241–298.

Omura T, Sato R (1964a). The carbon monoxide-binding pigment of liver microsomes. 1. Evidence for its hemoprotein nature. *J Biol Chem* 239, 2370–2378.

Omura T, Sato R (1964b). The carbon monoxide-binding pigment of liver microsomes. 2. Solubilization, purification, and properties. *J Biol Chem* 239, 2379–2385.

O'Neil WM, Bilfix BM, Markoglou N, Di Girolamo A, Tsoukas CN, Wainer IW (2000). Genotype and phenotype of cytochrome P-450 2D6 in human immunodeficiency virus-positive patients and patients with acquired immunodeficiency syndrome. *Eur J Clin Pharmacol* 56, 231–240.

Ozdemir V, Kalow W, Tang BK et al. (2000). Evaluation of the genetic contribution to CYP3A4 activity in vivo: a repeated drug administration method. *Pharmacogenetics* 10, 373–388.

Pantuck EJ, Pantuck CB, Min BH et al. (1989). Stimulatory effect of brussels sprouts and cabbage on human drug metabolism. *Clin Pharmacol Ther* 35, 88–95.

Penno MB, Dvorchik BH, Vesell ES (1981). Genetic variation in rates of antipyrine metabolite formation: a study in uninduced twins. *Proc Natl Acad Sci, USA* 78, 5193–5196.

Pfost DR, Boyce-Jacino MT, Grant DM (2000). A SNP shot: pharmacogenetics and the future of drug therapy. *Trend Biotechnol* 18, 334–338.

Piscitelli SC, Burstein AH, Chaitt D, Alfaro RM, Falloon J (2000). Indinavir concentrations and St. John's wort. *Lancet* 12, 547–548.

Piscitelli SC, Burstein AH, Welden N, Gallicano K, Falloon J (2001). Garlic supplements decrease saquinavir plasma concentrations. *Abstracts of the 8th Annual Conference on Retroviruses and Opportunistic Infections*, Chicago, IL.

Pollock BG, Mulsant BH, Sweet RA, Rosen J, Altieri LP, Perel JM (1995). Prospective cytochrome P-450 phenotyping for neuroleptic treatment in dementia. *Psychopharmacol Bull* 31, 327–331.

Preskorn SH (1997). Clinically relevant pharmacology of selective serotonin reuptake inhibitors. An overview with emphasis on pharmacokinetics and effects on oxidative drug metabolism. *Clin Pharmacokinet* 32(Suppl 1), 1–21.

Renton KW (2000). Hepatic drug metabolism and immunostimulation. *Toxicology* 142, 173–178.

Renton KW, Mannering GJ (1976). Depression of the hepatic cytochrome P-450 mono-oxygenase system by administered tilorone (2, 7-bis(2-(diethylamino)ethoxy)fluoren-9-one dihydrochloride). *Drug Metab Dispos* 4, 223–231.

Ring BJ, Catlow J, Lindsay TJ et al. (1996). Identification of the human cytochromes P-450 responsible for the in vitro formation of the major oxidative metabolites of the antipsychotic agent olanzapine. *J Pharmacol Exp Ther* 276, 658–666.

Sachse C, Brockmoller J, Bauer S, Roots I (1999). Functional significance of a $C \rightarrow A$ polymorphism in intron 1 of the cytochrome P-450 CYP1A2 gene tested with caffeine. *Br J Clin Pharmacol* 47, 445–449.

Schmucker DL (1989). Is the rat a suitable model for ageing research? In Woodhouse KW, Yelland C, James OFW, eds. *The Liver: Metabolism and Aging*. Rijswijk, the Netherlands: Eurage, pp. 3–18.

Shedlofsky SI, Israel BC, McClain CJ, Hill DB, Blouin RA (1994). Endotoxin administration to humans inhibits hepatic cytochrome P-450-mediated drug metabolism. *J Clin Invest* 94, 2209–2214.

Shimada T, Yamazaki H, Mimura M et al. (1994). Interindividual variations in human liver cytochrome P-450 enzymes involved in the oxidation of drugs, carcinogens and toxic chemicals: studies with liver microsomes of 30 Japanese and 30 Caucasians. *J Pharmacol Exp Ther* 270, 414–423.

Sindrup SH, Brøsen K (1995). The pharmacogenetics of codeine hypoalgesia. *Pharmacogenetics* 5, 335–346.

Sindrup SH, Brøsen K, Gram LF et al. (1992). The relationship between paroxetine and the sparteine oxidation polymorphism. *Clin Pharmacol Ther* 51, 278–287.

Sjöqvist F (1999). The past, present and future of clinical pharmacology. *Eur J Clin Pharmacol* 55, 553–557.

Sjöqvist F (2000). Drug safety in relation to efficacy: the view of a clinical pharmacologist. *Pharmacol Toxicol* 86(Suppl 1), 30–32.

Steen VM, Lovlie R, MacEwan T et al. (1997). Dopamine D_3-receptor gene variant and susceptibility to tardive dyskinesia in schizophrenic patients. *Mol Psychiatry* 2, 139–145.

Streetman DS, Bertino JS Jr., Nafziger AN (2000a). Phenotyping of drug-metabolizing enzymes in adults: a review of in-vivo cytochrome P-450 phenotyping probes. *Pharmacogenetics* 10, 187–216.

Streetman DS, Bleakley JF, Kim JS et al. (2000b). Combined phenotypic assessment of CYP1A2, CYP2C19, CYP2D6, CYP3A, *N*-acetyltransferase-2, and xanthine oxidase with the "Cooperstown cocktail". *Clin Pharmacol Ther* 68, 375–383.

Svensson JO, Bertilsson L (1999). Rapid high-performance liquid chromatographic method for determination of debrisoquine and 4-hydroxy-debrisoquine in urine for CYP2D6 phenotyping. *Pharmacogenetics* 9, 529–531.

Tanaka E, Hisawa S (1999). Clinically significant pharmacokinetic drug interactions with psycho-active drugs: antidepressants and antipsychotics and the cytochrome P-450 system. *J Clin Pharm Ther* 24, 7–16.

Trenholme GM, Williams RL, Rieckmann KH, Frischer H, Carson PE (1976). Quinine disposition during malaria and during induced fever. *Clin Pharmacol Ther* 19, 459–467.

Vesell ES (1978). Twin studies in pharmacogenetics. *Hum Genet Suppl* 1, 19–30.

Vesell ES (1984). Noninvasive assessment in vivo of hepatic drug metabolism in health and disease. *Ann NY Acad Sci* 428, 293–307.

Vogel F (1959). Moderne Probleme der Human-genetik. *Ergebn Inn Med Kinderheilk* 12, 52–125.

von Moltke LL, Greenblatt DJ (2000). Drug transporters in psychopharmacology – are they important? *J Clin Psychopharmacol* 20, 291–294.

Wacher VJ, Wu CY, Benet LZ (1995). Overlapping substrate specificities and tissue distribution of cytochrome P-450 3A and P-glycoprotein: implications for drug delivery and activity in cancer chemotherapy. *Mol Carcinogen* 13, 129–134.

Walter-Sack I, Klotz U (1996). Influence of diet and nutritional status on drug metabolism. *Clin Pharmacokinet* 31, 47–64.

Watkins LR, Maier SF, Goehler LE (1995). Immune activation: the role of pro-inflammatory cytokines in inflammation, illness responses, and pathological pain states. *Pain* 63, 289–302.

Weber WW (1997). *Pharmacogenetics*. New York: Oxford University Press.

Wentworth JM, Agostini M, Love J, Schwabe JW, Chatterjee VKK (2000). St John's wort, a herbal antidepressant, activates the steroid X receptor. *J Endocrinol* 166, R11–R16.

Wilkinson GR (1997). The effects of diet, aging, and disease-states on presystemic elimination and oral drug bioavailability in humans. *Adv Drug Deliv Rev* 27:129–159.

Wooles WR, Borzelleca JF (1966). Prolongation of barbiturate sleeping time in mice by stimulation of the reticuloendothelial system (RES). *J Reticuloendothel Soc* 3, 41–47.

Yuan R, Parmelee T, Balian JD et al. (1999). In vitro metabolic interaction studies: experience of the food and drug administration. *Clin Pharmacol Ther* 66, 9–15.

9

Pharmacogenetics of chiral psychotropic drugs

Pierre Baumann and Chin B. Eap

University Department of Adult Psychiatry, Prilly-Lausanne, Switzerland

OVERVIEW

A recent editorial on metabolism and chirality in psychopharmacology stated that many investigations do not consider that many psychotropic drugs have one or more chiral centers, introducing steric factors that may make important contributions to their overall pharmacological or toxicological profile (Baker et al., 1994). Moreover, there is an increasing awareness that, besides environmental factors, genetic factors regulate the fate of drugs in the organism, and that polymorphic enzymes such as some cytochrome P-450 isozymes display stereoselectivity toward chiral substrates or in the formation of chiral metabolites from achiral parent compounds. Present knowledge about the pharmacogenetics of metabolism of psychotropic drugs is based mainly on the study of the polymorphic enzymes CYP2D6 and CYP2C19. This chapter summarizes present knowledge on the pharmacology, metabolism, pharmacokinetics, and pharmacogenetics of antidepressants, antipsychotics, and methadone.

Introduction

Numerous psychotropic drugs are chiral and have been introduced as racemates (Table 9.1). Chiral drugs are defined as having one or several asymmetric centers: at least one carbon (or sulfur) atom of their molecule has four different atoms or groups attached to it. For one asymmetric carbon atom, two enantiomers may exist and they are mirror images of each other. Sometimes, confusing terms, signs, and letters are used for their denomination. Polarized light is deviated by such a molecule and the direction of rotation is called levorotatory ($-$; l) (or anticlockwise) or dextrorotatory ($+$; d) (or clockwise). However, because rotation may depend on the solvent used, the absolute configuration of the chiral molecule relative to the enantiomers of glyceraldehyde as standards is indicated by the symbols L and R. Increasingly, for drugs, the symbols R and S are used, according to the Cahn–Ingold–Prelog system for the designation of absolute configurations (Wainer, 1993). Clarification of these terms is essential because, in many of the reports cited in this chapter, different terms are used to designate enantiomers.

Table 9.1. Metabolism of chiral antidepressants by CYP2D6 and CYP2C19

Generic name	Drug introduced as	Pharmacologically active enantiomer (eutomer)[a]	Eutomer: substrate[b] of CYP2D6	CYP2C19
Escitalopram	Enantiomer	(S)-Citalopram	+	++
Citalopram	Racemate	(S)-Citalopram	+	++
Fluoxetine	Racemate	(S)- and (R)-Fluoxetine	++	
Paroxetine	3S-trans-Paroxetine	3S-trans-Paroxetine	++	
Sertraline	(+)-cis-(1S,4S)-Sertraline	(+)-cis-(1S,4S)-Sertraline	−	
Mianserin	Racemate	(S)- and (R)-Mianserin	++	
Mirtazapine	Racemate	(S)- and (R)-Mirtazapine	++	
Trimipramine	Racemate	l-Trimipramine	++	
Bupropion	Racemate		−	
Milnacipran	Racemate		−	
Reboxetine	(R,R)- and (S,S)-Reboxetine	(S,S)-Reboxetine	−	
Venlafaxine	Racemate	(R)-Venlafaxine	++	+ (?)
Viloxazine	Racemate			

Notes:

[a] Some of the distomers may also have some clinically relevant pharmacological activity, which can differ from that of the eutomer quantitatively or qualitatively.

[b] Substrate metabolism: −, not by CYP2D6; +, minor conversion by CYP2D6; ++, CYP2D6 (or CYP2C19) alone or with other forms of cytochrome P-450 plays a major role (some of the distomers may also be substrates of CYP2D6).

Generally, one of the enantiomers is considered to be the eutomer, i.e., the pharmacologically (more) active compound, in contrast to the distomer, which displays a lower pharmacological activity. Stereoselectivity is often expressed as the eudismic ratio (ratio of activities of a pair of enantiomers). However, a particular enantiomer may be an eutomer for one type of pharmacological activity, and the distomer for another type. This classification, therefore, neglects situations in which the enantiomers have either an overlapping pharmacological profile or distinct pharmacological properties that can all contribute to the overall clinical activity, as has been demonstrated for mirtazapine. This is explained by the fact that, in order to exert maximal pharmacological activity, drugs have to fit optimally into receptor molecules, taking account of many steric conditions. Enantiomers of chiral psychotropic drugs may differ by their pharmacokinetic, pharmacogenetic, and pharmacodynamic properties (Baumann and Rochat, 1995; Lane and Baker, 1999; Baumann and Eap, 2001). Knowledge of the activity of enantiomers is, therefore, important for a better understanding of their mechanism of action. Moreover, in the clinical context, it could be relevant to use stereoselective assays for therapeutic drug monitoring.

Most psychotropic drugs have active metabolites (Rudorfer and Potter, 1997, 1999; Sanchez and Hyttel, 1999), and many achiral drugs give rise to chiral metabolites, the formation of which may be stereoselective and depend on the genotype of the patients.

Although genetic polymorphisms have been described for numerous enzymes implicated in drug metabolism (Ingelman-Sundberg, 1998), clinically relevant data about the pharmacogenetics of the metabolism of psychotropic drugs have only been reported in relation to CYP2D6 and CYP2C19, which are isozymes of cytochrome P-450 (Bertilsson and Dahl, 1996; Bertilsson et al., 1997; Ingelman-Sundberg et al., 1999; Coutts and Urichuk, 1999; Dahl and Sjöqvist, 2000; see also Ch. 8). For these two enzymes, genotyping methods are available, but subjects can also be phenotyped for CYP2D6 activity with dextromethorphan, debrisoquine or sparteine, and for CYP2C19 activity with mephenytoin. For CYP2D6, gene amplification has been described, giving rise to high enzyme activity in subjects presenting this genotype. They are generally considered to be ultrarapid metabolizers (UMs) (Bertilsson et al., 1993; Johansson et al., 1993; Lundqvist et al., 1999). Phenotyping procedures do not allow to discriminate between extensive metabolizers (EMs) and UMs.

Cytochrome P-450 enzyme systems implicated in conjugation of drugs and other enzymes have been shown to have steric preferences toward drugs, and this explains differences in the metabolism of enantiomers. The aim of this chapter is to present the pharmacology, metabolism, pharmacokinetics, and pharmacogenetics of chiral psychotropic drugs. The relative lack of adequate studies on their pharmacogenetics may partly be explained by technical difficulties in the stereoselective analysis of these types of compounds (Marzo and Balant, 1996), but also by a lack of availability of pure enantiomers of drugs or their metabolites. Drugs that have been introduced as pure enantiomers (e.g., paroxetine, sertraline) will not be discussed here, but data concerning their pharmacogenetics are summarized elsewhere (see Ch. 8).

Chiral antidepressants

Tricyclic antidepressants and related compounds

Mianserin

Mianserin, a chiral antidepressant, is known for its antagonistic effects at serotonin and presynaptic α_2-adrenoreceptors (Pinder, 1985). (S)-(+)-Mianserin is more potent than the (R)-(−)-enantiomer in displacing α_1- and α_2-ligands, and in inhibiting norepinephrine reuptake in the brain, while both enantiomers have a negligible effect on serotonin (5-HT) and dopamine reuptake. While (R)-(−)-mianserin has no effect on potassium-evoked release of norepinephrine in cortical slices, (S)-$(+)$-mianserin exerts a potent increase in potassium release. After chronic administration, (S)-$(+)$-mianserin but not (R)-$(-)$-mianserin produces functional supersensitivity at α_2-autoreceptors. The antidepressant effect of (S)-$(+)$-mianserin, in contrast to that of the (R)-enantiomer, is also evident from animal experiments using behavioral tests. Interestingly, (S)-$(+)$-mianserin has a higher affinity for 5-HT$_1$ and 5-HT$_2$ receptors than (R)-$(-)$-mianserin, but stereo-selectivity is inversed with regard to their affinity for 5-HT$_3$ receptors.

These observations suggest that (S)-mianserin is probably the eutomer. In humans, it is more readily 8-hydroxylated and N-oxidized than the distomer (R)-mianserin, but the latter is preferentially N-desmethylated (Koyama et al., 1996; Chow et al., 1999). 8-Hydroxylation of mianserin is controlled by CYP2D6, CYP2B6, CYP3A4, and CYP1A2, and N-desmethylation by CYP2B6, CYP2C19, CYP3A4, CYP1A2, and CYP2D6 (Koyama et al., 1996). CYP3A4 does not appear to metabolize preferentially the enantiomers of mianserin (Eap et al., 1999). CYP2D6 more readily 8-hydroxylates (S)-mianserin but it also N-desmethylates (R)-mianserin (Chow et al., 1999). In Japanese patients (of whom probably none was a poor metabolizer (PM)) treated with mianserin, the mean ratio of (S)-/(R)-mianserin was 1.9, but it varied interindividually between 0.5 and 4.8 (Tybring et al., 1995). In EMs of dextromethorphan (CYP2D6), the ratio of (S)-/(R)-mianserin and (S)-/(R)-desmethylmianserin was 1–4.6 and 0.19–0.64, respectively (Eap et al., 1994). In CYP2D6-phenotyped healthy volunteers treated with a single oral dose of mianserin, the area under the plasma concentration versus time curve (AUC) of (S)-$(+)$-mianserin but not (R)-$(-)$-mianserin correlated significantly with the metabolic ratio of debrisoquine; the ratio of the AUCs of (S)-/(R)-mianserin was higher in PMs than in EMs (Dahl et al., 1994). Desmethylmianserin is also metabolized by CYP2D6 but none of these compounds is apparently a substrate of CYP2C19. However, in clinical steady-state conditions, concentrations of the enantiomers of mianserin and desmethylmianserin did not differ spectacularly between homozygous and heterozygous EMs (CYP2D6), but the only PM had the highest ratio (S)-/(R)-mianserin in plasma (Eap et al., 1998). The hypothesis that (S)-mianserin rather than (R)-mianserin is a substrate of CYP2D6 is strengthened by an interaction study (Yasui et al., 1997) with depressive patients treated with mianserin and thioridazine, which is a strong CYP2D6 inhibitor (Baumann et al., 1992). Coadministration of thioridazine (40 mg/day) for 1 week doubled plasma concentrations of (S)-mianserin but was without effect on (R)-mianserin. Interestingly, thioridazine increased also both (S)-desmethylmianserin and (R)-desmethylmianserin. In conclusion, (S)-mianserin and (R)-desmethylmianserin, but not (R)-mianserin, have to be considered to be stereoselectively metabolized by CYP2D6.

In carriers of the *CYP2D6*10* allele, CYP2D6 activity is decreased. This explains why Japanese carriers of a *CYP2D6*10* allele had higher plasma concentrations of

(S)-mianserin. Interestingly, they were more likely to respond to the drug than depressive patients with a wild type/wild type genotype (Mihara et al., 1997).

Mirtazapine

Mirtazapine (ORG 3770) (Holm and Markham, 1999) differs from mianserin only by a N-atom replacing a C-atom in the ring structure. It is also a potent α_2-adrenoceptor antagonist, with little affinity for α_1-adrenoceptors and it does not block norepinephrine reuptake. (S)-(+)-Mirtazapine is several times more potent than (R)-(−)-mirtazapine as an α_2-autoreceptor antagonist, as shown both by neurochemical and by behavioral experiments. Only (S)-(+)- but not (R)-(−)-mirtazapine increases serotonergic raphe cell firing and 5-HT release (David and Wilde, 1996). During a chronic treatment, (R)-(−)-mirtazapine had a more pronounced effect on 5-HT$_{1A}$ receptor function than does the (S)-(+)-enantiomer. Mirtazapine also acted as an antagonist at 5-HT$_2$- and 5-HT$_3$-receptors (Holm and Markham, 1999). (R)-(−)-Mirtazapine is thought to be responsible for α_2-adrenergic heteroreceptor and 5-HT$_3$-receptor blockade (Kooyman et al., 1994; McGrath et al., 1998). Chronic treatment with (R)-(−)- but not with (S)-(+)-mirtazapine led to a decrease in the density of β_1-adrenoceptors in frontal cortex, as already described for many other antidepressant treatments, and both enantiomers decreased the density of 5-HT$_2$-receptors (McGrath et al., 1998). However, the authors conclude that, in their model, none of the enantiomers seems to be more active than racemic mirtazapine.

In patients of unknown phenotype who were treated with mirtazapine, plasma (+)-mirtazapine and (−)-mirtazapine concentrations varied interindividually between <5 and 69 ng/ml and 13 and 88 ng/ml, respectively; generally, trough levels of (+)-mirtazapine were one third or half of those of (−)-mirtazapine (Dodd et al., 2000). Dahl et al. (1997b) summarized the published studies on the pharmacokinetics of mirtazapine and its metabolism by cytochrome P-450. In vitro, using microsomes from cells expressing single cytochrome P-450 isoforms, the formation of 8-hydroxymirtazapine occurs mainly by CYP2D6, and to some extent by CYP1A2, while CYP3A4 is mainly implicated in N-2 desmethylation and N-2 oxidation. More recently, it was calculated, on the basis of in vitro experiments in human liver microsomes, that the overall metabolism of mirtazapine was 55% by 8-hydroxylation, 35% by N-desmethylation, and 10% by N-oxidation, at an extrapolated in vivo mirtazapine concentration of 2 μmol/l in liver. In these conditions, CYP2D6 contributed 65% of the hydroxylation of mirtazapine, CYP1A2 30% (Störmer et al., 2000a), while CYP2C8 and CYP2C9 contributed less than 10% to the overall mirtazapine biotransformation (Störmer et al., 2000a). At higher concentrations of mirtazapine (250 μmol/l), the contribution of CYP2D6 decreased to 20% and that of CYP1A2 increased to 50% (Störmer et al., 2000b).

Recently, an in vitro study with cDNA transfected human lymphoblast microsomes expressing CYP isoforms showed a preferential metabolism of (+)-mirtazapine by CYP2D6 in comparison with (−)-mirtazapine, while CYP1A2 and CYP3A4 show low activity towards both mirtazapine enantiomers. Moreover, CYP2C9 and CYP2C19 do not seem to be involved in the metabolism of this antidepressant (Dodd et al., 2001). It was, therefore, unexpected to find, in a panel study with healthy human volunteers, that the pharmacokinetics of mirtazapine and its N-desmethylated metabolite, as examined by an achiral analytical procedure, did not differ between PMs and EMs of debrisoquine (Dahl et al., 1997a). In humans (S)-(+)-mirtazapine has a half-life of 9.9 ± 3.1 h and is mainly metabolized by 8-hydroxylation followed by glucuronidation, while (R)-(−)-mirtazapine has a half-life of 18.0 ± 2.5 h and is preferentially and reversibly N-glucuronidated as a quaternary ammonium glucuronide. After admininistration of racemic mirtazapine, the elimination of (R)-mirtazapine occurs at a similar rate in EMs and PMs (CYP2D6), but (S)-mirtazapine has a longer half-life in PMs (18.8 ± 4.7 h) than in EMs ($13.2 \pm 4.$ h), as observed using a stereoselective method (Delbressine et al., 1998; Timmer et al., 2000).

Trimipramine

The pharmacology of the chiral antidepressant trimipramine differs from that of other typical tricyclic drugs in that its activity as a norepinephrine and serotonin reuptake inhibitor is weak, but its affinity for 5-HT$_2$- and dopamine receptors is pronounced. In this sense, trimipramine presents some similarities with atypical antipsychotics such as clozapine. L-Trimipramine rather than D-trimipramine has to be considered as the pharmacologically active compound, as shown in in vitro studies. L-Trimipramine displaced ligands at dopamine D$_1$, D$_2$ binding sites in striatal areas in pig brain and 5-HT$_2$ binding sites in cerebral cortex of rat more potently than did D-trimipramine (Gross et al., 1991). L-Trimipramine, inhibited potassium-induced uptake of calcium in rat brain synaptosomes more potently than did D-trimipramine (Beauchamp et al., 1992); however, depending on the model used and the brain region examined there is a loss of stereoselectivity (Lavoie et al., 1994). Preliminary studies suggest that in accordance with its pharmacological profile, trimipramine may have some therapeutic effect in acute schizophrenia (Eikmeier et al., 1990; Berger and Gastpar, 1996).

Trimipramine is N-desmethylated to desmethyltrimipramine and both compounds are hydroxylated. Measurements of plasma steady-state concentrations of the enantiomers of trimipramine and its metabolites suggest that the metabolism of this antidepressant occurs stereoselectively in patients (Eap et al., 1992a). The demonstration that trimipramine is a CYP2D6 substrate was made in a study with healthy volunteers in whom plasma half-life of trimipramine was doubled after coadministration of the strong CYP2D6 inhibitor quinidine. Moreover, electro-encephalograph modifications produced by trimipramine were more pronounced and longer lasting after addition of quinidine (Eap et al., 1992b). CYP2D6 hydroxylates trimipramine stereoselectively, as shown in a study with depressive patients presenting a CYP2D6 and CYP2C19 EM phenotype and treated with 300–400 mg/day trimipramine for 5 weeks. CYP2D6 was implicated in the 2-hydroxylation of ʟ-trimipramine, ʟ-desmethyltrimipramine and ᴅ-desmethyltrimipramine, but not of ᴅ-trimipramine; CYP2C19 with some stereoselectivity responsible for N-desmethylation of ᴅ-trimipramine. The only patient with a genetic deficiency of CYP2D6 (PM of dextromethorphan) had the highest dose- and weight-corrected concentrations of ʟ- and ᴅ-desmethyltrimipramine, while the only PM of mephenytoin (CYP2C19 deficiency) had the highest ʟ- and ᴅ-trimipramine concentrations (Eap et al., 2000a). CYP3A4 contributes also to the biotransformation of trimipramine.

Selective serotonin reuptake inhibitors

Citalopram

The chiral antidepressant drug citalopram is a potent and the most selective serotonin reuptake inhibitor (SSRI) available (Hyttel et al., 1995; Sanchez and Hyttel, 1999) (Fig. 9.1). In vitro 5-HT uptake inhibition studies with rat brain synaptosomes and behavioral experiments demonstrated that both the (S)-(+)-enantiomers of citalopram and, to a minor extent, its main metabolite desmethylcitalopram have to be considered as the pharmacologically active agents (Hyttel et al., 1992; Owens et al., 2001). Eudismic ratios for 5-HT uptake inhibition are 167 and 6.6 for citalopram and desmethylcitalopram, respectively. (S)-(+)-Citalopram (escitalopram), in contrast to (R)-(−)-citalopram, potentiated the effect of ʟ-5-hydroxytryptophan (ʟ-5-HTP) in mice (Hyttel et al., 1992). In depressive patients treated with citalopram, (S)-citalopram plasma concentrations were generally lower than those of (R)-citalopram (Rochat et al., 1995a,b; Bondolfi et al., 1996, 2000; Sidhu et al., 1997). Mean serum elimination half-life was found to be 47 h and 35 h for (R)-(−)- and (S)-(+)-citalopram, respectively, in healthy subjects with an EM phenotype (CYP2D6) (Sidhu et al., 1997). Escitalopram represents the first example in psychopharmacology of a "chiral switch," i.e., the introduction of a single enantiomeric form of a drug previously available in a racemate form (Tucker, 2000). Some clinical studies confirm the clinical efficacy of escitalopram in depression (Montgomery et al., 2001).

In vitro studies with human liver microsomes and complementary DNA (cDNA)-expressed human cytochrome P-450 isoforms, combined with in vitro interaction studies, showed that CYP2C19, CYP3A4, and CYP2D6 catalyzed

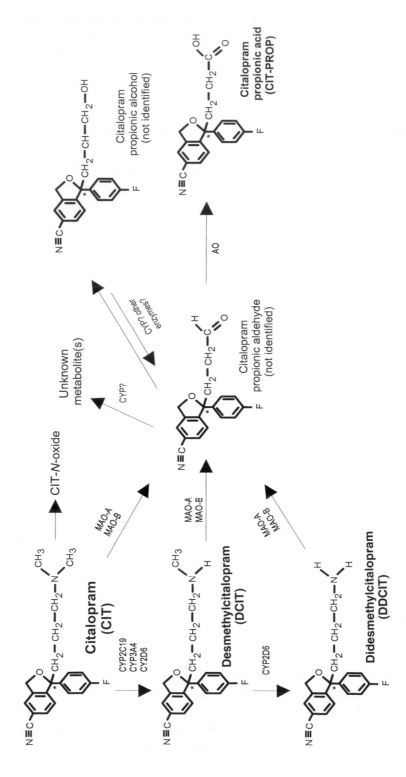

Fig.9.1.   Metabolic pathways of citalopram. MAO, monoamine oxidase; CYP, cytochrome P-450; AO, aldehyde oxidase.

N-desmethylation of citalopram to N-desmethylcitalopram (Kobayashi et al., 1997), while CYP1A2, CYP2A6, CYP2B6, CYP2C9, CYP2D6, and CYP2E1 were not involved (Fig. 9.1). In a panel study with CYP2C19 and CYP2D6 phenotyped healthy subjects, CYP2C19 controlled citalopram N-desmethylation to desmethyl-citalopram while CYP2D6 was involved in desmethylation of the latter to dides-methylcitalopram (Sindrup et al., 1993). In steady-state conditions, plasma concentration ratios of citalopram/desmethylcitalopram were found to be significantly higher in patients presenting a PM phenotype than in EMs (CYP2C19) (Baumann et al., 1996). However, in vitro, CYP2C19 and CYP3A4 show stereoselectivity towards (S)-citalopram, while some authors do not agree about a stereoselective activity of CYP2D6 towards citalopram (Rochat et al., 1997; Olesen and Linnet, 1999). Recent in vitro studies using human liver microsomes and expressed cytochromes carried out with escitalopram confirm the important role of CYP2C19, CYP2D6 and CYP3A4 in its N-demethylation (von Moltke et al., 2001).

Monoamine oxidase A and B (MAO-A and MAO-B) isoforms in human liver (Rochat et al., 1998) and in human brain (Kosel et al., 2002) metabolized citalo-pram stereoselectively (Fig. 9.1), but the pharmacogenetics of the metabolism of citalopram by polymorphic MAO has not yet been studied (Shih et al., 1999).

Fluoxetine

The chiral antidepressant fluoxetine and its metabolite, norfluoxetine, are both selective 5-HT uptake inhibitors. However, (S)-norfluoxetine (seproxetine) (Robertson et al., 1991) is considerably more potent than (R)-norfluoxetine as an eudismic ratio of 22 was found for 5-HT uptake inhibition in in vitro synaptoso-mal preparations (Wong et al., 1993). (S)-Norfluoxetine was also more potent than the (R)-enantiomer in blocking the in vivo depletion of 5-HT by p-chloroamphet-amine (Fuller et al., 1992) and it had a higher affinity than (R)-fluoxetine for opioid σ_1 receptors (Narita et al., 1996). (S)- and (R)-Fluoxetine, in contrast, do not notably differ in their inhibition of paroxetine binding at 5-HT uptake carrier sites (Wong et al., 1993) and in 5-HT uptake inhibition in vitro, in vivo, and ex vivo (Wong et al., 1990a). In contrast, (R)-norfluoxetine is more potent than the (S)-enantiomer in displacing ligands to the 5-HT_{1C} and 5-HT_2-receptors (Wong et al., 1993). As an anorectic agent in animals, (S)-fluoxetine is slightly more potent than (R)-fluoxetine (Wong et al., 1990b). Therefore, (S)- and (R)-fluoxetine and (S)-norfluoxetine, by their 5-HT uptake inhibition potency, are considered as the pharmacologically relevant enantiomers, in contrast to the less potent (R)-norfluoxetine.

After administration of the enantiomers of norfluoxetine, (S)-norfluoxetine was eliminated faster from rat brain than (R)-norfluoxetine (Fuller et al., 1992).

Separate injections (10 mg/kg intraperitoneally) of the enantiomers of fluoxetine in mice led to a longer persistance of 5-HT uptake inhibition by (S)-fluoxetine, despite the fact that its metabolite (S)-norfluoxetine is eliminated more rapidly than (R)-norfluoxetine after (R)-fluoxetine administration (Fuller and Snoddy, 1993). This is explained by the relative weakness of (R)-norfluoxetine as a 5-HT uptake inhibitor.

In vitro studies, using achiral analytical procedures, of N-desmethylation of fluoxetine to norfluoxetine in human liver microsomes and in microsomes from transfected cell lines expressing different cytochrome P-450 isoforms suggest that CYP2C9 is the main enzyme implicated. CYP2C19 and CYP3A4 play a minor role, while CYP2D6 is seemingly not implicated (von Moltke et al., 1997). However, in vitro, there is a significant correlation between microsomal immunodetectable CYP2D6 in human liver and N-desmethylation rates of (R)- and (S)-fluoxetine to their respective norfluoxetine metabolites. By comparison, CYP2D6 concentrations correlated better with bufuralol 1'-hydroxylation, which is a specific indicator for CYP2D6 activity, and quinidine only partly inhibited desmethylation of fluoxetine enantiomers. This suggests that other enzymes in addition to CYP2D6 largely contribute to the formation of norfluoxetine (Stevens and Wrighton, 1993).

Different results were obtained in vivo, using an achiral method, in a panel study with healthy human volunteers who were administered a single dose of fluoxetine. In this study, the terminal half-life of fluoxetine was considerably longer in PMs (76 h) than in EMs (24 h) of debrisoquine. The observation that partial metabolic clearance of fluoxetine into norfluoxetine was 10 times smaller in PMs than in EMs suggests that N-desmethylation of fluoxetine is at least partially controlled by CYP2D6 (Hamelin et al., 1996). Another panel study demonstrated clear evidence of a stereoselective elimination of fluoxetine and norfluoxetine by CYP2D6. A single oral dose of 60 mg fluoxetine was administered to six EMs and six PMs of debrisoquine and the elimination kinetics of fluoxetine, norfluoxetine and their enantiomers were measured over a period of 6 weeks. Oral clearance (plasma half-life) of (R)- and (S)-fluoxetine was 3.0 l/h (9.5 days) and 17 l/h (6.1 days), respectively, in the PMs, while the corresponding figures were 36 l/h (2.6 days) and 40 l/h (1.1 days) in the EMs (Fjordside et al., 1999). The plasma elimination half-lives of (R)- and (S)-norfluoxetine were the same in EMs (5.5 days), but were 6.9 days and 17.4 days, respectively in PMs (Fjordside et al., 1999). These data suggest that, at least partly, CYP2D6 controls the biotransformation of (R)- and of (S)-fluoxetine, and (S)-norfluoxetine, but not of (R)-norfluoxetine. However, a recent study with patients during a 3-week treatment with fluoxetine (20 mg/day) showed that only plasma concentrations of (S)-fluoxetine (Fig. 9.2a) and (S)-norfluoxetine (Fig. 9.3a) differed significantly between PMs and EMs, whereas those of (R)-fluoxetine (Fig. 9.2b) and (R)-norfluoxetine (Fig. 9.3b) did not (Eap et al., 2001a).

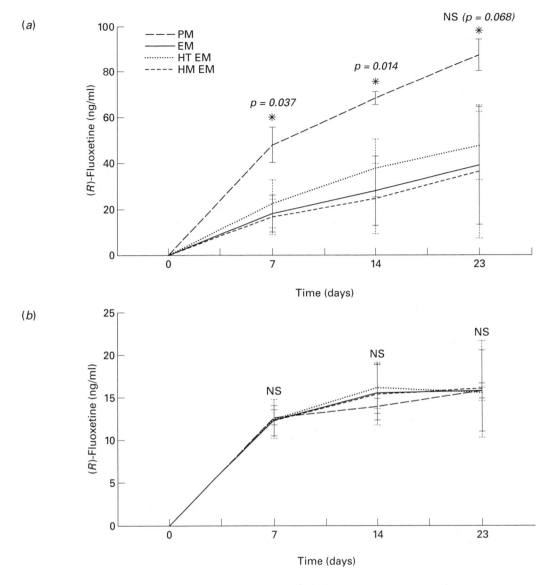

Fig. 9.2.   Trough plasma concentrations of (S)-fluoxetine (a) and (R)-fluoxetine (b) measured in three CYP2D6 poor metabolizers (PM), eight extensive metabolizers (EM), two heterozygous extensive metabolizers (HT EM) and six homozygous extensive metabolizers (HM EM) after administration of 20 mg racemic fluoxetine during 7, 14, and 23 days. The p values are given for comparison of poor metabolizers with extensive metabolizers; NS, not significant.

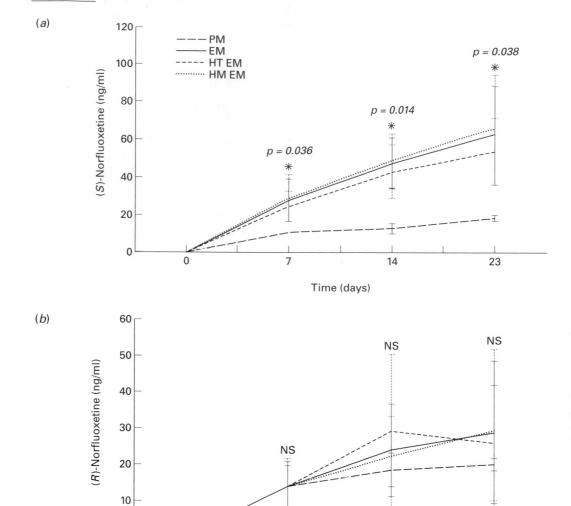

Fig. 9.3.   Trough plasma concentrations of (S)-norfluoxetine (a) and (R)-norfluoxetine (b) measured in three CYP2D6 poor metabolizers (PM), eight extensive metabolizers (EM), two heterozygous extensive metabolizers (HT EM) and six homozygous extensive metabolizers (HM EM) after administration of 20 mg racemic fluoxetine during 7, 14, and 23 days. The p values are given for comparison of poor metabolizers with extensive metabolizers; NS, not significant.

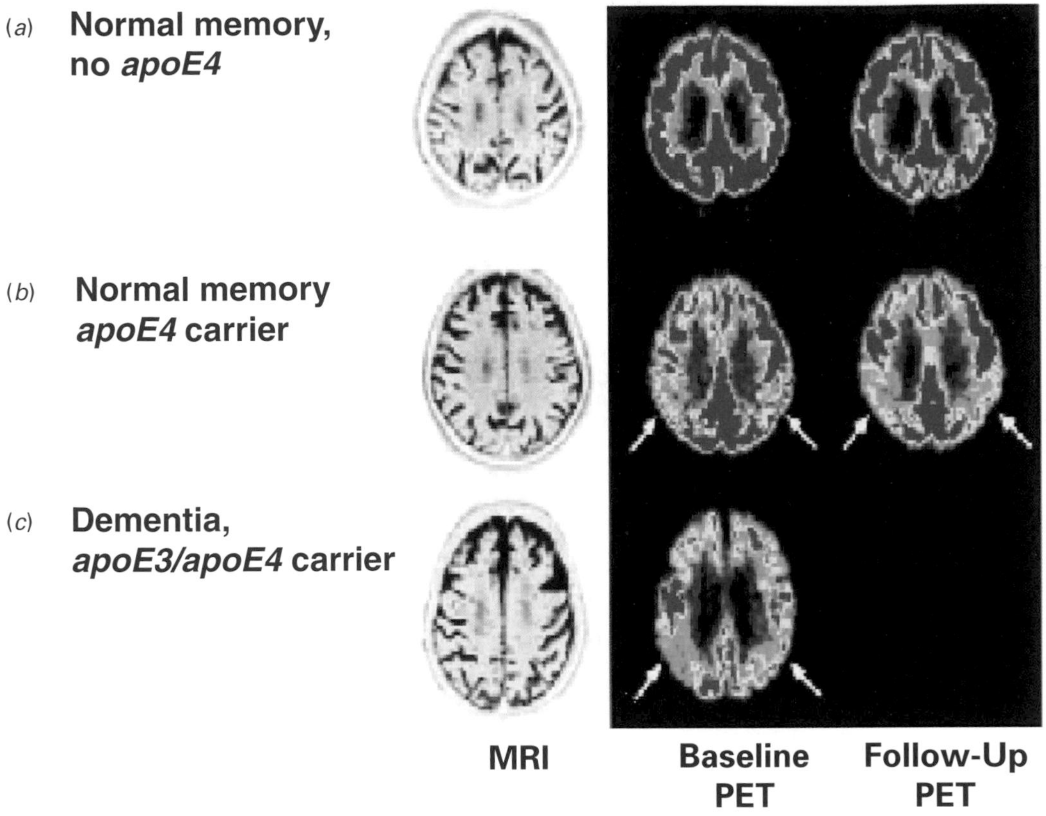

**(a) Normal memory,
no *apoE4***

**(b) Normal memory
apoE4 carrier**

**(c) Dementia,
apoE3/apoE4 carrier**

MRI   **Baseline
PET**   **Follow-Up
PET**

Fig. 19.1.   Examples of positron emission tomographic (PET) metabolic images coregistered with the magnetic resonance images (MRI) for three women: (*a*) 81-year-old with normal memory and apolipoprotein E (ApoE) *apoE3* genotype; (*b*) 76-year-old heterozygote with normal memory and carrying *apoE3/apoE4*; (*c*) 79-year-old with dementia of Alzheimer's disease carrying *apoE3/apoE4*. At baseline, inferior parietal cortical metabolism was 15% lower in (*b*) and 21% lower in (*c*) compared with the nondemented subject without ApoE4 (*a*). The demented woman also had more widespread metabolic dysfunction owing to disease progression. Two year follow-up scans showed minimal parietal decline for the woman without ApoE4 (*a*) but bilateral parietal cortical decline for the nondemented woman with ApoE4 (*b*) who also met clinical criteria for mild Alzheimer's disease at this follow-up. MRI scans were within normal limits. (Reproduced with permission from Small et al., 2000.)

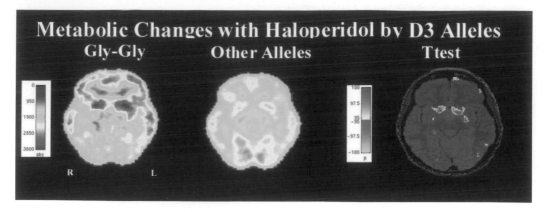

Fig. 19.2. Brain metabolism following haloperidol treatment by dopamine D_3 genotype (*DRD3*). The first two positron emission tomographic (PET) scans represent absolute metabolism following haloperidol treatment for 5 weeks. The flame scale indicates absolute glucose metabolism (mg/min per 100 g tissue): the red colors indicate more activity. The third scan (on the right) indicates the areas of significant difference between the subjects homozygous for *DRD3*gly and those carrying *DRD3*gly-ser or *DRD3*ser-ser (see text) following haloperidol treatment, superimposed on a magnetic resonance image. The flame scale is a p map in which red colors indicate areas where subjects have significantly higher metabolism following haloperidol treatment compared with other alleles, while blue colors indicate areas that have significantly lower metabolism. The patients with $D_{3gly-gly}$ have statistically significant metabolic increases in basal ganglia metabolism following haloperidol compared with patients carrying the other alleles.

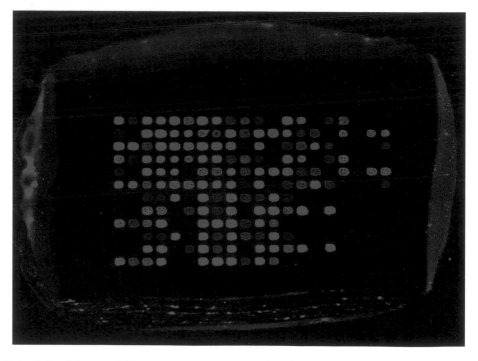

Fig. 19.3. Output of a chip containing 20 000 genes. An example of a SNP (single nucleotide polymorphism) chip with allelic typing on an individual's DNA is depicted. The brightly colored circles indicate which SNPs the individual's DNA contains. Gene chips the size of a thumbnail containing more than 20 000 genes are now available and can be combined with DNA from white blood cells to genotype an individual. The allelic typing can be used to predict clinical response and side effects to pharmacological treatment. (Courtesy of Dr Leena Peltonen.)

Recent antidepressants

Venlafaxine

Venlafaxine is an antidepressant characterized by its reuptake inhibiting properties for both 5-HT and norepinephrine in rat brain synaptosomes. The (R)-$(+)$-enantiomer is somewhat more potent than (S)-$(-)$-venlafaxine in inhibiting 5-HT reuptake, while there is little stereoselectivity with regard to norepinephrine reuptake inhibition. In this regard, nothing is known about the stereoselectivity concerning the active metabolite O-desmethylvenlafaxine, the plasma concentrations of which may exceed those of the parent compound in clinical steady-state conditions (Holliday and Benfield, 1995). After a single dose of venlafaxine in healthy volunteers, there was apparently no stereoselective elimination of venlafaxine enantiomers (Wang et al., 1992), but other studies are needed to confirm this finding (see below).

In vivo evidence for the metabolism of venlafaxine by CYP2D6 was shown in a panel study with healthy volunteers, who were treated with a single dose of venlafaxine. Mean oral clearance of venlafaxine was four times lower in PMs (23 ± 8 l/h) than in EMs (100 ± 62 l/h). Coadministration of the CYP2D6 inhibitor did not modify venlafaxine clearance in PMs but reduced it in EMs to the value observed in PMs (Lessard et al., 1999). In a plasma concentrations versus clinical effectiveness study with venlafaxine in CYP2D6-genotyped depressive patients, none of the three PMs (CYP2D6) were responders (Veefkind et al., 2000). In comparison with EMs, they showed some decreased biotransformation of venlafaxine to O-desmethylvenlafaxine and an increase of N-desmethylation to the minor metabolite N-desmethylvenlafaxine. In vitro studies with human liver microsomes confirmed that CYP2D6 and CYP3A4 control venlafaxine O-desmethylation and venlafaxine N-desmethylation, respectively (Otton et al., 1996). However, the question of stereoselectivity of this biotransformation appears to be complicated by the fact that, at high saturating concentrations, (R)-$(+)$-venlafaxine is mainly O-desmethylated, while at lower, non-saturating concentrations, the stereoselectivity is reversed. At any dose studied, (S)-$(-)$-venlafaxine is faster N-desmethylated than (R)-$(+)$-venlafaxine (Otton et al., 1996). In a clinical case study with an EM patient medicated with venlafaxine and other drugs differing by their CYP2D6-inhibiting potency, a similar dose-dependent influence of CYP2D6 in the stereoselective biotransformation of venlafaxine was observed (Eap et al., 2000b). Recent studies suggest that, besides CYP2C9 and CYP3A4, CYP2C19 may also contribute to N-desmethylation of venlafaxine, but no observations concerning stereoselectivity of this reaction are available (Fukuda et al., 2000).

Other recent chiral antidepressants

For other chiral antidepressants, such as bupropion, milnacipran, viloxazine, very few data are available with regard to a possible role of CYP2D6 or CYP2C19 in their metabolism or to some stereoselectivity in their fate (Rotzinger et al., 1999).

Milnacipran does not seem to have active metabolites, and the role of cytochrome P-450 in their formation is thought to be negligible (Puozzo and Leonard, 1996). The elimination of D-milnacipran seems to be slower than that of L-milnacipram (Spencer and Wilde, 1998).

Reboxetine, a selective norepinephrine reuptake-inhibiting antidepressant (Holm and Spencer, 1999), carries two asymmetric centers. A mixture of (R,R)-$(-)$- and (S,S)-$(+)$-reboxetine has been introduced in clinical practice. (S,S)-$(+)$-Reboxetine is more potent in inhibiting norepinephrine reuptake but plasma concentrations of (R,R)-$(-)$-reboxetine are generally twice as high as those of (S,S)-$(+)$-reboxetine, which is eliminated faster, as shown in single dose studies with healthy volunteers (Fleishaker et al., 1999). CYP3A4 is probably the main enzyme regulating their metabolism (Herman et al., 1999), while in vitro (Herman et al., 1999) and in vivo (Avenoso et al., 1999) studies suggest that reboxetine is not a substrate of CYP2D6, nor of other forms of cytochrome P-450.

No data are available on the role of cytochrome P-450 and on the stereoselective metabolism of the enantiomers of the antidepressant viloxazine (Rotzinger et al., 1999).

$(+)$-Bupropion is more potent than $(-)$-bupropion in uptake inhibition of norepinephrine and dopamine (Musso et al., 1993). CYP2B6 (Hesse et al., 2000) but not CYP2D6 (Pollock et al., 1996) appears to be the enzyme responsible for the hydroxylation of bupropion to its main metabolite, as shown by achiral methods.

Achiral antidepressants with chiral metabolites: amitriptyline and nortriptyline

The achiral antidepressant amitriptyline, its N-desmethylated metabolite nortriptyline and their 10-hydroxylated metabolites are all norepinephrine and 5-HT reuptake inhibitors (Nordin and Bertilsson, 1995). CYP2D6 is the main enzyme responsible for their hydroxylation, while CYP2C19, CYP3A4, CYP2C9, and CYP2D6 all contribute to N-desmethylation of amitriptyline to nortriptyline (Balant-Georgia et al., 1982; Mellström et al., 1983; Baumann et al., 1986; Breyer-Pfaff et al., 1992; Dahl et al., 1996; Schmider et al., 1996; Coutts et al., 1997; Ghahramani et al., 1997; Olesen and Linnet, 1997).

The introduction of a hydroxy group in the amitriptyline and nortriptyline molecules gives rise to two geometric isomers (E and Z) and four stereoisomers for each compound (Nusser et al., 1988) (Fig. 9.4), which differ in their molecular dynamics (Heimstad et al., 1992). They may undergo stereoselective glucuronidation before they are renally excreted, as shown for hydroxynortriptyline

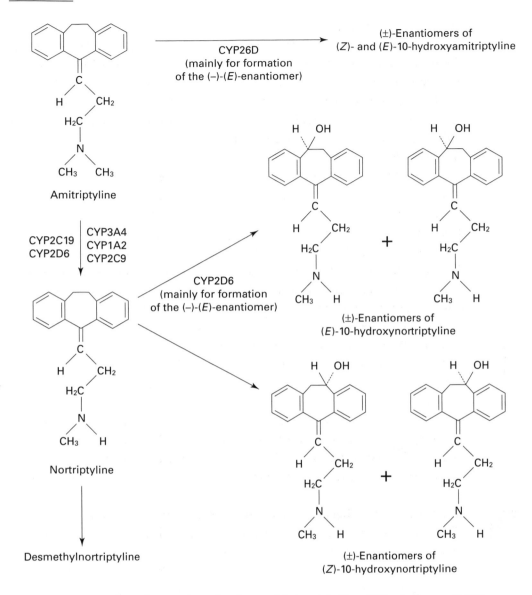

Fig. 9.4. Metabolic pathways of nortriptyline to chiral metabolites. CYP, cytochrome P-450.

(Dahl-Puustinen et al., 1989). After administration of nortriptyline or amitriptyline in humans, there is a preferential formation of (E)-(−)-10-hydroxymetabolites (Mellström et al., 1981; Young et al., 1988; Breyer-Pfaff et al., 1992). Pilot studies suggest that (E)-10-hydroxynortriptyline could be an antidepressant (Nordin et al., 1991). In the rat, (Z)-hydroxynortriptyline seems to be more cardiotoxic than (E)-hydroxynortriptyline.

Several reports demonstrate that, to a major extent, formation of (E)-$(-)$-10-hydroxyamitriptyline and (E)-$(-)$-10-hydroxynortriptyline, but not that of the other hydroxy metabolites, is stereoselectively controlled by CYP2D6 (Mellström et al., 1981; Dahl et al., 1991; Breyer-Pfaff et al., 1992; Pfandl et al., 1992; Nordin and Bertilsson, 1995). As an example, coadministration of the potent CYP2D6 inhibitor quinidine with nortriptyline decreased urinary excretion of (E)-$(-)$-10-hydroxynortriptyline but not that of (E)-$(+)$-10-hydroxynortriptyline, (Z)-$(+)$- and (Z)-$(-)$-10-hydroxynortriptyline in humans (Pfandl et al., 1992).

Antipsychotics

Chiral antipsychotics

Many antipsychotics are substrates of CYP2D6. At higher doses, which generally give rise to higher plasma concentrations, the risk for adverse effects of the extrapyramidal type increases. Therefore, many recent studies have dealt with the relationship between neuroleptic-induced movement disorders (Spina et al., 1992; Arthur et al., 1995; Andreassen et al., 1997; Armstrong et al., 1997; Chong, 1997; Sajjad, 1997) or a neuroleptic malignant syndrome (Ueno et al., 1996) and the CYP2D6 pharmacogenetic status of the patients.

Thioridazine

Thioridazine is one of the most frequently prescribed chiral antipsychotics, even though its use is related to the highest risks for cardiotoxicity (Reilly et al., 2000). This risk increases with increasing plasma concentrations of both the parent compound and some of its metabolites (Hartigan-Go et al., 1996). The metabolism of thioridazine is complicated by the fact that it is a racemic compound and because a second asymmetric center is introduced by its sulfoxidation to the active metabolite mesoridazine (thioridazine 2-sulfoxide) (Fig. 9.5). It is then further metabolized to sulforidazine (thioridazine 2-sulfone), which, together with thioridazine and mesoridazine, is also introduced as an antipsychotic agent in some countries. Thioridazine-ring sulfoxide (thioridazine 5-sulfoxide) is another important but cardiotoxic metabolite with four enantiomers (Gottschalk et al., 1978). Finally, the tertiary amine thioridazine and the sulfoxidized metabolites are also N-desmethylated.

(R)-$(+)$-Thioridazine (Patrick and Singletary, 1991) increased the turnover of dopamine in the striatum of rat brain 4.1 times more potently than (S)-$(-)$-thioridazine, despite both enantiomers being present in similar concentrations in the brain after peripheral administration of the enantiomers of thioridazine. In contrast, $(-)$-thioridazine is slightly more potent than the $(+)$-enantiomer in producing catalepsy and it seems also to be more toxic at higher doses. However, racemic

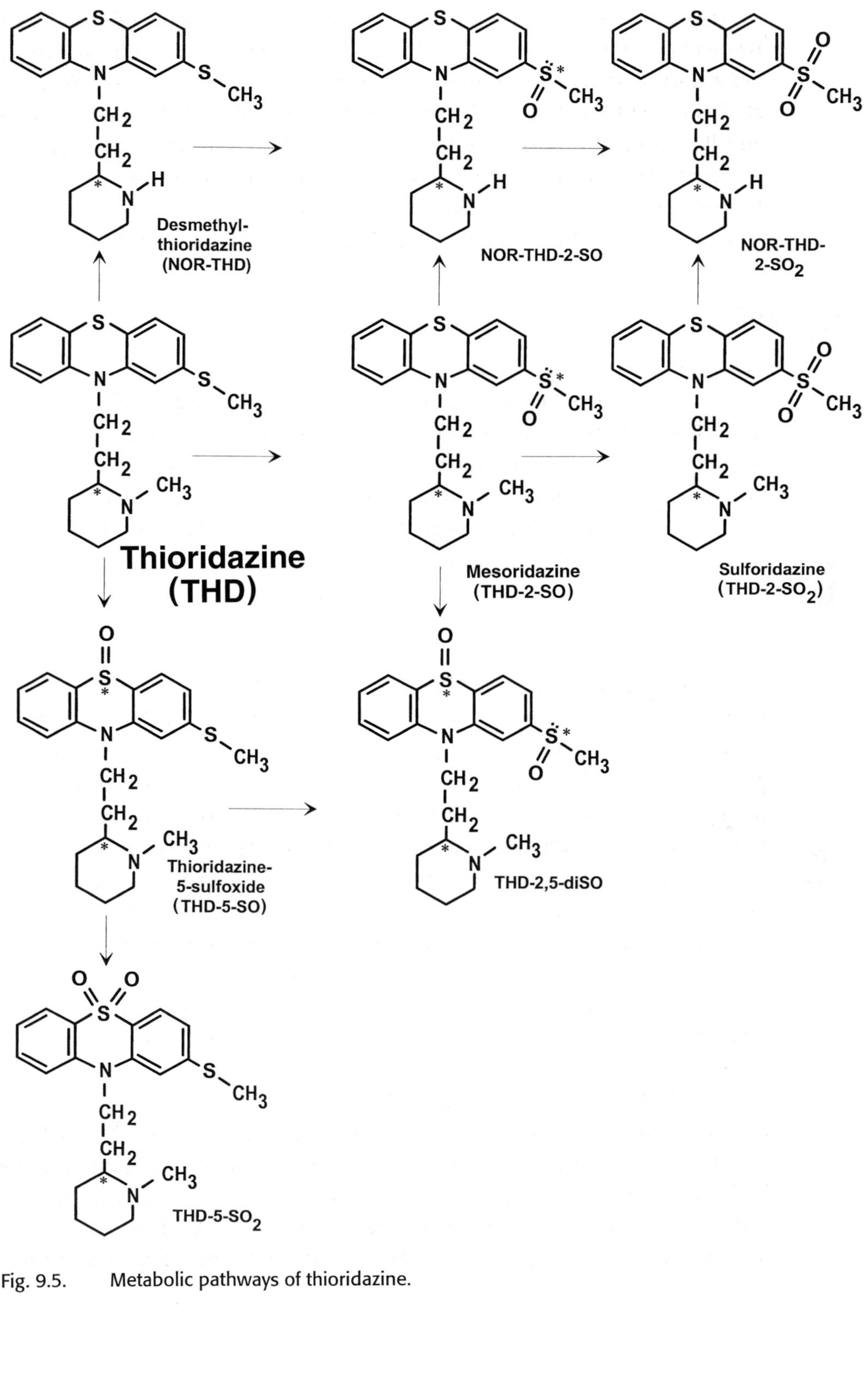

Fig. 9.5.   Metabolic pathways of thioridazine.

thioriazine appeared to be more cataleptogenic than either enantiomer alone, at equimolar concentrations. Both D_1 and D_2 receptors seem to be involved in this behavioral effect. Indeed, in vitro studies with rat forebrain tissues showed that the K_i-ratios ((+)-thioridazine/(−)-thioridazine) with regard to the affinity for different receptors were 2.71, 0.0978, 4.46, and 1.06 for D_2 receptors, D_1 receptors, α_1-adrenoceptors and muscarinic receptors, respectively (Svendsen et al., 1988). From these data, it seems difficult to define the eutomer clearly, as (+)-thioridazine and (−)-thioridazine appeared to be rather selective D_2 antagonists and D_1 antagonists, respectively. With regard to the risk of cardiotoxic effects, thioridazine 5-sulfoxide rather than thioridazine itself could be the arrhythmogenic compound, but this effect is probably not stereoselective (Hale and Poklis, 1996).

The pharmacogenetics of the metabolism of thioridazine in CYP2D6-phenotyped subjects was studied, using achiral methods, for the drug and its metabolites mesoridazine, sulforidazine, and thioridazine 5-sulfoxide (von Bahr et al., 1991). According to this study, the formation of mesoridazine, and partly that of the ring sulfoxide from thioridazine, appears to be controlled by CYP2D6. In a clinical study, only 1 of 25 schizophrenic and debrisoquine-phenotyped patients was a PM. They were treated with 400 mg/day thioridazine for 10 days, but the patient with a genetic CYP2D6 deficiency suffered from severe adverse effects and was a nonresponder. His daily dose of thioridazine was lowered to 100 mg, but in comparison with the other patients, his plasma levels of thioridazine were highest and those of mesoridazine and sulforidazine were lowest (Meyer et al., 1990). It was proposed to use the ratio of mesoridazine/thioridazine in plasma as a marker of CYP2D6 activity in subjects "phenotyped" with thioridazine (Llerena et al., 2000).

In a clinical study comparing the clinical effect of moclobemide/placebo versus moclobemide/thioridazine in 21 patients phenotyped with dextromethorphan and mephenytoin, the patients received orally 100 mg/day thioridazine for 14 days (Eap et al., 1996). Thioridazine, thioridazine 2-sulfoxide, thioridazine 2-sulfone, and thioridazine 5-sulfoxide in plasma were determined by a stereoselective high-pressure liquid chromatographic method. The results suggested that CYP2D6 is involved in the formation of two of the four enantiomers of mesoridazine, namely (S)-thioridazine 2-sulfoxide (a fast eluting band (FE)) and (R)-thioridazine 2-sulfoxide (a slow eluting band (SE)) and probably also in that of (S)-thioridazine 5-sulfoxide (FE), and (R)-thioridazine 5-sulfoxide (SE). (This denomination of stereoisomers is explained by the unavailability of pure enantiomers (Eap et al., 1991).) Unexpectedly, thioridazine was also found to be metabolized by CYP2C19. CYP2C19 activity, as measured with the mephenytoin test, correlated significantly with plasma concentrations of thioridazine, thioridazine 2-sulfone, thioridazine 2-sulfoxide (FE and SE) and thioridazine 5-sulfoxide (FE and SE).

Sulpiride

Both by affinity studies for the D_2 receptor and by behavioral tests in animals, (S)-(−)-sulpiride rather than (R)-(+)-sulpiride appears to be the antipsychotically active enantiomer (Rognan et al., 1990). The (S)-(−)-enantiomer is eight times more potent than racemic sulpiride in producing stimulation of prolactin in rats (Kakigi et al., 1992). (S)-(−)-Sulpiride, also called levosulpiride, has been introduced as an antipsychotic drug. After intravenous administration of racemic sulpiride, there is no evidence for stereoselective pharmacokinetics of this drug, the metabolism of which is probably not submitted to a genetically polymorphic metabolism (Wagstaff et al., 1994). After oral administration of sulpiride, the ratio L/D-sulpiride in serum of schizophrenic patients was <1 (range 0.66–0.97), in steady-state conditions (Müller et al., 2001).

Achiral antipsychotics with chiral metabolites

Haloperidol

The most important metabolic pathways of haloperidol implicate its glucuroconjugation and formation of reduced haloperidol, which is then partly backoxidized to the parent compound. CYP2D6 and CYP3A4 contribute to hydroxylation and dealkylation of haloperidol and reduced haloperidol (Kudo and Ishizaki, 1999). Reduced haloperidol lacks potent D_2 antagonism, but it has a high affinity for σ-receptors (Walker et al., 1990; Quirion et al., 1992; Bowen et al., 1995). Panel studies with haloperidol-treated PMs and EMs of debrisoquine showed that plasma half-life of haloperidol was significantly longer in PMs and its clearance was lower than in EMs (Llerena et al., 1992a). In the same study, plasma concentrations of reduced haloperidol were found to be higher in PMs than in EMs (Llerena et al., 1992b). Other authors excluded a leading role for CYP2D6 in the reversible interconversion between haloperidol and reduced haloperidol (Young et al., 1993), but, apparently, CYP3A4 could be involved in oxidation of reduced haloperidol (Kudo and Odomi, 1998; Pan et al., 1998).

All of these studies do not take account of the fact that reduced haloperidol has a chiral center, the enantiomers of which differ stereoselectively in their in vitro formation in human brain, liver, and blood: (S)-(−)-reduced haloperidol is formed almost exclusively (about 99%) (Eyles and Pond, 1992). However, in patients taking haloperidol, about 25% of reduced haloperidol excreted in urine is the (R)-enantiomer (Eyles et al., 1998). No data are available on the stereoselective backoxidation of reduced haloperidol to haloperidol, especially with regard to the contribution of cytochrome P-450.

Risperidone

The atypical antipsychotic drug risperidone and its chiral metabolite 9-hydroxyrisperidone are both potent D_2 and 5-HT$_2$ antagonists. Therefore, the sum of risperidone and 9-hydroxyrisperidone is considered to constitute the "active moiety" (Huang et al., 1993). This hypothesis is supported by proton emission tomographic studies carried out with PMs and EMs (CYP2D6) (Nyberg et al., 1995), but the antipsychotic effect of 9–hydroxyrisperidone given alone has not been evaluated in clinical studies.

In vitro studies with recombinant human cytochrome P-450 forms show that risperidone is metabolized both by CYP2D6 and by CYP3A4 to 9-hydroxyrisperidone. At least in the rat, CYP3A4 inducers can increase formation of 9-hydroxyrisperidone severalfold (Fang et al., 1999). Plasma half-life of risperidone was about 3 h and 22 h in EMs and PMs of debrisoquine, respectively, as shown in a small panel study. Plasma half-life of 9-hydroxyrisperidone is very similar in EMs and PMs (20–27 h) and that of the "active moiety" is also close to 20 h (Huang et al., 1993). In another study, dose-corrected concentrations of the "active moiety" were not higher in PMs than in EMs (Olesen et al., 1998). Therefore, it is thought that there is little need for adapting risperidone dose as a function of the pharmacogenetic status. However, a recent case study suggested that CYP2D6-deficient patients do not tolerate risperidone treatment well, despite "normal active moiety" concentrations (Bork et al., 1999). Data collected in UMs showed that dose-corrected plasma concentrations of risperidone were particularly low, compared with PMs and heterozygous EMs (Scordo et al., 1999). None of these studies considered the possibility that there are seemingly differences in the stereoselective hydroxylation of risperidone by CYP2D6 and CYP3A4 (L. Bertilsson et al., unpublished data), and there are no data available on the pharmacological profile of the individual enantiomers of 9-hydroxyrisperidone. However, in a recent in vitro study with human liver microsomes and recombinantly expressed enzymes, (+)-hydroxyrisperidone formation was found to be higher than that of the (−)-enantiomer. CYP2D6 preferentially formed (+)-hydroxyrisperidone, while CYP3A4 mainly catalyzed risperidone biotransformation to (8)-hydroxyrisperidone (Yasui-Furukori et al., 2001). In extensive metabolizers by CYP2D6, plasma concentrations of (+)-hydroxyrisperidone were higher than those of the (−)-hydroxy-enantiomer, in patients treated with risperidone.

Tranquillizers and hypnotic agents

Oxazepam

Oxazepam, a chiral anxiolytic drug, is mainly metabolized by glucuronidation. A stereoselective analysis of the metabolism of oxazepam appears to be a very difficult task as its enantiomers racemize spontaneously and rapidly (Yang and Lu, 1989).

Zopiclone

Zopiclone is a racemic hypnotic drug, of which the (−)-enantiomer has a 50 times higher affinity for the benzodiazepine receptor-binding site than the (+)-enantiomer (Blaschke et al., 1993). After a single dose of zopiclone, peak concentrations of (+)-zopiclone in plasma of volunteers appeared to be higher than those of (−)-zopiclone. The former enantiomer is eliminated more slowly than the (−)-enantiomer (Fernandez et al., 1993). No pharmacogenetic data are available, as CYP3A4 and CYP2C8, in contrast to CYP2C19 and CYP2D6, are found to metabolize zopiclone in vitro (Becquemont et al., 1999). The chiral benzodiazepines zopiclone and oxazepam represent examples of compounds that, at least to some extent, undergo spontaneous racemization in aqueous solutions (Fernandez et al., 1995).

Stimulants and illicit drugs

The metabolism of dexfenfluramine was examined in a panel study with healthy CYP2D6-phenotyped subjects after administration of a dose of 30 mg of this anorectic drug (Gross et al., 1996). Mean plasma AUC was about twice as high in PMs than in EMs. The apparent oral clearance was higher in EMs, but there was no difference between the groups for renal clearance. The data suggest that CYP2D6 mediates N-desmethylation of dexfenfluramine to nordexfenfluramine as apparent nonrenal clearance of the metabolite was considerably lower in PMs than in EMs. PMs were more likely to experience serotonergic adverse effects, such as nausea and vomiting, than were EMs.

Amphetamine derivatives such as MDMA (Ecstasy) and MDE (Eve) present a chiral structure. Their main metabolic pathways are desmethylation and N-dealkylation. Besides other forms of cytochrome P-450, CYP2D6 contributes to their metabolism (Maurer et al., 2000). Very little is known about the stereoselective metabolism and pharmacogenetics of these and other illicit drugs (Quinn et al., 1997).

Opioid substituents

Methadone, an opioid agonist, is used for the treatment of opioid dependence. In vitro binding experiments have shown that the necessary concentration of (R)- or l-methadone to inhibit by 50% the binding of [³H]-naloxone to whole rat brain homogenate is 10 times less than that of (S)- or d-methadone (Pert and Snyder, 1973). A 10-fold difference of affinity has also been found between the two enantiomers for the μ_1 and μ_2 receptors (concentrations for 50% inhibition (IC_{50}) of 3.0 and 6.9 nmol/l, respectively, for (R)-methadone and 26.4 and 88 nmol/l, respectively, for (S)-methadone for the μ_1- and μ_2-receptors, respectively), using preparations from bovine caudate nucleus (Kristensen et al., 1995). In humans, (R)-methadone is about 50 times as analgesically potent as the (S)-form (Scott et al., 1948) and it accounts for the large majority, if not all, of opioid effects of racemic methadone. Both enantiomers of methadone exhibit similar affinities for the N-methyl-D-aspartate (K_i of 3.4 and 7.4 µmol/l for (R)- and (S)-methadone, respectively) (Gorman et al., 1997).

Methadone is extensively metabolized in the body, mainly at the level of the liver, but probably also by intestinal CYP3A4. Its main metabolite (2-ethylidene-1, 5-dimethyl-3,3-diphenylpyrrolidine or EDDP) is inactive: it is formed by N-desmethylation and subsequent spontaneous cyclization (Sullivan and Due, 1973). However, urinary excretion of methadone plus EDDP only accounted for 17–57% of the given dose and, in addition to methadone, seven metabolites (including EDDP) have been isolated and identified in urine (Ånggard et al., 1975). In vitro and in vivo studies have shown that CYP3A4 (Iribarne et al., 1996, 1998; Moody et al., 1997; Foster et al., 1999) and CYP2D6 (Yue et al., 1995; Eap et al., 1997) are involved in methadone metabolism. Other isoforms, such as CYP1A2 (Yue et al., 1995; Eap et al., 1997), CYP2C9 (Foster et al., 1999), and CYP2C19 (Foster et al., 1999) might also be implicated, but their in vivo relevance has still to be demonstrated. Methadone N-desmethylation, which is mediated principally by CYP3A4, is probably not stereoselective (Foster et al., 1999). However, CYP2D6, which is probably involved in another metabolic pathway, might preferentially metabolize the (R)-enantiomer, as suggested by in vivo inhibition studies with fluoxetine and paroxetine, two strong CYP2D6 inhibitors, and by a panel study with CYP2D6 PMs and EMs, which showed a significantly lower partial metabolic clearance of (R)-methadone in the PMs compared with the EMs (Yue et al., 1995; Eap et al., 1997). In a very recent clinical study, the pharmacokinetic and pharmacogenetic data obtained suggest that the CYP2D genotype partly codetermines clinical response to methadone. (R)-Methadone plasma concentrations were significantly lower in ultrarapid metabolizers than in poor metabolizers (Eap et al., 2001b). A detailed review on the pharmacokinetics, pharmacodynamics, and pharmacogenetics of methadone can be found elsewhere (Eap et al., 2001).

Conclusions

Chiral psychotropic drugs represent a useful tool for the study of neuropharmacological mechanisms and of the function of metabolizing enzymes. Many widely used drugs are introduced as racemic compounds, the enantiomers of which clearly differ in their pharmacology, metabolism, and pharmacogenetics. With regard to their fate in the organism, this presentation is centered exclusively on metabolic aspects. It should be considered, however, that other aspects such as drug plasma protein binding may also be genetically and stereoselectively determined. As an example, the enantiomers of methadone stereoselectively bind to α_1-acid glycoprotein, of which one particular variant (A) preferentially binds basic drugs (Eap et al., 1990; Eap and Baumann, 1990; Jolliet-Riant et al., 1998). This genetically determined variant A may partially control transfer of drugs from blood to brain.

This overview confirms that the use of achiral analytical procedures can lead to erroneous conclusions with regard to the pharmacogenetics of metabolism of psychotropic drugs (Nation, 1994), as shown by the example of mirtazapine. As a consequence, pharmacogenetic studies should include the use of stereoselective methods to analyze the fate of chiral psychotropic drugs in the organism.

Acknowledgements

We gratefully acknowledge the editorial assistance of Mrs C. Bertschi, Mrs K. Powell, and the bibliographic help of Mrs E. Ponce.

REFERENCES

Andreassen OA, MacEwan T, Gulbrandsen A-K, McCreadie RG, Steen VM (1997). Nonfunctional CYP2D6 alleles and risk for neuroleptic-induced movement disorders in schizophrenic patients. *Psychopharmacology* 131, 174–179.

Armstrong M, Daly AK, Blennerhassett R, Ferrier N, Idle JR (1997). Antipsychotic drug-induced movement disorders in schizophrenics in relation to CYP2D6 genotype. *Br J Psychiatry* 170, 23–26.

Arthur H, Dahl M-L, Siwers B, Sjöqvist F (1995). Polymorphic drug metabolism in schizophrenic patients with tardive dyskinesia. *J Clin Psychopharmacol* 15, 211–216.

Avenoso A, Facciolì G, Scordo MG, Spina E (1999). No effect of the new antidepressant reboxetine on CYP2D6 activity in healthy volunteers. *Ther Drug Monit* 21, 577–579.

Ånggard E, Gunne L-M, Holmstrand J, McMahon RE, Sandberg C-G, Sullivan HR (1975). Disposition of methadone in methadone maintenance. *Clin Pharmacol Ther* 17, 258–266.

Baker GB, Coutts RT, Holt A (1994). Metabolism and chirality in psychopharmacology. *Biol Psychiatry* 36, 211–213.

Balant-Georgia AE, Schulz P, Dayer P et al. (1982). Role of the oxidation polymorphism on blood and urine concentrations of amitriptyline and its metabolites in man. *Arch Psychiatr Nervenkrank* 232, 215–222.

Baumann P, Eap CB (2001). Enantiomeric antidepressant drugs should be considered on individual merit. *Hum Psychopharmacol Clin Exp* 16, S85–S92.

Baumann P, Rochat B (1995). Comparative pharmacokinetics of selective serotonin reuptake inhibitors: a look behind the mirror. *Int Clin Psychopharmacol* 10(Suppl 1), 15–21.

Baumann P, Jonzier-Perey M, Koeb L, Küpfer A, Tinguely D, Schöpf J (1986). Amitriptyline pharmacokinetics and clinical response: II. Metabolic polymorphism assessed by hydroxylation of debrisoquine and mephenytoin. *Int Clin Psychopharmacol* 1, 102–112.

Baumann P, Meyer JW, Amey M et al. (1992). Dextromethorphan and mephenytoin phenotyping of patients treated with thioridazine or amitriptyline. *Ther Drug Monit* 14, 1–8.

Baumann P, Nil R, Souche A et al. (1996). A double-blind, placebo-controlled study of citalopram with and without lithium in the treatment of therapy-resistant depressive patients: a clinical, pharmacokinetic, and pharmacogenetic investigation. *J Clin Psychopharmacol* 16, 307–314.

Beauchamp G, Lavoie P-A, Elie R (1992). Effect of trimipramine on depolarization-induced and Na^+–Ca^{2+} exchange-induced ^{45}calcium uptake in synaptosomes from the cortex of the rat brain. *Neuropharmacology* 31, 229–234.

Becquemont L, Mouajjah S, Escaffre O, Beaune P, Funck-Brentano C, Jaillon P (1999). Cytochrome P-450 3A4 and 2C8 are involved in zopiclone metabolism. *Drug Metab Dispos* 27, 1068–1073.

Berger M, Gastpar M (1996). Trimipramine: a challenge to current concepts on antidepressives. *Eur Arch Psychiatry Clin Neurosci* 246, 235–239.

Bertilsson L, Dahl M-L (1996). Polymorphic drug oxidation – relevance to the treatment of psychiatric disorders. *CNS Drugs* 5, 200–223.

Bertilsson L, Dahl M-L, Sjöqvist F et al. (1993). Molecular basis for rational megaprescribing in ultrarapid hydroxylators of debrisoquine. *Lancet* 341, 63.

Bertilsson L, Dahl M-L, Tybring G (1997). Pharmacogenetics of antidepressants: clinical aspects. *Acta Psychiatr Scand* 96(Suppl 391), 14–21.

Blaschke G, Hempel G, Müller WE (1993). Preparative and analytical separation of the zopiclone enantiomers and determination of their affinity to the benzodiazepine receptor binding site. *Chirality* 5, 419–421.

Bondolfi G, Chautems C, Rochat B, Bertschy G, Baumann P (1996). Non-response to citalopram in depressive patients: pharmacokinetic and clinical consequences of a fluvoxamine augmentation. *Psychopharmacology* 128, 421–425.

Bondolfi G, Lissner C, Kosel M, Eap CB, Baumann P (2000). Fluoxetine augmentation in citalopram nonresponders: pharmacokinetic and clinical consequences. *Int J Neuropsychopharmacol* 3, 55–60.

Bork JA, Rogers T, Wedlund PJ, de Leon J (1999). A pilot study on risperidone metabolism: the role of cytochromes P-450 2D6 and 3A. *J Clin Psychiatry* 60, 469–476.

Bowen WD, Bertha CM, Vilner BJ, Rice KC (1995). CB-64D and CB-184: ligands with high sigma(2) receptor affinity and subtype selectivity. *Eur J Pharmacol* 278, 257–260.

Breyer-Pfaff U, Pfandl B, Nill K et al. (1992). Enantioselective amitriptyline metabolism in patients phenotyped for two cytochrome P-450 isozymes. *Clin Pharmacol Ther* 52, 350–358.

Chong S-A (1997). Tardive dyskinesia and CYP2D6 polymorphism in Chinese. *Br J Psychiatry* 171, 586.

Chow T, Hiroi T, Imaoka S, Chiba K, Funae Y (1999). Isoform-selective metabolism of mianserin by cytochrome P-450 2D. *Drug Metab Dispos* 27, 1200–1204.

Coutts RT, Urichuk LJ (1999). Polymorphic cytochromes P-450 and drugs used in psychiatry. *Cell Mol Neurobiol* 19, 325–354.

Coutts RT, Bach MV, Baker GB (1997). Metabolism of amitriptyline with CYP2D6 expressed in a human cell line. *Xenobiotica* 27, 33–47.

Dahl M-L, Sjöqvist F (2000). Pharmacogenetic methods as a complement to therapeutic monitoring of antidepressants and neuroleptics. *Ther Drug Monit* 22, 114–117.

Dahl-Puustinen ML, Dumont E, Bertilsson L (1989). Glucuronidation of E-10-hydroxynortriptyline in human liver, kidney, and intestine. *Drug Metab Dispos* 17, 433–436.

Dahl M-L, Nordin C, Bertilsson L (1991). Enantioselective hydroxylation of nortriptyline in human liver microsomes, intestinal homogenate, and patients treated with nortriptyline. *Ther Drug Monit* 13, 189–194.

Dahl M-L, Tybring G, Elwin C-E et al. (1994). Stereoselective disposition of mianserin is related to debrisoquine hydroxylation polymorphism. *Clin Pharmacol Ther* 56, 176–183.

Dahl M-L, Bertilsson L, Nordin C (1996). Steady-state plasma levels of nortriptyline and its 10-hydroxy metabolite: relationship to the CYP2D6 genotype. *Psychopharmacology* 123, 315–319.

Dahl M-L, Voortman G, Alm C et al. (1997a). *In vitro* and *in vivo* studies on the disposition of mirtazapine in humans. *Clin Drug Invest* 13, 37–46.

Dahl M-L, Voortman G, Alm C et al. (1997b). *In vitro* and *in vivo* studies on the disposition of mirtazapine in humans. *Clin Drug Invest* 13, 37–46.

Dalén P, Dahl M-L, Bernal Ruiz ML, Nordin J, Bertilsson L (1998). 10-Hydroxylation of nortriptyline in white persons with 0, 1, 2, 3, and 13 functional *CYP2D6* genes. *Clin Pharmacol Ther* 63, 444–452.

David R, Wilde MI (1996). Mirtazapine – a review of its pharmacology and therapeutic potential in the management of major depression. *CNS Drugs* 5, 389–402.

Delbressine LPC, Moonen MEG, Kaspersen FM et al. (1998). Pharmacokinetics and biotransformation of mirtazapine in human volunteers. *Clin Drug Invest* 15, 45–55.

Dodd S, Burrows GD, Norman TR (2000). Chiral determination of mirtazapine in human blood plasma by high-performance liquid chromatography. *J Chromatogr B* 748, 439–443.

Dodd S, Boulton DW, Burrows GD, de Vane CL, Norman TR (2001). In vitro metabolism of mirtazapine enantiomers by human cytochrome P450 enzymes. *Hum Psychopharmacol* 6, 541–544.

Eap CB, Baumann P (1990). Pharmacogenetics of drug binding to albumin and alpha1-acid glycoprotein. In Belpaire F, Bogaert M, Tillement J-P, Verbeeck R, eds. *Plasma Binding of Drugs and its Consequences.* Ghent: Academia Press, pp. 69–82.

Eap CB, Cuendet C, Baumann P (1990). Binding of *d*-methadone, *l*-methadone, and *dl*-methadone to proteins in plasma of healthy volunteers: role of the variants of alpha1-acid glycoprotein. *Clin Pharmacol Ther* 47, 338–346.

Eap CB, Souche A, Koeb L, Baumann P (1991). Light-induced racemization: artifacts in the analysis of the diastereoisomeric pairs of thioridazine 5-sulfoxide in the plasma and urine of patients treated with thioridazine. *Ther Drug Monit* 13, 356–362.

Eap CB, Koeb L, Holsboer-Trachsler E, Baumann P (1992a). Plasma levels of trimipramine and metabolites in four patients: determination of the enantiomer concentrations of the hydroxy metabolites. *Ther Drug Monit* 14, 380–385.

Eap CB, Laurian S, Souche A et al. (1992b). Influence of quinidine on the pharmacokinetics of trimipramine and on its effect on the waking EEG of healthy volunteers – a pilot study on two subjects. *Neuropsychobiology* 25, 214–220.

Eap CB, Powell K, Campus-Souche D et al. (1994). Determination of the enantiomers of mianserin, desmethylmianserin, and 8-hydroxymianserin in the plasma and urine of mianserin-treated patients. *Chirality* 6, 555–563.

Eap CB, Guentert TW, Schäublin-Loidl M et al. (1996). Plasma levels of the enantiomers of thioridazine, thioridazine 2-sulfoxide, thioridazine 2-sulfone, and thioridazine 5-sulfoxide in poor and extensive metabolizers of dextromethorphan and mephenytoin. *Clin Pharmacol Ther* 59, 322–331.

Eap CB, Bertschy G, Powell K, Baumann P (1997). Fluvoxamine and fluoxetine do not interact in the same way with the metabolism of the enantiomers of methadone. *J Clin Psychopharmacol* 17, 113–117.

Eap CB, de Mendonça Lima CA et al. (1998). Steady state concentrations of the enantiomers of mianserin and desmethylmianserin in poor and in homozygous and heterozygous extensive metabolizers of debrisoquine. *Ther Drug Monit* 20, 7–13.

Eap CB, Yasui N, Kaneko S, Baumann P, Powell K, Otani K (1999). Effects of carbamazepine coadministration on plasma concentrations of the enantiomers of mianserin and of its metabolites. *Ther Drug Monit* 21, 166–170.

Eap CB, Bender S, Gastpar M et al. (2000a). Steady state plasma levels of the enantiomers of trimipramine and of its metabolites in CYP2D6-, CYP2C19- and CYP3A4/5-phenotyped patients. *Ther Drug Monit* 22, 209–214.

Eap CB, Bertel-Laubscher R, Zullino D, Amey M, Baumann P (2000b). Marked increase of venlafaxine enantiomer concentrations as a consequence of metabolic interactions: a case report. *Pharmacopsychiatry* 33, 112–115.

Eap CB, Bondolfi G, Zullino D, Savary L, Powell K, Kosel M, Baumann P (2001a). Concentrations of the enantiomers of fluoxetine and norfluoxetine after multiple dose of fluoxetine in cytochrome P-4502D6 poor and extensive metabolizers. *J Clin Psychopharmacol* 21, 330–334.

Eap CB, Broly F, Mino A et al. (2001b). Cytochrome P450 *2D6* genotype and methadone steady-state concentrations. *J Clin Psychopharmacol* 21, 229–234.

Eikmeier G, Muszynski K, Berger M, Gastpar M (1990). High-dose trimipramine in acute schizophrenia. *Pharmacopsychiatry* 23, 212–214.

Eyles DW, Pond SM (1992). Stereospecific reduction of haloperidol in human tissues. *Biochem Pharmacol* 44, 867–8712.

Eyles DW, McGrath JJ, Stedman TJ, Pond SM (1998). Chirality of reduced haloperidol in humans. *Eur Neuropsychopharmacol* 8, 127–129.

Fang J, Bourin M, Baker GB (1999). Metabolism of risperidone to 9-hydroxyrisperidone by human cytochromes P-450 2D6 and 3A4. *Naunyn-Schmiedeberg's Arch Pharmacol* 359, 147–151.

Fernandez C, Maradeix V, Gimenez F, Thuillier A, Farinotti R (1993). Pharmacokinetics of zopiclone and its enantiomers in Caucasian young healthy volunteers. *Drug Metab Dispos* 21, 1125–1128.

Fernandez C, Gimenez F, Mayrargue J, Thuillier A, Farinotti R (1995). Degradation and racemization of zopiclone enantiomers in plasma and partially aqueous solutions. *Chirality* 7, 267–271.

Fjordside L, Jeppesen U, Eap CB, Powell K, Baumann P, Brøsen K (1999). The stereoselective metabolism of fluoxetine in poor and extensive metabolizers of sparteine. *Pharmacogenetics* 9, 55–60.

Fleishaker JC, Mucci M, Pellizzoni C, Poggesi I (1999). Absolute bioavailability of reboxetine enantiomers and effect of gender on pharmacokinetics. *Biopharm Drug Dispos* 20, 53–57.

Foster DJR, Somogyi AA, Bochner F (1999). Methadone N-demethylation in human liver microsomes: lack of stereoselectivity and involvement of CYP3A4. *Br J Clin Pharmacol* 47, 403–412.

Fukuda T, Nishida Y, Zhou Q, Yamamoto I, Kondo S, Azuma J (2000). The impact of the CYP2D6 and CYP2C19 genotypes on venlafaxine pharmacokinetics in a Japanese population. *Eur J Clin Pharmacol* 56, 175–180.

Fuller RW, Snoddy HD (1993). Drug concentrations in mouse brain at pharmacologically active doses of fluoxetine enantiomers. *Biochem Pharmacol* 45, 2355–2358.

Fuller RW, Snoddy HD, Krushinski JH, Robertson DW (1992). Comparison of norfluoxetine enantiomers as serotonin uptake inhibitors in vivo. *Neuropharmacology* 31, 997–1000.

Ghahramani P, Ellis SW, Lennard MS, Ramsay LE, Tucker GT (1997). Cytochromes P-450 mediating the N-demethylation of amitriptyline. *Br J Clin Pharmacol* 43, 137–144.

Gorman AL, Elliott KJ, Inturrisi CE (1997). The *d*- and *l*-isomers of methadone bind to the noncompetitive site on the N-methyl-D-aspartate (NMDA) receptor in rat forebrain and spinal cord. *Neurosci Lett* 223, 5–8.

Gottschalk LA, Dinovo E, Biener R, Nandi BR (1978). Plasma concentrations of thioridazine metabolites and EEG abnormalities. *J Pharm Sci* 67, 155–157,

Gross G, Xin X, Gastpar M (1991). Trimipramine: pharmacological reevaluation and comparison with clozapine. *Neuropharmacology* 30, 1159–1166.

Gross AS, Phillips AC, Rieutord A, Shenfield GM (1996). The influence of the sparteine/debrisoquine genetic polymorphism on the disposition of dexfenfluramine. *Br J Clin Pharmacol* 41, 311–317.

Hale P, Poklis A (1996). Thioridazine cardiotoxicity. *Clin Toxicol* 34, 127–128.

Hamelin BA, Turgeon J, Vallée F, Bélanger P-M, Paquet F, Lebel M (1996). The disposition of fluoxetine but not sertraline is altered in poor metabolizers of debrisoquine. *Clin Pharmacol Ther* 60, 512–521.

Hartigan-Go K, Bateman DN, Nyberg G, Martensson E, Thomas SHL (1996). Concentration-related pharmacodynamic effects of thioridazine and its metabolites in humans. *Clin Pharmacol Ther* 60, 543–553.

Heimstad E, Edvardsen O, Dahl SG (1992). Molecular structure and dynamics of the four 10-hydroxynortriptyline isomers. *Neuropsychopharmacology* 6, 137–144.

Herman BD, Fleishaker JC, Brown MT (1999). Ketoconazole inhibits the clearance of the enantiomers of the antidepressant reboxetine in humans. *Clin Pharmacol Ther* 66, 374–379.

Hesse LM, Venkatakrishnan K, Court MH et al. (2000). CYP2B6 mediates the in vitro hydroxylation of bupropion: potential drug interactions with other antidepressants. *Drug Metab Dispos* 28, 1176–1183.

Holliday SM, Benfield P (1995). Venlafaxine – a review of its pharmacology and therapeutic potential in depression. *Drugs* 49, 280–294.

Holm KJ, Spencer CM (1999). Reboxetine – a review of its use in depression. *CNS Drugs* 12, 65–83.

Holm KJ, Markham A (1999). Mirtazapine – a review of its use in major depression. *Drugs* 57, 607–631.

Huang M-L, van Peer A, Woestenborghs R et al. (1993). Pharmacokinetics of the novel antipsychotic agent risperidone and the prolactin response in healthy subjects. *Clin Pharmacol Ther* 54, 257–268.

Hyttel J, Arnt J, Sanchez C (1995). The pharmacology of citalopram. *Rev Contemp Pharmacother* 6, 271–285.

Hyttel J, Bøgesø KP, Perregaard J, Sanchez C (1992). The pharmacological effect of citalopram resides in the (S)-(+)-enantiomer. *J Neural Transm* 88, 157–160.

Ingelman-Sundberg M (1998). Functional consequences of polymorphism of xenobiotic metabolising enzymes. *Toxicol Lett* 102 – 103, 155–160.

Ingelman-Sundberg M, Oscarson M, McLellan RA (1999). Polymorphic human cytochrome P-450 enzymes: an opportunity for individualized drug treatment. *Trends Pharmacol Sci* 20, 342–349.

Iribarne C, Berthou F, Baird S et al. (1996). Involvement of cytochrome P-450 3A4 enzyme in the N-demethylation of methadone in human liver microsomes. *Chem Res Toxicol* 9, 365–373.

Iribarne C, Picart D, Dréano Y, Berthou F (1998). In vitro interactions between fluoxetine or fluvoxamine and methadone or buprenorphine. *Fundam Clin Pharmacol* 12, 194–199.

Johansson I, Lundqvist E, Bertilsson L, Dahl M-L, Sjöqvist F, Ingelman-Sundberg M (1993). Inherited amplification of an active gene in the cytochrome P-450 *CYP2D* locus as a cause of ultrarapid metabolism of debrisoquine. *Proc Natl Acad Sci, USA* 90, 11825–11829.

Jolliet-Riant P, Boukef MF, Duché J-C, Simon N, Tillement JP (1998). The genetic variant A of human alpha 1-acid glycoprotein limits the blood to brain transfer of drugs it binds. *Life Sci* 62, PL219–PL226.

Kakigi T, Maeda K, Tanimoto K, Kaneda H, Shintani T (1992). Effect of substituted benzamides on prolactin secretion in the rat. *Biol Psychiatry* 31, 827–831.

Kelder J, Funke C, de Boer T, Delbressine L, Leysen D, Nickolson V (1997). A comparison of the physicochemical and biological properties of mirtazapine and mianserin. *J Pharm Pharmacol* 49, 403–411.

Kobayashi K, Chiba K, Yagi T et al. (1997). Identification of cytochrome P-450 isoforms involved in citalopram N-demethylation by human liver microsomes. *J Pharmacol Exp Ther* 280, 927–933.

Kooyman AR, Zwart R, van der Heijden PML, van Hooft JA, Vijverberg HPM (1994). Interaction between enantiomers of mianserin and ORG3770 at 5-HT(3) receptors in cultured mouse neuroblastoma cells. *Neuropharmacology* 33, 501–507.

Kosel M, Gnerre C, Voirol P et al. (2002). In vitro biotransformation of the selective serotonin reuptake inhibitor citalopram, its enantiomers and demethylated metabolites by monoamine oxidase in rat and human brain preparations. *Mol Psychiatry* 7, 181–188.

Koyama E, Chiba K, Tani M, Ishizaki T (1996). Identification of human cytochrome P-450 isoforms involved in the stereoselective metabolism of mianserin enantiomers. *J Pharmacol Exp Ther* 278, 21–30.

Kristensen K, Christensen CB, Christrup LL (1995). The mu1, mu2, delta, kappa opioid receptor binding profiles of methadone stereoisomers and morphine. *Life Sci* 56, 45–50.

Kudo S, Ishizaki T (1999). Pharmacokinetics of haloperidol – an update. *Clin Pharmacokinet* 37, 435–456.

Kudo S, Odomi M (1998). Involvement of human cytochrome P-450 3A4 in reduced haloperidol oxidation. *Eur J Clin Pharmacol* 54, 253–259.

Lane RM, Baker GB (1999). Chirality and drugs used in psychiatry: nice to know or need to know? *Cell Mol Neurobiol* 19, 355–372.

Lavoie P-A, Beauchamp G, Elie R (1994). Absence of stereoselectivity of some tricyclic antidepressants inhibition of depolarization-induced calcium uptake in rat cingulate cortex synaptosomes. *J Psychiatry Neurosci* 19, 208–212.

Lessard E, Yessine M-A, Hamelin BA, O'Hara G, LeBlanc J, Turgeon J (1999). Influence of CYP2D6 activity on the disposition and cardiovascular toxicity of the antidepressant agent venlafaxine in humans. *Pharmacogenetics* 9, 435–443.

Llerena A, Alm C, Dahl M-L, Ekqvist B, Bertilsson L (1992a). Haloperidol disposition is dependent on debrisoquine hydroxylation phenotype. *Ther Drug Monit* 14, 92–97.

Llerena A, Dahl M-L, Ekqvist B, Bertilsson L (1992b). Haloperidol disposition is dependent on the debrisoquine hydroxylation phenotype – increased plasma levels of the reduced metabolite in poor metabolizers. *Ther Drug Monit* 14, 261–264.

Llerena A, Berecz R, de la Rubia A, Norberto M-J, Benitez J (2000). Use of the mesoridazine/thioridazine ratio as a marker for CYP2D6 enzyme activity. *Ther Drug Monit* 22, 397–401.

Lundqvist E, Johansson I, Ingelman-Sundberg M (1999). Genetic mechanisms for duplication and multiduplication of the human *CYP2D6* gene and methods for detection of duplicated *CYP2D6* genes. *Gene* 226, 327–338.

Marzo A, Balant LP (1996). Investigation of xenobiotic metabolism by CYP2D6 and CYP2C19: importance of enantioselective analytical methods. *J Chromatogr B: Biomed Appl* 678, 73–92.

Maurer HH, Bickeboeller-Friedrich J, Kraemer T, Peters FT (2000). Toxicokinetics and analytical toxicology of amphetamine-derived designer drugs ("Ecstasy"). *Toxicol Lett* 112, 133–142.

McGrath C, Burrows GD, Norman TR (1998). Neurochemical effects of the enantiomers of mirtazapine in normal rats. *Eur J Pharmacol* 356, 121–126.

Mellström B, Bertilsson L, Säwe J, Schulz H-U, Sjöqvist F (1981). *E*- and *Z*-10-hydroxylation of nortriptyline: relationship to polymorphic debrisoquine hydroxylation. *Clin Pharmacol Ther* 30, 189–193.

Mellström B, Bertilsson L, Sjöqvist F (1983). Amitriptyline metabolism: relationship to polymorphic debrisoquine hydroxylation. *Clin Pharmacol Ther* 34, 516–520.

Meyer JW, Woggon B, Baumann P, Meyer UA (1990). Clinical implication of slow sulphoxidation of thioridazine in a poor metabolizer of the debrisoquine type. *Eur J Clin Pharmacol* 39, 613–614.

Mihara K, Otani K, Tybring G, Dahl M-L, Bertilsson L, Kaneko S (1997). The CYP2D6 genotype and plasma concentrations of mianserin enantiomers in relation to therapeutic response to mianserin in depressed Japanese patients. *J Clin Psychopharmacol* 17, 467–471.

Montgomery SA, Loft H, Sanchez C, Reines EH, Papp M (2001). Escitalopram (*S*-enantiomer of citalopram): clinical efficacy and onset of action predicted from a rat model. *Pharmacol Toxicol* 88, 282–286.

Moody DE, Alburges ME, Parker RJ, Collins JM, Strong JM (1997). The involvement of cytochrome P-450 3A4 in the N-demethylation of L-α-acetylmethadol (LAAM), norlaam, and methadone. *Drug Metab Dispos* 25, 1347–1353.

Müller MJ, Härtter S, Köhler D, Hiemke C (2001). Serum levels of sulpiride enantiomers after oral treatment with racemic sulpiride in psychiatric patients: a pilot study. *Pharmacopsychiatry* 34, 27–32.

Musso DL, Mehta NB, Soroko FE, Ferris RM, Hollingsworth EB, Kenney BT (1993). Synthesis and evaluation of the antidepressant activity of the enantiomers of bupropion. *Chirality* 5, 495–500.

Narita N, Hashimoto K, Tomitaka S, Minabe Y (1996). Interactions of selective serotonin reuptake inhibitors with subtypes of σ receptors in rat brain. *Eur J Pharmacol* 307, 117–119.

Nation RL (1994). Chirality in new drug development – clinical pharmacokinetic considerations. *Clin Pharmacokinet* 27, 249–255.

Nordin C, Bertilsson L (1995). Active hydroxymetabolites of antidepressants: Emphasis on *E*-10-hydroxynortriptyline. *Clin Pharmacokinet* 28, 26–40.

Nordin C, Bertilsson L, Dahl M-L, Resul B, Toresson G, Sjöqvist F (1991). Treatment of depression with *E*-10-hydroxynortriptyline – a pilot study on biochemical effects and pharmacokinetics. *Psychopharmacology* 103, 287–290.

Nusser E, Nill K, Breyer-Pfaff U (1988). Enantioselective formation and disposition of (*E*)- and (*Z*)-10-hydroxynortriptyline. *Drug Metab Dispos* 16, 509–511.

Nyberg S, Dahl M-L, Halldin C (1995). A PET study of D_2 and 5-HT_2 receptor occupancy induced by risperidone in poor metabolizers of debrisoquin and risperidone. *Psychopharmacology* 119, 345–348.

Olesen OV, Linnet K (1997). Metabolism of the tricyclic antidepressant amitriptyline by cDNA-expressed human cytochrome P-450 enzymes. *Pharmacology* 55, 235–243.

Olesen OV, Linnet K (1999). Studies on the stereoselective metabolism of citalopram by human liver microsomes and cDNA-expressed cytochrome P-450 enzymes. *Pharmacology* 59, 298–309.

Olesen OV, Licht RW, Thomsen E, Bruun T, Viftrup JE, Linnet K (1998). Serum concentrations and side effects in psychiatric patients during risperidone therapy. *Ther Drug Monit* 20, 380–384.

Otton SV, Ball SE, Cheung SW, Inaba T, Rudolph RL, Sellers EM (1996). Venlafaxine oxidation in vitro is catalysed by CYP2D6. *Br J Clin Pharmacol* 41, 149–156.

Owens MJ, Knight DL, Nemeroff CB (2001). Second-generation SSRIs: human monoamine transporter binding profile of escitalopram and *R*-fluoxetine. *Biol Psychiatry* 50, 345–350.

Pan LP, de Vriendt C, Belpaire FM (1998). In-vitro characterization of the cytochrome P-450 isoenzymes involved in the back oxidation and N-dealkylation of reduced haloperidol. *Pharmacogenetics* 8, 383–389.

Patrick KS, Singletary JL (1991). Relative configuration of thioridazine enantiomers. *Chirality* 3, 208–211.

Pert CB, Snyder SH (1973). Opiate receptor: demonstration in nervous tissue. *Science* 179, 1011–1014.

Pfandl B, Morike K, Winne D, Schareck W, Breyer-Pfaff U (1992). Stereoselective inhibition of nortriptyline hydroxylation in man by quinidine. *Xenobiotica* 22, 721–730.

Pinder RM (1985). Adrenoreceptor interactions of the enantiomers and metabolites of mianserin: are they responsible for the antidepressant effect? *Acta Psychiatr Scand* 72(Suppl 320), 1–9.

Pollock BG, Everett G, Perel JM (1992). Comparative cardiotoxicity of nortriptyline and its isomeric 10-hydroxymetabolites. *Neuropsychopharmacology* 6, 1–10.

Pollock BG, Sweet RA, Kirshner M, Reynolds CF, III (1996). Bupropion plasma levels and CYP2D6 phenotype. *Ther Drug Monit* 18, 581–585.

Puozzo C, Leonard BE (1996). Pharmacokinetics of milnacipran in comparison with other antidepressants. *Int Clin Psychopharmacol* 11(Suppl 4), 15–27.

Quinn DI, Wodak A, Day RO (1997). Pharmacokinetic and pharmacodynamic principles of illicit drug use and treatment of illicit drug users. *Clin Pharmacokinet* 33, 344–400.

Quirion R, Bowen WD, Itzhak Y et al. (1992). Meeting report. A proposal for the classification of sigma binding sites. *Trends Pharmacol Sci* 13, 85–86.

Reilly JG, Ayis SA, Ferrier IN, Jones SJ, Thomas SHL (2000). QTc-interval abnormalities and psychotropic drug therapy in psychiatric patients. *Lancet* 355, 1048–1052.

Ring BJ, Eckstein JA, Gillespie JS, Binkley SN, Vandenbranden M, Wrighton SA (2001). Identification of the human cytochromes P450 responsible for in vitro formation of *R*- and *S*-norfluoxetine. *J Pharmacol Exp Ther* 297, 1044–1050.

Robertson DW, Krushinski JH, Bymaster FP, Reid LR, Wong DT (1991). Seproxetine: absolute configurations and stereospecific interactions of the enantiomers of norfluoxetine with the serotonin uptake carrier. *Pharmacologist* 33, 219.

Rochat B, Amey M, Baumann P (1995a). Analysis of enantiomers of citalopram and its demethylated metabolites in plasma of depressive patients using chiral reverse-phase liquid chromatography. *Ther Drug Monit* 17, 273–279.

Rochat B, Amey M, van Gelderen H, Testa B, Baumann P (1995b). Determination of the enantiomers of citalopram, its demethylated and propionic acid metabolites in human plasma by chiral HPLC. *Chirality* 7, 389–395.

Rochat B, Amey M, Gillet M, Meyer UA, Baumann P (1997). Identification of three cytochrome P-450 isozymes involved in N-demethylation of citalopram enantiomers in human liver microsomes. *Pharmacogenetics* 7, 1–10.

Rochat B, Kosel M, Boss G, Testa B, Gillet M, Baumann P (1998). Stereoselective biotransformation of the selective serotonin reuptake inhibitor, citalopram, and its demethylated metabolites by monoamine oxidases in human liver. *Biochem Pharmacol* 56, 15–23.

Rognan D, Sokoloff P, Mann A et al. (1990). Optically active benzamides as predictive tools for mapping the dopamine D2 receptor. *Eur J Pharmacol* 189, 59–70.

Rotzinger S, Bourin M, Akimoto Y, Coutts RT, Baker GB (1999). Metabolism of some "second" – and "fourth"- generation antidepressants: iprindole, viloxazine, bupropion, mianserin, maprotiline, trazodone, nefazodone and venlafaxine. *Cell Mol Neurobiol* 19, 427–442.

Rudorfer MV, Potter WZ (1997). The role of metabolites of antidepressants in the treatment of depression [review]. *CNS Drugs* 7, 273–312.

Rudorfer MV, Potter WZ (1999). Metabolism of tricyclic antidepressants. *Cell Mol Neurobiol* 19, 373–409.

Sajjad SHA (1997). CYP2D6 genotype and tardive dyskinesia. *Br J Psychiatry* 170, 580.

Sanchez C, Hyttel J (1999). Comparison of the effects of antidepressants and their metabolites on reuptake of biogenic amines and on receptor binding. *Cell Mol Neurobiol* 19, 467–489.

Schmider J, Greenblatt DJ, Harmatz JS, Shader RI (1996). Enzyme kinetic modelling as a tool to analyse the behaviour of cytochrome P-450 catalysed reactions: application to amitriptyline N-demethylation. *Br J Clin Pharmacol* 41, 593–604.

Scordo MG, Spina E, Facciola G, Avenoso A, Johansson I, Dahl ML (1999). Cytochrome P-450 2D6 genotype and steady-state plasma levels of risperidone and 9-hydroxyrisperidone. *Psychopharmacology* 147, 300–305.

Scott CC, Robbins EB, Chen KK (1948). Pharmacological comparison of the optical isomers of methadone. *J Pharmacol Exp Ther* 92, 282–286.

Shih JC, Chen K, Ridd MJ (1999). Monoamine oxidase: from genes to behavior. *Ann Rev Neurosci* 22, 197–217.

Shin JG, Kane K, Flockhart DA (2001). Potent inhibition of CYP2D6 by haloperidol metabolites: stereoselective inhibition by reduced haloperidol. *Br J Pharmacol* 51, 45–52.

Sidhu J, Priskorn M, Poulsen M, Segonzac A, Grollier G, Larsen F (1997). Steady-state pharmacokinetics of the enantiomers of citalopram and its metabolites in humans. *Chirality* 9, 686–692.

Sindrup SH, Brøsen K, Hansen MGJ, Aaes-Jørgensen T, Fredricson Overø K, Gram LF (1993). Pharmacokinetics of citalopram in relation to the sparteine and the mephenytoin oxidation polymorphisms. *Ther Drug Monit* 15, 11–17.

Smith DF (ed.) (1984). *CRC Handbook of Stereoisomers: Drugs in Psychopharmacology*. Boca Raton, FL: CRC Press, pp. 1–475.

Spencer CM, Wilde MI (1998). Milnacipran – a review of its use in depression. *Drugs* 56, 405–427.

Spina E, Ancione M, Di Rosa AE, Meduri M, Caputi AP (1992). Polymorphic debrisoquine oxidation and acute neuroleptic-induced adverse effects. *Eur J Clin Pharmacol* 42, 347–348.

Stevens JC, Wrighton SA (1993). Interaction of the enantiomers of fluoxetine and norfluoxetine with human liver cytochromes P-450. *J Pharmacol Exp Ther* 266, 964–971.

Störmer E, von Moltke LL, Greenblatt DJ (2000a). Scaling drug biotransformation data from cDNA-expressed cytochrome P-450 to human liver: a comparison of relative activity factors and human liver abundance in studies of mirtazapine metabolism. *J Pharmacol Exp Ther* 295, 793–801.

Störmer E, von Moltke LL, Shader RI, Greenblatt DJ (2000b). Metabolism of the antidepressant mirtazapine in vitro: contribution of cytochromes P-450 1A2, 2D6, and 3A4. *Drug Metab Dispos* 28, 1168–1175.

Sullivan HR, Due SL (1973). Urinary metabolites of *dl*-methadone in maintenance subjects. *J Med Chem* 16, 909–913.

Svendsen CN, Froimowitz M, Hrbek C et al. (1988). Receptor affinity, neurochemistry and behavioral characteristics of the enantiomers of thioridazine: evidence for different stereoselectivities at D_1 and D_2 receptors in rat brain. *Neuropharmacology* 27, 1117–1124.

Timmer CJ, Sitsen JMA, Delbressine LP (2000). Clinical pharmacokinetics of mirtazapine. *Clin Pharmacokinet* 38, 461–474.

Tucker GT (2000). Chiral switches. *Lancet* 355, 1085–1087.

Tybring G, Otani K, Kaneko S, Mihara K, Fukushima Y, Bertilsson L (1995). Enantioselective determination of mianserin and its desmethyl metabolite in plasma during treatment of depressed Japanese patients. *Ther Drug Monit* 17, 516–521.

Ueno S, Otani K, Kaneko S et al. (1996). Cytochrome P-450 *2D6* gene polymorphism is not associated with neuroleptic malignant syndrome. *Biol Psychiatry* 40, 72–74.

Veefkind AH, Haffmans PMJ, Hoencamp E (2000). Venlafaxine serum levels and *CYP2D6* genotype. *Ther Drug Monit* 22, 202–208.

von Bahr C, Movin G, Nordin C et al. (1991). Plasma levels of thioridazine and metabolites are influenced by the debrisoquin hydroxylation phenotype. *Clin Pharmacol Ther* 49, 234–240.

von Moltke LL, Greenblatt DJ, Duan SX et al. (1997). Human cytochromes mediating N-demethylation of fluoxetine in vitro. *Psychopharmacology* 132, 402–407.

von Moltke LL, Greenblatt DJ, Giancarlo GM, Granda BW, Harmatz JS, Shader RI (2001). Escitalopram (*S*-citalopram) and its metabolites in vitro: cytochromes mediating biotransformation, inhibitory effects, and comparison to *R*-citalopram. *Drug Metab Dispos* 29, 1102–1109.

Wagstaff AJ, Fitton A, Benfield P (1994). Sulpiride – a review of its pharmacodynamic and pharmacokinetic properties, and therapeutic efficacy in schizophrenia. *CNS Drugs* 2, 313–333.

Wainer IW (1993). *Drug Stereochemistry. Analytical Methods and Pharmacology*, 2nd edn, revised and expanded. New York: Marcel Dekker.

Walker JM, Bowen WD, Walker FO, Matsumoto RR, De Costa B, Rice KC (1990). Sigma receptors: biology and function. *Pharmacol Rev* 42, 355–403.

Wang CP, Howell SR, Scatina J, Sisenine SF (1992). The disposition of venlafaxine enantiomers in dogs, rats, and humans receiving venlafaxine. *Chirality* 4, 84–90.

Wong DT, Fuller RW, Robertson DW (1990a). Fluoxetine and its two enantiomers as selective serotonin uptake inhibitors. *Acta Pharm Nord* 2, 171–179.

Wong DT, Reid LR, Threlkeld PG (1990b). Suppression of food intake in rats by fluoxetine: comparison of enantiomers and effects serotonin antagonists. *Pharmacol Biochem Behav* 31, 475–479.

Wong DT, Bymaster FP, Reid LR, Mayle DA, Krushinski JH, Robertson DW (1993). Norfluoxetine enantiomers as inhibitors of serotonin uptake in rat brain. *Neuropsychopharmacology* 8, 337–344.

Wood MD, Thomas DR, Watkins CJ, Newberry NR (1993). Stereoselective interaction of mianserin with 5-HT$_3$ receptors. *J Pharm Pharmacol* 45, 711–714.

Yang SK, Lu X-L (1989). Racemization kinetics of enantiomeric oxazepams and stereoselective hydrolysis of enantiomeric oxazepam 3-acetates in rat liver microsomes and brain homogenate. *J Pharm Sci* 78, 10, 789–795.

Yasui N, Tybring G, Otani K et al. (1997). Effects of thioridazine, an inhibitor of CYP2D6, on the steady-state plasma concentrations of the enantiomers of mianserin and its active metabolite, desmethylmianserin, in depressed Japanese patients. *Pharmacogenetics* 7, 369–374.

Yasui-Furukori N, Hidestrand M, Spina E, Facciola G, Scordo MG, Tybring G (2001). Different enantioselective 9-hydroxylation of risperidone by the two human CYP2D6 and CYP3A4 enzymes. *Drug Metab Dispos* 29, 1263–1268.

Young RC, Dhar AK, Kutt H, Alexopoulos GS (1988). Isomers of 10-hydroxynortriptyline in geriatric depression. *Ther Drug Monit* 10, 164–167.

Young D, Midha KK, Fossler MJ et al. (1993). Effect of quinidine on the interconversion kinetics between haloperidol and reduced haloperidol in humans. Implications for the involvement of cytochrome P-450IID6. *Eur J Clin Pharmacol* 44, 433–438.

Yue QY, Svensson JO, Bertilsson L, Säwe J (1995). Racemic methadone kinetics in relation to the debrisoquine hydroxylation polymorphism in man. *Therapie Suppl*, 88.

Part V

Specific psychotropic drugs and disorders

10

Clozapine response and genetic variation in neurotransmitter receptor targets

David A. Collier[1], Maria J. Arranz[2], Sarah Osborne[2], Katherine J. Aitchison[2], Janet Munro[2], Dalu Mancama[2], and Robert W. Kerwin[2]

Section of Genetics[1] and Section of Clinical Neuropharmacology[2], Institute of Psychiatry, London, UK

OVERVIEW

Clozapine is an atypical antipsychotic drug with unique clinical features, particularly in treatment resistant schizophrenia. Between 10 and 60% of patients resistant or intolerant to treatment with other antipsychotic drugs respond to clozapine. Reliable genetic prediction of which patients will respond would have major economic, clinical, and safety implications. Candidate genes of potential utility in pharmacogenetic tests can be identified from clozapine's neurotransmitter targets. Clozapine has a complex pattern of interaction with neurotransmitter receptors, with high affinity for dopamine D_4, serotonin (5-HT) 1A, 2A, 2C, 6, and 7, histamine H_1, muscarinic M_1 and α_1- and α_2-adrenoceptors. Exactly which of these receptors mediates clozapine's clinical efficacy is unknown, but the involvement of 5-HT is very likely. Despite the lack of formal evidence from genetic epidemiology, it is reasonable to hypothesize that genetic variation in these receptors influences clinical response to clozapine by altering receptor function in some way. At most of these receptors, clozapine is a neutral antagonist, but at others, such as 5-HT_{2C}, it has inverse agonist activity. Further complexity comes from the unusual regulation of several of these receptors, with evidence for functional alternative splicing of 5-HT_{2C}, polymorphic imprinting of 5-HT_{2A}, and unusual downregulation of at least three 5-HT receptors through clozapine-induced cellular internalization. Most of clozapine's receptor targets have been tested in some way for association with clinical response using a case-control allelic association design. Polymorphisms in two genes, for 5-HT_{2A} and dopamine D_3, have been implicated in more than one study. However, there is a general lack of large, powerful prospective studies using multiple measures of response, and many polymorphisms in potentially relevant genes, such as that for α-aminobutyric acid type A (GABA-A), have not yet been examined. A novel epistatic approach, simultaneously examining genetic variation in multiple genes that encode clozapine's neurotransmitter targets has been piloted, but needs replication in a prospective study. To predict fully clinical response to clozapine treatment in schizophrenia, it will be necessary to take account of many variables in addition to genetic influence on clozapine's pharmacokinetics, including social, demographic, and clinical factors (e.g., compliance, social support, and history of birth trauma); genetic vulnerability to side effects such as weight gain and sedation; and the influence of genetic susceptibility factors for psychosis, which may define subtype and symptomatology. This chapter will concentrate on the genetics of response to the antipsychotic drug clozapine, focusing mainly on pharmacodynamic factors related to clozapine's receptor binding.

Introduction

Pharmacogenetics

There are two broad reasons for treatment failure: adverse reaction (i.e., "one which is noxious and unintended and which occurs at doses used in man for prophylaxis and treatment" (World Health Organization)) and lack of efficacy (Price-Evans, 1993). Drugs may fail to elicit a clinical response because of failure to reach a sustained therapeutic concentration (pharmacokinetics) or fail to elicit a response because of altered receptor binding or coupling (pharmacodynamics). In addition, differences in the pathophysiology of heterogeneous and complex diseases such as schizophrenia may affect response.

Historically, pharmacogenetics has not used classical epidemiological methods such as twin studies to analyze the heritability of drug effects, but instead has relied on biochemical genetics. Biotransformation was initially identified as being genetically variable because of the interindividual variability in the effects of certain drugs, with classical bi- or trimodal differences in drug breakdown across individuals. This indicates the existence of simple genetic effects such as a defective or overactive enzyme. Since the 1960s, progress has been much faster in understanding the genetics of drug metabolism than in the study of the genetic phenomena of drug receptors (Price-Evans, 1993), presumably because of the relative simplicity of understanding families of related enzymes rather than individual (and often unknown) drug targets. The field of receptor-based pharmacogenetics is just re-emerging.

Clozapine

Clozapine is a tricyclic dibenzodiazepine (Fig. 10.1) first developed in the 1960s and 1970s. It was known to have an atypical profile with a low incidence of extrapyramidal side effects (EPS) (Gerlach et al., 1974; Nair et al., 1977) but was withdrawn in 1975 after a cluster of cases of agranulocytosis in Finland (Amsler et al., 1977). It was later reintroduced with strict hematological monitoring because of its effective antipsychotic, antiaggressive and anxiolytic properties. In most of the world, clozapine is used in treatment-refractory or intolerant patients, i.e., those who are unresponsive to two or more classes of antipsychotic or are intolerant of their neurological side effects. In this group, about 37% are responsive to clozapine treatment after 6 weeks and about 81% after 1 year (Meltzer, 1992), although in one

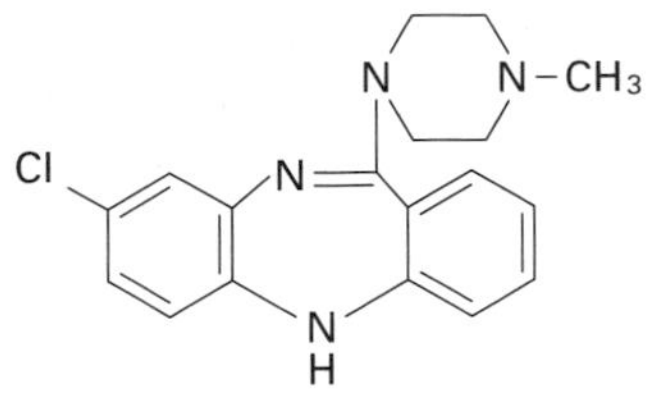

Fig. 10.1.   The chemical structure of clozapine, a tricyclic dibenzodiazepine.

study of strictly defined treatment-refractory schizophrenia or schizoaffective disorder only 10% responded (Simpson et al., 1999). Clozapine is used as a first line of treatment in several countries, notably Switzerland and the People's Republic of China. Treatment response to clozapine in first-onset psychosis exceeds 80%.

Clozapine is given at various doses from 50 to 900 mg per day, depending on how well the patient tolerates the drug. Dose is usually titrated to about 150 mg over 2 weeks and then in 25–50 mg increments to a maximum of 900 mg per day over several weeks (although usual clinical doses are lower). Although early research appeared to indicate that clozapine serum level was not important in response (reviewed by Fitton and Heel (1990)), more recent research indicates that a plasma serum concentration of clozapine of at least 350 μg/l and as high as 420 μg/l is required to optimize response (reviewed in Lieberman et al. (1995a)). For example Potkin et al. (1994) found that after 12 weeks 73% of patients with serum levels $\leq$420 μg/l responded to clozapine compared with only 29% of those with $\leq$420 μg/l. Its clinical efficacy is thought to be associated principally with its action at 5-HT neurotransmitter receptors, particularly 5-HT_{1A}, 5-HT_{2A}, and 5-HT_{2C}, but also at dopamine. It also has affinity for a variety of other neurotransmitter receptors, including high-affinity binding to muscarinic receptors and α-adrenoceptors.

What influences clinical response to antipsychotic medication?

The factors that influence response to antipsychotic medication are a largely unknown mixture of genetic and environmental factors. Clinical and social factors associated with good response to antipsychotics include compliance, family support during treatment, less severe delusions and hallucinations and better attention at baseline, male sex, fewer obstetric complications, less than 9 years of illness, and later age at onset (Wilcox and Nasrallah, 1987; Robinson et al., 1999).

The development of side effects influences treatment response, since a proportion of patients will be unable to tolerate a particular drug. For typical antipsychotics, these will include the development of EPS, and for clozapine side effects include neutropenia, sedation, seizures, and tachycardia. These are, in part, a result of heritable variability in drug metabolism: poor metabolizers of a given drug will develop dose-dependent side effects more easily since peak plasma concentrations of drugs will be much higher for a given dose. Other reasons may include genetic susceptibility to specific side effects.

However, the major reason for antipsychotic treatment failure is lack of efficacy for unknown reasons. There is almost no information from twin or family studies on the heritability of clinical responsiveness (i.e., improvement in disease symptoms) to antipsychotic drugs, aside from a few case reports of concordant twins (Vojvoda et al., 1996; Mata et al., 2001). While it is reasonable to assume that there is a pharmacogenetic influence on response to clozapine, there is an urgent need to clarify this by genetic epidemiological study.

Clinical response to clozapine might be mediated by variation in receptor density (through changes in gene expression, protein stability, or transport), altered kinetics of dimer or multimer formation, variation in efficiency of coupling to second messenger systems, or alterations in ligand affinity or allosteric modulator binding. It is important to note, however, that a pharmacogenetic effect is dependent on functional genetic variation; for some genes, there may be no genetic variation that affects clozapine's action.

Research methodology

What is response to clozapine?

Deciding on the criteria most useful for judging response to clozapine is difficult, since there are multiple ways to judge response ranging from specific neurophysiological measures such as P50 sensory gating through to quality-of-life measures. Furthermore, patients taking this drug in most parts of the world are likely to be resistant or intolerant to treatment with other antipsychotics, have worse illness, and a complex treatment history. Consequently, patients taking clozapine may have more severe symptoms, more chronic illness, and be more sensitive to side effects than schizophrenic patients in general. These factors must be borne in mind when generalizing pharmacogenetic findings to other antipsychotic drugs when clozapine has been used as a model.

The two most important considerations for judging clinical response are the instrument used and the time scale of measurement. The use of multiple but compatible measures has been recommended (Masellis et al., 2000) and consensus methods to judge clinical response have been proposed. Clearly, a double-blind prospective study of clozapine response, in the same manner as a drug trial, is the best method of analysis since good baseline data and detailed response criteria can be collected over a defined time period. Retrospective analysis, where a judgement of response is made based on case notes and/or the opinion of the treating medical staff, cannot be as good since it will necessarily produce less detailed clinical data and cannot follow patients from a defined baseline at the commencement of clozapine therapy. However retrospective analysis has practical advantages since substantial numbers of patients can be assessed relatively quickly. Retrospective methodology may be necessary for twin or family study of response since it will be difficult to ascertain a significant number of twins prospectively.

The Global Assessment Scale (known as GAS, GAF, or GAFS) (Endicott et al., 1976; see also Tress and Patton, 1994) is an improvement of the Health Rating Scale of Luborsky (1962) and the simplest and quickest scale used to assess global response to antipsychotic drugs. It is scored from 1 to 100 (individuals with minimal psychopathology score above 71), with ten anchor points divided into deciles. It has been used in a series of retrospective analyses of clozapine response (Arranz et al., 1998a). Response is usually defined as a 20-point increase in GAS score but can also be used as a continuous or quantitative scale in regression analysis. The Brief Psychiatric Rating Scale (BPRS) (Overall and Gorham, 1962; see also Tress and Patton, 1994), and the Positive and Negative Symptom Scale (PANSS) (Kay et al., 1992) are more detailed and the most often used for prospective studies of clozapine response (see Masellis et al., 1998, 2001). The PANSS measures positive and negative symptoms of schizophrenia and general psychopathology. Response according to both BPRS and PANSS is usually defined as a 20% decrease in score, but some clinical trials use a 40% decrease. An alternative measure, the Clinical Global Impression scale (CGI) (Guy, 1976), measures the impression of the severity of illness on a seven category scale. The CGI Improvement scale (CGI-I; 0–7) is widely used in clinical trials but has only been used in one pharmacogenetic study of clozapine response to augment BPRS criteria (Masellis et al., 1998). Improvement on at least one category (CGI-I score of 1 or 2) has been widely used to define response. Other methods used include the clinical classification of patients into four response groups, taking into account minimum clozapine dose (Noethen et al., 1995) or into three groups (Kohn et al., 1997). The Bunney–Hamburg Global Psychosis rating scale has also been used (Rao et al., 1994).

Other approaches, such as the measurement of specific symptomatology or quality of life, have been considered. Scales which measure specific symptomatology in more detail, such as PANSS may be useful, as severity of delusions and hallucinations predicts responsiveness and may be more sensitive measures for pharmacogenetic studies. Quality-of-life scales, such as the Lehman Quality of Life Interview and the Heinrichs–Carpenter scale (reviewed in Lehman et al. (1993)) or the WHOQOL-100 may also be useful. The WHOQOL-100 (Skevington and Wright, 2001) appears closely correlated with the effectiveness of antidepressant drugs, with 96% of facets responsive to perceived change in clinical depression. Quality of life may be the most important treatment outcome, for the patient, as well as being a sensitive indicator of drug action.

The use of neuropsychology or neurophysiology to assess treatment response in schizophrenia is a new area of investigation. Neuropsychological deficits appear to be established at the onset of illness, and indeed in childhood (Meltzer and McGurk, 1999; Bilder et al., 2000). A large generalized neuropsychological deficit and more subtle executive and attentional deficits are seen in first episode psychosis, mark the more severely ill patients, and have been postulated to predict poor outcome (Bilder et al., 2000). The use of neuropsychological tests to analyze treatment response may be particularly powerful as there is evidence that atypical drugs such as clozapine have the ability to improve various aspects of cognitive function, which is not seen for typical drugs (Meltzer and McGurk, 1999). For example, clozapine appears to improve verbal ability, attention, and some types of executive function, and these variables appear different in comparison with other drugs such as olanzapine (Meltzer and McGurk, 1999). Neurophysiological measures may also be powerful; clozapine corrects the P50 sensory gating deficit seen in the majority of schizophrenics (Nagamoto et al., 1996; Light et al., 2000).

How long does the response take?

The time needed to see the full spectrum of clinical response to clozapine is unclear, but, in general, 37% of patients are thought to respond after 6 weeks and 81% after 1 year (Meltzer, 1992). Evidence suggests that any prospective study of clozapine response should use a minimum time period of at least 12 weeks, since several trials have shown that this time length is necessary for response in most patients (Breier et al., 1994; Lieberman et al., 1994a, b; Potkin et al., 1994). Some patients may take 12 months to show good response, but the probable optimum is between 12 and 24 weeks (Lieberman et al., 1994b). Positive symptoms have been seen to improve after 8 weeks (Tandon et al., 1993) and improvement in negative symptoms may lag about 7 weeks behind (Lieberman et al., 1994b). Up to 9 months has been suggested as necessary to see the full benefits of clozapine (Meltzer, 1995), but some observers suggest that all of clozapine's differential beneficial effects (i.e., advantages over typical drugs) occur during the first 6 weeks (Rosenheck et al., 1999). However, it is important to note that clozapine is titrated up to a therapeutic dose and this may delay response.

Defining candidates genes: the pharmacology of clozapine and results of genetic analysis

The ability of clozapine to improve the symptoms of psychosis is dependent on its antagonist and reverse agonist activities at neurotransmitter receptors. Clozapine's affinity for some of its most important neurotransmitter receptors is shown in Table 10.1. The serum level of clinical doses of clozapine is estimated at 20 nmol (Seeman, 1992), so receptors with K_i values substantially more than this will not be fully occupied. Its affinity for the dopamine D_2 receptor is relatively weak compared

Table 10.1. The affinity of antipsychotic drugs for neurotransmitter receptors

Receptor	Binding constant K_i (nmol/l)					
	Haloperidol	Clozapine	Risperidone	Olanzapine	Ziprazidone	Quetiapine
Dopamine						
D_1	120	141	75	31	130	455
D_2	1.3	83	3.1	11	3.1	160
D_3	3.2	200	9.6	50	7.2	940
D_4	2.3	20	7	27	32	2200
Serotin						
$5\text{-}HT_{1A}$	>1000	6.46	488	>1000	2.5	>1000
$5\text{-}HT_{2A}$	78	2.5	0.16	5	0.39	295
$5\text{-}HT_{2C}$	>1000	8.6	25.8	11.3	0.72	>1000
$5\text{-}HT_{3}$	>1000	95	>1000	57	–	>1000
$5\text{-}HT_{6}$	6000	11	2000	10	76	4100
Histamine						
H_1	>1000	23	155	7	47	11
Muscarinic						
M_1	>1000	1.9	>1000	1.9	5100	120
Adrenergic						
α_1	46	39	2	19	13	7
α_2	360	11.6	3	228	310	87

with the affinity of typical antipsychotics such as haloperidol, which may provide some of the explanation for its reduced propensity to cause movement disorders. Its affinity for other dopamine receptors is also unexceptional (Shaikh et al., 1997), but it is a potent antagonist for 5-HT receptors (Meltzer, 1999), particularly 5-HT_{1A}, 5-HT_{2A}, and 5-HT_{2C}. The ratio D_2:5-HT affinity may be a key feature of atypical antipsychotic action. D_4 receptor binding (particularly D_2:D_4 and D_4:5-HT_{2A} binding ratios) may also be important for clozapine's action (Seeman, 1992; Shaikh et al., 1997; Kulkarni and Ninan, 2000; Kapur and Remington, 2001).

Genetic variation in clozapine's receptor targets is a potential source of pharmacodynamic influence on drug response, by altering drug action. It is not clear exactly which of clozapine's numerous receptor targets is responsible for its clinical action. Proof that genetic variation in a particular receptor affects clozapine's clinical efficacy is proof of that receptor's role in drug action. This would represent an important pharmacological finding in itself, in addition to the potential for genetic testing and the individualization of treatment.

Dopamine receptors

Dopamine D$_1$ and D$_5$ receptors

Clozapine is a weak antagonist at both D$_1$ and D$_5$ receptors (Table 10.1), with an approximately twofold lower affinity for D$_1$ and D$_5$ compared with D$_2$. Consequently, the D$_1$ receptor has not been thought to be a significant mediator of clozapine's clinical effects. However, it is the most abundant dopamine receptor and is far more prevalent than D$_2$ receptors in areas that have been implicated in schizophrenia, such as the prefrontal cortex and nucleus accumbens (Missale et al., 1998). The D$_5$ receptor is expressed at much lower levels in the brain, principally in hippocampus, cerebral cortex and lateral thalamus. Both D$_1$ and D$_5$ receptors have pre- and postsynaptic localization, and although they have similar pharmacology, they are not functionally redundant because of differences in expression patterns and cellular localization (Missale et al., 1998).

Both D$_1$ and D$_5$ receptors are downregulated in the prefrontal cortex but not the striatum by treatment with many commonly used antipsychotic drugs, including clozapine, which reduces cortical D$_1$ and D$_5$ expression by 30–40% (Lidow et al., 1997). There is evidence that this regional downregulation may be a consequence of D$_2$ antagonism rather than direct binding to D$_1$/D$_5$. This effect may be important for clinical efficacy of antipsychotics, including clozapine, as D$_1$-specific antagonists have been reported to improve negative symptoms in schizophrenia. However, D$_1$ blockade may diminish working memory (Williams and Goldman-Rakic, 1995). There is some evidence that clozapine is, in fact, a direct D$_1$ agonist (Ahlenius, 1999). Clozapine binds weakly to D$_5$ receptors with a K_i of 320.

The gene *DRD1* is not highly polymorphic, with no common missense variants in the coding region (Cichon et al., 1996). Several variants are known in the 5′ region and promoter (-48A/G, -2218T/C, -2102C/A, -2030T/C, -1992G/A, -1251G/C, and -800T/C) (Cichon et al., 1996) but these do not appear to be in regions critical for gene regulation. The *DRD5* coding region is more polymorphic (Sobell et al., 1995; Feng et al., 1998), producing Leu88Phe in the putative second transmembrane domain, Ala269Val in the third intracellular 100p, Pro330Gln in the third extracellular loop, Asn351Asp in the seventh transmembrane domain, Ser453Cys in the C-terminal domain, Cys335Stop in the third extracellular loop, and several silent polymorphisms. Most of these are uncommon and they have not been examined in clozapine response.

Dopamine D$_2$ receptor

The "D$_2$-like" receptors D$_2$, D$_3$ and D$_4$ differ from D$_1$/D$_5$ in that they have three introns, a long third cytoplamic loop, and a short C-terminal tail; they also inhibit rather than stimulate the enzyme adenylyl cyclase. Clozapine and other atypical antipsychotic drugs are notable because their clinical efficacy is not dependent on high affinity for the dopamine D_2 receptor, unlike D_2-specific drugs such as haloperidol (Snyder, 1981; Roth et al., 1994). Clozapine has affinity for D_2 receptors that is at least an order of magnitude lower than that for 5-HT_{1A}, 5-HT_{2A}, or 5-HT_{2C} receptors, and this is perhaps the reason atypical antipsychotics such as clozapine act without causing EPS. However, it is likely that D_2 binding, albeit weak, is important for clozapine's efficacy (Meltzer, 1994) and there is evidence for limbic over striatal selectivity based on assessment of D_2 occupancy using positron emission tomography neuroimaging (Pilowsky et al., 1997). The affinity of antipsychotics for D_2 receptors is dependent on the rate at which they dissociate from the receptor (K_{off}; Kapur and Seeman, 2000). Drugs such as clozapine with a higher K_{off} will dissociate from receptors faster and, once the receptors are unblocked, will provide more access to surges in dopamine transmission. A higher K_{off} for the D_2 receptor has been proposed by Kapur and Seeman (2000) as a mechanism for "atypical" antipsychotic effect.

There are multiple polymorphisms in *DRD2*, including -241A/G, Δ-141C, the "*TaqI A*" polymorphism, and that giving rise to Ser311Cys. One of these, the functional promoter variant Δ−141C, has been examined in a retrospective sample of clozapine responders and nonresponders and was associated with response in one study (Malhotra et al., 1998) but not in a second (Arranz et al., 1998b).

Dopamine D_3 receptor

Clozapine has relatively weak affinity for the dopamine D_3 receptor (K_i 200 nmol/l) and is likely to have low occupancy of this receptor in vivo, suggesting that this receptor may not be of major importance to clozapine's action. The D_3 receptor is about 100-fold less abundant than D_2 receptors in the brain, but the expression of D_3 in limbic areas, especially the nucleus accumbens, makes an attractive target for antipsychotic drugs (Schwartz et al., 1993). Malmberg et al. (1998) have shown that clozapine is a partial inverse agonist at D_3.

The D_3 receptor is coupled to several signaling pathways, including G_i/G_0-proteins and the c-*fos* system, but intracellular responses are relatively weak (Sokoloff et al., 1992). The ability of clozapine to induce c-*fos* mRNA, an index of receptor coupling, is not altered in transgenic mice lacking the DRD3, also indicating that D_3 is not an important mediator of clozapine's clinical effects. However D_3 has attracted interest as a potential genetic risk factor for schizophrenia, and elevated D_3 mRNA has been seen in lymphocytes from patients with schizophrenia (Ilani et al., 2001).

There are four known polymorphisms in *DRD3*: noncoding −712G/C and −205A/G and coding polymorphisms resulting in Ser9Gly and Ala38Thr (Crocq et al., 1992; Ishiguro et al., 2000). Homozygosity for one of these, giving Ser9Gly, has been associated with schizophrenia (Crocq et al., 1992; Shaikh et al., 1996) and tardive dyskinesia during treatment with typical neuroleptics (Steen et al., 1997; Basile et al., 1999; Segman et al., 1999, 2000; Eichhammer et al., 2000; Lovlie et al., 2000; Ozdemir et al., 2001). It has also been implicated as a pharmacogenetic factor for clozapine response in a retrospectively assessed sample using GAFS (Shaikh et al., 1996). Although this association with clozapine response was not replicated in subjects from a double-blind clinical trial of clozapine (Malhotra et al., 1998), a subsequent study in Pakistani patients showed a significant association with the allele producing Gly9 (Scharfetter et al., 1999). A combined analysis of these three reports was also significant ($p = 0.004$). Therefore, despite the low affinity of clozapine for D_3 receptors, there is now good evidence for a pharmacogenetic influence on clozapine response.

Dopamine D_4 receptor

The D_4 receptor has similar pharmacology to the D_2 and D_3 receptors except that its affinity for clozapine is 10–20-fold higher (van Tol et al., 1991). This switch in specificity appears to be the result of a change in just a few amino acid residues in the second, third, and seventh transmembrane segments, which form a binding site crevice (Simpson et al., 1999). *DRD4* is expressed in regions of the brain particularly relevant to schizophrenia, especially the frontal cortex, amygdala, and hippocampus, and also the hypothalamus and mesencephalon, but at low levels in the basal ganglia (reviewed in Missale et al. (1998)).

Based on estimates that the therapeutic plasma concentration of clozapine is 20 nmol/l, D_4 is expected to be the only dopamine receptor occupied at physiological concentration (Seeman, 1992). However it is not clear whether D_4 mediates any of clozapine's therapeutic actions: in a clinical trial the D_4-specific antagonist L-745870 did not improve psychotic symptoms and, if anything, made them worse (reviewed in Bristow et al. (1997)).

DRD4 is unusually variable. A 48 bp tandem repeat in exon 3 of the gene, with alleles ranging from 1 to 12 repeats, was hypothesized to influence clozapine response since it appeared to modulate clozapine's affinity for the receptor (van Tol et al., 1992). However a series of genetic association studies of clozapine response, using both prospective and retrospective methods, failed to find association between *DRD4* VNTR (variable number tandem repeats) alleles and clozapine response (Shaikh et al., 1993, 1995; Rao et al., 1994; Rietschel et al., 1996; Kohn et al., 1997; Cohen et al., 1999; Kaiser et al., 2000). It subsequently became evident that there were only minor pharmacological differences between different alleles of the 48 bp VNTR (Jovanovic et al., 1999), although an effect from the extensive internal sequence variation of the repeats themselves cannot be ruled out (Lichter et al., 1993).

A number of other variants also occur in *DRD4*, including a -11C/T in the 5′ untranslated region; a 12 bp repeat which adds four amino acid residues and a 21 bp deletion which deletes seven amino acid residues, both in exon 1; base changes giving rise to Gly11Arg and Val194Gly; and a 13 bp nonsense mutation in the region encoding transmembrane region 2 which results in a non-functional protein. None of these has been associated with clozapine response (reviewed in Shaikh et al. (1997)). More recently, a series of polymorphisms in the promoter region (-1217G ins/del, -809G/A, -616C/G, -603T ins/del, -602(G)8–9, and -521C/T) has been identified (Okuyama et al., 1999). The polymorphism -521C/T is functional in vitro in that it reduces receptor expression by 40% in in vitro assays. These polymorphisms have not been tested in clozapine response.

Serotonin receptors

Serotonin 5-HT$_{1A}$ receptors

Because of its expression in regions of the brain thought to be relevant to schizophrenia, such as the hippocampus dorsal raphe nucleus and the neocortex, and its pharmacological properties, 5-HT$_{1A}$ is a strong candidate for a pharmacogenetic influence on clozapine's clinical efficacy (Masellis et al., 2001). In contrast to other receptors, at which clozapine is an antagonist, clozapine acts as a partial agonist at 5-HT$_{1A}$ receptors, along with other atypical drugs such as ziprasidone (Newman-Tancredi et al., 1998). There is good evidence to suggest that 5-HT$_{1A}$ agonism is an important component of the therapeutic action of clozapine; 5-HT$_{1A}$ receptor stimulation appears to increase dopamine release in the prefrontal cortex (Kuroki et al., 1999; Ichikawa and Meltzer, 2000) and also to be partly responsible for a reduction in 5-HT efflux in the rat ventral hippocampus (Bengtsson et al., 1998). Agonism at 5-HT$_{1A}$ receptors appears to have many of the same effects as 5-HT$_{2A}$ antagonism (Meltzer, 1999). Antagonism at 5-HT$_{2A}$ receptors (or D$_2$ antagonism) concurrent with 5-HT$_{1A}$ agonism has a synergistic effect in animal models of antipsychotic activity (Wadenberg and Ahlenius, 1991; Zifa and Fillion, 1992).

There a several known polymorphisms in *5-HT1A*: -51T/C, -152C/G, -321G/C, -480delA, -581C/A. and -1018C/G in the 5′ untranslated region and 294G/A, and 549C/T plus changes resulting in Gly272Asp and Pro16Leu in the coding region (Erdmann et al., 1995; Nakhai et al., 1995; Bergen et al., 1996; Kawanishi et al., 1998; Wu and Comings, 1999). Most of these polymorphisms are uncommon and consequently not informative; one of these polymorphisms (Pro16Leu) originally detected in Japan, has been tested for association with clozapine response in Americans but was not polymorphic in that population (Masellis et al., 2001).

Serotonin 5-HT$_{2A}$ and 5-HT$_{2C}$ receptors

Clozapine and other atypical antipsychotics are potent ligands for 5-HT$_{2A}$ (K_i 2.5) and 5-HT$_{2C}$ (K_i 8.6) and consequently these receptors have attracted the most attention as mediators of clozapine's clinical action (Roth et al., 1994). However, there is no clear correlation between 5-HT$_{2A}$ and 5-HT$_{2C}$ affinity and atypical antipsychotic action, and some typical drugs, such as chlorpromazine, have high affinity for 5-HT$_{2C}$. Both 5-HT$_{2A}$ and 5-HT$_{2C}$ receptors are linked to the stimulation of intracelluar inositol phosphate levels via G-protein coupling.

The 5-HT$_{2A}$ receptor is highly expressed in many areas of the cortex, the neocortex, parts of the limbic system, and the basal ganglia. Detailed studies of the macaque cortex revealed that the most intense 5-HT$_{2A}$ expression is in pyramidal neurons of the cortex, where expression is both pre- and postsynaptic (Jakab and Goldman-Rakic, 1998). The "hot-spot" for expression is in the apical dendrite field proximal to the pyramidal cell soma, where the receptors may participate in sensory gating to regulate working memory and the related process latent inhibition. Both of these are relevant to dysfunctional states in psychosis, and clozapine may act specifically to improve sensory gating. The 5-HT$_{2C}$ receptor is expressed in the globus pallidus and substantia nigra of the basal ganglia, the choroid plexus and limbic system (reviewed in Hoyer (1994)).

Constitutively active forms of both 5-HT$_{2A}$ and 5-HT$_{2C}$ receptors have been produced by site-directed mutagenesis (Herrick-Davies et al., 1997; Egan et al., 1998) and this has led to the reclassification of many drugs, including atypical drugs, as 5-HT$_{2A}$/5-HT$_{2C}$ inverse agonists (Egan et al., 1998; Herrick-Davies et al., 1998, 2000). The mRNA for 5-HT$_{2C}$, but not 5-HT$_{2A}$, undergoes RNA editing to produce multiple isoforms differing at just a few amino acids (Burns et al., 1997). These isoforms are widely distributed in the brain and differ in the level of constitutive activity, with RNA editing tending to silence it (Herrick-Davies et al., 1999; Niswender et al., 1999). In this model, the unedited 5-HT$_{2C}$ receptor exists in conformational equilibrium shifted toward the active form in the absence of ligand. Atypical antipsychotics such as clozapine shift the equilibrium to favor the inactive conformation, rather than being classical neutral antagonists. Thus atypical antipsychotics have unique functional effects on 5-HT$_{2C}$; these effects mediate some of the clinical efficacy of clozapine, then regulation of RNA editing may be an important factor in the pharmacogenetics of clozapine response.

Both 5-HT$_{2A}$ and 5-HT$_{2C}$ receptors are also unusual in that they have another unusual mode of regulation, since both agonists and antagonists (including clozapine) induce their post-translational downregulation, mainly by internalization of the receptor (Newton and Elliot, 1997; Bhatnagar et al., 2001). Clozapine induces 5-HT$_{2A}$ internalization via an arrestin-independent endosome-mediated pathway (Bhatnagar et al., 2001). This internalization process may be central to clozapine's clinical efficacy.

The gene *5-HT2A* has multiple polymorphic variants in both the coding region (102T/C, 516C/T and giving rise to Thr25Asn, Ala447Val, and His452Tyr; Warren et al., 1993; Erdmann et al., 1996) and the 5' sequence/promoter region ($-$1438A/G, $-$1421C/T; Spurlock et al., 1998). An initial report of association between a *5-HT2A* variant, 102T/C, and clozapine response (Arranz et al., 1995) was not replicated in several independent studies (Masellis et al., 1995, 1998; Noethen et al., 1995; Malhotra et al., 1996a). However, a meta-analysis showed a trend of association between this polymorphism and response (Arranz et al., 1998a). In addition, Arranz et al. (1998c) and Masellis et al. (1998) found association between His452Tyr and clozapine response. The meta-analysis by Arranz et al. (1998a) also investigated the relation between His452Tyr polymorphism and clozapine response, confirming the apparent association. These results constitute the strongest evidence of association between receptor variants and treatment response and suggest an important role for the 5-HT$_{2A}$ receptors in mediating the therapeutic activity of clozapine.

5-HT2C has two polymorphisms, one giving rise to Ser23Cys and the other a complex GT/CT repeat region (Deckert et al., 1997; Arranz et al., 2000a). Both of these have been examined for association with clozapine response. The Ser23-producing allele has been associated with good clozapine response in a retrospective analysis (Sodhi et al., 1995) but this has not been replicated (Malhotra et al., 1996b; Rietschel et al., 1997; Masellis et al., 1998). The promoter GT/CT repeat has also been associated with clozapine response (Arranz et al., 2000a); however, since it is in strong linkage disequilibrium with the polymorphism giving Ser23Cys, this may reflect linkage disequilibrium between the two polymorphisms.

Serotonin 5-HT$_3$ receptors

Clozapine is a functional antagonist for 5-HT$_3$ receptors and binds with moderate affinity (Watling et al., 1990; Brunello et al., 1995) with a K_i value of about 123 nmol/l (Hermann et al., 1996). Unlike other 5-HT receptors, 5-HT$_3$ is a ligand-gated ion channel with structural features in common with GABA-A and glycine and nicotinic acetylcholine receptors (Maricq et al., 1991). It is expressed in the area postrema and mesolimbic system in the brain, which acts as an interface between limbic and motor structures. It has been suggested that 5-HT$_3$ can mediate anxiolytic (Broekkamp et al., 1989) and atypical antipsychotic properties (Warburton et al., 1994). There is also neurochemical evidence against clozapine's antipsychotic effects being dependent on 5-HT$_3$ (Squires and Saederup, 1999). Two different 5-HT$_3$ isoforms, 5-HT$_{3A}$ and 5-HT$_{3B}$, encoded by separate genes, have been cloned, both of which map close together on chromosome 11q23 (Weiss et al., 1995; Davies et al., 1999). *5-HT3A* has been screened for polymorphisms in schizophrenic and bipolar patients but these are rare and not associated with disease (Niesler et al., 2001). One study has examined 5-HT$_{3B}$ in clozapine response using a retrospectively assessed GAFS score (Arranz et al., 2000a). Two silent polymorphisms, 178C/T and 1596G/A, were examined but no association was found.

Serotonin 5-HT$_{5A}$ receptors

The 5-HT$_{5A}$ receptor does not have a high affinity for antipsychotic drugs such as clozapine (Waeber et al., 1998). It is expressed exclusively in the brain, mainly in the cerebral cortex (especially layers II–III and V–VI of the neocortex), hippocampus (dentate gyrus and pyramidal cell layer of CA1 and CA3), and cerebellum. This distribution indicates that 5-HT$_{5A}$ may be involved in higher cortical and limbic functions (Pasqualetti et al., 1998), and the receptor is thus a good candidate for etiological involvement in psychiatric disorders. One study has examined 5-HT$_{5A}$ receptors in clozapine response using a retrospectively assessed GAFS score (Birkett et al., 2000). Two silent polymorphisms, -19G/C and 12A/T, were examined but no association was found.

Serotonin 5-HT$_6$ receptors

Clozapine is a high-affinity antagonist for the 5-HT$_6$ receptor (Roth et al., 1994) and in rat brain the 5-HT$_6$ receptor may represent up to 40% of specific receptor binding (Glatt et al., 1995). The 5-HT$_6$ receptor is widely distributed in the human brain and is expressed most prominently in the caudate nucleus, at significant levels in the hippocampus and the amygdala, and at lower levels in the thalamus, subthalamic nucleus, and substantia nigra (Kohen et al., 1996). It stimulates adenylyl cyclase through G$_s$-protein (Barnes and Sharp, 1999). The human 5-HT$_6$ receptor is structurally (89% amino acid identity) and functionally similar to that in the rat, and on the basis of the affinity of the receptor for clozapine is expected to be substantially occupied at therapeutic doses in humans (Kohen et al., 1996). Clozapine appears to have a potent effect on 5-HT$_6$ expression as it can reduce 5-HT$_6$-binding sites (B_{max}) by as much as 62% in serum-free HeLa cells transfected with the rat receptor (Zhukovskaya and Neumaier, 2000). Downregulation of a receptor by an antagonist is unusual but has also been seen for the 5-HT$_{2A}$ and 5-HT$_{2C}$ receptors, where internalization is triggered by atypical antipsychotic drugs including clozapine (Willins et al., 1999). This indicates that 5-HT$_{2A}$, 5-HT$_{2C}$, and 5-HT$_6$ may be similar in that they share "paradoxical" downregulation by clozapine. The high affinity of clozapine for 5-HT$_6$ and its effect on expression indicates that it may be an important site for clinical action.

The gene *5-HT6* has six polymorphic variants (Vogt et al., 2000), 126G/T, 267C/T, 873+30C/T, 873+128A/C, 1128G/C, and 1376T/G, none of which change the amino acid sequence of the protein. One of these (267C/T) has been examined for association with clozapine response, and a weak association was found (Yu et al., 1999), but this was not replicated in a sample from the USA (Masellis et al., 2001).

Serotonin 5-HT$_7$ receptors

Clozapine is also a high-affinity agonist for the 5-HT$_7$ receptor (Roth et al., 1994). This receptor is expressed in midline, thalamic, and limbic structures in the brain (Eglen et al., 1997; Vanhoenacker et al., 2000) where it is thought to regulate cranial vasodilatation, emotion, and circadian rhythms. In contrast to 5-HT$_6$, it is not downregulated by clozapine (Zhukovskaya and Neumaier, 2000). One polymorphism is known in *5HT7*, giving rise to Pro279Leu (Pesonen et al., 1998) and this has not been associated with clozapine response (Masellis et al., 2001).

Serotonin transporter

The transporter 5-HT (5-HTT) has also been postulated to influence response to clozapine, as functional variation in the gene may affect the efficacy of antipsychotic drugs that act through the 5-HT system (Lesch, 1998). *5-HTT* gene knockout results in marked desensitization of 5-HT$_{1A}$ autoreceptors in the dorsal raphe nucleus without altering postsynaptic 5-HT$_{1A}$ receptor functioning in the hippocampus (Cour et al., 2001). One study has examined two polymorphisms in *5-HTT* (a polymorphic repetitive element upstream of the transcription start site (5-HTTLPR) and a VNTR in intron 2) for association with clozapine response (Arranz et al., 2000b), one of these, the functional 5-HTTLPR, showed a trend toward association with clozapine response but failed to reach statistical significance.

Histamine receptors

With the recent discovery of a novel histamine receptor gene *HHR4* (Nakamura et al., 2000; Oda et al., 2000; Liu et al., 2001; Morse et al., 2001; Nguyen et al., 2001), there are now four known receptors (H$_1$–H$_4$) encoded by four separate genes (Hough, 2001). All are G$_0$ protein-coupled receptors, transducing signals via G$_q$ (H$_1$), G$_s$ (H$_2$), and G$_i$/$_0$ (H$_3$, H$_4$). Both H$_1$ and H$_2$ receptors are expressed in the caudate, putamen, neocortex, and hippocampus, whereas H$_3$ receptors are expressed in the basal ganglia and globus pallidus and H$_4$ receptors in peripheral tissues (eosinophils and bone marrow) but not the brain (Nakamura et al., 2000). However RNAse protection assays indicate that some H$_4$ receptors may, in fact, be present in the brain (Liu et al., 2001). Clozapine is an agonist at all of these except the H$_3$ receptor ($K_i > 10\,000$ nmol/l), with strongest affinity for H$_1$ ($K_i = 2.8$ nmol/l) and only moderate affinity for H$_2$ ($K_i = 100$ nmol/l), and H$_4$ ($K_i = 510$–693 nmol/l). H$_1$ is the only receptor likely to be significantly occupied at physiological concentrations of clozapine.

H1 and *H2* genes have been screened for polymorphisms and tested for an influence on clozapine response (Mancama et al., 2000). Five polymorphisms (giving Lys19Asn, Asp349Glu, A1068G, ΔPhe358 and Leu449Ser) are known in H$_1$ and only one (G543A) in H$_2$. However, no evidence of a role in influencing clozapine response was found.

Cholinergic muscarinic receptors

There are five known cholinergic muscarinic receptors, encoded by five separate intronless genes, *CHRM1* through to *CHRM5*. Clozapine binds with high affinity to all of these receptors in in vitro binding studies (Bymaster et al., 1999), with K_i values 1.4 nmol/l (M_1) to 10 nmol/l (M_2), very close to those for olanzapine. However, there is evidence from binding studies in intact cells that these measures may be overestimates, with the true range nearer to 31 nmol/l (M_1) to 204 nmol/l (M_2) (Bymaster and Falcone, 2000). Risperidone and typical drugs such as haloperidol have low muscarinic affinity.

Historically, the cholinergic system was one of the first to be investigated in the pharmacological treatment of schizophrenia, where the use of anticholinesterase agents such as physostigmine and cholinergic stimulation with acetylcholine and arecoline showed some efficacy. A role for hypercholinergia has been postulated for psychosis, and there is also evidence that atypical antipsychotic action may be mediated by muscarinic receptors. For example the M_1/M_4 agonist xanomeline, which has little or no affinity for dopamine receptors, has antipsychotic-like activity in rats and mice (Shannon et al., 2000).

Genetic variation within the five muscarinic receptors has been proposed to contribute toward the differences in treatment response observed amongst patients. To-date four polymorphic loci have been identified within *CHMR1*: 267C/A, 1044G/A, 1221C/T and 1353C/T, while single polymorphisms have been identified in *CHMR3* (193G/A) and *CHMR4* (1338C/T). However, none of these have been found to influence clozapine response (D. Mancama, personal communication).

Alpha-adrenoceptors

There are seven α-adrenoceptors, encoded by separate genes (*ADRA1A–1D* and *ADRA2A–2C*). Pharmacologically, these receptors are broadly divided into α_1- and α_2-adrenoceptors, and clozapine is a high-affinity antagonist for both these classes, with a K_i of between 4 and 12 nmol/l. There is little information on the affinity of clozapine for individual receptor subtypes.

Central α_1-noradrenergic neurotransmission has been shown to be an important complement of dopaminergic transmission in the control of motor activity. The α_{1A}-adrenoceptor is widespread throughout the rat central nervous system, with high levels in olfactory regions, hypothalamic nuclei, brainstem, and spinal cord, particularly in areas related to motor function. The mRNA for α_{1B}-receptors is highly expressed in the pineal gland, most thalamic nuclei, lateral nucleus of the amygdala, and dorsal and median raphe nuclei, with moderate expression levels noted throughout the cerebral cortex and other regions. The α_{1D}-adrenoceptor is expressed in the olfactory bulb, cerebral cortex, hippocampus, reticular thalamic nucleus, regions of the amygdala, motor nuclei of the brainstem, inferior olivary complex and spinal cord. From studies of transgenic mice, the α_{1B}-adrenoceptor has been implicated in memory consolidation and fear-motivated exploratory behaviors (Knauber and Muller, 2000), which are both relevant to the cognitive and social deficits in schizophrenia, as well as having peripheral involvement in vascular and blood pressure responses (Cavalli et al., 1997).

The α_2-adrenoceptor subtypes inhibit adenylyl cyclase, are G-protein coupled and are widely expressed in human tissues, including brain (Eason and Liggett, 1993). Both the α_{2A}- and α_{2C}-adrenoceptors are required for normal presynaptic control of neurotransmitter release from central noradrenergic neurons (Hein et al., 1999). Antagonism of α_2-adrenoceptors enhances adrenergic transmission and reinforces frontocortical dopaminergic transmission, whereas blockade of α_1-adrenoceptors inhibits dorsal raphe-derived serotonergic pathways. This profile of activity may contribute to the antipsychotic properties of atypical drugs such as clozapine.

One study has examined adrenoreceptor genes in clozapine response (Bolonna et al., 2000). One polymorphism in *ADRA1A* (Arg492Cys) and two polymorphisms in the promoter region of *ADRA2A* (-1291C/G and -261G/A) were investigated in a sample of clozapine-treated schizophrenic patients scored retrospectively for response using the GAS. However, there were no differences between the responder and nonresponder groups, suggesting that these polymorphisms do not play an important role in determining antipsychotic response.

GABA receptors

Although dopamine, 5-HT, cholinergic muscarinic, histamine and adreno receptors are thought to be the major receptors for clozapine in the brain, other systems may play an important role in clozapine's action. Clozapine is a weak antagonist at GABA-A receptors (Squires and Saederup, 1997, 1998), can reverse the inhibitory effect of GABA on the binding of an inhibitory antagonist at GABA receptors (Squires and Saederup, 1991) and shows a preference for specific combinations of α- and β-subtypes (Korpi et al., 1995). This evidence suggests that clozapine can reduce GABA receptor activation; more recent work suggests that functional antagonism occurs at physiological concentrations of the drug (Michel and Trudeau, 2000). However, GABA receptors have not been tested for association with clozapine response as yet.

Interaction between genes

Clozapine's complex array of receptor binding makes it likely that multiple receptors contribute to the clinical action of this drug. It is, therefore, easy to imagine that genetic variation in several of the genes encoding these receptors will influence clinical response to clozapine. Additive genetic analysis of combinations of these polymorphisms should, therefore, improve the pharmacogenetic prediction of clozapine response over that considering only single gene variants. Arranz et al. (2000a) have attempted to test this approach using a series of polymorphisms from genes previously tested in a retrospectively assessed sample for association with clozapine. From 19 polymorphisms tested, a combination of six (5-HT$_{2C}$ 102T/C and His452Tyr; 5-HT$_{2C}$ −330G/T/−244C/T and Ser23Cys; *5-HTTLPR*; and H$_2$ −1018G/A) were selected on the basis that they showed a *p* value of <0.09 for association with response to clozapine. This combination gave a positive "predictive" value of 0.76 and a negative predictive value of 0.82, with a *p* value overall of 0.0001. A criticism of this approach is that it is a post hoc analysis of a series of polymorphisms not all of which have been shown to be individually associated with clozapine response but which have been selected for *p* values below an arbitrary level (0.09). This finding should be regarded as exploratory and needs careful replication in a prospectively assessed sample. However, it points the way forward to the prospect of combined analysis of multiple polymorphisms to provide accurate predictive information on clozapine response.

Conclusions

The aim of pharmacogenetic research is to define composite genetic tests that can be used to predict the outcome of drug treatment. This outcome can be defined in several ways and includes clinical response to treatment (reduction or elimination of disease symptomatology), vulnerability to side effects, or improvement in more specific disease-related measures such as cognitive performance. Such tests will provide benefits to the patient by identifying treatments likely to be successful early on in the disease process; early intervention appears to be important for long-term prognosis in schizophrenia. In addition, drug safety will be improved, as those patients most vulnerable to side effects can be identified in advance and either carefully monitored or given alternative therapy. Finally, these tests will have economic benefit in a climate of treatment rationing as the rate of unsuccessful treatment with costly drugs such as atypical antipsychotics will be avoided.

Clozapine therapy has been used as a model system for pharmacogenetic research into antipsychotic drugs. This is largely for the historical reasons that it has high affinity for the dopamine D$_4$ receptor, which shows extensive genetic variability, but also because its pharmacology is well understood. Although polymorphisms in two genes, *5-HT2A* and dopamine D$_3$, have been implicated in more than one study as influencing response to clozapine, research into its pharmacogenetics is still in its infancy, particularly with respect to genetic influence on side effects.

A novel epistatic approach, simultaneously examining genetic variation in multiple genes that encode clozapine's neurotransmitter targets, has been performed, and this points the way to analysis of the future. However, there is still a general lack of large, powerful prospective studies using multiple measures of response, and many polymorphisms in potentially relevant genes, such as *GABA-A*, have not yet been examined.

It is also important to note that pharmacogenetic tests will not be clinically useful if they only apply to a single drug such as clozapine. A genetic test will be most valuable in choosing which drug will be, on balance, most efficacious and least risky from a panel of suitable choices. This will require extensive pharmacogenetic analysis of a variety of antipsychotic drugs, both typical and atypical.

To predict fully clinical response to antipsychotic treatment in schizophrenia, it will be necessary to take account of many variables in addition to genetic influence on clozapine's pharmacokinetics and pharmacodynamics, including social, demographic, and clinical factors (e.g., compliance, social support, and history of birth trauma); genetic vulnerability to side effects such as weight gain and sedation; and the influence of genetic susceptibility factors for psychosis, which may define subtype and symptomatology. When this is achieved, a simple and reliable process for the individualization of treatment will be attainable.

REFERENCES

Ahlenius S (1999). Clozapine: dopamine D_1 receptor agonism in the prefrontal cortex as the code to decipher a Rosetta stone of antipsychotic drugs. *Pharmacol Toxicol* 84, 193–196.

Amsler HA, Teerenhovi L, Barth E, Harjula K, Vuopio P (1977). Agranulocytosis in patients treated with clozapine. A study of the Finnish epidemic. *Acta Psychiatr Scand* 56, 241–248.

Arranz M, Collier D, Sodhi M et al. (1995). Association between clozapine response and allelic variation in 5-HT_{2A} receptor gene. *Lancet* 346, 281–282.

Arranz MJ, Munro J, Sham P et al. (1998a). Meta analysis of studies on variation in 5HT_{2A} receptors and clozapine response. *Schizophr Res* 32, 93–99.

Arranz MJ, Li T, Munro J et al. (1998b). Lack of association between a polymorphism in the promoter region of the dopamine-2 receptor gene and clozapine response. *Pharmacogenetics* 8, 481–484.

Arranz MJ, Munro J, Owen MJ et al. (1998c). Evidence for association between polymorphisms in the promoter and coding regions of the 5-HT_{2A} receptor gene and response to clozapine. *Mol Psychiatry* 3, 61–66.

Arranz MJ, Munro J, Birkett J et al. (2000a). Pharmacogenetic prediction of clozapine response. *Lancet* 355, 1615–1616.

Arranz MJ, Bolonna AA, Munro J, Curtis CJ, Collier DA, Kerwin RW (2000b). The serotonin transporter and clozapine response. *Mol Psychiatry* 5, 124–125.

Barnes NM, Sharp T (1999). A review of central 5-HT receptors and their function. *Neuropharmacology* 38, 1083–1152.

Basile VS, Masellis M, Badri F et al. (1999). Association of the *MscI* polymorphism of the dopamine D_3 receptor gene with tardive dyskinesia in schizophrenia. *Neuropsychopharmacology* 21, 17–27.

Bengtsson HJ, Kullberg A, Millan MJ, Hjorth S (1998). The role of 5-HT$_{1A}$ autoreceptors and alpha1-adrenoceptors in the modulation of 5-HT release – III. Clozapine and the novel putative antipsychotic S 16924. *Neuropharmacology* 37, 349–356.

Bergen A, Wang CY, Nakhai B, Goldman D (1996). Mass allele detection (MAD) of rare *5-HT1A* structural variants with allele-specific amplification and lectrochemiluminescent detection. *Hum Mutat* 7, 135–143.

Bhatnagar A, Willins DL, Gray JA, Woods J, Benovic JL, Roth BL (2001). The dynamin-dependent, arrestin-independent internalization of 5-hydroxytryptamine 2A (5-HT$_{2A}$) serotonin receptors reveals differential sorting of arrestins and 5-HT$_{2A}$ receptors during endocytosis. *J Biol Chem* 276, 8269–8277.

Bilder RM, Goldman RS et al. (2000). Neuropsychology of first-episode schizophrenia: initial characterization and clinical correlates. *Am J Psychiatry* 157, 549–559.

Birkett JT, Arranz MJ, Munro J, Osborne S, Kerwin RW, Collier DA (2000). Association analysis of the *5-HT5A* gene in depression, psychosis and antipsychotic response. *Neuroreport* 11, 2017–2020.

Bolonna AA, Arranz MJ, Munro J et al. (2000). No influence of adrenergic receptor polymorphisms on schizophrenia and antipsychotic response. *Neurosci Lett* 280, 65–68.

Breier A, Buchanan RW, Irish D, Carpenter, WT Jr. (1993). Clozapine treatment of outpatients with schizophrenia: outcome and long-term response patterns. *Hosp Community Psychiatry* 44, 1145–1149.

Bristow LJ, Kramer MS, Kulagowski J, Patel S, Ragan CI, Seabrook GR (1997). Schizophrenia and L-745, 870, a novel dopamine D_4 receptor antagonist. *Trend Pharmacol Sci* 18, 186–188.

Broekkamp CL, Berendsen HH, Jenck F, van Delft AM (1989). Animal models for anxiety and response to serotonergic drugs. *Psychopathology* 22(Suppl 1), 2–12.

Brunello N, Masotto C, Steardo L, Markstein R, Racagni G (1995). New insights into the biology of schizophrenia through the mechanism of action of clozapine. *Neuropsychopharmacology* 13, 177–213.

Burns CM, Chu H, Rueter SM et al. (1997). Regulation of serotonin-2C receptor G-protein coupling by RNA editing. *Nature* 387, 303–308.

Bymaster FP, Falcone JF (2000). Decreased binding affinity of olanzapine and clozapine for human muscarinic receptors in intact clonal cells in physiological medium. *Eur J Pharmacol* 390, 245–248.

Bymaster FP, Nelson DL, DeLapp NW et al. (1999). Antagonism by olanzapine of dopamine D_1, serotonin 2, muscarinic, histamine H_1 and alpha1-adrenergic receptors in vitro. *Schizophr Res* 37, 107–122.

Cavalli A, Lattion AL, Hummler E et al. (1997). Decreased blood pressure response in mice deficient of the alpha1b-adrenergic receptor. *Proc Natl Acad Sci, USA* 94, 11589–11594.

Cichon S, Nothen MM, Stober G et al. (1996). Systematic screening for mutations in the 5′-regulatory region of the human dopamine D_1 receptor (*DRD1*) gene in patients with schizophrenia and bipolar affective disorder. *Am J Med Genet* 67, 424–428.

Cohen BM, Ennulat DJ, Centorrino F et al. (1999). Polymorphisms of the dopamine D4 receptor and response to antipsychotic drugs. *Psychopharmacology (Berl)* 141, 6–10.

Cour CM, Boni C, Hanoun N, Lesch KP, Hamon M, Lanfumey L (2001). Functional consequences of 5-HT transporter gene disruption on 5-HT1A receptor-mediated regulation of dorsal raphe and hippocampal cell activity. *J Neurosci* 21, 2178–2185.

Crocq MA, Mant R, Asherson P et al. (1992). Association between schizophrenia and homozygosity at the dopamine D_3 receptor gene. *J Med Genet* 29, 858–860.

Davies PA, Pistis M, Hanna MC et al. (1999). The 5-HT_{3B} subunit is a major determinant of serotonin-receptor function. *Nature* 397, 359–363.

Deckert J, Catalano M, Heils A et al. (1997). Functional promoter polymorphism of the human serotonin transporter: lack of association with panic disorder. *Psychiatr Genet* 7, 45–47.

Eason MG, Liggett SB (1993). Human alpha-2-adrenergic receptor subtype distribution: widespread and subtype-selective expression of alpha-2–C10, alpha-2–C4, and alpha-2–C2 mRNA in multiple tissues. *Mol Pharmacol* 44, 70–75.

Egan C, Herrick-Davis K, Teitler M (1998). Creation of a constitutively activated state of the 5-HT_{2A} receptor by site-directed mutagenesis: revelation of inverse agonist activity of antagonists. *Ann NY Acad Sci* 861, 136–139.

Eglen RM, Jasper JR, Chang DJ, Martin GR (1997). The 5-HT_7 receptor: orphan found. *Trend Pharmacol Sci* 18, 104–107.

Eichhammer P, Albus M, Borrmann-Hassenbach M et al. (2000). Association of dopamine D_3-receptor gene variants with neuroleptic induced akathisia in schizophrenic patients: a generalization of Steen's study on *DRD3* and tardive dyskinesia. *Am J Med Genet* 96, 187–191.

Endicott J, Spilzer RL, Fless JL, Cohen J (1976). The global assessment scale. *Arch Gen Psychiatry* 33, 766–772.

Erdmann J, Shimron-Abarbanell D, Cichon S et al. (1995). Systematic screening for mutations in the promoter and the coding region of the *5-HT1A* gene. *Am J Med Genet* 60, 393–399.

Erdmann J, Shimron-Abarbanell D, Rietschel M et al. (1996). Systematic screening for mutations in the human serotonin-2A (*5-HT2A*) receptor gene: identification of two naturally occurring receptor variants and association analysis in schizophrenia. *Hum Genet* 97, 614–619.

Feng J, Sobell JL, Heston LL, Cook EH Jr., Goldman D, Sommer SS (1998). Scanning of the dopamine D_1 and D_5 receptor genes by REF in neuropsychiatric patients reveals a novel missense change at a highly conserved amino acid. *Am J Med Genet* 81, 172–178.

Fitton A, Heel RC (1990). Clozapine: a review of its pharmacological properties, and therapeutic use in schizophrenia. *Drugs* 40, 722–747.

Gerlach J, Koppelhus P, Helweg E, Monrad A (1974). Clozapine and haloperidol in a single-blind cross-over trial: therapeutic and biochemical aspects in the treatment of schizophrenia. *Acta Psychiatr Scand* 50, 410–424.

Glatt CE, Snowman AM, Sibley DR, Snyder SH (1995). Clozapine: selective labeling of sites resembling 5HT_6 serotonin receptors may reflect psychoactive profile. *Mol Med* 1, 398–406.

Guy W (1976). *ECDEU Assessment Manual for Psychopharmacology*, revised edn. Bethesda, MD: US Department of Health, Education and Welfare, pp. 217–222.

Hein L, Altman JD, Kobilka BK (1999). Two functionally distinct alpha-2-adrenergic receptors regulate sympathetic neurotransmission. *Nature* 402, 181–184.

Hermann B, Wetzel CH, Pestel E, Zieglgansberger W, Holsboer F, Rupprecht R (1996). Functional antagonistic properties of clozapine at the 5-HT$_3$ receptor. *Biochem Biophys Res Commun* 225, 957–960.

Herrick-Davis K, Egan C, Teitler M (1997). Activating mutations of the serotonin 5-HT$_{2C}$ receptor. *J Neurochem* 69, 1138–1144.

Herrick-Davis K, Grinde E, Gauthier C, Teitler M (1998). Pharmacological characterization of the constitutively activated state of the serotonin 5-HT$_{2C}$ receptor. *Ann NY Acad Sci* 861, 140–145.

Herrick-Davis K, Grinde E, Niswender CM (1999). Serotonin 5-HT$_{2C}$ receptor RNA editing alters receptor basal activity: implications for serotonergic signal transduction. *J Neurochem* 73, 1711–1717.

Herrick-Davis K, Grinde E, Teitler M (2000). Inverse agonist activity of atypical antipsychotic drugs at human 5-hydroxytryptamine 2C receptors. *J Pharmacol Exp Ther* 295, 226–232.

Hough LB (2001). Genomics meets histamine receptors: new subtypes, new receptors. *Mol Pharmacol* 59, 415–419.

Hoyer D (1988). Molecular pharmacology and biology of 5-HT$_{1C}$ receptors. *Trends Pharmacol Sci* 9, 89–94.

Ichikawa J, Ishii H, Bonaccorso S, Fowler WL, O'Laughlin IA, Meltzer HY (2001). 5-HT(2A) and D(2) receptor blockade increases cortical DA release via 5-HT(1A) receptor activation: a possible mechanism of atypical antipsychotic-induced cortical dopamine release. *J Neurochem* 76, 1521–1531.

Ichikawa J, Meltzer HY (2000). The effect of serotonin (1A) receptor agonism on antipsychotic drug-induced dopamine release in rat striatum and nucleus accumbens. *Brain Res* 858, 252–263.

Ilani T, Ben-Shachar D, Strous RD et al. (2001). A peripheral marker for schizophrenia: increased levels of D$_3$ dopamine receptor mRNA in blood lymphocytes. *Proc Natl Acad Sci, USA* 98, 625–628.

Ishiguro H, Okuyama Y, Toru M, Arinami T (2000). Mutation and association analysis of the 5′ region of the dopamine D$_3$ receptor gene in schizophrenia patients: identification of the Ala38Thr polymorphism and suggested association between *DRD3* haplotypes and schizophrenia. *Mol Psychiatry* 5, 433–438.

Jakab RL, Goldman-Rakic PS (1998). 5-Hydroxytryptamine 2A serotonin receptors in the primate cerebral cortex: possible site of action of hallucinogenic and antipsychotic drugs in pyramidal cell apical dendrites. *Proc Natl Acad Sci. USA* 95, 735–740.

Jovanovic V, Guan HC, van Tol HH (1999). Comparative pharmacological and functional analysis of the human dopamine D4.2 and D4.10 receptor variants. *Pharmacogenetics* 9, 561–568.

Kaiser R, Konneker M, Henneken M et al. (2000). Dopamine D$_4$ receptor 48-bp repeat polymorphism: no association with response to antipsychotic treatment, but association with catatonic schizophrenia. *Mol Psychiatry* 5, 418–424.

Kapur S, Remington G (2001). Atypical antipsychotics: new directions and new challenges in the treatment of schizophrenia. *Annu Rev Med* 52, 503–517.

Kapur S, Seeman P (2000). Antipsychotic agents differ in how fast they come off the dopamine D$_2$ receptors: implications for atypical antipsychotic action. *J Psychiatr Neurosci* 25, 161–166.

Kawanishi Y, Harada S, Tachikawa H, Okubo T, Shiraishi H (1998). Novel mutations in the promoter and coding region of the human 5-HT$_{1A}$ receptor gene and association analysis in schizophrenia. *Am J Med Genet* 81, 434–439.

Kay SR, Opler LA, Fiszbein A (1992). *Positive and Negative Symptom Scale (PANSS)*. Niagra Falls, NY: Multi-Health Systems.

Knauber J, Muller WE (2000). Decreased exploratory activity and impaired passive avoidance behaviour in mice deficient for the alpha(1b)-adrenoceptor. *Eur Neuropsychopharmacol* 10, 423–427.

Kohen R, Metcalf MA, Khan N et al. (1996). Protein, nucleotide, OMIM cloning, characterization, and chromosomal localization of a human 5-HT$_6$ serotonin receptor. *J Neurochem* 66, 47–56.

Kohn Y, Ebstein RP, Heresco-Levy U et al. (1997). Dopamine D$_4$ receptor gene polymorphisms: relation to ethnicity, no association with schizophrenia and response to clozapine in Israeli subjects. *Eur J Neuropsychopharmacol* 7, 39–43.

Korpi ER, Wong G, Luddens H (1995). Subtype specificity of gamma-aminobutyric acid type A receptor antagonism by clozapine. *Naunyn-Schmiedeberg Arch Pharmacol* 352, 365–373.

Kulkarni SK, Ninan I (2000). Dopamine D4 receptors and development of newer antipsychotic drugs. *Fund Clin Pharmacol* 14, 529–539.

Kuroki T, Meltzer HY, Ichikawa J (1999). Effects of antipsychotic drugs on extracellular dopamine levels in rat medial prefrontal cortex and nucleus accumbens. *J Pharmacol Exp Ther* 288, 774–781.

Lehman AF, Postrado LT, Rachuba LT (1993). Convergent validation of quality of life assessments for persons with severe mental illnesses. *Qual Life Res* 2, 327–333.

Lesch KP (1998). Hallucinations: psychopathology meets functional genomics. *Mol Psychiatry* 3, 278–281.

Lichter JB, Barr CL, Kennedy JL, van Tol HH, Kidd KK, Livak KJ (1993). A hypervariable segment in the human dopamine receptor D$_4$ (*DRD4*) gene. *Hum Mol Genet* 2, 767–773.

Lidow MS, Elsworth JD, Goldman-Rakic PS (1997). Down-regulation of the D$_1$ and D$_5$ dopamine receptors in the primate prefrontal cortex by chronic treatment with antipsychotic drugs. *J Pharmacol Exp Ther* 281, 597–603.

Lieberman JA, Kane JM, Safferman AZ et al. (1994a). Predictors of response to clozapine. *J Clin Psychiatry* 55(Suppl B), 126–128.

Lieberman JA, Safferman AZ, Pollack S et al. (1994b). Clinical effects of clozapine in chronic schizophrenia: response to treatment and predictors of outcome. *Am J Psychiatry* 151, 1744–1752.

Light GA, Geyer MA, Clementz BA, Cadenhead KS, Braff DL (2000). Normal P50 suppression in schizophrenia patients treated with atypical antipsychotic medications. *Am J Psychiatry* 157, 767–771.

Liu C, Wilson SJ, Kuei C, Lovenberg TW (2001). Comparison of human, mouse, rat, and guinea pig histamine H$_4$ receptors reveals substantial pharmacological species variation. *J Pharmacol Exp Ther* 299, 121–130.

Lovlie R, Daly AK, Blennerhassett R, Ferrier N, Steen VM (2000). Homozygosity for the Gly-9 variant of the dopamine D$_3$ receptor and risk for tardive dyskinesia in schizophrenic patients. *Int J Neuropsychopharmacol* 3, 61–65.

Luborsky L (1962). Clinician's judgement of mental health. *Arch Gen Psychiatry* 7, 407–417.

Malhotra AK, Goldman D, Ozaki N, Breier A, Buchanan R, Pickar D (1996a). Lack of association between polymorphisms in the 5-HT$_{2A}$ receptor gene and the antipsychotic response to clozapine. *Am J Psychiatry* 153, 1092–1094.

Malhotra AK, Goldman D, Ozaki N et al. (1996b). Clozapine response and the 5HT$_{2C}$ Cys23Ser polymorphism. *Neuroreport* 7, 2100–2102.

Malhotra AK, Goldman D, Buchanan RW et al. (1998). The dopamine D$_3$ receptor (*DRD3*) Ser9Gly polymorphism and schizophrenia: a haplotype relative risk study and association with clozapine response. *Mol Psychiatry* 3, 72–75.

Malmberg A, Mikaels A, Mohell N (1998). Agonist and inverse agonist activity at the dopamine D$_3$ receptor measured by guanosine 5'-gamma-thio-triphosphate–35S-binding. *J Pharmacol Exp Ther* 285, 119–126.

Mancama D, Arranz MJ, Munro J, Makoff A, Kerwin R (2000). The histamine H$_1$ and histamine H$_2$ genes: candidates for schizophrenia and clozapine drug response. *GeneScreen* 1, 29–34.

Maricq AV, Peterson AS, Brake AJ, Myers RM, Julius D (1991). Primary structure and functional expression of the 5HT$_3$ receptor, a serotonin-gated ion channel. *Science* 254, 432–437.

Masellis M, Paterson AD, Badri F et al. (1995). Genetic variation of 5-HT$_{2A}$ receptor and response to clozapine. *Lancet* 346, 1108.

Masellis M, Basile V, Meltzer HY et al. (1998). Serotonin subtype 2 receptor genes and clinical response to clozapine in schizophrenia patients. *Neuropsychopharmacology* 19, 123–132.

Masellis M, Basile VS, Ozdemir V, Meltzer HY, Macciardi FM, Kennedy JL (2000). Pharmacogenetics of antipsychotic treatment: lessons learned from clozapine. *Biol Psychiatry* 47, 252–266.

Masellis M, Basile VS, Meltzer HY et al. (2001). Lack of association between the T→C267 serotonin 5-HT$_6$ receptor gene (*HTR6*) polymorphism and prediction of response to clozapine in schizophrenia. *Schizophr Res* 47, 49–58.

Mata I, Madoz V, Arranz MJ, Sham P, Murray RM (2001). Olanzapine: concordant response in monozygotic twins with schizophrenia. *Br J Psychiatry* 178, 86.

Meltzer HY (1992). Dimensions of outcome with schizophrenia. *Br J Psychiatry* 160(Suppl 17), 46–53.

Meltzer HY (1994). An overview of the mechanism of action of clozapine. *J Clin Psychopharmacol* 55 (Suppl B), 47–52.

Meltzer HY (1995). The role of serotonin in schizophrenia and the place of serotonin-dopamine antagonist antipsychotics. *J Clin Psychopharmacol* 15(Suppl 1), 2S-3S.

Meltzer HY (1999). The role of serotonin in antipsychotic drug action. *Neuropsychopharmacology* 2(Suppl), 106S–115S.

Meltzer HY, McGurk SR (1999). The effects of clozapine, risperidone, and olanzapine on cognitive function in schizophrenia. *Schizophr Bull* 25, 233–255.

Michel FJ, Trudeau LE (2000). Clozapine inhibits synaptic transmission at GABAergic synapses established by ventral tegmental area neurones in culture. *Neuropharmacology* 39, 1536–1543.

Missale C, Nash SR, Robinson SW, Jaber M, Caron MG (1998). Dopamine receptors: from structure to function. *Physiol Rev* 78, 189–225.

Morse KL, Behan J, Laz TM et al. (2001). Cloning and characterization of a novel human histamine receptor. *J Pharmacol Exp Ther* 296, 1058–1066.

Nagamoto HT, Adler LE, Hea RA, Griffith JM, McRae KA, Freedman R (1996). Gating of auditory P50 in schizophrenics: unique effects of clozapine. *Biol Psychiatry* 40, 181–188.

Nair NP, Zicherman V, Schwartz G (1977). Dopamine and schizophrenia. A reappraisal in the light of clinical studies with clozapine. *Can Psychiatr Assoc J* 22, 285–293.

Nakamura T, Itadani H, Hidaka Y, Ohta M, Tanaka K (2000). Protein, nucleotide molecular cloning and characterization of a new human histamine receptor, HH4R. *Biochem Biophys Res Commun* 279, 615–620.

Nakhai B, Nielsen DA, Linnoila M, Goldman D (1995). Two naturally occurring amino acid substitutions in the human 5-HT$_{1A}$ receptor: glycine 22 to serine 22 and isoleucine 28 to valine 28. *Biochem Biophys Res Commun* 210, 530–536.

Newman-Tancredi A, Gavaudan S, Conte C et al. (1998). Agonist and antagonist actions of antipsychotic agents at 5-HT$_{1A}$ receptors: a [^{35}S]GTPgammaS binding study. *Eur J Pharmacol* 355, 245–256.

Newton RA, Elliott JM (1997). Mianserin-induced down-regulation of human 5-hydroxytryptamine 2A and 5-hydroxytryptamine 2C receptors stably expressed in the human neuroblastoma cell line SH-SY5Y. *J Neurochem* 69, 1031–1038.

Nguyen T, Shapiro DA, George SR et al. (2001). Discovery of a novel member of the histamine receptor family. *Mol Pharmacol* 59, 427–433.

Niesler B, Weiss B, Fischer C et al. (2001). Serotonin receptor gene *HTR3A* variants in schizophrenic and bipolar affective patients. *Pharmacogenetics* 11, 21–22.

Niswender CM, Copeland SC, Herrick-Davis K, Emeson RB, Sanders-Bush E (1999). RNA editing of the human serotonin 5-hydroxytryptamine 2C receptor silences constitutive activity. *J Biol Chem* 274, 9472–9478.

Noethen MM, Rietschel M, Erdmann J et al. (1995). Genetic variation of the 5-HT$_{2A}$ receptor and response to clozapine. *Lancet* 346, 908–909.

Oda T, Morikawa N, Saito Y, Masuho Y, Matsumoto S (2000). Molecular cloning and characterization of a novel type of histamine receptor preferentially expressed in leukocytes. *J Biol Chem* 275, 36781–36786.

Okuyama Y, Ishiguro H, Toru M, Arinami T (1999). A genetic polymorphism in the promoter region of DRD4 associated with expression and schizophrenia. *Biochem Biophys Res Commun* 258, 292–295.

Overall JE, Gorham DR (1962). The brief psychiatric rating scale. *Psychol Rep* 10, 799–812.

Ozdemir V, Basile VS, Masellis M, Kennedy JL (2001). Pharmacogenetic assessment of antipsychotic-induced movement disorders: contribution of the dopamine D$_3$ receptor and cytochrome P-450 *1A2* genes. *J Biochem Biophys Meth* 47, 151–157.

Pasqualetti M, Ori M, Marazziti D, Castagna M, Nardi I (1998). Distribution of 5-HT$_{2C}$ and 5-HT$_{5A}$ receptor mRNA in human brain. *Ann NY Acad Sci* 861, 245.

Pesonen U, Koulu M, Bergen A et al. (1998). Mutation screening of the 5-hydroxytryptamine 7 receptor gene among Finnish alcoholics and controls. *Psychiatry Res* 77, 139–145.

Pilowsky LS, Mulligan RS, Acton PD, Ell PJ, Costa DC, Kerwin RW (1997). Limbic selectivity of clozapine. *Lancet* 350, 490–491.

Potkin SG, Bera R, Gulasekaram B et al. (1994). Plasma clozapine concentrations predict clinical response in treatment-resistant schizophrenia. *J Clin Psychiatry* 55(Suppl B), 133–136.

Price-Evans DA (1993). *Genetic Factors in Drug Therapy: Clinical and Molecular Pharmacogenetics.* Cambridge, UK: Cambridge University Press.

Rao PA, Pickar D, Gejman PV, Ram A, Gershon ES, Gelernter J (1994). Allelic variation in the D_4 dopamine receptor (*DRD4*) gene does not predict response to clozapine. *Arch Gen Psychiatry* 51, 912–917.

Rietschel M, Naber D, Oberlander H et al. (1996). Efficacy and side-effects of clozapine: testing for association with allelic variation in the dopamine D_4 receptor gene. *Neuropsychopharmacology* 15, 491–496.

Rietschel M, Naber D, Fimmers R, Moller HJ, Propping P, Nothen MM (1997). Efficacy and side-effects of clozapine not associated with variation in the $5\text{-}HT_{2C}$ receptor. *Neuroreport* 8, 1999–2003.

Robinson DG, Woerner MG, Alvir JM et al. (1999). Predictors of treatment response from a first episode of schizophrenia or schizoaffective disorder. *Am J Psychiatry* 156, 544–549.

Rosenheck R, Evans D, Herz L et al. (1999). How long to wait for a response to clozapine: a comparison of time course of response to clozapine and conventional antipsychotic medication in refractory schizophrenia. *Schizophr Bull* 25, 709–719.

Roth BL, Craigo SC, Choudhary MS et al. (1994). Binding of typical and atypical antipsychotic agents to 5-hydroxytryptamine-6 and 5-hydroxytryptamine-7 receptors. *J Pharmacol Exp Ther* 268, 1403–1410.

Scharfetter J, Chaudhry HR, Hornik K et al. (1999). Dopamine D_3 receptor gene polymorphism and response to clozapine in schizophrenic Pakistani patients. *Eur Neuropsychopharmacol* 10, 17–22.

Schwartz JC, Levesque D, Martres MP, Sokoloff P (1993). Dopamine D3 receptor: basic and clinical aspects. *Clin Neuropharmacol* 16, 295–314.

Seeman P (1992). Dopamine receptor sequences. Therapeutic levels of neuroleptics occupy D_2 receptors, clozapine occupies D_4. *Neuropsychopharmacology* 7, 261–284.

Segman R, Neeman T, Heresco-Levy U et al. (1999). Genotypic association between the dopamine D_3 receptor and tardive dyskinesia in chronic schizophrenia. *Mol Psychiatry* 4, 247–253.

Segman RH, Heresco-Levy U, Finkel B et al. (2000). Association between the serotonin 2C receptor gene and tardive dyskinesia in chronic schizophrenia: additive contribution of 5-HT2Cser and DRD3gly alleles to susceptibility. *Psychopharmacology* (*Berl*) 152, 408–413.

Shaikh S, Collier D, Kerwin RW et al. (1993). Dopamine D_4 receptor subtypes and response to clozapine. *Lancet* 341, 116.

Shaikh S, Collier DA, Sham P et al. (1995). Analysis of clozapine response and polymorphisms of the dopamine D_4 receptor gene (*DRD4*) in schizophrenic patients. *Am J Med Genet* 60, 541–545.

Shaikh S, Collier DA, Sham PC et al. (1996). Allelic association between a Ser-9–Gly polymorphism in the dopamine D_3 receptor gene and schizophrenia. *Hum Genet* 97, 714–719.

Shaikh S, Makoff A, Collier DA, Kerwin RW (1997). Dopamine D_4 receptors. Potential therapeutic implications in the treatment of schizophrenia. *CNS Drugs* 8, 1–11.

Shannon HE, Rasmussen K, Bymaster FP et al. (2000). Xanomeline, an M(1)/M(4) preferring muscarinic cholinergic receptor agonist, produces antipsychotic-like activity in rats and mice. *Schizophr Res* 42, 249–259.

Simpson GM, Josiassen RC, Stanilla JK, de Leon J et al. (1999). Double-blind study of clozapine dose response in chronic schizophrenia. *Am J Psychiatry* 156, 1744–1750.

Skevington SM, Wright A (2001). Changes in the quality of life of patients receiving antidepressant medication in primary care: validation of the WHOQOL-100. *Br J Psychiatry* 178, 261–267.

Snyder SH (1981). Dopamine receptors, neuroleptics, and schizophrenia. *Am J Psychiatry* 138, 460–446.

Sobell JL, Lind TJ, Sigurdson DC et al. (1995). The D_5 dopamine receptor gene in schizophrenia: identification of a nonsense change and multiple missense changes but lack of association with disease. *Hum Mol Genet* 4, 507–514.

Sodhi MS, Arranz MJ, Curtis D et al. (1995). Association between clozapine response and allelic variation in the 5-HT$_{2C}$ receptor gene. *Neuroreport* 7, 169–172.

Sokoloff P, Andrieux M, Besancon M et al. (1992). Pharmacology of human D_3 receptor expressed in a mammalian cell line: comparison with D_2 receptor. *Eur J Pharmacol* 225, 331–337.

Spurlock G, Heils A, Holmans P et al. (1998). A family based association study of T102C polymorphism in *5HT2A* and schizophrenia plus identification of new polymorphisms in the promoter. *Mol Psychiatry* 3, 42–49.

Squires RF, Saederup E (1991). A review of evidence for GABAergic predominance/glutamatergic deficit as a common etiological factor in both schizophrenia and affective psychoses: more support for a continuum hypothesis of "functional" psychosis. *Neurochem Res* 16, 1099–1111.

Squires RF, Saederup E (1997). Clozapine and some other antipsychotic drugs may preferentially block the same subset of GABA(A) receptors. *Neurochem Res* 22, 151–116.

Squires RF, Saederup E (1998). Clozapine and several other antipsychotic/antidepressant drugs preferentially block the same "core" fraction of GABA(A) receptors. *Neurochem Res* 23, 1283–129.

Squires RF, Saederup E (1999). Clozapine's antipsychotic effects do not depend on blockade of 5-HT$_3$ receptors. *Neurochem Res* 24, 659–667.

Steen VM, Lovlie R, MacEwan T, McCreadie RG (1997). Dopamine D_3-receptor gene variant and susceptibility to tardive dyskinesia in schizophrenic patients. *Mol Psychiatry* 2, 139–145.

Tandon R (1993). Neuropharmacologic basis for clozapine's unique profile. *Arch Gen Psychiatry* 50, 158–159.

Tress KH, Patton G (1994). The assessment of change in psychopathology. In Barnes TRE, Nelson HE, eds. *The Assessment of Psychosis: A Practical Handbook*. London: Chapman & Hall.

van Tol HH, Bunzow JR, Guan HC et al. (1991). Cloning of the gene for a human dopamine D_4 receptor with high affinity for the antipsychotic clozapine. *Nature* 350, 610–614.

van Tol HH, Wu CM, Guan HC et al. (1992). Multiple dopamine D_4 receptor variants in the human population. *Nature* 358, 149–152.

Vanhoenacker P, Haegeman G, Leysen JE (2000). 5-HT$_7$ receptors: current knowledge and future prospects. Review. *Trend Pharmacol Sci* 21, 70–77.

Vogt IR, Shimron-Abarbanell D, Neidt H et al. (2000). Investigation of the human serotonin 6 [5-HT6] receptor gene in bipolar affective disorder and schizophrenia. *Am J Med Genet* 96, 217–221.

Vojvoda D, Grimmell K, Sernyak M, Mazure CM (1996). Monozygotic twins concordant for response to clozapine. *Lancet* 61, 347.

Wadenberg ML, Ahlenius S (1991). Antipsychotic-like profile of combined treatment with raclopride and 8-OH-DPAT in the rat: enhancement of antipsychotic-like effects without catalepsy. *J Neural Transm Genet Sect* 83, 43–53.

Waeber C, Grailhe R, Yu XJ et al. (1998). Putative 5-HT$_5$ receptors: localization in the mouse CNS and lack of effect in the inhibition of dural protein extravasation. *Ann NY Acad Sci* 861, 85–90.

Warburton EC, Joseph MH, Feldon J, Weiner I, Gray JA (1994). Antagonism of amphetamine-induced disruption of latent inhibition in rats by haloperidol and ondansetron: implications for a possible antipsychotic action of ondansetron. *Psychopharmacology (Berl)* 114, 657–664.

Warren JT Jr., Peacock ML, Rodriguez LC, Fink JK (1993). An *MspI* polymorphism in the human serotonin receptor gene (*HTR2*): detection by DGGE and RFLP analysis. *Hum Mol Genet* 2, 338.

Watling KJ, Beer MS, Stanton JA, Newberry NR (1990). Interaction of the atypical neuroleptic clozapine with 5-HT$_3$ receptors in the cerebral cortex and superior cervical ganglion of the rat. *Eur J Pharmacol* 182, 465–472.

Weiss B, Mertz A, Schrock E, Koenen M, Rappold G (1995). Assignment of a human homolog of the mouse *htr3* receptor gene to chromosome 11q23.1–q23.2. *Genomics* 29, 304–305.

Wilcox JA, Nasrallah HA (1987). Perinatal insult as a risk factor in paranoid and nonparanoid schizophrenia. *Psychopathology* 20, 285–287.

Williams GV, Goldman-Rakic PS (1995). Modulation of memory fields by dopamine D$_1$ receptors in prefrontal cortex. *Nature* 376, 572–575.

Willins DL, Berry SA, Alsayegh L et al. (1999). Clozapine and other 5-hydroxytryptamine-2A receptor antagonists alter the subcellular distribution of 5-hydroxytryptamine-2A receptors in vitro and in vivo. *Neuroscience* 91, 599–606.

Wu S, Comings DE (1999). A common C−1018G polymorphism in the human *5-HT1A* receptor gene. *Psychiatr Genet* 9, 105–106.

Yu YW, Tsai SJ, Lin CH, Hsu CP, Yang KH, Hong CJ (1999). Serotonin-6 receptor variant (C267T) and clinical response to clozapine. *Neuroreport* 10, 1231–1233.

Zhukovskaya NL, Neumaier JF (2000). Clozapine downregulates 5-hydroxytryptamine 6 (5-HT$_6$) and upregulates 5-HT$_7$ receptors in HeLa cells. *Neurosci Lett* 288, 236–240.

Zifa E, Fillion G (1992). 5-Hydroxytryptamine receptors. *Pharmacol Rev* 44, 401–458.

11

Genetic factors underlying drug-induced tardive dyskinesia

Ronnen H. Segman and Bernard Lerer

Department of Psychiatry, Hadassah-Hebrew University Medical Center, Jerusalem, Israel

OVERVIEW

Tardive dyskinesia (TD) affects about one fifth of schizophrenia patients following chronic exposure to dopamine receptor antagonist drugs. Spontaneous dyskinesia has been reported in unmedicated schizophrenia patients and patients with TD have been reported to show distinct clinical features, suggesting a common underlying phenotype that may bear a distinct genetic predisposition. Drug- and patient-related risk factors for the development of TD have received much research attention but appear to predict only a minor part of the variance in the incidence of TD. Genetically determined individual variability in factors affecting drug levels, as well as compensatory responses to chronic dopaminergic antagonism, may account for a major portion of the variance in the incidence of TD. To-date, however, there has been a conspicuous lack of studies exploring a genetic predisposition to TD. Current data stem from sporadic clinical observations and from supportive, albeit indirect, evidence from rodent studies showing strain differences in behavioral and phamacodynamic models for drug-induced TD. Despite the lack of an established genetic contribution or mode of inheritance for vulnerability to develop TD, in recent years a number of groups have ventured to examine directly a possible contribution of specific candidate genes to TD, employing case-control association design in chronically medicated schizophrenia patients. Such studies report direct association of candidate polymorphic genes with drug-induced TD, providing further support for the existence of a genetic contribution and suggesting the likelihood of a polygenic, multi-factorial inheritance for such vulnerability. These studies open a window for improved understanding of drug-induced extrapyramidal reactions, as well as a more selective schizophrenia phenotype. The current chapter will review this rapidly developing field, incorporating recently available molecular genetic tools for a renewed exploration of the biological basis of TD.

Introduction

Human evidence supporting a genetic basis for tardive dyskinesia

Tardive dyskinesia (TD) is an irreversible, debilitating adverse drug reaction characterized by the delayed appearance of involuntary choreoathetotic movements in patients chronically exposed to dopamine receptor antagonists. Prevalence estimates are confounded by factors such as a considerable rate of spontaneous dyskinesias, as well as masking of TD by concurrent neuroleptic administration (Koller, 1988). Kane and Smith (1982) reviewed 50 prevalence studies conducted over a 20-year period and calculated a mean prevalence rate of 20%. Risk factors for the development of TD include older age and female gender. Other factors, less consistently confirmed, include duration and intensity of prior neuroleptic exposure, organic brain abnormalities and the existence of affective disorder (Burke et al., 1989). *As drug-related variables predict only a minor part of the variance in the incidence of TD, a predominant pharmacogenetic component appears plausible.* To-date, however, there has been a conspicuous lack of studies exploring a genetic predisposition to TD.

In a retrospective comparison of patients with chronic schizophrenia patients, those exhibiting TD showed a significantly increased rate of family history of psychiatric disorder, as well as a reduced rate of obstetric complications, suggesting the importance of a genetic predisposition (O'Callaghan et al., 1990). Also, there are case reports of concordance for TD in siblings exposed to neuroleptics, pointing to the importance of conducting systematic family studies (Weinhold et al., 1981; Muller et al., 1998a).

Three studies examined the correlation of TD with human leukocyte antigen (HLA) subtypes. HLA-B44 was associated with increased incidence of TD in one study (Canoso et al., 1986), but this finding was not replicated in two other studies (Meltzer et al., 1990; Brown and White, 1991). HLA-DR4 was found to increase the relative risk for TD to 3.04 in a group of 53 patients with chronic schizophrenia (Meltzer et al., 1990).

Recently, increasing research efforts have directly examined the genetic make-up of patients exhibiting spontaneously occurring extrapyramidal disorders, such as Parkinson's disease and the dystonias. Whereas single major loci have been implicated with familial forms of Parkinson's disease (Gasser, 2000) and dystonia (Muller et al., 1998b), the more prevalent form of sporadic Parkinson's disease has been hypothesized to relate to a multifactorial polygenetic etiology where multiple small-effect loci may increase the risk for neurotoxin-induced nigral degeneration depending on combined effects of environmental exposure and interactions with other genetic susceptibility factors. Importantly, such loci were found to contribute a small proportion to the risk for incurring spontaneous sporadic Parkinson's disease (Tan et al., 2000), pointing to the relevance of a candidate gene association design in such a context.

Animal data supporting a genetic basis for tardive dyskinesia

Studies in rats chronically exposed to neuroleptics found different strains to show significant differences in animal behavioral and biochemical models of TD, suggesting the importance of a genetic component. Repetitive jaw movement following withdrawal of chronic neuroleptic treatment was found to be significantly different in different strains of selectively bred rats (Rosengarten et al., 1994). Similarly, the appearance of vacuous chewing movements following chronic haloperidol administration was found to differ markedly in various rat strains (Tamminga et al., 1990). One of the seminal theories regarding the pathophysiology of TD proposes underlying dopamine receptor supersensitivity in the basal ganglia (Klawans et al., 1977). The mean rise in caudate dopamine receptor populations in 10 different mouse strains chronically exposed to haloperidol was found to be significantly different, again pointing to the importance of genetic factors mediating this pharmacodynamic property in mice (Belmaker et al., 1981).

Genetic strategies

General considerations

While the level of exposure to the offending agent (the cumulative dosage and duration of chronic neuroleptic exposure) appears to bear some correlation with the incidence of these idiosyncratic reactions, as yet undefined, genetically based patient factors are likely to play an important role. It is likely that heritable individual variability in factors affecting drug levels, as well as those regulating endogenous dopamine levels and compensatory responses to dopaminergic antagonism, may account for a major portion of the variance in the incidence of TD.

Association approach for locating actual genes involved

The fact that prolonged exposure to D_2 receptor antagonist drugs is necessary to unravel the clinical phenotype limits the usefulness of classical family studies for determining the degree of heritability and mode of inheritance of drug-induced TD. Similarly, the use of linkage-based studies for locating involved genes is limited by the difficulty in ascertaining family members sharing a similar exposure to neuroleptics.

A candidate gene association design is a useful alternative. Genes coding for known drug targets can be directly explored for involvement in TD susceptibility. Allelic association is a widely used strategy for the detection of quantitative trait loci (QTL), as it provides the statistical power required for detection of genes accounting for a relatively small percentage of the variance (Owen and McGuffin, 1993). Association studies are most meaningful when they employ candidate genes that make a priori sense based on current knowledge of brain chemistry. The majority of polymorphic regions and mutations described in genes coding for key proteins in neurotransmitter systems are silent (nonfunctional) intronic sites or rare mutations. The focus should be on polymorphic regions exhibiting prevalent allelic variants and possessing functional significance. Common functional variability resulting from polymorphic sites in genes encoding key proteins in relevant candidates can be directly explored for increased prevalence among patients with TD compared with schizophrenic patients not expressing TD despite a similar neuroleptic exposure.

Candidate genes for drug-induced tardive dyskinesia

Examples of such candidates include relevant neurotransmitter systems, such as dopamine, serotonin (5-HT), and α-aminobutyric acid (GABA), and enzymes involved in drug metabolism, which may both influence the level of exposure to drugs and neutralize neurotoxic metabolites (see below). Interaction between allelic variation in such small-effect genetic loci may increase or decrease the risk for TD in a cumulative or epistatic manner. Such risk-modifying loci may act through several putative mechanisms, as detailed in the following examples.

Dopaminergic enzymes and receptors

Dopaminergic enzymes and receptors may be implicated in several ways. Genetic polymorphisms in key *synthetic* and *metabolic enzymes* responsible, respectively, for the production and degradation of dopamine may influence individual variability in endogenous dopamine levels, as well as the capacity for compensatory adaptation of dopamine levels in response to chronic dopamine receptor antagonist administration. Genetic variability in *dopamine receptors* may predict functional differences in response patterns to neuroleptic agents and may be relevant to the expression of idiosyncratic reactions.

Other neurotransmitters

Other neurotransmitter systems may be implicated as risk-modifying factors. The reported lack of TD with clozapine treatment has been attributed, among other theories, to its potent serotonergic action as a 5-HT$_{2A/C}$ antagonist at A-9 neurons. Genetic variation in the functional status of these receptors may result in individual differences in their response to endogenous serotonergic tone.

Metabolizing enzymes

Metabolizing enzymes may act through modifying the risk for neural damage following exposure to environmental agents such as toxins and drugs. In the case of drug-induced TD, polymorphic forms of the cytochrome P-450/debrisoquine hydroxylation system, resulting in individual variability in the metabolic clearance of neuroleptic drugs, may be directly implicated.

Analytic strategies and phenotype definition

Association of polymorphic candidate genes with risk for TD can be pursued by comparing unrelated ethnically matched patients exposed to neuroleptic drugs, some of whom develop TD and some of whom remain unaffected, despite similar exposure. Two alternative analytic strategies can be employed in the context of such a model. The first strategy assigns a dichotomous threshold division to patients as affected or nonaffected and examines the relative prevalence of alleles and genotypes in the two groups. The other strategy investigates continuous measures of dyskinesia in all drug-exposed patients grouped according to allelic status. As pointed out by Plomin et al. (1991), phenotypic associations with QTL can be utilized to explore the relationship between continuous variation in the clinical phenotype and the putative pathogenic genotype. This approach does not force reliance solely on a single, dichotomous diagnostic category but utilizes all available information, which may correlate more readily with candidate QTL.

Diagnostic assessment for genetic studies

A major hindrance to the application of a case-control, association design to the study of drug-induced TD is the verification of the clinical status of both affected and control subjects. Individuals harboring a genetic make-up that may predispose to TD may be included in the control group because they have not been exposed to a dosage and duration of neuroleptic treatment sufficient for phenotypic expression. Similarly, individuals suffering from milder manifestations of TD may be missed, owing to symptom masking by current neuroleptic administration. A case-control design must, therefore, employ well-evaluated patients demonstrating established TD, compared with ethnically matched patients who do not exhibit TD despite a similar heavy neuroleptic exposure in terms of both dosage and duration. Importantly, drug exposure must be comparable in terms of D_2 receptor affinity for different neuroleptic drugs. It is customary to compare dosages against a conventional reference drug in terms of chlorpromazine equivalent units. In order to avoid common false-positive diagnoses of TD, assessment must take place following a prolonged period of stability in both antipsychotic and anticholinergic drug dose to avoid confounding transient withdrawal dyskinesia. In the elderly, pseudodyskinetic manifestations of edentulousness must be ruled out.

Candidate gene studies of drug-induced tardive dyskinesia

Starting with the study of Arthur et al. (1995), a number of groups chose to explore specific genetic contributions to TD directly. Given the above considerations, these studies have employed a candidate genetic association approach, bypassing the difficult to apply steps of establishing heritability through family studies. Following is a review of the current state of data regarding principal genes investigated to date.

Dopaminergic genes

Dopamine D_3 receptor gene

The gene for the dopamine D_3 receptor (*DRD3*) has recently attracted considerable interest as a site of action of antipsychotic drugs and for its potential role in the pathogenesis of schizophrenia (Schwartz et al., 2000). The human *DRD3* gene has been localized to chromosome 3q13.3 by in situ hybridization. The D_3 receptor readily binds classical and also atypical antipsychotic drugs but differs from other dopamine receptor subtypes in that it is primarily localized to limbic regions, which may be particularly important in the regulation of emotions and in the pathogenesis of schizophrenia (Sokoloff et al., 1990; Zahm and Brog, 1992). *DRD3* contains a polymorphic site in the first exon that gives rise to a serine to glycine substitution in the N-terminal extracellular domain of the receptor protein (Lannfelt et al., 1993). The in vivo functional significance of the polymorphic Ser9Gly site is unknown. DRD_3 receptor-binding analysis of Chinese hamster ovary (CHO) cells infected with Semliki Forest virus to express the wild-type complementary DNA (cDNA), a recombinant DNA producing Ser9Gly, or both showed similar pharmacological properties for several D_3 receptor ligands. However, the *DRD3*gly-gly homozygote showed a significantly higher binding affinity for dopamine whereas heterozygotes (i.e., doubly infected cells) were not significantly different from the wild type. In addition, both DRD*3* gly-gly homozygotes and *DRD3* ser-gly heterozygotes showed significantly higher binding affinity for the selective D_3 ligand GR99841 compared with the wild-type receptor (Lundstrom and Turpin, 1996). While these results do not allow a straightforward extrapolation with regard to the biological significance of heterozygote versus homozygote status, they support either examining *DRD3*gly-gly homozygotes against all other genotypes or grouping *DRD3*gly-gly homozygotes and *DRD3*ser-gly heterozygotes against wild-type homozygotes. Such extrapolations should be made with caution, however, as these results were obtained in an in vitro recombinant system not necessarily reflecting in vivo receptor status in the brain. A clearer understanding of the functional significance of the Ser9Gly site must await more detailed studies employing in vivo radioligand binding, as well as postmortem brain and in vitro receptor studies.

Steen et al. (1997) first reported association of *DRD3* allele *2* (*DRD3*gly) and TD in schizophrenic patients and a significant excess of alleles *2/2* (*DRD3*gly-gly) homozygotes. This finding was subsequently supported by the observations of Segman et al. (1999), Basile et al. (1999), and Lovlie et al. (2000) but not by Rietschel et al. (2000). In line with a small-effect cumulative polygenetic model described above, a significant small increase in the Abnormal Involuntary Movement Scale (AIMS) total and subscores can be seen among schizophrenic patients carrying the *DRD3*gly allele as opposed to those homozygotic for *DRD3*ser (Fig. 11.1).

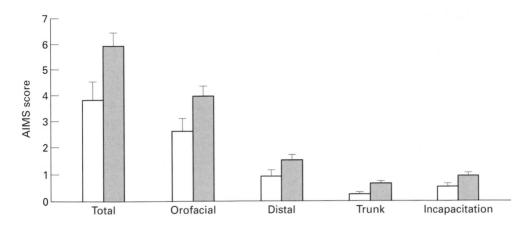

Fig. 11.1.   Abnormal Involuntary Movement Scale (AIMS) total and subscale scores in schizophrenia patients grouped according to the structure of the polymorphic site in the dopamine D_3 receptor: *DRD3*ser–ser (□)or *DRD3*ser–gly/ser–gly(■). A small but significant ($p<0.05$) increase in AIMS total score and in trunk and incapacitation subscale scores can be seen among schizophrenia patients carrying the *DRD3*-gly allele compared with the *DRD3*-ser homozygotes among schizophrenia patients. (Data from Segman et al., 1999.)

The findings of Steen et al. (1997) suggest that previous reports of an association of *DRD3* with schizophrenia may have been confounded by variable rates of TD-prone subjects in the samples examined. This explanation would be particularly relevant to studies that found an association between schizophrenia and allele *2* of *DRD3* (*DRD3*gly) (Kennedy et al., 1995; Ebstein et al., 1997). An association between neurocognitive deficits and TD has been described, and it has also been suggested that patients with more pronounced negative symptoms may be more vulnerable to TD, and that these features may represent associated aspects of a particular schizophrenic subtype (Kane, 1995). Whereas our results (Segman et al., 1999) do not show a direct association of *DRD3* genotype with Positive and Negative Syndrome Scale (PANSS) score, AIMS and PANSS scores were significantly correlated only in patients with the *DRD3*ser-gly or *DRD3*gly (alleles 1/2 and alleles 2/2, respectively) genotypes. The correlation was not limited to negative or cognitive symptoms but encompassed positive features as well. Among patients with the *DRD3*ser-ser (alleles 1/1) genotype, AIMS total was not significantly correlated with PANSS total nor with any of the PANSS subscales. Although preliminary, these results may be interpreted to support a genetic contribution of *DRD3* genotype to a subtype of schizophrenia characterized by greater severity across a range of symptoms as well as predisposition to TD. Previous inconclusive results of attempts to associate *DRD3* genotype and schizophrenia may have been confounded by differing rates of patients prone to TD in the samples, as proposed by Steen et al. (1997). A useful approach to address this possibility further would be to dissect schizophrenic patient samples clinically according to *DRD3* genotype, with our findings predicting higher TD and PANSS scores in patients carrying the *DRD3*gly (2) allele.

Dopamine D$_2$ receptor gene

The gene for the dopamine D$_2$ receptor (*DRD2*) is the main target for classical antipsychotic drugs and a natural candidate for investigation of its role as a putative risk modifier of drug-induced TD. The only published study to-date, examined a *Taq-I* restriction polymorphism at the *DRD2* locus located on 11q23. *A1* allelic status at this polymorphic site has been linked with lower DRD$_2$ binding potential in vivo in positron emission tomographic (Pohjalainen et al., 1998) and single photon emission computed tomographic (Thompson et al., 1997) studies, although not by all studies (Laruelle et al., 1998). If the *A1* allele is associated with reduced DRD$_2$ binding, it may be through linkage disequilibrium with another functional polymorphism in the *DRD2* gene. Chen et al. (1997) examined the relative frequency of *Taq-I A* alleles among 93 patients with TD compared with 84 controls without TD. They found increased frequency of *A2* homozygotes and carriers among TD patients, although *A2* allelic frequency was significantly increased only for female patients with TD in the sample divided according to gender. Independent replication of these preliminary findings as well as investigation of other, functional polymorphic sites in *DRD2* are warranted.

Serotonergic genes

Serotonin 2A receptor gene

The 5-HT$_{2A}$ receptor is a site of action for atypical antipsychotic agents and has been implicated with their added efficacy as well as their reduced extrapyramidal side effect profile (Meltzer, 1999). Atypical antipsychotic agents such as clozapine (Tamminga et al., 1994; Casey, 1998) and olanzapine (Glazer, 2000) have been shown to induce much lower rates of TD compared with conventional antipsychotic drugs, and this has been attributed to a protective effect of their high 5-HT$_2$ receptor-blocking activity relative to D$_2$ receptor blockade (Glazer, 2000). The 5-HT$_{2A}$ receptor is distributed in striatal brain areas that modulate motor activity (Marazziti et al., 1997). This receptor has been shown to interact with dopaminergic neurotransmission in brain regions relevant to antipsychotic drug action (Schmidt et al., 1995). Rodent studies suggest that high occupation of 5-HT$_{2A}$ receptors with lower D$_2$ receptor occupancy might be involved in the absence of upregulation of D$_2$ receptors after treatment with atypical antipsychotic drugs (Kusumi et al., 2000). This may be relevant to the documented lower rates of TD with atypical agents, given the classical hypothesis implicating D$_2$ receptor supersensitivity with pathogenesis of drug-induced TD (Rubovits and Klawans, 1972). Furthermore, pretreatment with atypical antipsychotic agents has been shown to reduce repetitive jaw movements in a rat model for TD (Rosengarten et al., 1999) and 5-HT$_{2A}$ receptor antagonists have been shown to attenuate apomorphine-induced stereotypic oral movements in rats (Barwick et al., 2000). Finally, long-term elevations in 5-HT$_{2A}$ receptor binding and mRNA expression in neostriatal regions have been documented in response to ontogenetic loss of dopamine neurons following 6-hydroxydopamine administration (Kostrzewa et al., 1998), suggesting that such changes may similarly be relevant to pathogenetic processes related to neuroleptic-induced TD. Taken together, the above clinical and basic data, suggest a protective role for 5-HT$_{2A}$ receptor blockade in TD. We hypothesized that a genetically variant 5-HT$_{2A}$ receptor may alter risk for TD in schizophrenia patients following chronic exposure to antipsychotic drugs.

The gene for 5-HT$_{2A}$ receptor (*5-HTR2A*) is located on chromosome 13q14–21 (Hsieh et al., 1990). A number of polymorphic sites have been described in *5-HTR2A* (Waren et al., 1993; Erdmann et al., 1996; Ozaki et al., 1996; Collier et al., 1997; Ohara et al., 1997). Of these, three sites, including the 102T/C, −1438A/G, and His452Tyr, are common variations in the population. A number of studies have shown a small but significant contribution of the 102T/C and, more recently, the A-1438G polymorphisms to risk for schizophrenia (Tay et al., 1997; Williams et al., 1997; Spurlock et al., 1998) but several other studies could not replicate these findings (Hawi et al., 1997; Shinkai et al., 1998; Kouzmenko et al., 1999; Ohara et al., 1999). A number of studies, including a meta-analysis, have found association of the His452Tyr polymorphism with response to clozapine in schizophrenic patients (Arranz et al., 1998; Masellis et al., 1998) whereas both positive (Arranz et al., 1998) and negative (Malhotra et al., 1996; Masellis et al., 1998) results have been found for the 102T/C polymorphism. Given their respective localization, the A-1438G polymorphism may be expected to alter the transcriptional activity of the receptor whereas the silent T102C site is likely to reflect the impact of the promoter site through linkage disequilibrium; however, A-1438G was not found to affect promoter activity in HeLa cells (Spurlock et al., 1998) and correlations with receptor density are inconclusive (Kouzmenko et al., 1999; Turecki et al., 1999). Further studies are required to establish the functional impact of these polymorphic sites.

Given the above, we examined the possibility that these common *5-HTR2A* polymorphic sites influence the tendency to express TD following prolonged antipsychotic drug exposure in schizophrenic patients (Segman et al., 2001). Two polymorphisms were examined in the coding region of *5-HTR2A*, the conservative T102C and that producing His452Tyr, and the A-1438G in the promoter. The T102C and the A-1438G polymorphisms were in complete linkage disequilibrium. There was a significant excess of 102C and −1438G alleles (62.7%) in the patients with TD compared with the patients without TD (41.1%) and matched normal control subjects (45.9%; $\chi^2 = 12.8$; df 2; $p = 0.002$; odds ratio (OR) 2.41; 95% confidence interval (CI) 1.43–3.99) and of 102CC and -1438GG genotypes (schizophrenia with TD 42.4%, schizophrenia without TD 16.1%; controls 20.8%; $\chi^2 = 13.3$; df 4, $p = 0.01$). The 102CC and the -1438GG genotypes were associated with significantly higher AIMS trunk dyskinesia scores ($F = 3.9$; df 2, 116; $p = 0.02$) and more incapacitation ($F = 5.0$; df 2, 115; $p = 0.006$). In contradistinction, the His452Tyr polymorphism showed no association at all with TD. These findings suggest that *5-HTR2A* is significantly associated with susceptibility to TD in patients with chronic schizophrenia (Segman et al., 2001). Previously reported association of the T102C and A-1438G polymorphisms in *5-HTR2A* with schizophrenia may reflect association of a subgroup of patients with a susceptibility to abnormal involuntary movements related to antipsychotic drug exposure.

It is noteworthy that Basile et al. (2001) did not find an association of *5-HTR2A* with TD. Their clinical sample of schizophrenic patients was approximately 20 years younger than that of Segman et al. (2001). Based on a further analysis of their data, Segman and Lerer (2001) demonstrated that the association of *5-HTR2A* with abnormal involuntary movements is age related. Older patients (>49 years) showed a significant association while younger patients did not. This effect could explain the discrepant findings of Segman et al. (2001) and Basile et al. (2001) in regard to the association of TD with *5-HTR2A*.

Serotonin 2C receptor gene

The 5-HT$_{2C}$ receptor is distributed in nigrostriatal brain areas that modulate motor activity (Abramowski et al., 1995). Functional studies on serotonin-mediated phosphoinositide hydrolysis in the caudate nucleus in rats demonstrated a prominent role for this receptor subtype, different from that of 5-HT$_{2A}$ receptor-mediated activity (Wolf and Schultz, 1997). Additionally, 5-HT$_{2C}$ agonists were shown to decrease locomotor activity, whereas 5-HT$_{2A}$ agonists increased such activity (Wolf and Schultz, 1997). The 5-HT$_{2C}$ receptor has been shown to interact with dopaminergic neurotransmission in basal ganglia in rodents; 5-HT$_{2C}$ receptors are upregulated following 6-hydroxydopamine lesioning in rats, and 5-HT$_{2C}$ antagonist administration reduces dyskinetic movements in these rats (Fox et al., 1988). Interestingly, excessive stimulation of 5-HT$_{2C}$ receptors in the caudate and subthalamic nuclei elicits orofacial dyskinesias resembling those seen in patients following chronic neuroleptic exposure (Erble-Wang et al., 1996). Both systemic and local subthalamic infusion of the 5-HT$_{2C}$ receptor agonist, *m*-chlorophenylpiperazine (mCPP), has been shown to elicit orofacial dyskinesias, and this effect was blocked by 5-HT$_{2C}$ antagonism (Erble-Wang et al., 1996). Based on the above data, it has been suggested that the 5-HT$_{2C}$ receptor may be responsible for some of the dyskinetic effects of antipsychotic drugs (Wolf and Schultz, 1997).

The human 5-HT$_{2C}$ receptor gene (*HTR2C*) has been localized to chromosome Xq24. It contains a common C–G transversion at nucleotide 68 of the coding sequence that gives rise to a cysteine to serine substitution in the N-terminal extracellular domain of the receptor protein (Lappalainen et al., 1995). The pharmacological profile and in vivo significance of the mutant receptor protein is unknown; however, preliminary reports point to an altered binding affinity to mCPP in vitro (Lappalainen et al., 1995). To-date only two studies have examined some functional aspects of the *5-HT2C* serine/cysteine polymorphic site in humans, both reporting a functional significance. Higher concentrations of cerebrospinal fluid 3-methoxy-4-hydroxyphenylglycol were reported in Finnish, alcoholic violent offenders and population control males who were hemizygotes for the serine genotype (Lappalainen et al., 1999). This finding is of interest to the extent that it can be generalized to other populations. Also, unaltered endocrine/thermic responses to mCPP but a reduced hypophagic response were observed in a small group of normal female subjects comprising *5-HT2C* serine/cysteine heterozygotes and serine homozygotes compared with wild-type cysteine homozygote female subjects (Quested et al., 1999).

Given the above, we sought to examine the possibility that the *HTR2C* polymorphic site influences the tendency to manifest TD following prolonged antipsychotic drug exposure in schizophrenia patients (Segman et al., 2000). We found a significant excess of *5-HTR2C*ser alleles in schizophrenic patients with TD (27.2%) compared with patients without TD (14.6%) and normal controls (14.2%; $\chi^2 = 6.4$; df 2; $p = 0.03$), which was owing to the female patients ($\chi^2 = 8.6$; df 2; $p = 0.01$). Among the female TD patients, there was an excess of Cys-Ser and Ser-Ser genotypes ($\chi^2 = 11.9$; df 4; $p = 0.02$). Analysis of covariance controlling for age at first antipsychotic treatment revealed a significant effect of *5-HTR2C* genotype on orofacial dyskinesia scores ($F = 3.47$; df 2; $p = 0.03$). In a stepwise multiple regression analysis, *5-HTR2C* and *DRD3* genotype (*5-HTR2C*ser and *DRD3*gly allele carriage), respectively, contributed 4.2% and 4.7% to the variance in orofacial dyskinesia scores. These findings support a small but significant contribution of the *HTR2C* and *DRD3* to susceptibility to TD, which is additive in nature.

Serotonin transporter gene

The serotonin transporter (5-HTT) is the rate-limiting factor in terminating the synaptic action of 5-HT, and is the molecular target for selective serotonin reuptake inhibitors (SSRIs). SSRIs have been reported to cause TD (Dubovsky and Thomas, 1996; Leo, 1996). Nigrostriatal dopaminergic neurons are tonically inhibited by dorsal raphe serotonergic projections (Nedergaard et al., 1988). SSRIs have been suggested to act via these connections in reducing the release of synaptic dopamine in the nigrostriatal system. Chronic decreases in dopaminergic transmission may, in turn, facilitate hypersensitivity of the postsynaptic dopamine receptors, thereby giving rise to TD (Chong et al., 2000). An insertion/deletion polymorphism has been reported in the promoter region of the *5-HTT* gene (5-HTT linked polymorphic region: 5-HTTLPR) (Heils et al., 1996) localized to 17q11.1–12. The short variant of the polymorphism has been shown to reduce the in vitro transcriptional efficiency of the 5-HTT gene promoter, resulting in decreased 5-HTT expression and 5-HT uptake in lymphoblasts (Heils et al., 1996). Chong et al. (2000) examined the 5-HTTLPR site in 188 schizophrenic patients and found no correlation of allelic status with AIMS score or with TD diagnosis. We have observed similar results (R. H. Segman et al., unpublished data).

Metabolic enzymes

Cytochrome P-450 system

Cytochrome P-450 (CYP) enzymes may be related to the pathogenesis of TD either through a pharmacokinetic effect of altering neuroleptic drug levels or through neutralization of putative secondary neurotoxic factors.

Cytochrome P-450 2D6

The metabolism of many drugs including several common neuroleptic drugs is influenced by polymorphisms of *CYP2D6* located on 22q13.1, which encodes the CYP2D6 enzyme debrisoquine/sparteine hydroxylase. Approximately 5–10% of European Caucasians lack the enzyme CYP2D6 and are designated poor metabolizers (PM). Given standard drug therapy, PM subjects are likely to achieve higher than average concentrations of neuroleptic drugs in plasma, with an increased risk of extrapyramidal side effects, possibly including TD. A number of studies investigated association of *CYP2D6* alleles with TD. Arthur et al. (1995) first investigated *CYP2D6* allele frequencies among 16 schizophrenic patients with TD and found only one PM subject, suggesting no increased rate of PM compared with normal population rates. Armstrong et al. (1997) examined 76 schizophrenic patients and reported a trend for increased movement disorder ratings and TD among the five PM subjects in the group. Andreasen et al. (1997) examined a group of 100 schizophrenia patients 10% of whom were PM. They reported a nonsignificant trend for increased rate of TD among PM subjects. Ohmori et al. (1999) found no correlation of *CYP2D6* alleles with AIMS scores or TD diagnosis among 99 schizophrenic patients. Taken together, these studies do not support the likelihood of a major contribution of *CYP2D6* alleles to risk for neuroleptic-induced TD. However, the small number of TD subjects in each study is insufficient to exclude a small effect of this locus, given the low population prevalence of the PM allele.

Cytochrome P-450 1A2

Although CYP1A2 has a lower affinity for typical antipsychotic agents than the high affinity CYP2D6, it is much more abundant in the liver and is further induced by smoking, making it a clinically important metabolic clearance pathway for typical antipsychotics. CYP1A2 activity in vivo shows an over 10-fold variability and is under significant genetic control (Kalow and Tang, 1991). A C-to-A substitution has been described in intron 1 of *CYP1A2* located on 15q22–qter (Sachse et al., 1999). Among healthy Caucasians, smokers with the C/C genotype had, on average, 40% lower CYP1A2 activity as measured by a caffeine metabolic ratio ([1, 7-dimethylxanthine + 1, 7-dimethyluric acid]/[caffeine]), in comparison with those homozygous for the variant A. In contrast, the C-to-A genetic polymorphism in *CYP1A2* did not importantly contribute to variability in CYP1A2 activity in non-smokers (Sachse et al., 1999). Basile et al. (2000) investigated a sample of 85 schizo-phrenic patients assessed for TD severity using AIMS for association with the C-to-A polymorphism in *CYP1A2*. The mean AIMS score in patients with the C/C genotype (associated with reduced CYP1A2 inducibility) was 2.7- and 3.4-fold greater than in those with the A/C or A/A genotype, respectively (F = 7.4; df 2, $p =$ 0.0007). A subanalysis in the 44 known smokers in the sample revealed a more pro-nounced effect. The mean AIMS score in smokers was 5.4– and 4.7-fold greater in C/C homozygotes when compared with heterozygotes and A/A homozygotes, respectively (F = 3.7; df = 2, 41; $p = 0.008$). These data suggest that the C-to-A genetic polymorphism in *CYP1A2* may serve as a genetic risk factor for the devel-opment of TD in patients with schizophrenia. Independent replication of these findings is warranted.

Manganese superoxide dismutase

Impaired free radical detoxification has been previously implicated in schizophre-nia (Reddy et al., 1991). In addition, data supporting increased free radical burden have been reported following neuroleptic treatment (Pall et al., 1987), and increased free radical activity in patients with TD has also been reported (Lohr et al., 1990). Based on the above, Hori et al. (2000) investigated a role in TD for man-ganese superoxide dismutase (MnSOD), the gene for which is located on 6q25.3. They examined a biallelic polymorphism (Ala9Val) in the mitochondrial targeting sequence of human MnSOD, which was previously reported to associate with risk for Parkinson's disease (Shimoda-Matsubayashi et al., 1996). The study included 192 schizophrenic patients, 39 with TD and 153 without TD, and 141 normal con-trols. No significant differences were found in the allelic or genotypic distribution between schizophrenics and controls. A significantly reduced rate of the rare 9Ala carriers (homozygote and heterozygotes) was found among patients with TD com-pared with schizophrenia patients without TD ($p = 0.03$), and decreased 9Ala allele was found among patients with TD ($p = 0.02$; OR 0.29; 95% CI 0.10–0.83). They conclude that the allele giving 9Ala may correlate with higher MnSOD activity and may play a role in protecting against susceptibility to TD in schizophrenics.

Additive small gene effects

From the data reviewed above, a polygenic contribution of several small-effect genetic loci is suggested. In such case, the additive contribution of multiple such loci in an individual will dictate the consequent response to the external event (e.g., long-term neuroleptic exposure, in terms of the propensity to express TD. In theory, such contributing loci may have an additive contribution operating to increase the risk in a simple additive or in a synergistic pattern. Conversely, some loci may instead operate to lower the risk, if they play a protective effect.

The first evidence for such additive effect of different loci in TD has been reported for the *5-HTR2C* and *DRD3* loci (Segman et al., 2000). In a stepwise multiple regression analysis, *5-HTR2C* and *DRD3* genotypes (*5-HTR2C*ser and *DRD3*gly allele carriage, respectively) contributed independently 4.2% and 4.7% to the variance in orofacial dyskinesia scores. In Fig. 11.2, the additive significance of allele carriage in the two contributing loci can be seen.

Such an additive effect is well based in current neurochemical understanding of dopamine–5-HT interactions. As noted above, the 5-HT$_{2C}$ receptor has been shown to interact with dopaminergic neurotransmission in basal ganglia. The 5-HT$_{2C}$ receptors are upregulated following 6-hydroxydopamine lesioning in rats and 5-HT$_{2C}$ antagonist administration reduces dyskinetic movements in these rats (Fox et al., 1988). It may be hypothesized that 5-HT$_{2C}$ receptor upregulation may also occur in response to neurotoxic damage, which may be mediated by the accumulation of neurotoxins such as 6-hydroxydopamine following prolonged exposure to dopamine receptor antagonist drugs. The additive effect of genetically determined endogenous differences in 5-HT$_{2C}$ and D$_3$ receptor reactivity may, therefore, contribute in a cumulative manner to clinical differences in resultant expression of TD.

Conclusions

Genetic association studies of TD have proven to be a fruitful approach for locating predisposing molecular mechanisms, despite the lack of family-based evidence for heritability and mode of inheritance (Table 11.1). This is largely because targets of drug action pose direct hypotheses implicating candidate genes that may be directly tested for involvement in risk determination. The *DRD3* gene is by far the most robust finding to date, with four of five independent studies confirming association. Other promising findings, including the reported associations with

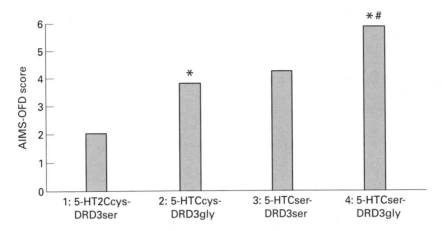

Fig. 11.2.   Adjusted mean Abnormal Involuntary Movement Scale-Oro-Facial-Digital (AIMS-OFD) scores (derived from ANCOVA) of patients with chronic schizophrenia carrying varying alleles for the serotonin (5-HT) 2C receptor (*5-HT2C*) and the dopamine D_3 receptor (*DRD3*). 1, both wild type (WT); 2, WT plus mutant; 3, mutant + WT; 4, mutant plus mutant. By ANCOVA with age at first antipsychotic treatment as covariate: main effect 5-HT2C, $F = 5.38$ (df 1: 110), $p = 0.02$; main effect *DRD3*, $F = 7.28$ (df 1:110), $p = 0.008$; interaction, $F = 10.06$ (df 1:110), $p = 0.81$. * $p < 0.05$ compared with alleles 1; $p < 0.05$ compared with alleles 2 (univariate planned comparisons). An additive contribution can be seen where pathogenic allele carriers for both loci (i.e. *5-HT2C*ser and *DRD3*gly) show highest AIMS-OFD scores. Wild-type carriers for both loci (i.e., *5-HT2C*cys and *DRD3*ser) show the lowest scores, and carriers of a pathogenic allele in just one of the loci show an intermediate AIMS score. (With permission, from Segman et al., 2000.)

5-HTR2A and *5-HTR2C* and *MnSOD* genetic polymorphic sites, require independent replications. Such findings open a window for understanding the molecular basis of drug-induced TD, and possibly other extrapyramidal disorders. In addition they may aid in the prediction of susceptibility to neuroleptic-induced TD before drug exposure, as well as help to direct the development of safer and more specific antipsychotic drugs. Genetic susceptibility to TD may mark a more specific phenotype of schizophrenia, with selective prognostic course and drug-response profile, and may prove instrumental for improving phenotype definition in genetic studies of schizophrenia.

Future research of the genetic causes of TD may employ a number of methodological strategies. The currently utilized case-control candidate genetic association design may be served by larger samples of phenotypically well-defined TD patients and controls sharing similar drug exposure. A superior approach entails the use of transmission disequilibrium analysis, employing parental genotypes of TD subjects, as this methodology is immune both to the problem of ethnic stratification

Table 11.1. Genetic association findings in tardive dyskinesia

Gene polymorphism	Chromosomal location	Association	Replication	Nonreplication
DRD3 Ser9Gly	3q13.3	Positive: Steen et al., 1997	Segman et al., 1999; Basile et al., 1999; Lovlie et al., 2000 (trend)	Rietschel et al., (2000)
DRD2 Taq-I	11q23	Positive in female patients with TD: Chen et al., 1997	NA	NA
5-HTR2A: T102C/A-, 1438G, his452tyr	13q14–21	Segman et al., 2000; positive for T102C/A− and 1438G; negative for His452Tyr	NA	Basile et al., 2001 (*Note:* discrepancy may be explained by age effect – Segman and Lerer, 2002)
*5-HTR2C*cys-ser	Xq24	Positive: Segman et al., 2000	NA	NA
5-HTT promoter I/D	17q11.1–12	Negative: Chong et al., 2000	NA	NA
CYP2D6 (PM allele)	22q13.1	Trend; Arthur et al., 1995; Andreasen et al., 1997	NA	Armstrong et al., 1997; Ohmori et al., 1999
CYP1A2 intron 1 C/A	15q22-qter	Positive: Basile et al., 2000	NA	NA
MnSOD Ala9Val	6q25.3	Hori et al., 2000	NA	NA

Notes:

NA, not available; TD, tardive dyskinesia; PM, poor metabolizer.

among patients and controls and of false-negative diagnoses of TD status among medicated control schizophrenic subjects, who may either develop TD upon a more prolonged exposure or have latent TD masked by the concurrent use of neuroleptics at the time of assessment.

The alternative approach of exploration of unknown genes through genome scan can be implemented through one of two routes. Routine inclusion of antipsychotic drug exposure and response quantification and dyskinesia assessments in large-scale linkage studies for schizophrenia would allow utilization of pharmacogenetic information for sharpening of the biological schizophrenia phenotype, possibly improving its diagnostic specificity as well as allowing a linkage-based search for genetic loci predisposing for TD. Alternatively, single nucleotide polymorphism (SNP) genome mapping may be employed for larger groups of unrelated with TD patients and medicated schizophrenia controls. Finally, comparative global expression patterns of mRNA transcripts may be utilized for matching relevant brain areas from autopsy brain specimens of patients with TD and medicated schizophrenia controls.

TD constitutes a sharply defined pharmacogenetic phenotype, which may continue to serve as a model for implementing accumulating genetic molecular tools for locating genotype–phenotype correlations in complex phenotypes.

Acknowledgements

This work was supported in part by grants from the Yisumi Fund of Hadassit Research and Development Corporation and the National Institute for Psychobiology in Israel to RS. The Biological Psychiatry Laboratory, Hadassah Hebrew University Medical Center, is supported by the Harry Stern Family Foundation.

REFERENCES

Abramowski D, Rigo M, Duc D, Hoyer D, Staufenbiel M (1995). Localization of the 5-hydroxytryptamine 2C receptor protein in human and rat brain using specific antisera. *Neuropharmacology* 34, 1635–1645.

Andreasen OA, MacEwan T, Gulbrandsen AK, McCreadie RG, Steen VM (1997). Non-functional CYP2D6 alleles and risk for neuroleptic-induced movement disorders in schizophrenic patients. *Psychopharmacology (Berl)* 131, 174–179.

Armstrong M, Daly AK, Blennerhassett R, Ferrier N, Idle JR (1997). Antipsychotic drug-induced movement disorders in schizophrenics in relation to CYP2D6 genotype. *Br J Psychiatry* 170, 23–26.

Arthur H, Dahl ML, Siwers B, Sjoqvist F (1995). Polymorphic drug metabolism in schizophrenic patients with tardive dyskinesia. *J Clin Psychopharmacol* 15, 211–216.

Arranz MJ, Munro J, Sham P (1998). Meta-analysis of studies on genetic variation in 5-HT$_{2A}$ receptors and clozapine response. *Schizophr Res* 32, 93–99.

Barwick VS, Jones DH, Richter JT, Hicks PB, Young KA (2000). Subthalamic nucleus microinjections of 5-HT$_2$ receptor antagonists suppress stereotypy in rats. *Neuroreport* 11, 267–270.

Basile VS, Masellis M, Badri F et al. (1999). Association of the *MscI* polymorphism of the dopamine D$_3$ receptor gene with tardive dyskinesia in schizophrenia. *Neuropsychopharmacology* 21, 17–27.

Basile VS, Ozdemir V, Masellis M et al. (2000). A functional polymorphism of the cytochrome P-450 1A2 (*CYP1A2*) gene: association with tardive dyskinesia in schizophrenia. *Mol Psychiatry* 4, 410–417.

Basile VS, Ozdemir V, Masellis M et al. (2001). Lack of association between serotonin-2A receptor gene (*HTR2A*) polymorphisms and tardive dyskinesia in schizophrenia. *Mol Psychiatry* 6, 230–234.

Belmaker RH, Bannet J, Brecher-Fried E, Yanai J, Ebstein RP (1981). The effect of haloperidol feeding on dopamine receptor number in ten mouse strains. *Clin Genet* 19, 353–356.

Brown KW, White T (1991). HLA and TD. *Br J Psychiatry* 158, 270–272.

Burke RE, Kangh UJ, Jankovic J (1989). Tardive akathisia: an analysis of clinical features and response to open therapeutic trials. *Mov Disord* 4, 157–175.

Canoso RT, Romero JA, Yunis EJ (1986). Immunogenetic markers in chlorpromazine induced TD. *J Neuroimmunol* 12, 247–252.

Casey DE (1998). Effects of clozapine therapy in schizophrenic individuals at risk for tardive dyskinesia. *J Clin Psychiatry* 59 (Suppl 3), 31–37.

Chen CH, Wei FU, Koong FJ, Hsiao KJ (1997). Association of Taq-I A polymorphism of dopamine D_2 receptor gene and tardive dyskinesia in schizophrenia. *Biol Psychiatry* 41, 827–829.

Chong SA, Tan EC, Tan CH, Mahendren R, Tay AHN, Chua HC (2000). Tardive dyskinesia is not associated with the serotonin gene polymorphism (5-HTTLPR) in Chinese. *Am J Med Genet (Neuropsychiatr Genet)* 96, 712–715.

Collier DA, Arranz MJ, Li T, Mupita D, Brown N, Treasure J (1997). Association between *5-HT2A* gene promoter polymorphism and anorexia nervosa. *Lancet* 350, 412.

Dubovsky SL, Thomas M (1996). Tardive dyskinesia associated with fluoxetine. *Psychiatr Serv* 47, 991–993.

Ebstein RP, Macciardi F, Blaine D, Serretti A, Gur E, Verga M (1997). Evidence for an association between the dopamine D_3 receptor gene (*DRD3*) and schizophrenia. *Hum Hered* 47, 6–16.

Erble-Wang K, Lucki I, Chesselet MF (1996). A role for the subthalamic nucleus in the 5-HT$_{2C}$ induced oral dyskinesia. *Neuroscience* 72, 117–128.

Erdmann J, Shimron-Abarbanell D, Rietschel M (1996). Systematic screening for mutations in the human serotonin-2A (5-HT$_{2A}$) receptor gene: identification of two naturally occurring receptor variants and association analysis in schizophrenia. *Hum Genet* 97, 614–619.

Fox SH, Moser B, Brotchie M (1988). Behavioral effects of 5-HT$_{2C}$ receptor antagonism in the substantia nigra zona reticulata of the 6-hydroxydopamine-lesioned rat model of Parkinson's disease. *Exp Neurol* 151, 35–49.

Glazer WM (2000). Expected incidence of tardive dyskinesia associated with atypical antipsychotics. *J Clin Psychiatry* 61, 21–26.

Gasser T (2000). Autosomal-dominantly inherited forms of Parkinson's disease. *J Neural Transm Suppl* 58, 31–40.

Hawi Z, Myakishev MV, Straub RE (1997). No association or linkage between the 5-HT2A/T102C polymorphism and schizophrenia in Irish families. *Am J Med Genet* 74, 370–373.

Heils A, Teufel A, Petri S et al. (1996). Allelic variation of human serotonin transporter gene expression. *J Neurochem* 66, 2621–2624.

Hori H, Ohmori O, Shinkai T (2000). Manganese superoxide dismutase dene polymorphism and schizophrenia: relation to tardive dyskinesia. *Neuropsychopharmacology* 23, 170–177.

Hsieh CL, Bowcock AM, Farrer LA et al. (1990). The serotonin receptor subtype 2 locus *HTR2* is on chromosome 13 near genes for esterase D and retinoblastoma and on mouse chromosome 14. *Somat Cell Genet* 16, 567–574.

Kalow W, Tang BK (1991). Use of caffeine metabolite ratios to explore CYP1A2 and xanthine oxidase activities. *Clin Pharmacol Ther*, 50, 508–519.

Kane JM (1995). Tardive dyskinesia: epidemiological and clinical presentation. In Bloom FE, Kupfer DJ, eds. *Psychopharmacology: The 4th Generation of Progress*. Raven Press: New York, pp. 1485–1495.

Kane JM, Smith JM (1982).Tardive dyskinesia. *Arch Gen Psychiatry* 37, 473–481.

Kennedy JL, Billett E, Macciardi FM, Verga M, Parsons T, Meltzer HY (1995). Association study of the dopamine D_3 receptor gene and schizophrenia. *Am J Med Genet* (*Neuropsychiatr Genet*) 60, 558–562.

Klawans HL, Hitri A, Nausieda PA, Wiener WL (1977). In Hanin IR, Usdin E, eds. *Animal Models of Dyskinesia in Psychiatry and Neurology*, Oxford, Pergamon Press, pp. 351–363.

Koller WC (1988). Idiopathic oral facial dyskinesia. *Adv Neurol* 149, 225–237.

Kostrzewa RM, Reader TA, Descarries L (1998). Serotonin neural adaptations to ontogenetic loss of dopamine neurons in rat brain. *J Neurochem* 70, 889–898.

Kouzmenko AP, Scaffidi A, Pereira AM, Hayes WL, Copolov DL, Dean B (1999). No correlation between A(-1438)G polymorphism in 5-HT_{2A} receptor gene promoter and the density of frontal cortical 5-HT_{2A} receptors in schizophrenia. *Hum Hered* 49, 103–105.

Kusumi I, Takahashi Y, Suzuki K, Kameda K, Koyama T (2000). Differential effects of subchronic treatments with atypical antipsychotic drugs on dopamine D_2 and serotonin 5-HT_{2A} receptors in the rat brain. *J Neur Transm* 107, 295–302.

Lannfelt L, Sokoloff P, Martres MP et al. (1993). Amino acid substitution in the dopamine D_3 receptor as a useful polymorphism for investigating psychiatric disorders. *Psychiatr Genet* 2, 249–256.

Lappalainen J, Zhang L, Dean M et al. (1995). Identification expression and pharmacology of a Cys23–Ser23 sustitution in the human 5-HT_{2C} receptor gene (HTR2C). *Genomics* 27, 274–279.

Lappalainen J, Long JC, Virkkunen M, Ozaki N, Goldman D, Linnoila M (1999). HTR2C Cys23Ser polymorphism in relation to CSF monoamine metabolite concentrations and DSM-III-R psychiatric diagnoses. *Biol Psychiatry* 46, 821–826.

Laruelle M, Gelernter J, Innis RB (1998). D_2 receptors binding potential is not affected by *Taq1* polymorphism at the D_2 receptor gene. *Mol Psychiatry* 3, 261–265.

Leo RJ (1996). Movement disorders associated with the serotonin selective reuptake inhibitors. *J Clin Psychiatry* 57, 449–454.

Lohr JB, Kuczenski R, Bracha HS, Moir M, Jeste DV (1990). Increased indices of free radical activity in the cerebrospinal fluid of patients with tardive dyskinesia. *Biol Psychiatry* 28, 535–539.

Lovlie R, Daly AK, Blennerhassett R, Ferrier N, Steen VM (2000). Homozygosity for Gly-9 variant of the dopamine D_3 receptor and risk for tardive dyskinesia in schizophrenic patients. *Int J Neuropsychopharmacol* 3, 61–66.

Lundstrom K, Turpin MP (1996). Proposed schizophrenia related gene polymorphism: expression of the Ser9Gly mutant human dopamine D_3 receptor with the Semliki Forest virus system. *Biochem Biophys Res Commun* 225, 1068–1072.

Malhotra AK, Goldman D, Ozaki N, Breier A, Buchanan R, Pickar D (1996). Lack of association between polymorphisms in the 5-HT$_{2A}$ receptor gene and the antipsychotic response to clozapine. *Am J Psychiatry* 153, 1092–1094.

Marazziti D, Rossi A, Palego L (1997). [^{3}H]Ketanserin binding in human brain postmortem. *Neurochem Res* 22, 753–757.

Masellis M, Basile V, Meltzer HY (1998). Serotonin subtype 2 receptor genes and clinical response to clozapine in schizophrenia patients. *Neuropsychopharmacology* 19, 123–132.

Meltzer HY (1999). The role of serotonin in antipsychotic drug action. *Neuropsychopharmacology* 21(Suppl), 106–115.

Meltzer WS, Newton JE, Steele RW (1990). HLA antigens in tardive dyskinesia. *J Neuroimmunol* 26, 179–181.

Muller DJ, Ahle G, Alfter D et al. (1998a). Familial occurrence of tardive dyskinesia. *Am J Med Genet* 81, 527.

Muller U, Steinberger D, Nemeth AH (1998b). Clinical and molecular genetics of primary dystonias. *Neurogenetics* 1, 165–177.

Nedergaard S, Bolam JP, Greenfield SA (1988). Facilitation of a dendritic calcium conductance by 5-hydroxytryptamine in the substantia nigra. *Nature* 333, 174–177.

O'Callaghan E, Larkin C, Kinsella A, Wadington JL (1990). Obstetric complications, the putative familial sporadic distinction and TD in schizophrenia. *Br J Psychiatry* 157, 578–584.

Ohara K, Ino A, Ishigaki T, Tani K, Tsukamoto T, Nakamura Y (1997). Analysis of the 5′-flanking promoter region of the *5-HT2A* receptor gene in schizophrenia. *Neuropsychopharmacology* 17, 274–278.

Ohara K, Nagai M, Tani K, Tsukamoto T (1999). Schizophrenia and the serotonin-2A receptor promoter polymorphism. *Psychiatr Res* 85, 221–224.

Ohmori O, Kojima H, Shinkai T, Terao T, Suzuki T, Abe K (1999). Genetic association analysis between CYP2D6*2 allele and tardive dyskinesia in schizophrenic patients *Psychiatr Res* 87, 239–244.

Owen MJ, McGuffin P (1993). Association and linkage: complementary strategies for complex disorders. *Am J Med Genet* 30, 578–584.

Ozaki N, Rosenthal NE, Pesonen U (1996). Two naturally occurring amino acid substitutions of the 5-HT$_{2A}$ receptor: similar prevalence in patients with seasonal affective disorder and controls. *Biol Psychiatry* 40, 1267–1272.

Pall HS, Williams AC, Blake DR, Lunec J (1987). Evidence of enhanced lipid peroxidation in the cerebrospinal fluid of patients taking phenothiazines. *Lancet* ii, 596–599.

Plomin R, McClearn GE, Gora-Maslak G, Neiderhiser JM (1991). Use of recombinant inbred strains to detect quantitative trait loci associated with behavior. *Behav Genet* 21, 99–116.

Pohjalainen T, Rinne JO, Nagren K et al. (1998). The A1 allele of the human D$_2$ dopamine receptor gene predicts low D$_2$ receptor availability in healthy volunteers. *Mol Psychiatry* 3, 256–260.

Quested DJ, Whale R, Sharpley AL et al. (1999). Allelic variation in the 5-HT$_{2C}$ receptor and functional response to the 5-HT$_{2C}$ receptor antagonist mCPP. *Psychopharmacology* 144, 306–307.

Reddy R, Sahebarao MP, Mukherjee S, Murthy JN (1991). Enzymes of the antioxidant defense system in chronic schizophrenic patients. *Biol Psychiatry* 30, 409–412.

Rietschel M, Krauss H, Muller DJ et al. (2000). Dopamine D_3 receptor variant and tardive dyskinesia. *Eur Arch Psychiatry Clin Neurosci* 250, 31–35.

Rosengarten H, Schiweitzter JW, Friedhoff AJ, (1994). Possible genetic factors underlying the pathophysiology of TD. *Pharmacol Biochem Behav* 49, 633–667.

Rosengarten H, Schweitzer JW, Friedhoff AJ (1999). The effect of novel antipsychotics in rat oral dyskinesia. *Prog Neuropsychopharmacol Biol Psychiatry* 23, 1389–1404.

Rubovits R, Klawans HL Jr. (1972). Implications of amphetamine induced stereotyped behavior as a model for tardive dyskinesia. *Arch Gen Psychiatry* 27, 502–507.

Sachse C, Brockmoller J, Bauer S, Roots I (1999). Functional significance of a C→A polymorphism in intron 1 of the cytochrome P-450 *CYP1A2* gene tested with caffeine. *Br J Clin Pharmacol* 47, 445–449.

Schmidt CJ, Sorensen SM, Kehne JH, Carr AA, Palfreyman MG (1995). The role of 5-HT$_{2A}$ receptors in antipsychotic activity. *Life Sci* 56, 2209–2222.

Schwartz JC, Diaz J, Pilon C, Sokoloff P (2000). Possible implications of the dopamine D(3) receptor in schizophrenia and in antipsychotic drug actions. *Brain Res Rev* 2–3, 277–287.

Segman RH, Lerer B (2002). Age and the relationship of dopamine D_3, serotonin 2C and serotonin 2A receptor genes to abnormal involuntary movements in chronic schizophrenia. *Mol Psychiatry* 6, 225–229.

Segman R, Neeman T, Heresco-Levy U et al. (1999). Genotypic association between the dopamine D_3 receptor gene and tardive dyskinesia in chronic schizophrenia. *Mol Psychiatry* 4, 247–253.

Segman R, Heresco-Levy U, Finkel B et al. (2000). Association between the serotonin 2C receptor gene and tardive dyskinesia in chronic schizophrenia: additive contribution of *5-HT2C*ser and *DRD3*gly to susceptibility. *Psychopharmacology* (*Berl*) 152, 408–413.

Segman RH, Heresco-Levy U, Finkel B et al. (2001). Association between the serotonin 2A receptor gene and tardive dyskinesia in chronic schizophrenia. *Mol Psychiatry* 6, 225–229.

Shimoda-Matsubayashi S, Matsumine H, Kobayashi T, Naka-gawara-Hattori Y, Shimizu Y, Mizuno Y (1996). Structural dimorphism in the mitochondrial targeting sequence in the human manganese superoxide dismutase gene. *Biochem Biophys Res Commun* 226, 561–565.

Shinkai T, Ohmori O, Kojima H, Terao T, Suzuki T, Abe K (1998). Negative association between T102C polymorphism of the 5-HT$_{2A}$ receptor gene and schizophrenia in Japan. *Hum Hered* 48, 212–215.

Sokoloff P, Giros B, Martres MP, Bouthenet ML, Schwartz JC (1990). Molecular cloning and characterization of a novel dopamine receptor (D3) as a target for neuroleptics. *Nature* 347, 146–151.

Spurlock G, Heils A, Holmans P et al. (1998). A family based association study of T102C polymorphism in *5HT2A* and schizophrenia plus identification of new polymorphisms in the promoter. *Mol Psychiatry* 3, 42–49.

Steen VM, Lovelie R, MacEwan T, McCreadie RG (1997). Dopamine D_3-receptor gene variant and susceptibility to tardive dyskinesia in schizophrenic patients. *Mol Psychiatry* 21, 139–145.

Tamminga CA, Dale JM, Goodman L, Kaneda H, Kaneda N (1990). Neuroleptic induced vacuous chewing movements as an animal model of tardive dyskinesia; a study in 3 rat strains. *Psychopharmacology* 102, 474–478.

Tamminga CA, Thaker GK, Moran M, Kakigi T, Gao XM (1994). Clozapine in tardive dyskinesia: observations from human and animal model studies. *J Clin Psychiatry* 55(Suppl B), 102–106.

Tan EK, Khajavi M, Thornby JI, Nagamitsu S, Jankovic J, Ashizawa T (2000). Variability and validity of polymorphism association studies in Parkinson's disease. *Neurology* 55, 533–538.

Tay AH, Lim LC, Lee WL, Wong KE, Wong LY, Tsoi WF (1997). Association between allele *1* of T102C polymorphism, 5-hydroxytryptamine 2A receptor gene and schizophrenia in Chinese males in Singapore. *Hum Hered* 47, 298–300.

Thompson J, Thomas N, Singleton A et al. (1997). D_2 dopamine receptor gene (*DRD2*) *Taq1 A* polymorphism: reduced dopamine D_2 receptor binding in the human striatum associated with the *A1* allele. *Pharmacogenetics* 7, 479–484.

Turecki G, Briere R, Dewar K (1999). Prediction of level of serotonin 2A receptor binding by serotonin receptor 2A genetic variation in postmortem brain samples from subjects who did or did not commit suicide. *Am J Psychiatry* 156, 1456–1458.

Waren JT, Peacock ML, Rodriguez LC, Fink JK (1993). An *MspI* polymorphism in the human serotonin receptor gene: detection by DGGE and RFLP analysis. *Hum Mol Genet* 2, 338.

Weinhold P, Wegner JT, Kane JM (1981). Familial occurrence of tardive dyskinesia. *J Clin Psychiatry* 42, 165–166.

Williams J, McGuffin P, Nothen M, Owen MJ (1997). Meta-analysis of association between the 5-HT_{2A} receptor T102C polymorphism and schizophrenia. European Multicentre Association Study of Schizophrenia Collaborative Group [letter]. *Lancet* 349, 1221.

Wolf A, Schultz LJ (1997). The serotonin 5-HT_{2C} receptor is a prominent serotonin receptor in basal ganglia: evidence from functional studies on serotonin mediated phosphoinositide hydrolysis. *J Neurochem* 69, 1449–1458.

Zahm DS, Brog JS (1992). On the significance of subterritories in the "accumbens" part of the rat ventral striatum. *Neuroscience* 50, 761–767.

12

Functional gene-linked polymorphic regions in pharmacogenetics

Marco Catalano

IRCCS H. San Raffaele, Department of Neuropsychiatric Sciences, Milan, Italy

OVERVIEW

Starting from the complexity of neural pathways and their close integration, this chapter focuses on the possible advantages of investigating polymorphisms involved in the regulation of gene expression or in variation of enzymatic activity, using examples related to neurotransmitter pathway modulation (namely, uptake and metabolism). These examples (i.e., serotonin transporter-linked polymorphic region, monoamine oxidase A (MAO-A) promoter region, and catechol-O-methyltransferase (COMT)) are also used to support the hypothesis that quantitative variations of expression and functional levels would be better than structural changes at single receptor sites to identify differences in both treatment response and, likely, psychopathology. The possible influence of the serotonin (5-HT) transporter variants on the efficacy of fluvoxamine, paroxetine, pindolol augmentation, and on the effects of total sleep deprivation, is described in depression. The possible importance of this functional polymorphism in obsessive-compulsive disorder (OCD), stress reactivity and panic disorder (PD) is also discussed. Variations in MAO-A activity in female patients are discussed in relation to the pharmacogenetics of panic disorder, together with some hypotheses regarding the chromosomal location of the gene. Some preliminary results are described linking a functional polymorphism in the coding sequence of the gene *COMT* and antidepressant response in unipolar depression and bipolar mood disorder. Finally, the expected impact of new approaches (i.e., orphan receptor research, nucleic acid chips, and single nucleotide polymorphisms) is discussed in terms of the advantages and pitfalls (e.g., many new exciting data but also a stronger need for very careful replications and analysis). Ethical considerations are also outlined in that pharmacogenomics undoubtedly bears scientific promise but also raises ethical concerns for the conduct of research with human subjects, particularly with respect to confidentiality, risk–benefit analysis, DNA banking, and pharmacoeconomic issues.

Introduction

Neurotransmission and neuromodulation represent the final result of a complex series of events involving transmitters, receptors, transporters, transducers, enzymes, and other molecules for the fine tuning of many (if not all) physiological processes in most living organisms.

In Vertebrata, moreover, all neural pathways are closely integrated; consequently, an event at a given point can have consequences at many other points sideways, upwards or downwards. Early biological psychiatry was compelled by the knowledge of those times into restricted, simplistic views and limited to the "synecdochaic fallacy." For many years, the broad and rough concept of neurotransmitter pathway dysfunction ("one receptor–one dysfunction–one disorder") as the most important causal factor for psychopathology has been a leading "dogma" in biological psychiatry. The therapeutic effect of many psychotropic drugs was exclusively attributed to their ability to block or enhance these altered pathways, thus supporting, in turn, a sort of crystallized view (i.e., one pathway–one disease) (Hyman and Nestler, 1996). This, for example, gave rise to the dopaminergic hypothesis of schizophrenia and the noradrenergic–serotonergic dichotomy of mood disorders. More recently, serotonergic hypotheses have gained a great popularity for a (maybe too) wide spectrum of psychiatric disorders, ranging from mood to anxiety, to OCDs.

The advent of molecular biology techniques, and their application to the complex issue of central nervous system (CNS) functioning, has contributed to a substantial modification of these limited views. The many findings they have allowed have highlighted the limits of traditional psychiatric nosology and have had impact on knowledge and clinical practice. Consequently, diagnostic research has not seemed to keep pace with advances in molecular neurobiology, and the rate-limiting step in identifying susceptibility genes for psychiatric disorders has become phenotype definition. Therefore, the success of psychiatric genetics may require the development of a "genetic nosology" that can classify individuals in terms of the heritable aspects of psychopathology (van Praag 1997; Smoller and Tsuang, 1998).

Molecular techniques, indeed, have played a fundamental role in revealing some aspects of the real complexity of the CNS. They have enabled, for example, a more precise definition of receptor families and subtypes and allowed the development of more sophisticated genome-based pharmacogenetic approaches, thus offering more opportunities than views and studies based only on peripheral phenotypes. Furthermore, the growing interest in regulatory regions and post-transcriptional regulatory mechanisms is offering not only interesting findings but also new incentives for a more open-minded molecular psychiatry. Quantitative variations of expression (regardless of their pre- or post-transcriptional origin) could explain the complexity of CNS functioning better and may be better for explaining both psychopathology and clinical response to psychotropic drugs than structural variations that resemble a type of "on/off model." These advances can justify increased optimism about the future of psychopharmacogenetics, and it is reasonable to believe that clinical applications will follow in the next few years, albeit limited to some psychiatric disorders.

The serotonin transporter

The serotonin transporter (5-HTT) plays a pivotal role in regulating serotonergic transmission by removing 5-HT from the synaptic cleft. 5-HTT represents a prime target for the widely used serotonin reuptake inhibitors, both selective and not (SSRIs and SRIs, respectively). The 5-HTT is encoded by a single gene located on chromosome 17 and organized in 14 exons spanning about 35 kilobases (kb). A mutation screening study of the whole coding region of the gene gave no exciting result (Di Bella et al., 1996) but a functional polymorphism in the promoter site (the 5-HTT gene-linked polymorphic region (5-HTTLPR)) has opened the doors to some interesting studies. This polymorphism consists of the insertion or deletion of a 44 bp sequence (Heils et al., 1996) and gives rise to two variants: long (*l*), and short (*s*). These variants showed different transcriptional efficiencies, resulting in different 5-HTT protein expression (the basal transcriptional activity of the *l* variant being more than twice that of the *s* variant) and functional levels. In fact, in vitro studies showed that the differences in 5-HTT mRNA synthesis resulted in different 5-HTT expressions and 5-HT cellular uptake (Lesch et al., 1996). Moreover, 5-HTTLPR genotypes seem to affect significantly 5-HTT-binding sites and mRNA levels in postmortem human brain tissue (Little et al., 1998). Therefore, the 5-HTT locus could represent a good candidate for psychiatric genetics.

Many studies have been performed on the possible role of this locus in conferring genetic susceptibility for different psychiatric disorders, with interesting (even if sometimes controversial) results suggesting, as a whole, a possible link to the anxiety–depression spectrum (for a review see Lesch and Mössner (1998)). However, since psychiatric disorders are likely multifactorial and oligo- or polygenic, a gene (or genes) with a minor or even null contribution in conferring susceptibility to a given disease could play a significant role in determining the response to treatment. Briefly, it could influence pharmacokinetic and/or pharmacodynamic parameters, act directly at a target site, or condition onset and/or intensity of side effects (Kalow, 1997; Iyer and Ratain, 1998; Nebert, 1999; Masellis et al., 2000). Indeed, interesting results have been produced using this polymorphism in pharmacogenetic approaches.

Two consecutive studies by the same research group have suggested a relationship between the antidepressant efficacy of two SSRIs, fluvoxamine (Smeraldi et al., 1998) and paroxetine (Zanardi et al., 2000), and allelic variation within the 5-HTTLPR, at equivalent drug plasma levels. In both studies, *l/l* homozygotes

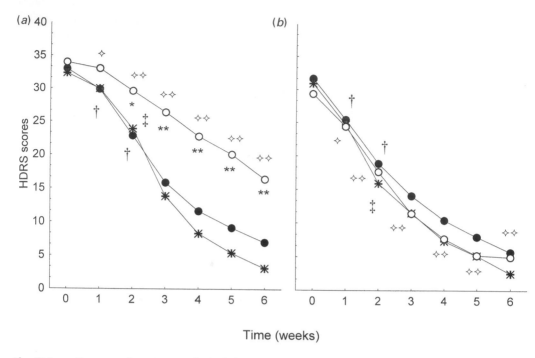

Fig. 12.1.   Patterns of symptomatological change as shown by HDRS (Hamilton Depression Rating Scale) score during treatment with fluvoxamine alone (*a*) or fluvoxamine plus pindolol (*b*) in groups carrying long (*l*) or short (*s*) variants of the serotonin transporter linked polymorphic region (5-HTTLPR). Genotypes were *l/l* (●; *n* = 15), *l/s* (✳; *n* = 23), and *s/s* (○; *n* = 15 (*a*), *n* = 8 (*b*) (see text)). *s/s* versus *l/l* and *l/s*: **p* < 0.05; ** *p* < 0.0001. *s/s* treated with fluvoxamine plus placebo (*a*) versus *s/s* treated with fluvoxamine plus pindolol (*b*): ◦ *p* < 0.01; ◦◦, *p* < 0.0001. *l/s* treated with fluvoxamine plus placebo (*a*) versus *l/s* treated with fluvoxamine plus pindolol (*b*): † *p* < 0.0001. *l/l* treated with fluvoxamine plus placebo (*a*) versus *l/l* treated with fluvoxamine plus pindolol, *p* < 0.01. (With permission from Smeraldi et al. (1998). Polymorphism within the promoter of the serotonin transporter gene and antidepressant efficacy of fluvoxamine. *Molecular Psychiatry* 3, 508–511.)

showed a more prompt and better antidepressant response than *l/s* and *s/s* individuals (Figs. 12.1 and 12.2). Even more interestingly, the former study was performed on a particular type of depression, delusional depression. This is a very severe form of mood disorder, often also characterized by refractoriness to antidepressant treatments. In these cases, it is common to use augmentation therapy with the addition of pindolol (a mixed β-adrenergic and 5-HT$_{1A}$ antagonist) to boost antidepressant effect by preventing inhibition of serotonergic firing by activation of somatodendritic autoreceptors. Unfortunately, side effects are not uncommon, mainly because of the β-adrenergic antagonism. Consequently, the possibility of identifying a subset of patients who may benefit from pindolol augmentation could

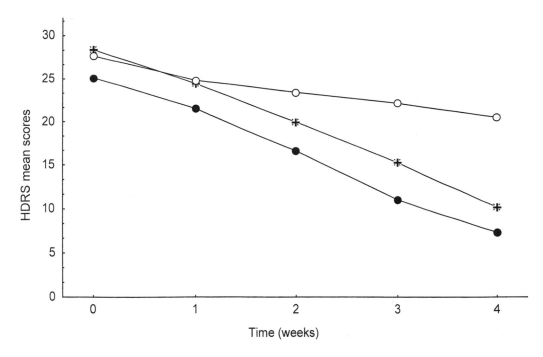

Fig. 12.2. Paroxetine plasma levels in patients with different genotypes for the serotonin transporter in the linked polymorphic region 5-HTTLPR: *l/l* (●; *n* = 16); *l/s* (✳, *n* = 26); *s/s* (○, *n* = 16). A two-way repeated measures ANOVA (MANOVA) on HDRS (Hamilton Depression Rating Scale) scores (with time as the within subjects factor, genotype as the between subjects factor, and paroxetine plasma levels as covariate) showed a highly significant effect of genotype ($F = 10.62$; df 2, 54; $p = 0.0001$), and of genotype $\times$ time interaction ($F = 9.06$; df 8, 220; $p < 0.0001$). Within-cell regression showed no significant effects of paroxetine plasma levels. Post hoc comparisons (Newman–Keuls test) showed that group *l/l* had significantly better scores than group *l/s* and *s/s* from week 2 to week 4; while group *l/s* had significantly better scores than group *s/s* from week 2 to week 4. (IRCCS Hospital San Raffaele, Department of Neuropsychiatric Science, unpublished figure. Ref. paper: Zanardi et al., 2000.)

represent a significant advance in the treatment of this severe form of depression. In fact, our finding showed that the addition of pindolol abolished the genotype effect on fluvoxamine response. In other words, in the group of patients treated with fluvoxamine plus pindolol, all the genotypes acted like the *l/l* homozygotes treated with fluvoxamine alone, suggesting that only the *s/s* homozygotes should be particularly amenable to pindolol addition.

These findings have been recently confirmed by a submitted study performed on an independent sample of 155 depressed patients using the same design (Serretti, personal communication). In this case too, *l/l* homozygotes showed a better response to fluvoxamine, and pindolol augmentation ameliorated the outcome in

5-HTTLPR s/s homozygotes, again reducing the difference in the response rate among the genotypes. Another study (Pollock et al., 2000) obtained interesting results using paroxetine in a group of elderly depressed patients. The findings suggested a prompter antidepressant effect only in subjects bearing the *l/l* alleles suggesting a significant relationship between 5-HTTLPR and acute response to SSRI therapy. SSRI plasma levels were also used as variable in the data analysis in this study. All these results suggest that genotyping at 5-HTTLPR could represent a promising approach to individualize the treatment of depression.

However, a recent study in patients of Asiatic descent indicated a better antidepressant response in *s/s* homozygotes (Kim et al., 2000). This raises the possibility that other factors, such as ethnic differences or population stratification, could act as confounders in pharmacogenetic protocols. This last study differed from the ones suggesting a better response for *l/l* homozygotes in several ways. The main difference resided in the assessment protocol, as the authors used an end-point analysis instead of repeated measures: using the dichotomous variable "responder/nonresponder" instead of a time course assessment of depressive symptoms. There was also the possible presence of placebo responders (to be suspected also in the study by Pollock and associates (2000)). This could be an important issue, given the possibility that 5-HTTLPR variants might have significant effects on personality features (Hamer et al., 1999; Greenberg et al., 2000; Osher et al., 2000), which in turn, could condition a different psychological attitude toward medication. Last, but not least, results in the study of Kim et al. (2000) were not corrected for the estimated bioavailability of the drug. This is a difficult issue in that even the exclusion of outliers for plasma levels of the given SSRI is not a guaranteed method, although it would protect results from influences owing to extreme variations in bioavailability. Unfortunately, to the best of my knowledge, only one study exists on the plasma/CNS ratio of SSRIs (Strauss et al., 1998). Nevertheless, despite these differences, all the studies seem to confirm the possible importance of the 5-HTTLPR in the pharmacogenetics of serotonergic antidepressants.

SRIs and SSRIs are also used to treat OCD and PD. In OCD, two studies seem to exclude any significant influence of 5-HTT variant on the response rate to usual SRIs treatment protocols (Billet et al., 1997; Catalano et al., 2000), suggesting that in this disorder other etiopathogenetic factors could predominate. In other words, it cannot be excluded that different biochemical pathways could subtend or condition the efficacy of SRIs in different disorders, and there may be different etiopathogenetic mechanisms. This hypothesis seems to fit with the well-known differences between depression and OCD in latency of therapeutic effect and dose regimen (Montgomery, 1994; Tollefson et al., 1994; Greist et al., 1995; Blier and de Montigny, 1998).

By comparison, a preliminary result from an Italian sample of PD seems to suggest a significant relationship between the 5-HTTLPR *l* allele and positive response to treatment with SSRIs (citalopram and paroxetine) but not with SRIs (clomipramine). This study also suggested the presence of a gender difference with regard to both response and some clinical features, as indicated in a previous study on PD that will be discussed later in this chapter (Deckert et al., 1999). A higher frequency of the *l* allele was significantly associated with a positive response to treatment, as well as with the absence of agoraphobia, only in the female subsample (Bosi, 2000). This last finding seems to be in agreement with results from Wichems and associates (2000), who found increases in anxiety and stress responses to be more prominent in female than in male *5-HTT* knockout mice.

Two further studies on 5-HTTLPR deserve mention as they suggest other possible roles of 5-HTT. In the first, cerebrospinal fluid (CSF) 5-hydroxyindoleacetic acid (5-HIAA) and blood pressure plus heart rate were used as indices of 5-HT turnover and stress reactivity, respectively. All these parameters showed a significant increase in subjects bearing one or two copies of the 5-HTTLPR *l* allele (Williams et al., 2001). The second study described the effects of total sleep deprivation (TSD) in bipolar patients and showed a significantly better response (expressed as higher perceived mood levels after TSD) in *l/l* homozygotes for 5-HTTLPR (Benedetti et al., 1999) (Fig. 12.3). Taken together, these results seem to support the hypothesis of 5-HT as a "wide-spectrum" modulating neurotransmitter (as also suggested by its multiple pre- and postsynaptic receptor subtypes) with different roles in different backgrounds. In other words, if there was a significant influence of 5-HTTLPR variants it would indicate a more direct role of 5-HT in a given situation (for example, depression and treatment response); a nonsignificant or negligible effect could suggest a more indirect role or no role at all.

Obviously, these data must be cautiously interpreted, and their further replication is critical. However, they seem to confirm the possible importance of this functional polymorphism not only as a pharmacogenetic tool but also as an auxiliary tool to develop a more precise genetic nosology in psychiatry.

Neurotransmitter metabolism

Neurotransmitter metabolism is another "hot-spot" both for psychiatric genetics and psychopharmacogenetics. Differences in enzymatic activity can condition different rates of neurotransmitter degradation, which, in turn, can condition different functional consequences. Two classes of enzyme play a fundamental role in neurotransmitter catabolism: the MAOs and COMT.

Two MAO isozymes are known, A and B, which differ in molecular weight and immunological properties. Two adjacent genes, mapped on the 11.23–11.4 region of the X chromosome, encode the isozymes. Norepinephrine and 5-HT are the

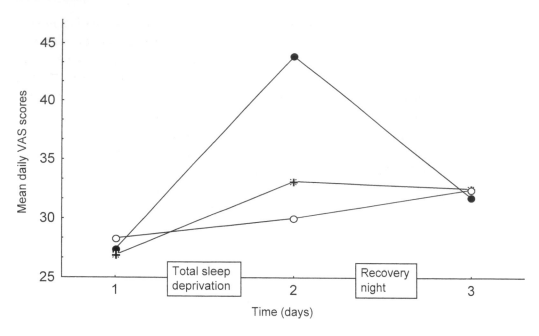

Fig. 12.3.   The effect of genotype for the serotonin transporter in the linked polymorphic region (*5-HTTLPR*) on the response to total sleep deprivation in bipolar patients. *l/l* (●; $n = 20$); *l/s* (✳; $n = 35$); *s/s* (○; $n = 13$). Self-ratings of mood (scores 0, 50, 100, correspond to depression, euthymia, and euphoria) before and after sleep deprivation were analyzed using a two-way repeated measures ANCOVA, with time ($p = 0.0008$) and genotype (not significant) as independent factors (time × genotype interaction: $p = 0.05$) and age at onset as covariate (not significant). (IRCCS. Hospital San Raffaele, Department of Neuropsychiatric Science unpublished figure. Ref. paper: Benedetti et al., 1999.)

preferential substrates of MAO-A, while MAO-B preferentially oxidizes phenyl-ethylamine and dopamine.

Monoamine oxidase A

Inhibitors of MAO-A can be both reversible and irreversible in action and have antidepressant properties; they have been shown to be effective in the treatment of PD. Therefore, the gene *MAO-A* might be considered a candidate for genetic or pharmacogenetic studies.

A novel repeat polymorphism in the promoter of *MAO-A* has been examined for association with PD in two independent samples of different descent (German and Italian). This polymorphism consists of a 30 bp motif that repeats two (very rare) to five times. An additional allele, named "3a" was shown to contain three full repeats plus 18 bp of the repeated motif. Functional characterization of the polymorphism using luciferase assay showed that constructs containing the longer repeats (3a, 4, and 5) had a higher transcriptional activity than the shorter (i.e.,

3 repeats, since the 2 repeats variant was not tested, given its rareness), thus suggesting increased MAO-A activity in subjects bearing the longer alleles. There was a significantly higher frequency of the longer alleles among females with PD than among control females, whereas no significant difference was observed between male patients with PD and male controls (Deckert et al., 1999). The finding could simply suggest that increased MAO-A activity is a risk factor for PD in female patients, perhaps also explained by epigenetic hormonal influences on the disease; however, the chromosomal location of the gene made the situation more intriguing. In fact, in females, one allele should have been randomly silenced because of X-inactivation. Accordingly, "long/long" females should have behaved like male hemizygotes bearing only a long allele. It is possible that the differences observed were by chance because of the size differences between the two subsamples. If this is not the case then several hypotheses could be invoked to explain it. It is possible that genomic imprinting has occurred in which the imprint silences the allele from one parent. In this case, the males with PD might bear a silenced *MAO-A* gene. However, the issue of X-linked imprinting is still very controversial, and the possibility of a living organism without any MAO-A activity would actually be surprising. A further possibility is skewed random X inactivation, which has been reported, as has the tendency for male offspring of skewed mothers to inherit alleles from the inactive X chromosome in the region from Xp11 to Xq22 (Naumova et al., 1995). Alternatively, as X inactivation silences most but not all of the genes on one of the two X chromosomes in mammalian females, women with PD could bear two active *MAO-A* alleles.

Albeit interesting, these hypotheses are largely speculative. Nevertheless, a different study on clinical psychopharmacology using an artificial neural network (Politi et al., 1999) has suggested a possible profile of a good responder to moclobemide (a reversible MAO-A inhibitor) as a female with prominent anxiety symptoms. While these results should be assessed cautiously, these data could suggest MAO-A inhibitors as a good choice in the treatment of females with PD.

Interestingly, a sexually dimorphic effect for MAO-A has been shown in two studies, although involving different disorders and the opposite direction. The first study, by Karayiorgou and associates (1999) used a different, intragenic polymorphism but suggested an association between a high activity *MAO-A* allele and male OCD probands. The second, very preliminary, showed a similar finding (i.e., a higher frequency of more active alleles in males) in a group of bipolar patients using the MAO-A promoter polymorphism (Casorati, 1999).

Catechol-*O*-methyltransferase

COMT, along with MAO, represents the major mammalian enzymatic system involved in the degradation of catecholamines. A gene mapped to 22q11.1–q11.2 encodes the enzyme (Grossman et al., 1992). Variation in COMT enzyme activity is a common finding in humans. This variation is attributable to a functional poly-morphism within the coding region of the gene. It consists of a G-to-A transition at codon 158 of the gene, and gives rise to two variants with huge differences in enzymatic activity (i.e., a three- to fourfold variation between the high- and low-activity alleles) (Lachmann et al., 1996a).

This metabolic role, together with findings regarding behavioral and psychiatric consequences of the 21q11 microdeletion (Shprintzen et al., 1992; Pulver et al., 1994; Lachmann et al., 1996b; Papolos et al., 1996), has suggested *COMT* as a can-didate gene and has prompted several psychiatric genetic studies, all with contrast-ing results (Kirov et al., 1998, 1999; Mynett-Johnson et al., 1998; de Chaldee et al., 1999; Wei and Hemmings, 1999; Geller and Cook, 2000; Henderson et al., 2000; Li et al., 2000). Consequently, it is still unclear whether *COMT* has any role in confer-ring susceptibility to psychiatric disorders. However, some findings suggesting a possible interaction between 5-HTTLPR and *COMT* polymorphisms (Benjamin et al., 2000 a,b) prompted a study of COMT in relation to fluvoxamine antidepress-ant response despite the affinity profile of the enzyme. In fact, COMT does not degrade 5-HT, having mainly dopamine and norepinephrine as substrates.

A very recent unpublished study on 94 unipolar depressed and 65 bipolar patients in which the time course of response to fluvoxamine was assessed by *COMT* genotype suggested a less favorable response to the antidepressant only in unipolar depressed patients homozygous for the higher activity variant of the gene (Tentoni, 2000). Obviously, the possibility of a chance finding, despite statistical significance, cannot be discarded a priori, and application to clinical practice is clearly premature. Moreover, as ethnic differences in both erythrocyte COMT activity and *COMT* gene alleles have been previously demonstrated (McLeod et al., 1998; Palmatier et al., 1999), population-linked effects may produce false-positive results. Nevertheless, this finding could support proposed biological differences between bipolar and unipolar disease and, if confirmed, could offer a new pharma-cogenetic tool for the treatment of depression. First, it could allow the identifica-tion of unipolar patients who might be particularly amenable to fluvoxamine (or other SSRIs) treatment and, second, even suggest COMT inhibitors as adjuvant drugs (as in Parkinson's disease).

Conclusions

Regulatory regions and metabolism of neurotransmitters seem to have something to offer psychopharmacogenetics. Indeed, quantitative variations of expression provide better explanations of both psychopathological variations and response to treatment than do mutations leading to alterations at receptor sites. Pharmacogenetic studies are also providing data to support the hypothesis that

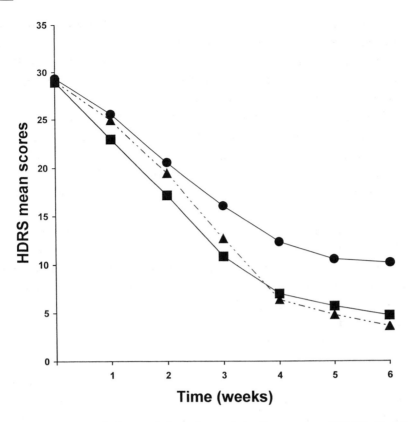

Fig. 12.4.   Influence of catechol-*O*-methyltransferase (COMT) genotypes (*HH* (●), *HL* (■), and *LL*
(▲); where *H* indicates higher activity and *L* lower activity) on response to fluvoxamine in
unipolar depression. A two-way repeated measures ANOVA (MANOVA) on HDRS
(Hamilton Depression Rating Scale) scores (with time as the within subjects factor,
genotype as the between subjects factor) showed a significant effect of genotype
($F = 3.41$; df 2, 91; $p = 0.0372$), of time ($F = 247.86$; df 6, 546; $p < 0.0001$), and of genotype
× time interaction ($F = 2.20$; df 12, 546; $p < 0.0107$). Post hoc analysis (Newman–Keuls
test) showed significant statistical differences starting from weeks 2 (*HH* versus *HL*) and 3
(*HH* versus *LL*). (Adapted from Tentoni, 2000.)

response to the same drug does not always mean that the treated disorders share
identical pathogenetic pathways. For example, SRIs are advantageous in treating
both depression and OCD, but a direct influence of 5-HTTLPR variant seems to be
specifically restricted to depression. Similarly, a lack of responsiveness to a given
drug does not always mean a misdiagnosis, since refractory patients are a reality,
and now we may hope to identify them in advance. Similar reasoning can be applied
to adverse reactions, as the real benefit of a treatment is always the fruit of a careful
balance between efficacy and side effects.

Obviously, genes with products that are prime targets of specific drugs are far more interesting, and screening for polymorphisms should include regulatory regions and/or sequences. On the pharmacological side, this means that, when possible, drugs that display a narrower range of targets are preferable starting points. Also, it is worth recalling that, since psychiatric disorders are likely multifactorial and oligo- or polygenic, a gene with a minor contribution in conferring susceptibility could play a significant role in determining the response to treatment. In other words, a single gene could contribute only a very minor part of the pathological variance but, at the same time, encode a protein of pivotal importance for the response to a given treatment. It could, for example, exert a significant influence on the metabolism of the drug, or represent a prime target for the drug.

Like all experimental results, psychopharmacogenetic findings need to be cautiously regarded and confirmed by independent replication. This holds particularly true now that new approaches can potentially offer significant new information together with a large number of data requiring explanation. For example, investigation of orphan receptors could lead to the discovery of many neuropeptides, which, in turn, could represent the starting points of new drug discovery programs (Civelli et al., 1999) and DNA and RNA chip technology could accelerate molecular research by allowing the simultaneous screening of thousand of genes.

Single nucleotide polymorphisms (SNPs) are another new area that has generated great excitement and SNPs are rapidly becoming the main focus of "new pharmacogenetics" (for a review see Pfost et al. (2000)). Prudent skepticism, at least for complex psychiatric disorders, is warranted. For many years, new possible tools and related promises and perspectives have excited interest, from restriction fragment length polymorphisms, through variable number of tandem repeats, high-throughput sequencing, microsatellites, etc. Although these techniques have allowed an enormous number of experiments worldwide and have required high investments, the practical results are quite unbalanced and thus disappointing. It is true that the increasing number of known SNPs could give psychopharmacogenetics new chances, but SNP discovery is not enough. SNP scoring is needed, and we know that correlating genotypes with clinical phenotypes is never easy in psychopharmacology. Nevertheless, if correctly managed, this approach could be helpful, particularly with regard to polymorphisms involved in post-transcriptional gene regulatory mechanisms, the importance of which has been described by Day and Tuite (1998) and in Chapter 7.

Finally, some ethical consideration and attention to doubts and criticism of so-called pharmacogenomics are needed, as these developments, although bearing scientific promise, raise ethical concerns for the conduct of research with human subjects, particularly with respect to confidentiality, risk–benefit analysis, DNA banking, and pharmacoeconomic issues (Issa, 2000).

Acknowledgements

The author gratefully acknowledges his colleagues at DSNP for collaboration and support, and Professor Bernard Lerer for valuable discussion and friendly advice.

REFERENCES

Benedetti F, Serretti A, Colombo C et al. (1999). Influence of a functional polymorphism within the promoter of the serotonin transporter gene on the effects of total sleep deprivation in bipolar depression. *Am J Psychiatry* 156, 1450–1452.

Benjamin J, Osher Y, Kotler M (2000a). Association between tridimensional personality questionnaire (TPQ) traits and three functional polymorphisms: dopamine receptor D_4 (*DRD4*), serotonin transporter promoter region (5-HTTLPR) and catechol *O*-methyltransferase (*COMT*). *Mol Psychiatry* 5, 96–100.

Benjamin J, Osher Y, Lichtenberg P et al. (2000b). An interaction between the catechol *O*-methyltransferase and serotonin transporter promoter region polymorphisms contributes to tridimensional personality questionnaire persistence scores in normal subjects. *Neuropsychobiology* 41, 48–53.

Billett EA, Richter MA, King N, Heils A, Lesch KP, Kennedy JL (1997). Obsessive compulsive disorder, response to serotonin reuptake inhibitors and the serotonin transporter gene. *Mol Psychiatry* 2, 403–406.

Blier P, de Montigny C (1998). Possible serotonergic mechanisms underlying the antidepressant and anti-obsessive-compulsive disorder responses. *Biol Psychiatry* 44, 313–323.

Bosi M (2000). Applicazione di tecniche molecolari alla genetica e farmacogenetica del disturbo di panico. Postgraduate Thesis, University of Milan School of Medicine.

Casorati P (1999). Applicazione di tecniche molecolari ai problemi della nosologia psichiatrica: ruolo di un polimorfismo funzionale nella regione regolatoria del gene codificante per le MAO-A. MD Graduate Thesis, University of Milan, School of Medicine.

Catalano M, Di Bella D, Erzegovesi S, Bellodi L (2000). Serotonin transporter polymorphisms and response to SSRIs in different psychiatric disorders: a mirror of etiopathogenetic differences? *Int J Neuropsychopharmacol* 3, S26.

Civelli O, Reinscheid RK, Nothacker H-P (1999). Orphan receptors, novel neuropeptides and reverse pharmaceutical research. *Brain Res* 848, 63–65.

Day DA, Tuite MF (1998). Post-transcriptional gene regulatory mechanisms in eukaryotes: an overview. *J Endocrinol* 157, 361–371.

de Chaldee M, Laurent C, Thibaut F et al. (1999). Linkage disequilibrium on the *COMT* gene in French schizophrenics and controls. *Am J Med Genet* 88, 452–457.

Deckert J, Catalano M, Syagailo YV et al. (1999). Excess of high activity monoamine oxidase A gene promoter alleles in female patients with panic disorder. *Hum Mol Genet* 8, 621–624.

Di Bella D, Catalano M, Balling U, Smeraldi E, Lesch K-P (1996). Systematic screening for mutations in the coding region of the human serotonin transporter (5-HTT) gene using PCR and DGGE. *Am J Med Genet* 67, 541–545.

Geller B, Cook EH Jr. (2000). Ultradian rapid cycling in prepubertal and early adolescent bipolarity is not in transmission disequilibrium with Val/Met *COMT* alleles. *Biol Psychiatry* 47, 605–609.

Greenberg BD, Li Q, Lucas FR et al. (2000). Association between the serotonin transporter promoter polymorphism and personality traits in a primarily female population sample. *Am J Med Genet* 96, 202–216.

Greist J, Chouinard G, DuBoff E et al. (1995). Double-blind parallel comparison of three dosages of sertraline and placebo in outpatients with obsessive-compulsive disorder. *Arch Gen Psychiatry* 52, 289–295.

Grossman MH, Emanuel BS, Budarf ML (1992). Chromosomal mapping of the human catechol-*O*-methyltransferase gene to 22q11.1–q11.2. *Genomics* 12, 822–825.

Hamer DH, Greenberg BD, Sabol SZ, Murphy DL (1999). Role of the serotonin transporter gene in temperament and character. *J Pers Disord* 13, 312–327.

Heils A, Teufel A, Petri S et al. (1996). Allelic variation of human serotonin transporter gene expression. *J Neurochem* 66, 2621–2624.

Henderson AS, Korten AE, Jorm AF et al. (2000). COMT and DRD3 polymorphisms, environmental exposures, and personality traits related to common mental disorders. *Am J Med Genet* 96, 102–107.

Hyman SE, Nestler EJ (1996). Initiation and adaptation: a paradigm for understanding psychotropic drug action. *Am J Psychiatry* 153, 151–162.

Issa AM (2000). Ethical considerations in clinical pharmacogenomics research. *Trend Pharm Sci* 21, 247–249.

Iyer L, Ratain MJ (1998). Pharmacogenetics and cancer chemotherapy. *Eur J Cancer* 34, 1493–1499.

Kalow W (1997). Pharmacogenetics in biological perspective. *Pharm Rev* 49, 369–379.

Karayiorgou M, Sobin C, Blundell ML et al. (1999). Family-based association studies support a sexually dimorphic effect of COMT and MAOA on genetic susceptibility to obsessive-compulsive disorder. *Biol Psychiatry* 45, 1178–1189.

Kim DK, Lim SW, Lee S et al. (2000). Serotonin transporter gene polymorphism and antidepressant response. *Neuroreport* 11, 215–219.

Kirov G, Murphy KC, Arranz MJ et al. (1998). Low activity allele of catechol-*O*-methyltransferase gene associated with rapid cycling bipolar disorder. *Mol Psychiatry* 3, 342–345.

Kirov G, Jones I, McCandless F, Craddock N, Owen MJ (1999). Family-based association studies of bipolar disorder with candidate genes involved in dopamine neurotransmission: *DBH, DAT1, COMT, DRD2, DRD3* and *DRD5*. *Mol Psychiatry* 4, 558–565.

Lachmann HM, Papolos DF, Saito T, Yu YM, Szumlanski CL, Weinshilboum RM (1996a). Human catechol-*O*-methyltransferase pharmacogenetics: description of a functional polymorphism and its potential applications to neuropsychiatric disorders. *Pharmacogenetics* 6, 243–250.

Lachmann HM, Morrow B, Shprintzen R et al. (1996b). Association of codon 108/158 catechol-*O*-methyltransferase gene polymorphism with the psychiatric manifestations of velo-cardio-facial syndrome. *Am J Med Genet* 67, 468–472.

Lesch K-P, Mössner R (1998). Genetically driven variation in serotonin uptake: is there a link to affective spectrum, neurodevelopmental, and neurodegenerative disorders? *Biol Psychiatry* 44, 179–192.

Lesch K-P, Bengel D, Heils A et al. (1996). Association of anxiety-related traits with a polymorphism in the serotonin transporter gene regulatory region. *Science* 274, 1527–1531.

Li T, Ball D, Zhao J et al. (2000). Family-based linkage disequilibrium mapping using SNP marker haplotypes: application to a potential locus for schizophrenia at chromosome 22q11. *Mol Psychiatry* 5, 77–84.

Little KY, McLaughlin DP, Zhang L et al. (1998). Cocaine, ethanol, and genotype effects on human midbrain serotonin transporter binding sites and mRNA levels. *Am J Psychiatry* 155, 207–213.

Masellis M, Basile VS, Ozdemir V et al. (2000). Pharmacogenetics of antipsychotic treatment: lessons learned from clozapine. *Biol Psychiatry* 47, 252–266.

McLeod HL, Syvanen AC, Githang'a J et al. (1998). Ethnic differences in catechol *O*-methyltransferase pharmacogenetics: frequency of the codon 108/158 low activity allele is lower in Kenyan than Caucasian or Southwest Asian individuals. *Pharmacogenetics* 8, 195–199.

Montgomery SA (1994). Pharmacological treatment of obsessive-compulsive disorder. In Hollander E, Zohar J, Marazziti D, Olivier B, eds. *Current Insights in Obsessive Disorder*. New York: John Wiley, pp. 215–226.

Mynett-Johnson LA, Murphy VE, Claffey E, Shields DC, McKeon P (1998). Preliminary evidence of an association between bipolar disorder in females and the catechol-*O*-methyltransferase gene. *Psychiatr Geneti* 8, 221–225.

Naumova AK, Olien L, Bird LM et al. (1995). Transmission-ratio distortion of X-chromosomes among male offspring of females with skewed X-inactivation. *Dev Genet* 17, 198–205.

Nebert DW (1999). Pharmacogenetics and pharmacogenomics: why is this relevant to the clinical geneticist? *Clin Genet* 56, 247–258.

Osher Y, Hamer D, Benjamin J (2000). Association and linkage of anxiety-related traits with a functional polymorphism of the serotonin transporter gene regulatory region in Israeli sibling pairs. *Mol Psychiatry* 5, 216–219.

Palmatier MA, Kang AM, Kidd KK (1999). Global variation in the frequencies of functionally different catechol-*O*-methyltransferase alleles. *Biol Psychiatry* 46, 557–567.

Papolos DF, Faedda GL, Veit S et al. (1996). Bipolar spectrum disorders in patients diagnosed with velo-cardio-facial syndrome: does a hemizygous deletion of chromosome 22q11 result in bipolar affective disorder? *Am J Psychiatry* 153, 1541–1547.

Pfost DR, Boyce-Jacino MT, Grant DM (2000). A SNPshot: pharmacogenetics and the future of drug therapy. *Trend Biotechnol* 18, 334–338.

Politi E, Balduzzi C, Bussi R, Bellodi L (1999). Artificial neural networks: a study in clinical psychopharmacology. *Psychiatry Res* 87, 203–215.

Pollock BG, Ferrell RE, Mulsant BH et al. (2000). Allelic variation in the serotonin transporter promoter affects onset of paroxetine treatment response in late-life depression. *Neuropsychopharmacology* 23, 587–590.

Pulver AE, Nestadt G, Goldberg R et al. (1994). Psycotic illness in patients diagnosed with velo-cardio-facial syndrome and their relatives. *J Nerv Mental Disord* 182, 476–478.

Shprintzen RJ, Goldberg RB, Golding-Kushner KJ, Marion RW (1992). Late onset psycosis in velo-cardio-facial syndrome. *Am J Med Genet* 42, 141–142.

Smeraldi E, Zanardi R, Benedetti F, Di Bella D, Perez J, Catalano M (1998). Polymorphism within the promoter of the serotonin transporter gene and antidepressant efficacy of fluvoxamine. *Mol Psychiatry* 3, 508–511.

Smoller JW, Tsuang MT (1998). Panic and phobic anxiety: defining phenotypes for genetic studies. *Am J Psychiatry* 155, 1152–1162.

Strauss WL, Layton ME, Dager SR (1998). Brain elimination half-life of fluvoxamine measured by ^{19}F magnetic resonance spectroscopy. *Am J Psychiatry* 155, 380–304.

Tentoni L (2000). Approccio molecolare alla farmacogenetica dei disturbi dell'umore. MD Graduate Thesis, University of Milan School of Medicine.

Tollefson GD, Ramprey AH Jr., Potvin JH et al. (1994). A multicenter investigation of fixed-dose fluoxetine in the treatment of obsessive-compulsive disorder. *Arch Gen Psychiatry* 51, 559–567.

van Praag HM (1997). Over the mainstream: diagnostic requirements for biological psychiatric research. *Psychiatry Res* 72, 201–212.

Wei J, Hemmings GP (1999). Lack of evidence for association between the COMT locus and schizophrenia. *Psychiatr Genet* 9, 183–186.

Wichems C, Li Q, Andrews A, Lesch KP, Murphy DL (2000). Serotonin transporter knockout mice show a spontaneous behavioural phenotype of increased "anxiety" and stress responses. *Int J Neuropsychopharmacol* 3, S47.

Williams RB, Marchuk DA, Gadde KM et al. (2001). Central nervous system serotonin function and cardiovascular responses to stress. *Psychosomat Med* 63, 300–305.

Zanardi R, Benedetti F, Di Bella D, Catalano M, Smeraldi E (2000). Efficacy of paroxetine in depression is influenced by a functional polymorphism within the promoter of serotonin transporter gene. *J Clin Psychopharmacol* 20, 105–107.

13

Alternative phenotypes and the pharmacogenetics of mood and anxiety disorders

Emanuela Mundo and James L. Kennedy

Centre for Addiction and Mental Health, University of Toronto, Canada

OVERVIEW

The biological mechanisms of action of the main classes of antidepressant compound involve the serotonin (5-HT) system. Consequently, genes of this system have been considered ideal candidates in pharmacogenetic studies of the antidepressant response. There are critical methodological issues created by the complexity of the definition of the phenotypes (i.e., categorical versus dimensional), the involvement of nongenetic factors in determining the clinical effect of antidepressants, and the different genetic strategies available to detect genetic susceptibility in complex traits (e.g., family-based association studies, transmission disequilibrium test for qualitative and quantitative traits). In this chapter, we present and discuss the most recent findings on genetic predictors of the response to antidepressants in mood and anxiety disorders. The need for a more homogeneous phenotype definition (e.g., including phenotypes related to the diagnosis such as rapid cycling course, psychotic symptoms, atypical features) is pointed out. We also propose and discuss the role of alternative phenotypes (side effects or non-desirable reactions) in pharmacogenetic studies focused on the prediction of the clinical effect of antidepressants. As an example, the phenomenon of antidepressant-induced mania, as an abnormal response to antidepressants, is described. The most recent data on the role of candidate genes (particularly for the 5-HT system, e.g., $5\text{-}HTT$, $5HT1D\beta$, $5HT2A$) in contributing to the risk of developing this phenotype are presented and discussed. In the conclusion, the importance of having stable (i.e., genetic) predictors of normal and abnormal responses to antidepressants is pointed out, as well as the role of molecular genetic strategies in the clinical management of psychiatric disorders requiring treatment with antidepressant compounds.

Introduction

Most of the known compounds with antidepressant activity have as a main target the monoaminergic systems. Tricyclic antidepressants (TCAs) block the reuptake of serotonin (5-HT) and/or norepinephrine, selective serotonin reuptake inhibitors (SSRIs) selectively block the reuptake of 5-HT, and monoamine oxidase inhibitors (MAOIs) interfere with the metabolism of 5-HT, norepinephrine, and dopamine. However, all these compounds, as well as other antidepressant strategies (e.g, electroconvulsive treatment and sleep deprivation), have in common as a final effect the enhancement of 5-HT transmission, although mediated via different mechanisms (Blier and de Montigny, 1998). For this reason, 5-HT system genes have been considered the ideal candidates for the study of the prediction of antidepressant response.

In a pharmacogenetic perspective, the response to antidepressant treatment should be considered a complex phenotype. This means that it is heterogeneous, that its mode of inheritance is unclear, that it is very likely to be controlled by more than one gene, and that it is influenced also by environmental factors (Hirschfeld et al., 1998). Therefore, a clear and careful definition of the phenotype represents a critical step in designing molecular genetic studies for the prediction of the response to antidepressants.

In comparative clinical trials, this phenotype is usually defined in a quantitative/dimensional fashion (i.e., the amount of symptom improvement). However, this kind of evaluation alone may lead to confounding conclusions as the "mean" effect of a drug may derive from the co-occurrence in the same treatment group of dramatic improvements and poor responses (or lack of response). By comparison, the inclusion also of a qualitative/categorical evaluation of the response (i.e., number of responders/nonresponders according to validated and "a priori" criteria), taking into consideration the variability within treatment groups, gives more precise information about the efficacy of the compounds tested.

In genetic studies, we need to adapt these definitions of the phenotype to the analytical strategies available to identify gene effects in complex traits. To-date, family-based association study designs are considered the most appropriate to detect genetic susceptibility for complex phenotypes, where single genes are thought to be of small effect (Risch and Merikangas, 1996). In these studies, the best strategy in the definition of the "pharmacological response" phenotype appear to be the combined use of a dimensional and a categorical approach (Macciardi and Mundo, 1999). The effect of the use of this strategy on the modeling and on the statistical power of pharmacogenetic studies is extensively addressed in Chapter 5.

Genetic predictors of the response to antidepressants in mood and anxiety disorders: the controversial role of the serotonin transporter gene

Despite a wide variety of compounds with antidepressant properties being available and commonly used, proserotonergic drugs are the ones that have received the most consideration in a pharmacogenetic perspective. SSRIs are commonly used to treat major depression (Potter, 1998) and some anxiety disorders, such as obsessive-compulsive disorder (OCD) (Greist et al., 1995; Mundo et al., 1997), panic disorder, and generalized anxiety disorder (Feighner, 1999; Zohar and Westenberg, 2000). The exact mechanism of action of SSRIs in inducing a clinical response is not completely known and it is very likely to be different in depression and OCD (Blier and de Montigny, 1998). However, all these compounds share the ability of blocking the serotonin transporter (5-HTT), although with different degrees of selectivity and potency (Hyttel, 1994).

The 5-HTT is located on the terminals of serotonergic neurons and its function is the reuptake of 5-HTT from the synaptic cleft into the cell. It is encoded by a gene (*SLC6A4*) located on chromosome 17, which spans 31 kilobases (kb) and consists of 14 exons. This gene has two known polymorphisms. One is within the promoter region and consists of a 44 base pair (bp) insertion/deletion (the *5-HTT* gene-linked polymorphic region, 5-HTTLPR) (Heils et al., 1996; Lesch et al., 1996). According to the results of functional studies (Collier et al., 1996; Heils et al., 1996; Lesch et al. (1996) the long variant (*l*) generates more gene expression than the short one (*s*): the uptake of 5-HT is up to 50% less in cells carrying one or two copies of the *s* allele than in cells homozygous for the *l* allele, and the *l/l* cells produce steady-state concentrations of 5-HTT mRNA that are up to 1.7 times the concentrations in both *l/s* and *ss* cells. These data support the presence of a dominant model, instead of a codominant one, for the effect of the *s* allele. Moreover, according to a recent report, the *s* variant of the 5-HTTLPR has been suggested to confer higher stability to 5-HT function. In the study of Hanna et al. (1998), the seasonal fluctuations of blood 5-HT concentrations in OCD families were enhanced in subjects homozygous for the *l* variant in comparison with subjects heterozygous or homozygous for the *s* allele.

The other polymorphism known for the *SLC6A4* is a variable number of tandem repeats (VNTR) located in the second intron of the gene, with three alleles (*Stin2.9*, *Stin2.10* and *Stin2.12*) known in humans (Ogilvie et al., 1995).

Given the critical role of the 5-HTT in 5-HT neurotransmission, the functional variants of *SLC6A4* have been considered ideal candidates for the prediction of the clinical response to pro-serotonergic compounds in both OCD and mood disorders (Table 13.1).

The serotonin transporter gene and the antiobsessional response

The relationship between the 5-HTTLPR and antiobsessional response was first investigated in a paper by Billett et al. (1997) in which 72 patients with OCD treated with pro-serotonergic agents (clomipramine or SSRIs) were subdivided into responders and nonresponders to the medication. The allele and genotype

Table 13.1. Summary of the main studies investigating the association between 5-HTTLPR variants and the response to antidepressants

Study	Treatment	Diagnosis	Association/variant
Billet et al., 1997	SSRIs, clomipramine	OCD	None
McDougle et al., 1998	SSRIs	OCD	Negative/*l*
Smeraldi et al., 1998	Fluvoxamine	BP, UP[a]	Positive/*l*
Smeraldi et al., 1998	Fluvoxamine + pindolol	BP, UP[a]	None
Benedetti et al., 1999	Sleep deprivation	BP	Positive/*l*
Zanardi et al., 2000	Paroxetine	BP, UP[a]	Positive/*l*
Pollock et al., 2000	Paroxetine	UP[b]	Positive/*l*
Pollock et al., 2000	Nortriptyline	UP[b]	None
Kim et al., 2000	Fluoxetine, paroxetine	UP	Positive/*s*

Notes:

SSRI, selective serotonin reuptake inhibitor; OCD, obsessive-compulsive disorder; BP, bipolar disorder; UP, unipolar disorder; *l*, long variant; *s*, short variant.

[a] All patients had a major depressive episode with psychotic features.

[b] Patients with major depressive episodes with psychotic features were excluded.

frequencies for the 5-HTTLPR were computed and compared between the two groups. No significant differences were found, apparently excluding the role of this polymorphism in predicting the antiobsessional response. However, no definitive conclusions could be drawn from this preliminary study as the definition of the phenotype (i.e., the evaluation of the pharmacological response) was done retrospectively, in a semiquantitative fashion according to a global clinician's rating, and without validation criteria.

A more recent study performed on a smaller sample of OCD patients (McDougle et al., 1998) suggested an association between the *l* allele of the 5-HTTLPR and the lack of antiobsessional response to SSRIs, defined by a more appropriate combination of several validated criteria. In this study, a patient was defined as a "responder" if he/she met all the following criteria: (i) an improvement $\geq 35\%$ on the scores of the Yale–Brown Obsessive-Compulsive scale (Y-BOCS) (Goodman et al., 1989), which is commonly used to rate the severity of OCD symptoms and the symptom subtypes; (ii) a total Y-BOCS score < 16; (iii) a global improvement rated as "much" or "very much" at the Clinical Global Impression (CGI) rating scale (Guy, 1976); and (iv) the consensus of the treating clinician and of two of the investigators that the clinical condition was improved. In addition, in the same study, a critical alternative phenotype was evaluated: the presence of comorbid tic disorders. The co-occurrence of chronic tics or Gilles de la Tourette syndrome has been considered one of the most relevant predictors of nonresponse to SSRIs in OCD

(McDougle et al., 1994; McDougle, 1997). Consequently, studies on the genetic predictors of the pharmacological response in this disorder should always take into account this variable as a possible confounding factor. According to the data reported by McDougle et al. (1998), the *l* variant of the 5-HTTLPR was significantly associated with a lack of response to SSRIs in OCD patients either with or without comorbid tic disorders. This suggests that the predictive role of the gene for the effect of the antiobsessional compounds is independent of the presence of one of the traits that usually confer pharmacological resistance in OCD. However, many other phenotypes alternative to the diagnosis of OCD (e.g., presence/absence of poor insight, specific symptom subtypes) could have accounted for the association found in this study and may be primarily related to the gene effect detected.

Finally, these studies (Billet et al., 1997; McDougle et al., 1998), despite having investigated a critical issue in the clinical management of OCD and having tried to identify stable (i.e., genetic) predictors of the treatment outcome, both present the limitation of having considered as homogeneous a category that may be not homogeneous. There is growing evidence that OCD is a heterogeneous diagnosis, including patients with different genetic susceptibilities, clinical characteristics, and different response to medication (McDougle, 1997; Alsobrook et al., 1999; Nestadt et al., 2000). These differences should be taken into account and stratified as possible confounding factors in determining genetic predictors of the antiobsessional response. To investigate this issue further, studies considering more homogeneous subgroups of OCD patients are warranted.

The serotonin transporter gene and antidepressant response

In the first controlled study published of *SLC6A4* and mood disorders, patients with major depression and with at least one copy of the *l* variant appeared to show a better response to the SSRI fluvoxamine than patients with the *s* variant only (Smeraldi et al., 1998). The investigation of another sample of patients with major depression and treated with paroxetine showed the same association between the *l* variant of the 5-HTTLPR and the antidepressant response (Zanardi et al., 2000). A similar result was reported in the paper by Pollock et al. (2000), where patients treated with paroxetine showed an association between the *l* variant of the polymorphism and antidepressant response. In the same study, an independent group of patients treated with the noradrenergic antidepressant nortriptyline showed no association with the variants of 5-HTTLPR, suggesting the specificity of this marker in predicting the response to serotonergic compounds. (See also Ch. 12.)

Similar results were obtained investigating a sample of depressed patients with bipolar disorder (BP) who underwent one night of total sleep deprivation. The mechanism of action of total sleep deprivation is still unclear, but there is evidence for a specific role of the 5-HT system (Smeraldi et al., 1999). In the study of Benedetti et al. (1999) the 5-HTTLPR was investigated as a genetic predictor of the antidepressant response to one night of total sleep deprivation. Patients homozygous for the *l* variant showed a better improvement of mood ratings than patients heterozygous or homozygous for the *s* allele.

However, in a recent report by Kim et al. (2000), a significant association was revealed between either homozygosity for the *Stin2.12* allele of the VNTR or homozygosity for the *s* allele of the 5-HTTLPR and the response to SSRIs. In particular, the absence of the *Stin2.12* allele was the most powerful predictor of nonresponse to treatment.

At present, the significance of these findings and the relationships between the variants of the 5-HTTLPR and antidepressant response remain unclear. It has been commented (Kelsoe, 1998) that subjects homozygous for the *s* variant have a lower number of 5-HTT sites and, thus, have higher 5-HT levels in the synaptic cleft. This situation induces a higher inhibition of 5-HT firing and release by 5-HT presynaptic autoreceptors, with the final result being a reduction of overall serotonergic neurotransmission, which in turn predisposes to a poorer response to SSRIs. This hypothesis is apparently confirmed by the evidence that patients treated with adjuvant pindolol (a selective blocker of the 5-HT$_{1A}$ autoreceptors) show no association between the antidepressant response to SSRIs and either of the 5-HTTLPR variants (Smeraldi et al., 1998; see also Ch. 12).

The rationale of administering pindolol together with SSRIs as an adjuvant treatment for major depression is rooted in both the mechanism of action of SSRIs and in the complex regulation mechanisms of 5-HT neurotransmission (Artigas et al., 1994; Blier and de Montigny, 1998). The administration of SSRIs induces, within hours, blockade of the 5-HTT and, as a consequence, increased availability of 5-HT in the synaptic cleft. This happens after the first administration of the compounds, with a latency that mostly depends on the time of absorption of the different SSRIs. The increased availability of 5-HT stimulates the presynaptic autoreceptors (5-HT$_{1A}$), which, as a compensatory mechanism to maintain homeostasis, reduce the firing of the 5-HT neurons, decreasing 5-HT transmission. This is one of the explanatory hypotheses of the 3–4 week latency of the clinical response to antidepressant compounds, the time needed for the appropriate downregulation of the 5-HT$_{1A}$ autoreceptors, which has been found to be shortened by the addition of pindolol (Artigas et al., 1994; Zanardi et al., 1998). However, the fact that *l/l*, *l/s*, and *ss* subjects who are given pindolol in addition to fluvoxamine respond in the same way regardless their genotype (Smeraldi et al., 1998) partially contradicts the explanatory hypothesis of the association between the *l/l* genotype and the response to SSRIs discussed above. In fact, if the presence of the *l* variant of the 5-HTTLPR, which implies a higher reuptake of 5-HT, was truly associated with a lower inhibition of the 5-HT$_{1A}$ presynaptic autoreceptors, the addition of pindolol to these subjects should result in a better and much faster response to SSRIs. Moreover, the situation appears to be even more controversial considering the recent report by Kim et al. (2000), which associates a good response to SSRIs alone with the *s/s* genotype instead of the *l/l* one. The fact that Kim et al. (2000) used an Asian population may have contributed to the discrepant results.

A critical review of these studies (Table 13.1) suggests that the involvement of genes other than *SLC6A4* in determining the variability of the effects of SSRIs is quite likely.

As for all complex phenotypes, it is likely that several genes interact to confer susceptibility to the antidepressant response, in a system in which each gene has a small effect. Consequently, the investigation of single candidates is unlikely to give unequivocal and definitive results. Statistical methods of modeling the way in which several genes may interact to determine the susceptibility to the response to pharmacological compounds are now being developed (Macciardi et al., 1999; see also Ch. 5). In this modeling the interaction of genes (e.g., additive, multiplicative) in influencing a given phenotype can be detected for both qualitative and quantitative traits.

Given the fundamental role of dendritic autoreceptors in determining the latency and the quality of the clinical response to pro-serotonergic drugs in mood disorders (Blier and de Montigny, 1998), the investigation of variants of the gene *5-HT1A* together with the variants of *SLC6A4* in patients who are responder or nonresponder to medication and tests of gene–gene interaction models appear to be the most appropriate strategies to deal with the complexity of the pharmacogenetics of antidepressant response. It should be also considered that several methodological issues might have contributed to the failure to obtain unequivocal results in studies carried out so far. All these investigations have examined the role of *SLC6A4* in predicting the phenotype of antidepressant response. However, several sources of heterogeneity, as well as interesting alternative phenotypes to the diagnosis, have not been controlled. First, the antidepressant response has been evaluated in different diagnostic groups, BP, unipolar disorder (UP), or both. The diagnostic category "major depression" includes different subgroups of patients with different clinical characteristics and biological substrata, which possibly implies different genetic susceptibilities. Second, some aspects of this heterogeneity appear to be critical in influencing the response to treatment. For instance, the presence of "atypical features" (McGrath et al., 2000), psychotic symptoms (Schatzberg and Rothshild, 1992; Coryell, 1998), "rapid cycling" course (Fujiwara et al., 1998), and some temperamental factors (Tome et al., 1997) have been found to confer different degrees of resistance to the antidepressant treatment. As a consequence, these are phenotypes alternative to, but strictly related to, the principal diagnosis and they should be considered independently when studying the possible genetic predictors of the antidepressant response.

Finally, in the different studies reviewed here, the response to antidepressants has been defined variably (e.g., with hetero- and self-administered ratings), and this also prevents an adequate integration of the different results. The variability in the definition of the phenotypes as well as in the methods of rating is very likely to have added complexity to a trait that is already intrinsically complex, and this is likely to be reflected in controversial results.

The genetic prediction of antidepressant response using alternative phenotypes

The methodological accuracy of molecular genetic studies for the prediction of response to antidepressants is largely dependent upon the complexity and the heterogeneity of the phenotype studied. As already discussed, the response to antidepressants implies several concurrent sources of complexity and variability. These include the genetic and biological heterogeneity observed across different diagnoses and within the same diagnostic category, and the variability of environmental factors that influence both the clinical features of the illness and the response to the medication. The best way to approach the problem of the complexity of phenotypes in pharmacogenetic studies on psychotropic drugs is to select simpler phenotypes, qualitatively defined as present/absent, for which the causal relationship with the drug is clearly detectable and for which the correlation genotype–phenotype could be more clear-cut. The occurrence of side effects (or nondesirable reactions) represents one such strategy, and it appears also to be relevant from a clinical perspective. Given that side effects are complex phenotypes, the investigation of more than one marker and the incorporation of nongenetic factors is advisable. This strategy of including more than one genetic predictor together with nongenetic variables in modeling the prediction of developing side effects from psychotropic medication has been already used successfully in the investigation of the genetic predictors of tardive dyskinesia in long-term neuroleptic-treated patients (Basile et al., 1999, 2000).

Antidepressant-induced mania and the predictive role of serotonin system genes

Epidemiological and clinical features of antidepressant-induced mania

The induction of mania during antidepressant treatment is not a rare phenomenon. It has been described to occur with different frequencies in patients with BP, UP, and OCD (Wehr and Goodwin, 1987; Solomon et al., 1990; Vieta and Bernardo, 1992; Mundo et al., 1993; Altshuler et al., 1995; Boerlin et al., 1998). In the past, the frequency of induction of mania during antidepressant treatment has been estimated to be 9.5–33%, varying across different mood disorder diagnostic categories (i.e., UP and BP) and different antidepressant treatments (Bunney, 1978; Lewis and Winkour, 1982). However, the phenomenon of antidepressant-induced mania appears to be strictly related to a diagnosis of BP, and in these patients the switch rate during antidepressant treatment is definitively higher than in UP patients (Angst, 1985). Therefore, in the 1990s, the rate of manic switches has been estimated separately for UP and BP patients, and researchers have been primarily focusing on the occurrence of the phenomenon in BP.

According to the report of Stoll et al. (1994) antidepressant-induced manic/hypomanic episodes appear to be clinically different from the spontaneous ones, usually having a shorter duration and less severe psychotic symptoms. Whether the type of antidepressant treatment can influence the risk of mood switches remains controversial. According to Solomon et al. (1990), a manic switch during antidepressant treatment occurs in approximately 20% of the inpatient admissions with a diagnosis of BP regardless of treatment status (TCAs, MAOIs, or electroconvulsive therapy). Other reports, however, show lower rates of antidepressant-induced manic switches in BP patients treated with SSRIs than in those treated with TCAs or MAOIs (Peet, 1994; Boerlin et al., 1998).

The impact of the occurrence of antidepressant-induced manic switches on the natural course and on the clinical management of BP is quite high (Wehr and Goodwin, 1987; Goodwin and Jamison, 1990). Several studies have focused on the possible clinical predictors of this phenomenon, and to-date, a higher number of previous manic or hypomanic episodes appears to be the only clinical variable affecting the risk for developing induced mania during antidepressant treatment (Angst, 1985; Boerlin et al., 1998).

Pharmacogenetics of antidepressant-induced mania

The pharmacogenetics of the antidepressant response is a rather new field of interest and, to-date, there are no systematic studies that have investigated the role of 5-HT system genes in predicting the induction of mania during antidepressant treatment. However, in a recent pilot report, an interesting association between the 5-HTTLPR and the induction of manic switches during antidepressant treatment was shown (Mundo et al., 2000). In this study, two groups of unrelated patients with BP were selected. The first group comprised patients with a positive history of antidepressant-induced mania, with the following characteristics: (i) a confirmed DSM-IV (American Psychiatric Association, 1994) diagnosis of bipolar I or bipolar II disorder; (ii) at least one depressive episode treated with pro-serotonergic antidepressants (i.e., fluoxetine, fluvoxamine, paroxetine, sertraline, nefazodone, moclobemide, imipramine, or clomipramine); and (iii) at least one episode

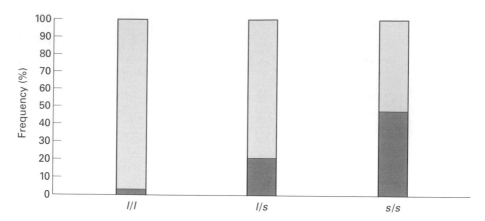

Fig. 13.1.   Frequency of genotypes (*l*, long allele; *s* short allele), for the serotonin transporter in the linked polymorphic region 5-HTTLPR in bipolar patients with (■; $n = 18$) and without (■; $n = 76$) antidepressant-induced mania. Statistical analysis: chi-square = 12.432; df 2; $p = 0.001$.

fulfilling the DSM-IV criteria for either mania or hypomania (American Psychiatric Association, 1994) developed *during* the antidepressant treatment. The second group consisted of patients with the following characteristics: (i) a confirmed diagnosis of bipolar I or bipolar II disorder; and (ii) no antidepressant-induced manic or hypomanic episodes. For all the subjects the 5-HTTLPR was genotyped under blind conditions with respect to the phenotype of occurrence of induced mania or not.

Allelic association analysis showed that among patients with antidepressant-induced mania there was an excess of the *s* allele (chi-square = 14.333; df = 1; $p = 0.0001$). The association analysis performed with the genotypes was also significant, showing a lower rate of homozygosity for the *l* variant and a higher rate of homozygosity for the *s* in the group of patients who experienced manic switches during antidepressant treatments (Fig. 13.1). More recently, these findings on the association between the 5-HTTLPR and antidepressant-induced mania have been replicated in a more controlled study including a larger group of BP subjects with a history of antidepressant-induced mania and a matched group of BP subjects who at no time experienced manic switches during treatment with pro-serotonergic compounds (Mundo et al., 2001).

Two additional genes (for the 5-HT$_{1D\beta}$ and the 5-HT$_{2A}$ receptor) have been investigated as possible predictors of the same phenotype (E. Mundo et al., unpublished data). The 5-HT$_{1D\beta}$ receptor is a terminal autoreceptor involved in the regulation of 5-HT release, and it is expressed mostly in the limbic regions and in the striatum. It is encoded by an intronless gene located on chromosome 6 (6q14–15)

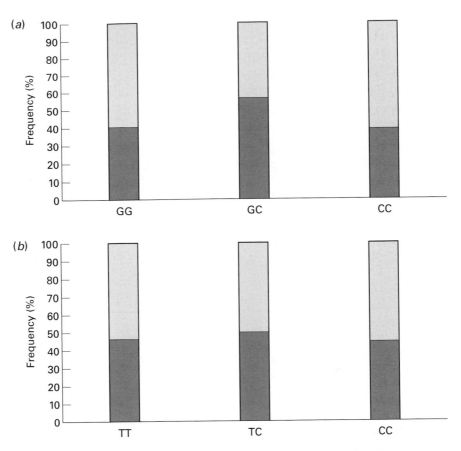

Fig. 13.2.   Genotype frequencies in bipolar patients with (■) and without (▨) antidepressant-induced mania. (*a*) G861C polymorphism (homozygotes GG and CC; heterozygote GC) of the gene for the 5-hydroxytryptamine (5-HT) 1DB receptor (*5-HT1Dβ*) (chi-square = 1.331; df 2; *p* = 0.514). (*b*) T102C polymorphisms (TT and CC homozygotes and TC heterozygote) of the gene for the 5HT2A receptor (chi-square = 0.115; df, 2; *p* = 0.925).

(Demchyshyn et al., 1992). The polymorphisms known for this gene are G861C, T−261G, and T371G (Nöthen et al., 1994; Lappalainen et al., 1995). 5-*HT2A* is located on chromosome 13q14–21 and its variants have been investigated as candidates in mood disorders, with mixed results (Gutierrez et al., 1995; Zhang et al., 1997; Enoch et al., 1999; Vincent et al., 1999).

In the sample of patients with antidepressant-induced mania described above and in a matched group of BP patients who never experienced manic or hypomanic episodes during antidepressant treatment with pro-serotonergic compounds, the G861C polymorphism of *5-HT1Dβ* and the T102C polymorphism of *5-HT2A* (Warren et al., 1993) were studied. No allelic or genotypic association (Fig. 13.2) was found with either of the two variants tested. These additional loci, which did not associate with the occurrence of antidepressant-induced mania, appear to confer specificity to the role of 5-HTTLPR in predicting this phenotype. One of the possible hypotheses to explain this specific finding is based on the functional characteristics of the polymorphism. According to the data reported by Lesch et al. (1996), subjects homozygous for the *s* variant have a lower gene expression and, thus, should have fewer 5-HTT sites. This could imply a higher sensitivity to either the block of 5-HT reuptake or the increase of 5-HT availability. Both these effects are commonly induced by the administration of pro-serotonergic compounds that directly or indirectly act on 5-HT neurotransmission (Blier and de Montigny, 1998).

However, if this hypothesis is true, patients with the *s/s* genotype should be more likely either to respond to pro-serotonergic antidepressants or to show a shorter latency for the response itself. As discussed in the previous section, most of the studies investigating the role of 5-HTTLPR in predicting the response to SSRIs have found a significant association between the antidepressant effect of these drugs and the *l* variant of the polymorphism, and not with the *s*. Further studies are needed to address the complexity of the biological mechanisms underlying the antidepressant response (Kelsoe, 1998). However, from the data here presented, we can reasonably hypothesize that the normal clinical response (i.e., the remission of depressive symptoms with return to euthymia) and the "abnormal" response (i.e., the induction of manic switches) to antidepressant medication are different phenomena, implying different biological mechanisms and different genetic susceptibilities.

The identification of specific predictors of these two phenotypes will lead to a substantial improvement in the understanding of the complex biological mechanisms that underlie the desirable and the nondesirable clinical effects of antidepressant compounds. Important information on the pathophysiology of depression and mania will be derived from a better understanding of the mechanism of action of antidepressants; moreover, such knowledge will contribute to the design of more specific, and thus more efficient, therapeutic strategies.

Conclusions

During the 1990s, there was a significant advance in understanding of the mechanism of action of antidepressants and the pathophysiology of the diseases successfully treated with these drugs. However, the identification of stable (i.e., genetic) predictors of treatment outcome, on which ideal pharmacological strategies for the clinical management of mood and anxiety disorders could be based, remains a difficult task. The heterogeneity of the definition of the phenotype "antidepressant response," the different meaning and clinical expression related to it across the different diagnoses and within the same diagnostic category, the complexity of the biological mechanisms involved in the clinical response itself, and the interaction between environmental and genetic factors in determining it, all prevent the possibility of observing a clear and unequivocal correlation between genotype and phenotype in pharmacogenetic studies. For these reasons it may be helpful to use simpler and more homogeneous alternative phenotypes (e.g., nondesirable side effects) and statistical genetic strategies that allow the modeling of complex interactions among different genes and between genetic and nongenetic factors. The utility of pharmacological tools in identifying biological heterogeneity and, thus, alternative phenotypes in complex disorders has been underlined recently by several studies conducted in mood and anxiety disorders. The future of pharmacogenetic studies oriented towards the identification of stable predictors of the response to antidepressants should follow the same direction, combining clinical pharmacological and genetic approaches. This strategy will be quite valuable to understand the biological basis of the heterogeneous effects of the different antidepressant compounds and the biological basis of psychiatric disorders and adverse reactions to medication, with the consequence of major improvements in the treatment and in the long-term outcome of these disorders.

REFERENCES

American Psychiatric Association (1994). *Diagnostic and Statistical Manual of Mental Disorders*, 4th edn. Washington, DC: American Psychiatric Association.

Alsobrook JP II, Leckman JF, Goodman WK, Rasmussen SA, Pauls DL (1999). Segregation analysis of obsessive-compulsive disorder using symptom-based factor scores. *Am J Med Genet* 88, 669–675.

Altshuler LL, Post RM, Leverich GS, Mikalauskas K, Rosoff A, Ackerman L (1995). Antidepressant-induced mania and cycle acceleration: a controversy revisited. *Am J Psychiatry* 152, 1130–1138.

Angst J (1985). Switch from depression to mania – a record survey over decades between 1920 and 1982. *Psychopathology* 18, 140–154.

Artigas F, Perez V, Alvarez E (1994). Pindolol induces a rapid improvement of depressed patients treated with serotonin reuptake inhibitors. *Arch Gen Psychiatry* 51, 248–251.

Basile VS, Masellis M, Badri F et al. (1999). Association of the *MscI* polymorphism of the dopamine D_3 receptor gene with tardive dyskinesia in schizophrenia. *Neuropsychopharmacology* 21, 17–27.

Basile VS, Ozdemir V, Masellis M et al. (2000). A functional polymorphism of the cytochrome P-450 *1A2* (*CYP1A2*) gene: association with tardive dyskinesia in schizophrenia. *Mol Psychiatry* 5, 410–417.

Benedetti F, Serretti A, Colombo C et al. (1999). Influence of a functional polymorphism within the promoter of the serotonin transporter gene on the effects of total sleep deprivation in bipolar depression. *Am J Psychiatry* 156, 1450–1452.

Billett EA, Richter MA, King N, Heils A, Lesch KP, Kennedy JL (1997). Obsessive-compulsive disorder, response to serotonin reuptake inhibitors and the serotonin transporter gene. *Mol Psychiatry* 2, 403–406.

Blier P, de Montigny C (1998). Possible serotonergic mechanisms underlying the antidepressant and the anti-obsessive-compulsive disorder responses. *Biol Psychiatry* 44, 313–323.

Boerlin HL, Gitlin MJ, Zoellner LA, Hammen CL (1998). Bipolar depression and antidepressant-induced mania: a naturalistic study. *J Clin Psychiatry* 59, 374–379.

Bunney WE (1978). Psychopharmacology of the switch process in affective process. In Lipton MA, Damascio A, Kellam KF, eds. *Psychopharmacology: a Generation of Progress.* New York: Raven Press, pp. 1249–1259.

Collier DA, Stober G, Li T et al. (1996). A novel functional polymorphism within the promoter of the serotonin transporter gene: possible role in susceptibility to affective disorders. *Mol Psychiatry* 1, 453–460.

Coryell W (1998). The treatment of psychotic depression. *J Clin Psychiatry* 60, 326–335.

Demchyshyn L, Sunahara RK, Miller K et al. (1992). A human serotonin 1D receptor variant (5-HT1Dbeta) encoded by an intronless gene on chromosome 6. *Proc Natl Acad Sci USA* 89, 5522–5526.

Enoch MA, Goldman D, Barnett R, Sher L, Mazzanti CM, Rosenthal NE (1999). Association between seasonal affective disorder and the *5-HT2A* promoter polymorphism, -1438G/A. *Mol Psychiatry* 4, 89–92.

Feighner JP (1999). Overview of antidepressants currently used to treat anxiety disorders. *J Clin Psychiatry* 60(Suppl 22), 18–22.

Fujiwara Y, Honda T, Tanaka Y, Aoki S, Kuroda S (1998). Comparison of early- and late-onset rapid cycling affective disorders: clinical course and response to pharmacotherapy. *J Clin Psychopharmacol* 18, 282–288.

Goodman WK, Price LH, Rasmussen SA et al. (1989). The Yale–Brown Obsessive-Compulsive Scale (Y-BOCS): Part I. Development, use, and reliability. Arch Gen Psychiatry 46, 1006–1011.

Goodwin FK, Jamison KR (1990). *Manic Depressive Illness.* New York: Oxford University Press.

Greist JH, Jefferson JW, Kobak KA, Katzelnick DJ, Serlin RC (1995). Efficacy and tolerability of serotonin transport inhibitors in obsessive-compulsive disorder: a meta-analysis. *Arch Gen Psychiatry* 52, 53–60.

Gutierrez B, Arranz M, Fananas L et al. (1995). 5-HT$_{2A}$ receptor gene and bipolar affective disorder. *Lancet* 346, 969.

Guy W (1976). ECDEU *Assessment Manual for Psychopharmacology.* [Publication 76–338.] Washington, DC: US Department of Health, Education and Welfare.

Hanna GL, Himle GA, Curtis GC et al. (1998). Serotonin transporter and seasonal variation in blood serotonin in families with obsessive-compulsive disorder. *Neuropsychopharmacology* 18, 102–111.

Heils A, Teufel A, Petri S et al. (1996). Allelic variation of human serotonin transporter expression. *J Neurochem* 66, 2621–2624.

Hirschfeld RM, Russel JM, Delgado PL et al. (1998). Predictors of response to acute treatment of chronic and double depression with sertraline or imipramine. *J Clin Psychiatry* 59, 669–675.

Hyttel J (1994). Pharmacological characterization of selective serotonin reuptake inhibitors (SSRIs). *Int Clin Psychopharmacol* 9(Suppl 1), 19–26.

Kelsoe JR (1998). Promoter prognostication: the serotonin transporter gene and antidepressant response. *Mol Psychiatry* 3, 475–476.

Kim DK, Lim SW, Lee S et al. (2000). Serotonin transporter gene polymorphism and antidepressant response. *Neuroreport* 11, 215–219.

Lappalainen J, Dean M, Charbonneau L, Virkkunen M, Linnoila M, Goldman D (1995). Mapping of the serotonin 5-HT1D beta autoreceptor gene on chromosome 6 and direct analysis for sequence variants. *Am J Med Genet* 60, 157–161.

Lesch KP, Bengel D, Heils A et al. (1996). Association of anxiety-related traits with a polymorphism in the serotonin transporter gene regulatory region. *Science* 274, 1527–1531.

Lewis JL, Winkour G (1982). The induction of mania. *Arch Gen Psychiatry* 39, 303–306.

Macciardi F, Mundo E (1999). Power of quantitative transmission disequilibrium test in evaluating the genetic components of pharmacological response in psychiatric disorders. *Abstracts of the 8th Annual Meeting of the International Genetic Epidemiology Society*, St. Louis, MO, USA, abstract 96.

Macciardi F, Basile VS, Kennedy JL (1999). Modeling gene–gene interaction in complex traits. *A J Hum Genet* 65(Suppl 4), A210.

McDougle CJ (1997). Update on pharmacologic management of OCD: agents and augmentation. *J Clin Psychiatry* 58(Suppl 12), 11–17.

McDougle CJ, Goodman WK, Leckman J, Lee N, Heninger G, Price LH (1994). Haloperidol addition in fluvoxamine-refractory obsessive-compulsive disorder. *Arch Gen Psychiatry* 51, 302–308.

McDougle CJ, Epperson CN, Price LH, Gelernter J (1998). Evidence for linkage disequilibrium between serotonin transporter gene (*SLC6A4*) and obsessive-compulsive disorder. *Mol Psychiatry* 3, 270–273.

McGrath PJ, Stewart JW, Petkova E et al. (2000). Predictors of relapse during fluoxetine continuation or maintenance treatment of major depression. *J Clin Psychiatry* 61, 518–524.

Mundo E, Ronchi P, Bellodi L (1993). Obsessive-compulsive patients at risk for antidepressant-induced mania. *Hosp Community Psychiatry* 44, 689–690.

Mundo E, Bianchi L, Bellodi L (1997). Efficacy of fluvoxamine, paroxetine and citalopram in the treatment of obsessive-compulsive disorder: a single-blind study. *J Clin Psychopharmacol* 17, 267–271.

Mundo E, Walker M, Tims H, Macciardi FM, Kennedy JL (2000). The role of serotonin transporter gene in antidepressant-induced mania in bipolar patients. *Biol Psychiatry* 47(Suppl 8), 135S.

Mundo E, Walker M, Cate T, Macciardi F, Kennedy JL (2001). The role of serotonin transporter protein gene in antidepressant-induced mania in bipolar disorder: preliminary findings. *Arch Gen Psychiatry* 58, 539–544.

Nestadt G, Lan T, Samuels J et al. (2000). Complex segregation analysis provides compelling evidence for major gene underlying obsessive-compulsive disorder and for heterogeneity by sex. *Am J Hum Genet* 67, 1611–1616.

Nötham MM, Erdmann J, Shimron-Abarbanell D, Propping P (1994). Identification of a genetic variation in the human serotonin 1D beta receptor gene. *Biochem Biophys Res Commun* 205, 1194–1200.

Ogilvie AD, Battersby S, Bubb VJ et al. (1995). Polymorphism in serotonin transporter gene associated with susceptibility to major depression. *Lancet* 347, 731–733.

Peet M (1994). Induction of mania with selective serotonin reuptake inhibitors and tricyclic antidepressants. *Br J Psychiatry* 164, 549–550.

Pollock BG, Ferrell RE, Mulsant BH et al. (2000). Allelic variation in the serotonin transporter promoter affects onset of paroxetine treatment response in late-life depression. *Neuropsychopharmacology* 23, 587–590.

Potter WZ (1998). Bipolar depression: specific treatments. *J Clin Psychiatry* 59(Suppl): 18, 30–36.

Risch N, Merikangas K (1996). The future of genetic studies on complex human diseases. *Science* 273, 1516–1517.

Schatzberg AF, Rothshild AJ (1992). Psychotic (delusional) major depression: should it be included as a distinct syndrome in DSM-IV? *Am J Psychiatry* 49, 733–745.

Smeraldi E, Zanardi R, Benedetti F, Di Bella D, Perez J, Catalano M (1998). Polymorphism within the promoter of the serotonin transporter gene and antidepressant efficacy of fluvoxamine. *Mol Psychiatry* 3, 508–511.

Smeraldi E, Benedetti F, Barbini B, Campori E, Colombo C (1999). Sustained antidepressant effect of sleep deprivation combined with pindolol in bipolar depression: a placebo-controlled trial. *Neuropsychopharmacology* 20, 380–385.

Solomon R, Rich CL, Darko DF (1990). Antidepressant treatment and occurrence of mania in bipolar patients admitted for depression. *J Affect Disord* 18, 253–257.

Stoll Al, Mayer PV, Kolbrener M et al. (1994). Antidepressant-associated mania: a controlled comparison with spontaneous mania. *Am J Psychiatry* 151, 1642–1645.

Tome MB, Cloninger CR, Watson JP, Isaac MT (1997). Serotonergic autoreceptor blockade in the reduction of antidepressant latency: personality variables and response to paroxetine and pindolol. *J Affect Disord* 44, 101–109.

Vieta E, Bernardo M (1992). Antidepressant-induced mania in obsessive-compulsive disorder. *Am J Psychiatry* 149, 1282–1283.

Vincent JB, Masellis M, Lawrence J et al. (1999). Genetic association analysis of serotonin system genes in bipolar affective disorder. *Am J Psychiatry* 156, 136–138.

Warren JT Jr., Peacock ML, Rodriguez LC, Fink JK (1993). An *MspI* polymorphism in the human serotonin receptor gene (*HTR2*): detection by DDGE and RFLP analysis. *Hum Mol Genet* 2, 338.

Wehr TA, Goodwin FK (1987). Can antidepressants cause mania and worsen the course of affective illness? *Am J Psychiatry* 144, 1403–1411.

Zanardi R, Franchini L, Gasperini M, Lucca A, Smeraldi E, Perez J (1998). Faster onset of action of fluvoxamine in combination with pindolol in the treatment of delusional depression: a controlled study. *J Clin Psychopharmacol* 18, 441–446.

Zanardi R, Benedetti F, Di Bella D, Catalano M, Smeraldi E (2000). Efficacy of paroxetine in depression is influenced by a functional polymorphism within the promoter of the serotonin transporter gene. *J Clin Psychopharmacol* 20, 105–107.

Zhang HY, Ishigaki T, Tani K et al. (1997). Serotonin 2A receptor gene polymorphism in mood disorders. *Biol Psychiatry* 41, 768–773.

Zohar J, Westenberg HG (2000). Anxiety disorders: a review of tricyclic antidepressants and selective serotonin reuptake inhibitors. *Acta Psychiatr Scand* 403, 39–49.

14

Pharmacogenetics of anxiolytic drugs and the GABA–benzodiazepine receptor complex

Smita A. Pandit, Spilios V. Argyropoulos, Patrick G. Kehoe, and David J. Nutt

Psychopharmacology Unit, School of Medical Sciences, Bristol, UK

OVERVIEW

The benzodiazepines (BDZ) have proven to be both effective and controversial in the treatment of anxiety. Whilst giving rapid relief of anxiety, they have undesirable characteristics, such as the development of tolerance, dependence, withdrawal symptoms, and alcohol potentiation. New insights into the genetics of the BD2 receptor system may lead to the development of new drugs that act on the γ-aminobutyric acid (GABA) receptor complex and are devoid of the problems associated with the classical BDZs. This pharmacotherapeutic approach has gathered impetus following the discovery of the various subunits of the GABA receptor, which are thought to play an important role in the regulation of anxiety and the actions of anxiolytics, and which demonstrate differential brain expression. There are a number of genetic variations in the GABA-A receptor and its subunits that can have an effect on the pharmacology of anxiolytic drugs. The various permutations of the subunits in the composition of these receptors impact on the activity and efficacy of these drugs. A second level of complexity is introduced with the genetic variations in each of these subunits. Such variations can result in amino acid replacements, deletions or imperfect subunit construction at a protein level, thereby resulting in different receptor combinations. This chapter discusses the above with reference to recent evidence from animal and human studies, as well as the implications for future anxiolytic treatment strategies.

Introduction

Clinical anxiety is a common cause of morbidity in the general population (Weiller et al., 1998). The current classification systems of mental disorders, ICD-10 (World Health Organization, 1992) and DSM-IV (American Psychiatric Association, 1994), use a categorical/nosological approach and divide the various anxiety states into specific syndromes, the anxiety disorders. Beyond the subjective distress these syndromes may cause, the importance of the associated social and occupational malfunctioning, as well as the financial implications, have become all too evident in recent years (Rice and Miller, 1998).

Despite the undoubted success of the existing treatments for anxiety, a substantial proportion of patients fail to respond to them. Since their introduction in the 1960s, the benzodiazepines (BDZs) have been the mainstay for the treatment of anxiety. More recently the newer serotonin reuptake inhibitor (SSRI) "antidepressants" are used increasingly, and cognitive behavior therapy has become the psychological therapy of choice. The available treatments are not without their problems. Long-term use of BDZs have well-documented difficulties, such as tolerance to the therapeutic effect, potential for abuse and dependence, and discontinuation syndrome (Lader, 1999). Antidepressants are slow to act and are not devoid of side effects. Psychological therapies are not easily transferred from the research context to clinical practice and properly trained therapists are in short supply, especially in the national health services. Therefore, the quest for effective ways of treating anxiety including novel pharmacological approaches to anxiety remains as pressing as ever.

Pharmacogenetics is one of the exciting new ideas arising from the recent boom in genetic research. The emerging combination of two strands of scientific inquiry – genetics and neurochemistry – into this new discipline promises to revolutionize our ways of developing and prescribing drugs. The first aim of pharmacogenetics is to study how genetic differences between subjects influence their variability in response to drugs. Furthermore, pharmacogenetics, by means of using specific genetic profiles, aims to be able to predict individual patient's responses to a particular compound (Roses, 2000). However, unlike the pharmacogenetic studies carried out in schizophrenia with clozapine (Arranz et al., 1995), studies in anxiety disorders with anxiolytic drugs are limited in number.

The genetics that underlie anxiety disorders are of a complex nature. Pathways consist of genes and their products (i.e., proteins), each of which is subject to genetic heterogeneity. Therefore, the functioning of such pathways may be modulated by genetic variation. The most obvious example of this is the role of metabolism and its associated genetic variation in the pharmacology of anxiolytic drugs. These drugs are metabolized by the P-450 enzyme complex in the liver, which is susceptible to genetic variations. Such genetic variations can result in individuals inheriting genes that influence the rates at which they metabolize drugs and thus the bioavailability of anxiolytics can vary among these individuals. Therefore, pharmacokinetic considerations are as important as pharmacodynamic ones. They are treated separately, in more detail, in Chapter 8.

Another target for a pharmacogenetic approach in anxiety is the pharmacodynamics of anxiolytic drugs. The neurochemistry of anxiety deals mainly with monoamine (serotonin (5-HT), norepinephrine, dopamine) neurotransmission, and the GABA – BDZ receptor complex (Sandford et al., 2000). Of the existing anxiolytics, the SSRIs are thought to exert their action through the 5-HT system, and polymorphisms of the gene (*SLC6A4*) for the serotonin transporter (5-HTT) have been shown to contribute to the expression of anxiety symptoms (Evans et al., 1997). The 5-HT system is also discussed in more detail elsewhere in this book (Chs. 6, 12, and 13). Low dopamine D_2 receptor expression and dopamine reuptake site density in the striatum of patients with social phobia has been reported (Tiihonen et al., 1997; Schneier et al., 2000) and this is, in all likelihood, under genetic control.

In this chapter we will focus on developments in the GABA–BDZ receptor field of research. Recent advances in molecular and neuroimaging techniques have given us greater insight into the structure of this receptor and its properties. Most of our understanding about this receptor and the ligands which act on it is based on studies conducted in animals. Based on our current knowledge of this receptor, future studies can be conducted in humans, focusing on the development of new drugs that could pave the way towards effective treatment of anxiety.

GABA, benzodiazepines, and anxiety

GABA is the main inhibitory neurotransmitter in the central nervous system. Depending on the brain region, 20–50% of all central synapses utilize GABA as their transmitter. Three types of GABA receptor have been identified, but most of the GABA activity in the brain involves the fast-signaling, ligand-gated GABA-A receptors, of which the BDZ site is an integral part. Inhibition of the GABAergic system results in enhanced alertness, reduced sleep, anxiety, restlessness and exaggerated reactions, even to harmless stimuli (Nutt and Malizia, 2001).

The mechanism of action of the BDZs was only discovered in the 1970s. It was shown that there was a highly specific potentiation of GABA by BDZs (Mohler and Okada, 1977; Squires and Braestrup, 1977). In the decade that followed, the binding site for BDZs in the brain, later shown to be a part of the GABA-A receptor complex, was discovered (Hafely, 1978), and the GABA-A receptor complex itself was isolated and sequenced (Schofield et al., 1987). The receptor complex was finally visualized by electron microscopy (Nayeem et al., 1994).

The GABA-A receptor is a protein complex made up of five protein subunits (Tallman and Gallager, 1985; Sieghart, 1989; Nayeem et al., 1994). The subunits are arranged like a rosette around a central pore that spans the cell membrane. When GABA binds with the receptor, there is a conformational change of the complex. This results in the opening of the central pore, a net influx to the cell of chloride ions, hyperpolarization of the cell, and inhibition of the excitability of the cell membrane. Other compounds such as barbiturates, anesthetics, alcohol, and

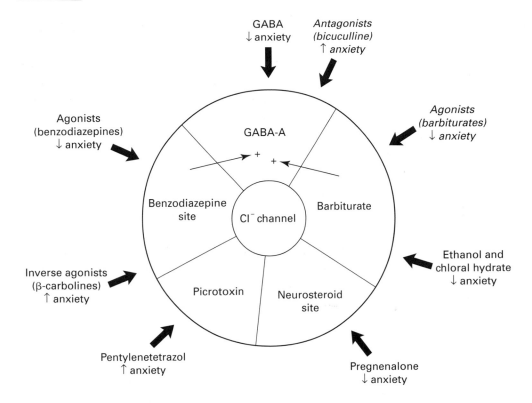

Fig. 14.1.   The γ-aminobutyric acid (GABA)–benzodiazepine receptor chloride ionophore complex.

neurosteroids also bind to the complex and directly open the chloride channels (Nutt and Malizia, 2001) (Fig. 14.1). BDZs, however, act by allosteric modulation of the GABA-A recognition site, thereby augmenting or diminishing its inhibitory effects without directly opening the chloride channel. This action of BDZs results in their distinct advantage over other drugs like barbiturates, chloral hydrate, and clormethiazole, all of which can, in high concentrations, cause sustained tonic opening of chloride ion channels, which in an overdose can result in respiratory depression and death.

Molecular biology of the GABA-A receptor

Molecular cloning studies have shown that the five subunits making up the GABA-A receptor are assembled from a family of at least 17 subunits. Each subunit is encoded by a different gene in mammals, and the complementary DNA (CDNA) and amino acid sequences have been characterized at a molecular level (Doble, 1999). Seven classes of subunit, with multiple isoforms, have been identified by their sequence homology (α_{1-6}, β_{1-3}, γ_{1-3}, δ, ε, π, $\rho_{1,2}$) (Fritschy and Mohler, 1995;

Mehta and Ticku, 1999; Whiting, 1999). Each subunit consists of four transmembrane domains; a long N-terminal exocytic domain with various glycosylation sites and to which ligands probably bind (Cockroft et al., 1990), a short C-terminal exocytic chain, and a intracellular loop susceptible to protein kinases. Amino acid sequence homology varies between different subunits from 30% to as much as 70% if they are of the same class.

In situ hybridization histochemistry experiments have shown that there is a variable distribution of GABA-A receptor subunits and that they can be quantified by the distribution of their mRNAs (Zhang et al., 1991a, b; Persohn et al., 1992; Wisden et al., 1992). For example, while α_1- and α_6-subunits are present predominantly in the cerebellum the α_5-subunit appears to be present only in the hippocampus, although in lower concentrations than the α_1- and α_2-subunits. The cerebral cortex has intermediate levels of α_{1-4}-subunits and low levels of α_5-subunit. The expression of the β-subunits is weaker in the substantia nigra (Sieghart et al., 1987; Sequier et al., 1988; Luddens et al., 1990; McLennan et al., 1991; Malizia and Nutt, 1995). Of the γ-subunits, the γ_1-subunit mRNA is predominantly expressed in the amygdala and septum and is probably the only one with this kind of distribution. The γ_2-subunit, however, is present in abundance in almost every region of the brain while the γ_3-subunit is present in the cortex and the basal nuclei (Ymer et al., 1990; Wisden et al., 1992; Wang et al., 1998).

Immunoprecipitation studies have shown that the most commonly found subunits in the brain are α_1, β_2, and γ_2 and these are present in 60–70% of GABA-A receptors (Benke et al., 1991a, 1994; Duggan et al., 1992; Ruano et al., 1994), while α_2-, α_3-, α_5-, β_3-, and δ-subunits are moderately present, each being found in 15–30% of GABA-A receptors (Duggan and Stephenson, 1990; Benke et al., 1991b, 1994; McKernan et al., 1991; Endo and Olsen, 1993; Marksitzer et al., 1993; Mertens et al., 1993). From the remaining subunits (i.e., α_4, α_6, β_1, γ_1 and γ_3), each is represented in only about 10% of GABA-A receptors (Fritschy et al., 1993; Quirk et al., 1994; Togel et al., 1994). The majority of GABA-A receptors contain at least one α_1-subunit variant along with β_2-, β_3- and γ_2-subunits (Fritschy and Mohler, 1995); the commonest permutation being $\alpha_1\beta_2\gamma_2$, which is found in 67% of receptors (Fritschy et al., 1992). Interestingly, the genes encoding for this particular combination of subunits are themselves located as a cluster of genes, all on chromosome 5 in humans and on chromosome 11 in mouse (Table 14.1). This begged the question whether there are certain proteins that preferentially help cluster specific subunits together? The proteins rapsyn (Yang et al., 1997) and gephrin (Essrich et al., 1998) were found to cluster some but not all GABA-A receptors. The amino acid sequence on subunits mediating clustering by rapsyn may be used in future to isolate proteins responsible for clustering of native receptors in the brain (Kardos, 1999). This also opens up new ways to look at the postsynaptic receptor structures

Table 14.1. Chromosomal localization of the genes that encode the various subunits of the α-aminobutyric acid GABA-A receptor in humans

Subunit	Human chromosome
α_1	5q32–5q33
α_2	4p13–4q11
α_3	Xq28
α_4	4p13–4q11
α_5	15q11–15q13
α_6	5q32–5q33
β_1	4p13–4q11
β_2	5q32–5q33
β_3	15q11–15q13
γ_1	4p13–4q11
γ_2	5q32–5q33
γ_3	15q11–15q13

Source: Adapted with permission from Doble, 1999.

that might use a single clustering protein and to construct different inhibitory and/or excitatory neurotransmitter-gated ion channels enabling the postsynaptic membrane to receive signals from different neurotransmitters (Jonas et al., 1998; Nicoll and Malenka, 1998; Kardos, 1999).

However, gene clustering is not the only factor that controls the assembly of the subunits in a specific receptor. For example, even though α_1- and α_6-subunits are colocalized in the same gene cluster on chromosome 5, the α_6-subunit is only expressed in the cerebellum while the α_1-subunit is present throughout the CNS. Therefore, there is some level of control on gene expression (Fritschy and Mohler, 1995), which suggests that the expression of GABA-A receptors may change in response to physiological or pathophysiological stimuli. This is supported by evidence that there is an alteration in GABA-A receptor expression in response to behavioral or pharmacological challenges such as stress, chronic alcohol administration, or visual deprivation (Mhatre et al., 1993; Huntsman et al., 1994; Mhatre and Ticku, 1994). This also opens up an interesting area for further research into the etiology of anxiety disorders and, more specifically, personality factors associated with the development of anxiety disorders. The expression of the various subunits may be affected by chronic administration of BDZs, thus leading to the phenomenon of dependence and tolerance. In generalized anxiety disorder, there is a tolerance of the sedative effect without the development of tolerance to the anxiolytic effect (Doble and Martin, 1996) and this could be a result of the differential expression of the subunits in different areas of the brain during chronic treatment with BDZs.

Putative functions of the GABA-A receptor subunits

GABA binds to the β-subunit. The BDZ site is localized at the interface of the α- and γ-subunits of the GABA-A receptor (Wong et al., 1992; Zezula et al., 1996), however, when hypnotics like zaleplon, zopiclone, and zolpidem and anxiolytic and anticonvulsant BDZs (as well as BDZ antagonists and inverse agonists) bind to the receptor, the actual binding is at the α-subunit (Sieghart, 1995; Johnstone, 1996). The α-subunit is essential to allow classical BZDs to bind to the receptor, but it is the γ_2-variant that has an influence on their pharmacological profiles (Pritchet et al., 1989a; Angelotti and MacDonald, 1993). However, when the γ_1- and γ_3- subunits are present, they result in receptors that have a low affinity for BDZs. GABA-gated chloride conductance is more enhanced when at least one α- and one β-subunit are present (Siegel et al., 1990; Verdoorn et al., 1990).

The functional properties of the receptors, including their sensitivity for GABA, degree of rectification and rate of desensitization, vary with the subunit combinations (Pritchett et al., 1989b; Saxena and MacDonald 1994; Verdoorn, 1994; Fritschy and Mohler, 1995). Thus different subtypes of GABA-A receptors have different sensitivities to BDZ receptor ligands (Doble, 1999). Initial attempts to classify GABA-A/BDZ receptors suggested the presence of two different types of receptor: type I receptors, which are present mainly in the cerebellum and are formed by the coexpression of α_1-, $\beta_{1,3}$-, and γ_2-subunits, and type II receptors, which are present mainly in the cortical structures and are formed by the coexpression of $\alpha_{2,3,5}$-, $\beta_{1,3}$-, and γ_2-subunits (Pritchett et al., 1989b). The receptors carrying an α_4-subunit have low affinity for classical BDZs like diazepam, while those carrying α_2- and β_3-subunits have a higher affinity for zolpidem. The α_6-subunit-containing receptor, which is exclusively expressed in cerebellar granule cells, is insensitive to all hypnotic drugs except Ro-154513 (Luddens et al., 1990; Pritchett and Seeburg, 1990; Wisden et al., 1991).

Smith et al. (1998) were able to show that the blockade of the GABA-A receptor α_4-subunit gene transcript prevented withdrawal properties of the endogenous neuroactive steroid allopregnanolone, which caused an increased susceptibility to seizures. Increased expression of α_4-subunit was seen in the hippocampus and cerebral cortex after chronic ethanol consumption in rats (Mathews et al., 1998). An understanding of the physiological role of the subunits and the changes in the expression of receptors in pathological conditions will determine which subunit-selective drugs may be developed to treat certain conditions (Kardos, 1999; Whiting, 1999).

Identification of the role of GABA-A subunits in anxiety, through molecular manipulation

Several approaches, including gene knockout (gene deletion) and gene knockin (gene mutation), have been used to try to establish the role of various subunits and the resulting receptor variants (Mehta and Ticku, 1999). Experiments with knock-out mice involve the prevention of expression of specific subunit genes in order to produce GABA-A receptors that are deficient in specific subunits. One of the first such experiments involved the gene for the γ_2-subunit (Gunther et al., 1995). Homozygous γ_2-subunit knockout mice, with both alleles knocked-out, were found to be not viable. By comparison, heterozygotes, with one active allele of the gene, survived to adulthood and bred. Interestingly, the GABA-A–BDZ receptors in these heterozygotes have only half the usual complement of γ_2-subunits and are less sensitive to BDZs like flunitrazepam and diazepam. The mice also exhibited symptoms of hypervigilance and anxiety. Therefore, this approach produces a system that can be seen as a genetically defined model of trait anxiety which reproduces molecular, pharmacological, and behavioral features akin to human anxiety disorders (Nutt and Malizia, 2001). Further, these mice exhibited decreased flumazenil binding throughout the brain, which was similar to the decreases shown in flumazenil binding found in panic disorder in humans (Malizia et al., 1998; Crestani et al., 1999). These findings also suggest that the GABA-A receptor dysfunction could be a causative factor for heightened harm avoidance behavior and a hypersensitivity to negative associations in patients (Crestani et al., 1999).

The knockout technique has been used to produce mice deficient in other types of subunit as well. When the gene for the β_3-subunit is knocked out, hyperactive mice demonstrating poor coordination, abnormal reflexes, and spontaneous seizures are produced (Homanics et al., 1997). The receptors in these mice have an attenuated response to GABA. Their pharmacological response to loreclazole indicate that the β_3-subunit has been replaced by a β_2-subunit (Krasowski et al., 1998). Reduced sensitivity to anesthetic agents, like halothane and midazolam, was also observed, thus linking these receptors with the effects of these drugs.

Knocking out the gene encoding the α_6-subunit produces mice that appear normal. However, there is a complete absence of BDZ-insensitive GABA-A receptors in the cerebellum. It also suppresses the expression of δ-subunit. The α_6-subunit was earlier implicated in the mediation of some of the CNS-depressant effects of alcohol (Ticku et al., 1988; Luddens et al., 1990). However, subsequent research has shown that the deletion of the α_6-encoding gene does not lead to any changes in sensitivity to alcohol in animals, nor does it have a role to play in the development of alcohol tolerance (Homanics et al., 1998). Despite the above, it has recently been reported that male children of male alcoholics have an increased likelihood of possessing a genetic variant of the α_6-subunit, which may explain their inherited subsensitivity to alcohol and BDZs (Schukit et al., 1999). Recent studies have shown that RO-154513 is a good ligand for characterization of α_6-containing-receptors in rats and humans by positron emission tomography (Feeney et al., 2000). The use of neuroimaging techniques can thus assist in delineating the role of subunits in humans.

More recently, the knockin technique has been used to produce mice where the α_1-subunit, following mutation, has become insensitive to BDZs but is still responsive to GABA (see next section). This results in the abolition of the sedative actions of BDZs, with preservation of the anxiolytic and anticonvulsant properties (Rudolph et al., 1999). Subsequent mutation of the two remaining α-subunits has shown that the anxiolytic effect is also lost if the α_2- but not the α_3-subunit is mutated (Low et al., 2000). The α_2-subunit is mainly localized to the limbic system. Therefore, the above finding further supports the role of this circuit in anxiety. The growing evidence for the specificity of the various BDZ actions being mediated via different receptor subtypes/subunit clusters is currently driving research into subunit-selective drugs, such as α_2- or α_3-agonists, as nonsedating anxiolytics and α_5 inverse agonists (which act mainly in the hippocampus) as memory enhancers.

Studies of mutation of individual amino acids

Although BDZs bind to the α-subunit, photoaffinity labeling experiments led to the hypothesis that this site may carry different binding domains for different chemical classes of drug (Mohler et al., 1980; Mohler, 1982). Other experiments evaluated the effect of treatment of GABA-A receptors with chemical reagents that would irreversibly modify particular amino acid groups on the receptor surface, and the residue histidine in the binding domain of the BDZs was incriminated (Doble et al., 1992). Based on this, a map of the GABA-A receptor surface with a pocket containing an histidyl group was proposed (Doble et al., 1995). In this model, it is proposed that the BDZs bind to the bottom of the pocket whereas zopiclone, as well as other cyclopyrrolones and probably flumazenil, bind to the rim of the pocket. If drugs bind to different domains on the receptor surface, this may have consequences for the different sorts of conformational change that the receptor can assume upon activation (Doble, 1999).

In an attempt to characterize the molecular determinants of clinically important drug targets, studies involving site-directed mutagenesis of the genes of individual amino acid residues in the receptor have identified essential residues in the binding of different molecules (Table 14.2). Tyrosine (Tyr)157, Threonine (Thr)160, Thr202 and Tyr205 amino acid residues of the β-subunit and phenylalanine (Phe)64 of the α_1-subunit are important for the binding of GABA in rats. Histidine (His)101 (His102 in humans), and glycine (Gly)200 (Gly201 in humans) of the α-subunit and Phe77, methionine (Met)130 and Thr142 of the γ-subunit are reported to be the key determinants for BDZ binding in the rat brain. Two tyrosine residues, Tyr159 and Tyr209, are also crucial for BDZ binding (Amin et al., 1997). The His102

Table 14.2. Site-directed mutagenesis of the α- and γ-subunits

Amino acid	Subunit	Effect
Histidine 101	α	Site of photolabeling; indispensable for benzodiazepine binding; irrelevant for flumazenil and zopiclone binding
Tyrosine 159	α	Indispensable for benzodiazepine binding
Glycine 200	α	Confers BZ_1/BZ_2 selectivity
Phenylalanine 77	γ	Indispensable for zolpidem and flumazenil binding; irrelevant for benzodiazepine binding
Methionine 130	γ	Indispensable for flumazenil and benzodiazepine binding
Threonine 142	γ	Irrelevant for benzodiazepine binding; important determinant of efficacy

Source: Adapted with permission from Doble, 1999.

residue of the α-subunit interacts directly with the phenyl group of diazepam, flunitrazepam, chlordiazepoxide, and other 5-phenyl BDZs. This His residue is absent in the α_4-subunit and is replaced by arginine (Arg)100 in the α_6-subunit of the human and rat GABA-A receptors. These changes make the GABA-A receptors containing α_4- and α_6-subunits insensitive to conventional BDZs like diazepam, flunitrazepam, and clonazepam. The replacement of Arg100 by the glutamine (Gln)100 in the α_6-subunit of alcohol-sensitive rat cerebellum alters the normal diazepam-insensitive GABA-A receptors into diazepam-sensitive ones. Mutations in the γ_2-subunit also affect BDZ activity. Thr142 determines efficacy (Mihic et al., 1994) and its mutation to serine increases the efficacy of BDZs and flumazenil but decreases that of imidazopyridines. These results are consistent with the idea that the BDZ binding pocket is in the interface between the α- and γ-subunits (Doble, 1999).

In the rat, variation in alcohol and BDZ sensitivity has been correlated with an inherited variant of the GABA-A α_6-receptor. The Pro385Ser genotype was implicated and studied in humans by studying saccadic eye movements in children of alcoholics (Iwata et al., 1999). They found that this genotype may play a role in BDZ sensitivity and conditions such as alcoholism and may be correlated with this trait. Similar studies in humans, translating results of animal studies, need to be carried out.

Possible interventions at the GAB-A receptor set-point

The BDZ receptor site is unique in having three different functional classes of ligand binding to it: agonists, inverse agonists, and antagonists. The current treatment of

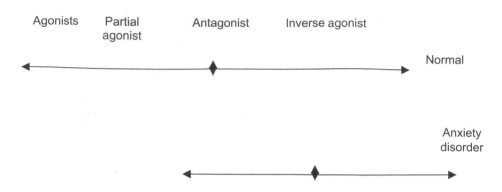

Fig. 14.2.   The γ-aminobutyric acid (GABA)–benzodiazepine receptor set-point.

anxiety disorders involves the use of BDZs, which are full agonists at most GABA-A receptor subtypes. The inverse agonists decrease the probability of the chloride channel opening in response to GABA and have stimulant and proconvulsant properties. The antagonists (like flumazenil) block the activities of both agonists and inverse agonists. These features indicate that the receptor manifests bidirectional agonism.

The GABA-A–BDZ receptor site has been hypothesized to play a regulatory role so that a protein conformation "fine tunes" GABA function, altering maximal efficacy or the rate of desensitization. The BDZ receptor spectrum is not fixed and the "set-point," where drugs bind, can be altered. Alterations in the set-point have been suggested as a possible mechanism to explain the phenomena of tolerance and dependence seen with BDZ treatment and rebound anxiety and insomnia on their withdrawal. It has been hypothesized that, with prolonged use, the set-point drifts in the inverse agonist direction, thus leading to a change in the receptor sensitivity and subsequent development of the above effects (Little et al., 1988; Nutt et al., 1992) (Fig. 14.2). This change in sensitivity can be explained by exchange of one subunit for another within the receptor. A model has been proposed according to which, with chronic BDZ treatment, the transcription of the gene cluster that encodes the prevalent $\alpha_1, \beta_2, \gamma_3$-receptor on chromosome 5 is downregulated while transcription of subunits encoded on chromosome 15 are upregulated; as a result the rarer subunits of chromosome 15 replace those of chromosome 5, leading to reduced sensitivity of the receptor (Holt et al., 1996, 1997a). This postulated change of the transcription rates is supported by the repression of the activity of the promoter sequence of the α_1-subunit gene seen after chronic treatment with lorazepam (Kang et al., 1994) and the decreased rate of transcription of the γ_2-subunit seen in diazepam-treated animals (Holt et al., 1997b).

This theory led to the development of variety of new drugs such as abecarnil (Holt et al., 1996), zopiclone, zolpidem (Holt et al., 1997a), and imidazenil (Pesold et al., 1997), which produce more restricted changes in subunit transcription.

These drugs also have less dependence potential compared with the classical BD2s (Lader, 1997, 1998; Doble, 1999). Also, chronic treatment with the inverse agonist FG7142 leads to opposite changes in GABA-A receptor subunit expression (Primus and Gallager, 1992). This postulated mechanism of transcription changes can thus provide a potentially useful animal model in which experimental treatment regimens can be identified to reset the receptor set-point in order to forestall the appearance of or attenuate or abolish established dependence (Doble and Martin, 1996). In epilepsy, studies have been conducted to 'reset the set-point' with the antagonist flumazenil. Such an approach reverses the tolerance to the anticonvulsant effect of clonazepam. While it is too early to say the same about BDZ dependence, studies in this area are needed.

Another strategy to prevent the development of dependence and tolerance is to initiate "drug holidays" (Doble and Martin, 1996). This may lead to changes in the set-point as well as changes in the expression of subunits. This hypothesis also requires further investigation, both in animals and humans.

Drug development: subtype selective ligands

The GABA-A receptor shows marked heterogeneity, and specific GABA-A receptors in particular brain regions with specific subunit assemblies are expressed to serve specific functions. Based on this hypothesis, subtype-selective ligands are being developed in the hope that they may have more precisely targeted therapeutic activity and fewer side effects. The major drawback of this attractive approach is that the physiological and pharmacological profiles of some relevant receptor assemblies are as yet unknown. Once this information becomes available, it would be theoretically possible to synthesize compounds selective for a particular receptor assembly so as to get a desired therapeutic effect, while the undesirable effects could be minimized.

Based on our current knowledge of the physiological and pharmacological role of various subunits of GABA-A receptors, the pharmacodynamic action of drugs like triazolopyridazine (CL218872), zolpidem, and abecarnil can be surmised. These drugs have been shown to bind with different affinities at different GABA-A receptors. CL218872 has a significantly higher affinity for the BDZ type I receptors than for type II receptors. It is thought to be anxiolytic without being sedative. Since type I receptors are present in the cerebellum, and type II receptors are present in the hippocampus, it was hypothesized that anxiolysis was mediated in the cerebellum. However, subsequent research does not support this. Zolpidem has a higher affinity for $\alpha_1\beta_2\gamma_2$-receptors. It has a 20-fold reduced affinity for the type II $\alpha_2\beta_2\gamma_2$-receptors and $\alpha_3\beta_3\gamma_3$-receptor subtypes but not to the type II $\alpha_5\beta_2\gamma_2$-receptor (Pritchett and Seeburg, 1990). Zolpidem produces sedation at lower doses than those producing anxiolysis, muscle relaxation, and anticonvulsant effects

(Darcourt et al., 1999). Abecarnil is a partial agonist at the GABA-A $\alpha_5\beta_2\gamma_2$-receptor and a full agonist at $\alpha_3\beta_2\gamma_3$-receptor. This is reflected in its therapeutic and side effect profile. Animal work with abecarnil has shown that it is an effective anxiolytic and anticonvulsant, with weak or insignificant effects on motor incoordination and a low propensity to cause dependence (Stephens et al., 1990). Further, it has no amnesic effects (Ozawa et al., 1994). In some (but not all) human studies, abecarnil was significantly better than placebo in the treatment of generalized anxiety disorder, and did not produce withdrawal effects upon abrupt discontinuation (Aufdembrinke, 1998).

Neurosteroids

Besides the GABA and BDZ sites, there are at least three other domains with binding sites on the GABA-A receptor: for picrotoxin, barbiturates, and anesthetic steroids (Gee et al., 1988; Turner et al., 1989). Unlike the BDZ site, the modulation of the GABA receptor by neurosteroids requires the presence of a β-subunit instead of a γ-subunit (Puia et al., 1990). The substitution of a γ_1- by γ_2-subunit greatly enhances the sensitivity of neuroactive steroids (Puia et al., 1991, 1993). The δ- and ε-subunits inhibit neurosteroid modulation of GABA-A receptors.

The natural steroid hormone progesterone is converted in the brain to 3α-hydroxy-5α-pregnan-20-one (allopregnenolone) (Morrow et al., 1987), which is sedative, decreases anxiety, and controls seizure activity by enhancing GABA function (Holzbauer, 1976; Crawley et al., 1986). During the premenstrual period, when the circulating levels of progesterone fall sharply, anxiety symptoms and susceptibility to seizures is known to occur. In an elegant experiment, Smith et al. (1998) produced a progesterone-withdrawal model in rats. Falling levels of the hormone led to insensitivity to BDZs and increased seizure susceptibility. These effects were mediated through the corresponding falling levels of allopregnenolone, which enhanced the transcription of the α_4-subunit. Blockade of the transcription of this subunit prevented these phenomena.

Ganaloxone is a synthetic neurosteroid with improved bioavailability compared with allopregnenolone. It may provide control of seizures that is superior to that of valproate, clonazepam, ethosuximide or diazepam, and it is currently undergoing clinical trials. Animal studies show that it may provide additional benefits by controlling anxiety, and mood changes associated with preseizure activity (Carter et al., 1997; Beekman et al., 1998).

Future research

There is a potential for further research into the development of compounds that effectively differentiate between the receptor subtypes of GABA-A receptor and target different subunits. Furthermore, research looking at modulation of differential expression in receptors, the specific physiological role of each subunit, the mechanisms influencing the clustering of subunit genes and their expression, and the different binding domains of receptors could lead to development of ligands that are effective anxiolytics.

Conclusions

Our understanding of the neurobiology of anxiety disorders and their treatment has been considerably increased in recent years following advances in neurochemistry and neuroimaging. The GABA-A receptor has been shown to play a pivotal role in mediating anxiety. There are a number of genetic variations in the GABA-A receptor and its subunits that can impact on the pharmacology of anxiolytic drugs. The various permutations of the subunits in the composition of these receptors have an effect on the activity and efficacy of these drugs. A second level of complexity is introduced with genetic variations in each of these subunits. Such variations can result in amino acid replacements, deletions, and imperfect subunit construction at a protein level, thereby resulting in different receptor combinations. Any such variations can strongly interfere with the pharmacokinetics of anxiolytic drugs. Developments in genetics and molecular biology have opened a window into the role of the GABA-A receptor subunits and the consequences of the heterogeneity of GABA-A receptors in different parts of the brain.

Exciting new research into pharmacogenetics will be based on our improving understanding of different drugs acting at this receptor. Future insights and research would pave the way for designing effective anxiolytic drugs with better safety profile and fewer side effects than the existing ones. If the pharmacogenetic approach were to prove clinically useful in the future, it will also enable us to predict the responsiveness of different patient populations to specific drugs. Then the vague recommendation of old to "tailor" each treatment regimen to the individual patient concerned may, finally, acquire a true meaning.

REFERENCES

American Psychiatric Association (1994). *Diagnostic and Statistical Manual of Mental Disorders*, 4th edn. Washington, DC: American Psychiatric Association.

Amin J, Brooks-Kayal A, Weiss DS (1997). Two tyrosine residues on the alpha subunit are crucial for benzodiazepine binding and allosteric modulation of gamma-aminobutyric acid-A receptors. *Mol Pharmacol* 51, 833–841.

Angelotti T, MacDonald RL (1993). Assembly of GABA-A receptor subunits $\alpha 1\beta 1$ and $\alpha 1\beta 1\gamma 2$ subunits produce unique ion channels with dissimilar single-channel properties. *J Neurosci* 13, 1429–1440.

Arranz MJ, Collier D, Sodhi M et al. (1995). Association between clozapine response and allelic variation in 5-HT$_{2A}$ receptor gene. *Lancet* 346, 281–282.

Aufdembrinke B (1998). Abercanil, a new beta-carboline, in the treatment of anxiety disorders. *Br J Psychiatry* 173(Suppl 34), 55–63.

Beekman M, Ungard JT, Gasior M et al. (1998). Reversal of behavioural effects of pentylenetetrazol by the neuroactive steroid ganoxolone. *J Pharmacol Exp Ther* 284, 868–877.

Benke DA, Mertens S, Trzeciak A, Gillessen D, Mohler H (1991a). GABA-A receptor display association of γ2-subunit with α1 and β2/3 subunits. *J Biol Chem* 266, 4478–4483.

Benke DA, Cicen-Sain A, Mertens S, Mohler H (1991b). Immunochemical identification of the α1 and α3 subunits of the GABA-A receptor in the rat brain. *J Receptor Res* 11, 407–424.

Benke D, Fritschy JM, Trzeciak A, Bannwarth W, Mohler H (1994). Distribution, prevalence and drug binding profile of gamma aminobutyric acid type A receptor subtypes differing in the beta subunit variant. *J Biol Chem* 269, 27100–27107.

Carter RB, Wood PL, Wieland S et al. (1997). Characterisation of the anticonvulsant properties of ganoloxone (CCD1042; 3-hydroxy-3beta-methyl-5alpha-pregnan-20-one), a selective high-affinity steroid modulator of the gamma-aminobutyric acid-A receptor. *J Pharmacol Exp Ther* 280, 1284–1295.

Cockroft VB, Osguthorpe DJ, Barnard EA, Lunt GG (1990). Modelling of agonist binding to the ligand gated ion channel superfamily of receptors. *Protein Struct Funct Genet* 8, 386G–397G.

Crawley JN, Glowa JR, Majewska MD, Paul SM (1986). Anxiolytic activity of an endogenous adrenal steroid. *Brain Res* 398, 382–385.

Crestani F, Lorez M, Baer K et al. (1999). Decreased GABA-A receptor clustering results in enhanced anxiety and a bias for threat cues. *Nat Neurosci* 2, 833–839.

Darcourt G, Pringuey D, Sallière D, Lavoisy J (1999). The safety and tolerability of zolpidem – an update. *J Psychopharmacol* 13, 81–93.

Doble A (1999). New insights into the mechanism of action of hypnotics. *J Psychopharmacol* 13 (Suppl 4:1), S11–S20.

Doble A, Martin II. (1996). *The GABA/Benzodiazepine Receptor as a Target for Psychoactive Drugs.* Austin, TX: RG Landes Company.

Doble A, Canton T, Piot O et al. (1992). The pharmacology of cyclopyrrolone derivatives acting at the GABA-A benzodiazepine receptor. *Adv Biochem Psychopharmacol* 47, 407–418.

Doble A, Canton T, Malgouris P (1995). The mechanism of action of zopiclone. *Eur Psychiatry* 10 (Suppl 3), 117S-128S.

Duggan M, Stephenson FA (1990). Biochemical evidence for the existence of gamma-aminobutyrate-A receptor iso-oligomers. *J Biol Chem* 265, 3831–3835.

Duggan M, Pollard S, Stephenson FA (1992). Quantitative immunoprecipitation studies with anti-gammaaminobutyric acid A receptor γ2 1–15 Cys antibodies. *J Neurochem* 58, 72–77.

Endo S, Olsen RW (1993). Antibodies specific for α-subunit subtypes of GABA-A receptors reveals brain heterogeneity. *J Neurochem* 60, 1388–1398.

Essrich C, Lorez M, Benson JA, Fritschy JM, Luscher B (1998). Postsynaptic clustering of major GABA-A receptor subtypes requires the γ2 subunit and gephrin. *Nat Neurosci* 1, 563–571.

Evans J, Battersby S, Ogilvie AD et al. (1997). Association of short alleles of a VNTR of the serotonin transporter gene with anxiety symptoms in patients presenting after deliberate self harm. *Neuropharmacology* 36, 439–443.

Feeney A, Lingford-Hughes A, Hume S et al. (2000). Characterisation of ^{11}C- RO 154513 as a PET ligand for limbic GABA-benzodiazepine receptors. *J Psychopharmacol* 14(Suppl), A30, P30.

Fritschy JM, Mohler H (1995). GABA-A receptor heterogeneity in the adult rat brain: differential regional and cellular distribution of seven major subunits. *J Comp Neurol* 359, 154–194.

Fritschy JM, Benke D, Mertens S, Oertel WH, Bachi T, Mohler H (1992). Five subtypes of type A gammaaminobutyric acid receptors identified in neurons by double and triple immunofluorescence staining with subunit specific antibodies. *Proc Natl Acad Sci, USA* 89, 6726–6730.

Fritschy JM, Benke D, Mertens S, Gao B, Mohler H (1993). Immunochemical distinction of GABA-A receptor subtypes differing in drug binding profiles and cellular distribution. *Soc Neurosci Abst* 19, 476.

Gee KW, Bolger MB, Brinton RE, Coirini H, McEwen BS (1988). Steroid modulation of the chloride ionophore in rat brain: structure–activity requirements, regional dependence and mechanism of action. *J Pharmacol Exp Ther* 246, 803–812.

Gunther U, Benson J, Benke D et al. (1995). Benzodiazepine-insensitive mice generated by targeted disruption of the gamma2 subunit of gamma-aminobutyric acid type A receptors. *Proc Natl Acad Sci, USA* 92, 7749–7753.

Hafeley WE (1978). Central action of the benzodiazepines: general introduction. *Br J Psychiatry* 133, 231–238.

Holt RA, Bateson AN, Martin IL (1996). Chronic treatment with diazepam or abecarnil differentially affects the expression of GABA-A receptor subunit mRNAs in the rat cortex. *Neuropharmacology* 35, 1457–1463.

Holt RA, Bateson AN, Martin IL (1997a). Chronic zolpidem treatment alters GABA-A receptor mRNA levels in the rat cortex. *Eur J Pharmacol* 329, 129–132.

Holt RA, Martin IL, Bateson AN (1997b). Chronic diazepam exposure decreases transcription of the rat GABA-A receptor gamma-2 subunit gene. *Mol Brain Res* 48, 164–166.

Holzbauer M (1976). Physiological aspects of steroids with anaesthetic properties. *Med Biol* 22, 97–102.

Homanics GE, Ferguson C, Quinlan JJ et al. (1997). Gene knockout of the α6 subunit of the GABA type A receptor: lack of effect on responses to ethanol, phenobarbital, and general anaesthetics. *Mol Pharmacol* 51, 588–596.

Homanics GE, Le NQ, Kist F, Mihalek R, Hart AR, Quinlan JJ (1998). Ethanol tolerance and withdrawal responses in GABA-A receptor alpha 6 subunit null allele mice and in inbred C57BL/6J and strain 129/SvJ mice. *Alcohol Clin Expl Res* 22, 259–265.

Huntsman NM, Isackson PJ, Jones EG (1994). Lamina-specific expression and activity-dependent regulation of seven G receptor subunit mRNAs in monkey visual cortex. *J Neurosci* 14, 2236–2259.

Iwata N, Cowley DS, Radel M, Roy-Byrne PP, Goldman D (1999). Relationship between a GABAA alpha6 Pro385Ser substitution and benzodiazepine sensitivity. *Am J Psychiatry* 156, 1447–1449.

Johnstone GA (1996). GABA-A receptor pharmacology. *Pharmacol Ther* 69, 173–198.

Jonas P, Bischofberger J, Sandkuhler J (1998). Corelease of two fast neurotransmitters at a central synapse. *Science* 281, 419–424.

Kang I, Lindquist DG, Kinane TB, Ercolani L, Pritchard GA, Miller LG (1994). Isolation and characterization of the promoter of the human GABA-A receptor 1 subunit gene. *J Neurochem* 62, 1643–1646.

Kardos J (1999). Recent advances in GABA research. *Neurochem Int* 34, 353–358.

Krasowski MD, Harrison NL, Firestone LL, Homanics GE (1998). A deficit of functional GABA-A receptors in neurons of beta3 subunit knockout mice. *Neurosc Lett* 240, 81–84.

Lader M (1997). Zopiclone: is there any dependence and abuse potential? *J Neurol* 244(Suppl 1), S18–S22.

Lader M (1998). Withdrawal reactions after stopping hypnotics in patients with insomnia. *CNS Drugs* 10, 425–440.

Lader MH (1999). Limitations on the use of benzodiazepines in anxiety and insomnia: are they justified? *Eur Neuropsychopharmacol* 9(Suppl 6), S399–S405.

Little HT, Gale R, Sellers N, Nutt DJ, Taylor SC (1988). Chronic benzodiazepine treatment increases the effects of the inverse agonist FG7142. *Neuropharmacology* 27, 381–383.

Low K, Crestani F, Keist R et al. (2000). Molecular and neuronal substrate for the selective attenuation of anxiety. *Science* 290, 131–134.

Luddens H, Pritcett DB, Kohler M et al. (1990). Cerebellar GABA-A receptor selective for a behavioural alcohol antagonist. *Nature* 346, 648–651.

Malizia AL, Nutt DJ (1995). Psychopharmacology of benzodiazepines – an update. *Hum Psychopharmacol* 1, S1–S14.

Malizia AL, Cunningham VJ, Bell CJ, Liddle PF, Jones T, Nutt DJ (1998). Decreased brain GABA-A-benzodiazepine receptor binding in panic disorder. Preliminary results from a quantitative PET study. *Arch Gen Psychiatry* 55, 715–720.

Marksitzer R, Benke D, Fritschy JM, Trzeciak A, Bannwarth W, Mohler H (1993). GABAA-receptors: drug binding profile and distribution of receptors con alpha 2-subunit in situ. *J Receptor Res* 13, 467–477.

Mathews DB, Devaud LL, Fritschy JM, Sieghart W, Morrow AL (1998). Differential regulation of GABA-A receptor gene expression by ethanol in the rat hippocampus versus cerebral cortex. *J Neurochem* 70, 1160–1166.

McKernan RM, Quirk K, Prince R et al. (1991). GABA-A receptor subtypes immunopurified from rat brain with α subunit specific antibodies have unique pharmacological properties. *Neuron* 7, 667–676.

McLennan A, Brecha N, Khrestchatisky M et al. (1991). Independent cellular and ontogenic expression of mRNA encoding alpha polypeptides of the rat GABA-A receptor. *Neuroscience* 43, 369–380.

Mehta AK, Ticku MK (1999). An update on GABA-A receptors. *Brain Res Rev* 29, 196–217.

Mertens S, Benke D, Mohler H (1993). GABA-A receptor populations with novel subunit combinations and drug binding profiles identified in brain by $\alpha5$ and δ-subunit specific immunopurification. *J Biol Chem* 268, 5965–5973.

Mhatre MC, Ticku MK (1994). Chronic ethanol treatment up-regulates the GABA-A receptor β subunit expression. *Mol Brain Res* 23, 246–252.

Mhatre MC, Pena G, Sieghart W, Ticku MK (1993). Antibodies specific for GABA-A receptor α subunits reveal that chronic alcohol treatment down-regulates α-subunit expression in rat brain regions. *J Neurochem* 61, 1620–1625.

Mihic SJ, Whiting PJ, Klein RL, Wafford KA, Harris RA (1994). A single amino acid of the human gamma-aminobutyric acid type A receptor gamma 2 subunit determines benzodiazepine efficacy. *J Biol Chem* 269, 32768–32773.

Mohler H (1982). Benzodiazepine receptors: differential interaction of benzodiazepine agonists and antagonists after photoaffinity labeling with flunitrazepam. *Eur J Pharmacol* 80, 435–436.

Mohler H, Okada T (1977). Benzodiazepine receptor: demonstration in the central nervous system. *Science* 198, 849–851.

Mohler H, Battersby MK, Richards JG (1980). Benzodiazepine receptor protein identified and visualised brain tissue by a photoaffinity label. *Proc Natl Acad Sci, USA* 77, 1666–1670.

Morrow AL, Suzdak PD, Paul SM (1987). Steroid hormone metabolites potentiate GABA receptor mediated chloride ion influx with nanomolar potency. *Eur J Pharmacol* 142, 483–485.

Nayeem N, Green TP, Martin IL, Barnard EA (1994). Quaternary structure of the native GABA-A receptor determined by electron microscopic image analysis. *J Neurochem* 62, 815–818.

Nicoll RA, Malenka RC (1998). A tale of two transmitters. *Science* 281, 360–361.

Nutt DJ, Malizia AL (2001). New insights into the role of the GABA-A-benzodiazepine receptor in psychiatric disorder. *Br J Psychiatry* 179, 390–396.

Nutt DJ, Smith CF, Bennett R, Jackson HC (1992). Investigations on the set-point theory of benzodiazepine receptor function. *Adv Biochem Psychopharmacol* 47, 419–429.

Ozawa M, Sugimachi K, Nakada-Kometani Y, Akai T, Yamaguchi M (1994). Chronic pharmacological activities of the novel anxiolytic β-carboline abecarnil in rats. *J Pharmacol Exp Ther* 269, 457–462.

Persohn E, Malherbe P, Richards JG (1992). Comparative molecular neuroanatomy of cloned GABA-A receptor subunits in the rat CNS. *J Comp Neurol* 326, 193–216.

Pesold C, Carruncho HJ, Impagnatiello F et al. (1997). Tolerance to diazepam and changes in the GABA-A receptor subunit expression in rat neocortical areas. *Neuroscience* 79, 477–487.

Primus RJ, Gallager DW (1992). GABA-A receptor subunit mRNA levels are differentially influenced by chronic FG 7142 and diazepam exposure. *Eur J Pharmacol* 226, 21–28.

Pritchett DB, Seeburg PH (1990). GABA-A receptor alpha 5 subunit creates novel type II benzodiazepine receptor pharmacology. *J Neurochem* 54, 1802–1804.

Pritchett DB, Luddens H, Seeburg PH (1989a). Type I and type II GABA-A–benzodiazepine receptors produced in transfected cells. *Science* 245, 1389–1392.

Pritchett DB, Sontheimer H, Shivers B et al. (1989b). Importance of a novel GABA-A receptor subunit for benzodiazepine pharmacology. *Nature* 338, 582–585.

Puia G, Santi M, Vicini S et al. (1990). Neurosteroids act on recombinant GABA-A receptors. *Neuron* 4, 759–765.

Puia G, Vicini S, Seeburg PH, Costa E (1991). Influence of recombinant GABA-A receptor subunit composition on the action of allosteric modulators of GABA-gated Cl$^-$ currents. *Mol Pharmacol* 39, 691–696.

Puia G, Ducic S, Vicini S, Costa E (1993). Does neurosteroid modulatory efficacy depend on GABA-A receptor subunit composition? *Receptors Channels* 1, 135–142.

Quirk K, Gillard NP, Ragan CI, Whiting PJ, McKernan RM (1994). GABA-type A receptors in the rat brain can contain both gamma2 and gamma3 subunits, but gamma1 does not exist in combination with another gamma subunit. *Mol Pharmacol* 45, 1061–1070.

Rice DP, Miller LS (1998). Health economics and cost implications of anxiety and other mental disorders in the United States. *Br J Psychiatry* 173(Suppl 34), 4–9.

Roses AD (2000). Pharmacogenetics and the practice of medicine. *Nature* 405, 857–865.

Ruano D, Araujo A, Machado A, Deblas AL, Vitorica J (1994). Molecular characterisation of type I GABA-A receptor complex from rat cerebral cortex and hippocampus. *Mol Brain Res* 25, 225–233.

Rudolph U, Crestani F, Benke D et al. (1999). Benzodiazepine actions mediated by specific gamma-aminobutyric acid (A) receptor subtypes. *Nature* 401, 796–800.

Sandford JJ, Argyropoulos SV, Nutt DJ (2000). The psychobiology of anxiolytic drugs. Part I: basic neurobiology. *Pharmacol Ther* 88, 197–212.

Saxena NC, MacDonald RL (1994). Assembly of GABA-A receptor subunits: role of the gamma subunit. *J Neurosci* 14, 7077–7086.

Schneier FR, Liebowitz MR, Abi-Dargham A, Zea-Ponce Y, Lin SH, Laruelle M (2000). Low dopamine D(2) receptor binding potential in social phobia. *Am J Psychiatry* 157, 457–459.

Schofield PR, Darlison MG, Fujita N et al. (1987). Sequence and functional expression of the GABA-A receptor shows a ligand-gated receptor super-family. *Nature* 328, 221–227.

Schukit MA, Mazzanti C, Smith TL, Ahmed U, Radel M, Iwata N, Goldman D (1999). Selective genotyping for the role of 5 HT2C and GABA alpha6 receptors and the serotonin transporter in the level of response to alcohol: a pilot study. *Biol Psychiatry* 45, 647–651.

Sequier JM, Richards JG, Malherbe P, Price GW, Mathews S, Mohler H (1988). Mapping of brain areas containing RNA homologous to cDNAs encoding the α and β subunits of the rat GABA-A receptor. *Proc Natl Acad Sci, USA* 85, 7815–7819.

Siegel E, Baur R, Trube G, Mohler H, Malherbe P (1990). The effect of subunit composition of rat brain GABA-A receptors on channel function. *Neuron* 5, 703–711.

Sieghart W (1989). Multiplicity of GABAA-benzodiazepine receptors. *Trend Pharm Sci* 10, 407–411.

Sieghart W (1995). Structure and pharmacology of GABA-A receptor subtypes. *Pharm Rev* 47, 181–234.

Sieghart W, Eichinger A, Richards JG, Mohler H (1987). Photoaffinity labeling of benzodiazepine receptor proteins with the partial inverse agonist [^{3}H]RO 15–4513: a biochemical and autoradiographic study. *J Neurochem* 48, 46–52.

Smith SS, Gong QH, Hsu FC, Markowitz RS, French-Mullen JMH, Li X (1998). GABA(A) receptor α4 subunit suppression prevents withdrawal properties of an endogenous steroid. *Nature* 392, 926–930.

Squires RF, Braestrup C (1977). Benzodiazepine receptors in rat brain. *Nature* 266, 732–734.

Stephens DN, Schneider HH, Kehr W et al. (1990). Abecarnil, a metabolically stable, anxioselective beta-carboline acting at benzodiazepine receptors. *J Pharmacol Exp Ther* 253, 334–343.

Tallman JF, Gallager DW (1985). The GABA-ergic system: a locus of benzodiazepine action. *Annu Rev Neurosci* 8, 21–44.

Ticku M, Mehta A, Lehoullier P (1988). Spinal cord cultured neurons: an in vitro model to study GABA synaptic pharmacology. In Biggio G, Costa E eds. *Adv Biochem Psychopharmacol: Chloride channels and their Modulation by Neurotransmitters and Drugs*, Vol 45. New York: Raven Press, pp. 151–159.

Tiihonen J, Kuikka J, Bergstrom K, Lepola U, Koponen H, Leinonen E (1997). Dopamine reuptake site densities in patients with social phobia. *Am J Psychiatry* 154, 239–242.

Togel M, Mossier B, Fuchs K, Sieghart W (1994). γ-Aminobutyric acid A receptors displaying association of γ3 subunits with β2/3 and different α-subunits exhibit unique pharmacological properties. *J Biol Chem* 269, 12993–12998.

Turner DM, Ransom RW, Yang JSJ, Olsen RW (1989). Steroid anaesthetics and naturally occurring analogs modulate the gamma-aminobutyric acid receptor complex at a site distinct from barbiturates. *J Pharmacol Exp Ther* 248, 960–966.

Verdoorn TA (1994). Formation of heteromeric γ-aminobutyric acid type A receptors containing two different α-subunits. *Mol Pharmacol* 45, 475–480.

Verdoorn TA, Draguhn A, Ymer S, Seeburg PH, Sakmann B (1990). Functional properties of recombinant rat GABA-A receptors depend upon subunit composition. *Neuron* 4, 919–928.

Wang, JB, Liu ZF, Kofuji P, Burt DR (1998). The GABA-A receptor gamma1 subunit in seizure prone (DBA/2) and resistant (C57BL/6) mice. *Brain Res Bulletin* 45, 421–425.

Weiller E, Bisserbe J-C, Maier W, Lecrubier Y (1998). Prevalence and recognition of anxiety symptoms in five European primary care settings: a report from the WHO study on psychological problems in general health care. *Br J Psychiatry* 173(Suppl 34), 18–23.

Whiting PJ (1999). The GABA-A receptor gene family: new targets for therapeutic intervention. *Neurochem Int* 34, 387–390.

Wisden W, Herb A, Wieland H, Kiennanen K, Luddens H, Seeburg PH (1991). Cloning, pharmacological characteristics and expression pattern of the rat GABA-A receptor α4 subunit. *FEBS Lett* 289, 227–230.

Wisden W, Laurie DJ, Moyner H, Seeburg PH (1992). The distribution of 13 GABA-A receptor subunit mRNAs in the rat brain. I. Telencephalon, diencephalon, mesencephalon. *J Neurosci* 12, 1040–1062.

Wong G, Sei Y, Skolnick P (1992). Stable expression of gamma-aminobutyric acid typeA/benzodiazepine receptors in transfected cell line. *Mol Pharmacol* 42, 996–1003.

World Health Organization (1992). *The Tenth Revision of the International Classification of Diseases and Related Health Problems (ICD-10)*. Geneva: World Health Organization.

Yang SH, Armson PF, Cha J, Philips WD (1997). Clustering of GABA-A receptors by rapsyn/43kD protein in vitro. *Mol Cell Neuroscience* 8, 430–438.

Ymer S, Draguhn A, Wisden W et al. (1990). Structural and functional characterisation of the subunit of GABA/benzodiazepine receptors. *EMBO J* 9, 3261–3267.

Zezula J, Slany A, Sieghart W (1996). Interaction of allosteric ligands with GABA-A receptors containing one, two, or three different subunits. *Eur J Pharmacol* 301, 207–214.

Zhang JH, Araki T, Sato M, Tohyma M (1991a). Distribution of GABA-A receptor α1 subunit gene expression in the rat forebrain. *Mol Brain Res* 11, 239–247.

Zhang JH, Sato M, Tohyma M (1991b). Region specific expression of the mRNAs encoding β-subunits (β1, β2 and β3) of GABA-A receptor in the rat brain. *J Comp Neurol* 303, 637–657.

15

Genetic factors and long-term prophylaxis in bipolar disorder

Martin Alda

Department of Psychiatry, Dalhousie University, Halifax, Canada

OVERVIEW

Response to long-term lithium treatment in bipolar disorder appears to be related to the family history of a patient. Conversely, some studies have indicated that treatment response could identify a subtype of bipolar disorder characterized by a stronger role of genetic factors and possibly by major-gene effects. Several research groups have now collected samples from patients treated with lithium and these are being studied by molecular genetic methods. These studies aim to identify genes associated with the treatment response or to map genes for bipolar disorder in homogeneous populations of treatment responders. Preliminary findings with a number of candidate genes have produced mostly negative findings, but several promising associations have been also identified, for instance, an association of lithium-responsive bipolar disorder with the gene for phospholipase $C\gamma1$. Further research will be needed to examine differences between genetic factors involved in treatment response as opposed to genes associated with the illness. One possible research strategy appears to be a study of pairs of relatives concordant for the illness but discordant for their treatment response. Other important areas of research are phenotype definition, especially definition of long-term prophylactic response, and studies of biochemical phenotypes and alterations in gene expression.

Introduction

Lithium is the standard treatment for bipolar disorder. In recent years, several other treatments have appeared promising, mainly anticonvulsants, but also calcium channel blockers and other drugs.

Response to lithium appears to identify a more homogeneous subtype of bipolar disorder with higher heritability. Recent data also suggest that treatment response itself may be a highly familial trait. Several groups have now conducted molecular genetic studies in order to identify genes contributing to the etiology of bipolar disorder as well as genes that may influence long-term treatment response.

There is limited evidence that the response to mood stabilizers could be individually specific (Post et al., 1984). Therefore, we will focus on individual treatments, in particular on lithium for which the most data are available.

Lithium

Family and family-history studies of lithium response

The relationship between family history and response to lithium has been the subject of investigations since the 1970s. These included studies where diagnostic information on most relatives was obtained indirectly (family-history studies) and studies where diagnostic information was obtained by interviewing in person as many relatives as possible (family studies). Arguably, the distinction is somewhat artificial and many studies used a combination of approaches to gather all available information. These studies are summarized in Table 15.1.

Mendlewicz et al. (1973) published a family study of 36 patients treated with lithium for 3 years. Those patients who did not relapse (24 out of 36) were classified as responders and, significantly more often, had a family history of bipolar disorder compared with those who relapsed on lithium (12 out of 36). Subsequently, several other studies found an association between prophylactic lithium response and a family history of bipolar disorder. These studies generally fall into one of two categories. Family-history studies often looked for factors predicting response to lithium. Family history would be typically included among other clinical variables. Their results are less clear-cut than those of family studies (discussed below). Some family-history studies found an association between a family history of bipolar disorder and treatment response (Prien et al., 1974; Svestka and Nahunek, 1975; Svestka, 1979; Maj et al., 1984); some also found an association with a family history of unipolar depression (Abou-Saleh and Coppen, 1986). Several other studies, however, were unable to confirm such findings (Dunner et al., 1976) or found the opposite: an association of family history of bipolar disorder and non-response to lithium (Misra and Burns, 1976; Strober et al., 1988). The latter two studies must be interpreted with caution as the first was based on a case series of seven nonresponders only, with no comparison group, and the second was a study of adolescent bipolar disorders. A more detailed review of these studies can be found in Grof et al. (1994).

Family studies, by comparison, provide a consistent support of the hypothesis of familial differences between responders and nonresponders. In addition to the study of Mendlewicz et al. (1973), several other investigations showed similar results (Zvolsky et al., 1974, 1979; Mendlewicz, 1979; Smeraldi et al., 1984; Grof et al., 1994). In our analysis of 121 families, we found, on the one hand, that responders to lithium had significantly higher rates of bipolar disorder among their

Table 15.1. Family/family-history studies and response to lithium

Study	Type	Design/outcome	Probands	Treatment duration	Results
Mendlewicz et al., 1973	F	Prevalence of family history of BD and UD	24 R, 12 NR	6–37 months	More frequent history of BD in families of R
Zvolsky et al., 1974	F	Prevalence of psychiatric disorders in first-degree relatives	58 BD	>2 years	Higher rates in relatives of complete and partial responders
Prien et al., 1974	FH	Response to treatment	48 R, 43 NR	2 years	Better response in subjects with FH of BD
Svestka and Nahunek, 1975	FH	Treatment outcome	55 R, 26 NR	1–7 years	FH of endogenous psychoses and suicide higher in R
Dunner et al., 1976	FH	Relapse rate on lithium	52 R, 44 NR	1–45 months	No effect of FH of BD or UD
Misra and Burns, 1977	FH	FH of AD	9 NR	2–8 years	7 out of 9 NR had FH of AD
Zvolsky et al., 1979	F	Prevalence of psychiatric disorders in first-degree relatives	26 R, 17 NR	>7 years	Higher rates in relatives of R compared with those of NR
Mendlewicz et al., 1979	F	Concordance rates in twins	24 R, 18 NR	>2 years	Higher concordance (both MZ and DZ) for R
Maj et al., 1984	FH	Frequency of FH of BD, UD, and other disorders	59 R, 41 NR	2 years	More frequent FH of BD in relatives of R
Smeraldi et al., 1984	F	Morbidity risks of AD in first-degree relatives	92 R, 53 NR	>3 years	Higher rates of AD in relatives of R
Abou-Saleh and Coppen, 1986	FH	Affective Morbidity Index (AMI) during lithium treatment	27 BP	2 years	Lower AMI in patients with FH of BD or UD
Shapiro et al., 1989	FH	Relapse rate on lithium	117	2 years	Relapse rate on lithium or imipramine unrelated to FH

Grof et al., 1994	F	Morbidity risks of BD, UD, SZ in first-degree relatives	71 R, 50 NR	3–20 years	Increased risk of BD in families of R, increased SZ in families of NR
Engstrom et al., 1997	F	Frequency of episodes on lithium	51 Fam, 47 nFam	13 ± 8 years 11 ± 8 years	0.32 ± 0.44 in nFam patients 0.58 ± 0.70 in Fam patients
Coryell et al., 2000	F and FH	Morbidity risks of BD, UD, SZ and alcoholism in relatives of probands with low, medium or high morbidity on Li	62 low, 55 medium, 69 high	7.8 ± 5.8 years 5.7 ± 4.1 years 5.5 ± 4.5 years	No major differences between the groups

Notes:

F, family study; FH, family-history study; R, responders; NR, nonresponders; BD, bipolar disorder; UD, unipolar depression; AD, affective disorder; SZ, schizophrenia; Fam, familial; nFam, non-familial (sporadic).

first-degree relatives, while nonresponders had higher rates of schizophrenia in their families (Grof et al., 1994). On the other hand, we did not find any difference between the two groups with respect to family history of alcoholism, and the prevalence of alcoholism in families of both groups of probands was quite low (Duffy et al., 1998b).

More recently, two studies, in particular, raised questions about the possible link between family history and treatment response. Engstrom et al. (1997) analyzed data from 90 families, 39 with positive and 51 with negative family histories of bipolar disorder. They found that the family-history-negative subjects had fewer episodes on lithium compared with those with positive family histories. This was a family-history study with at least one relative per family interviewed. The treatment response was not defined categorically but rather used as a quantitative variable (frequency of episodes on and off lithium). Therefore, it is not possible to compare the data with those from earlier studies. For instance, it is not clear how many responders (subjects with no activity of illness while treated) were in the sample.

In the second study, Coryell et al. (2000) reported psychiatric morbidity in relatives of probands subdivided according to their frequency of episodes in the course of prophylactic treatment. The diagnostic data on relatives were based on personal interviews with a majority of the relatives, who were also re-interviewed after 6 years. As in the study of Engstrom et al. (1997), Coryell et al. (2000) reported average frequencies of episodes on and off lithium. The study could not find any differences between the rates of bipolar disorder in families of patients divided into three groups according to their episode frequency in the course of lithium treatment (high–medium–low). The group with the highest morbidity on lithium had a higher frequency of family history positive for major depression. Again, it is not possible to tell whether the probands had actually responded to the treatment or whether the differences reflect the natural course of the illness with some "responders" being patients with slow cycling disorder. Even the responders had a noticeable activity of illness while in treatment. Finally, the interpretation of the findings is more difficult because the group with a low frequency of episodes on lithium also had significantly lower morbidity before the treatment.

Consequently, it is not clear to what extent these recent results are in conflict with the older ones. The earlier studies usually included subjects with large numbers of pretreatment episodes who, by definition, had to stay free of any recurrence for a specified length of time – a minimum of 3 years in Smeraldi et al. (1984) and in Grof et al. (1994). Finally, we have argued elsewhere that bipolar disorder is now diagnosed more liberally (Grof et al., 1995; Grof and Alda, 2000). This makes it more difficult to compare results obtained within studies that used a more conservative approach to diagnosis. This is also reflected in the huge increase in population prevalence of mood disorders, certainly not explained simply by period or cohort effects, and in the increase in morbidity risks in family studies (Grof et al., 1995; Duffy et al., 2000a).

Family studies are complemented by high-risk studies of the children of lithium responders and nonresponders. These studies show that the offspring of responders typically develop disorders in the affective spectrum, with little or no comorbidity and often high premorbid functioning. Their illness seems to be episodic with complete interepisodic recoveries. The children of nonresponders often develop multiple psychiatric problems that include nonaffective symptoms as well. Their illness seems to follow a more chronic course, characterized by incomplete remissions (Duffy et al., 1998a).

Mode of inheritance

Smeraldi et al. (1984) first applied segregation analysis to family data from responders and nonresponders to lithium. They found support for major-gene effects in the families of responders. Our data from responders are also consistent with a major-gene effect, specifically a gene of a recessive type (Alda et al., 1994). This result was replicated by our group in an independent sample (Alda et al., 1997). As segregation analyses typically test the mode of inheritance by fitting specific genetic models to family data, their results need to be viewed as approximate, providing leads for further research. Their application to lithium-responsive bipolar disorder suggests that this may be a suitable population for gene mapping studies.

Lithium response as a phenotype

It has been argued that lithium response identifies a more homogeneous genetically distinct subtype of bipolar disorder. Conversely, some authors view lithium response mainly as a continuum, determined to a large extent by good compliance and low (or no) comorbidity. It is also possible that lithium response is influenced by genetic factors, partially or completely independent from those contributing to the etiology of the illness.

Therefore, it is of interest to establish whether lithium response itself is familial. Only few studies have examined this issue in the past.

Several investigations of children treated with lithium suggested beneficial effects in a variety of conditions but primarily in affective symptoms (Annell, 1969; Delong, 1978; Youngerman and Canino, 1978; McKnew et al., 1981). One study of children of bipolar lithium responders suggested that they had a response concordant with that of their parents (McKnew et al., 1981). Indirect support for the familiality of lithium treatment response in the children of bipolar probands can also be found in a study by Duffy et al. (1998a), who described similarities between parents and children with respect to the episodicity of the clinical course, a hallmark of the lithium-responsive form of bipolar disorder (Grof et al., 1993). Most recently, in a study of 24 relatives of probands who responded unequivocally to lithium, 16 (67%) showed a clear-cut response (Grof et al., 2000). This is significantly higher than the response rate in a comparison sample in which only 9 out of 30 (30%) subjects responded according to the same criteria.

Admittedly, none of these results can differentiate between the two main possibilities, namely, that lithium response is determined by an independent genetic factor or that responders represent a subtype of the illness. Both would predict a trend towards familial clustering of the response. For the same reason, the results of association studies comparing responders and nonresponders cannot be interpreted one way or the other either. Ultimately, a comparison of nonresponders and responders from the same family could help in identifying genes associated with the response but not with the illness. In our experience, such pairs of relatives, with their response (or nonresponse) well established, are difficult to find.

Molecular genetic studies

Several research groups have established clinical samples of patients treated with lithium for the purpose of molecular genetic investigations. Some of these studies are aimed primarily at the identification of those loci influencing the response to the treatment. Other groups use treatment response as an additional phenotypic dimension or homogeneity criterion.

Studies of lithium responders as a homogeneous subtype of bipolar disorder

We have studied patients with bipolar disorder responsive to lithium in collaboration with the International Group for Study of Lithium (IGSLI). The group coordinates research efforts of centers in Austria, Canada, Czech Republic, Denmark, Germany, and Sweden. The cornerstone of our work has been the assumption that lithium-responsive bipolar disorder is a distinct, more genetically based subtype of bipolar disorder.

The initial association studies focused on the gene for tyrosine hydroxylase (Cavazzoni et al., 1996) and on markers on chromosome 18 (Turecki et al., 1996). Subsequently, candidate genes were analyzed that were thought to be relevant to the etiology of the illness and/or treatment response. Among these, there is a positive association with the gene for phospholipase $C\gamma1$ (Turecki et al., 1998). In a subset of unilineal families there was also suggestive linkage (lod = 1.45; $p = 0.004$). Phospholipase C is a promising candidate gene because of its role in the phosphoinositol cycle, a major target of lithium. No association was found with several other candidate genes: monoamine oxidase A (Turecki et al., 1999a), corticotropin-releasing hormone, proenkephalin (Alda et al., 2000), and several genes related to

GABAergic function (Duffy et al., 2000b). The hypothesis of anticipation and unstable trinucleotide repeats was tested by searching for polyglutamate protein sequences in lymphoblasts, using a specific antibody (Turecki et al., 1999c), and by studying association with markers known to contain CAG repeats (Turecki et al., 2000). Neither study supported the anticipation hypothesis.

These candidate gene association studies were usually complemented by linkage analyses of a related sample of moderately large families. Linkage was also tested to chromosome 18, at the time one of the most studied regions in bipolar disorder, with several independent reports of linkage (Berrettini et al., 1994; Stine et al., 1995; Freimer et al., 1996). Using a set of markers spanning the entire chromosome, no linkage could be demonstrated even after separating the families into those with maternal or paternal transmission of the illness (Turecki et al., 1999b). It is possible that linkage to chromosome 18 may be more common in subjects with atypical illness. This would also be consistent with the report of linkage of schizophrenia to chromosome 18 (Schwab et al., 1998).

Following these studies of candidate genes and candidate regions, a full genome scan was completed with several chromosomal regions showing lod scores in the 1.8 to 3.5 range, namely those on chromosomes 6, 7, 15, 21, and 22 (Turecki et al., 2001). The scan included a total of 247 subjects in 31 families identified through probands with bipolar disorder responsive to lithium. A total of 108 subjects in these families were affected with bipolar disorder or recurrent unipolar depression. These conditions were considered as a phenotype for the first set of analyses. For the genome scan, 378 markers spaced at approximately 10 cM intervals were used. The data were analyzed by parametric (lod score) and non-parametric (SimIBD) methods. There was evidence for linkage in the 15q14 region (marker ACTC lod = 3.46; locus-specific; $p = 0.000014$) and suggestive linkage for another marker on chromosome 7q11.2 (D7S1816; lod = 2.68; $p = 0.00011$). In the second set of analyses, treatment response was used as a phenotype; unaffected relatives and those not treated with lithium were considered "phenotype unknown" in the linkage analysis. The highest lod score for this phenotype was for the marker D7S1816 (lod = 1.53; locus-specific $p = 0.003$).

Studies comparing responders and nonresponders to lithium

Several research groups have initiated searches for genes associated with response (or no response) to lithium using association case-control strategies.

A sample of lithium-treated patients has been collected as a part of the European Collaborative Project on Affective Disorders. In a preliminary analysis of the sample with dopamine receptor genes and tyrosine hydroxylase, Lipp et al. (1997) reported equivocal results, with a trend towards the association of bipolar disorder with the D_2 receptor gene among nonresponders to lithium. Part of the sample collected at the University of Milan was analyzed separately and reported on in several papers. The association analyses included genes for dopamine D_3 receptor (Serretti et al., 1998), tryptophan hydroxylase (Serretti et al., 1999a), dopamine receptors D_2 and D_4 and γ-aminobutyric acid A (GABA-A) α_1-subunit (Serretti et al., 1999b), and serotonin receptors 2A, 2C, and 1A (Serretti et al., 2000). These analyses were based on a sample of up to 125 subjects with major affective disorders, both bipolar and unipolar. None of the markers tested gave any evidence of association.

The group of V. Steen has been focusing on genes controlling the phosphoinositol pathway (Steen et al., 1996; Sjoholt et al., 1997; Lovlie et al., 1999). They identified several polymorphisms in the gene for inositol polyphosphate 1-phosphatase. One of these polymorphisms was associated with lithium response in the Norwegian part of the sample, but not in the subjects from Israel (Steen et al., 1998).

Del Zompo et al. (1999) studied the gene for the serotonin transporter, in particular the polymorphism in the promoter region known to affect the transcriptional activity of the gene. They found a trend towards higher frequency of the *l* allele among lithium nonresponders, which contrasts with the reported association of nonresponse to several different serotonin reuptake inhibitors and the *ss* genotype (Smeraldi et al., 1998; Kim et al., 2000; Zanardi et al., 2000; see also Ch. 6.)

Other mood stabilizers

There is a relative paucity of data pertaining to family history and the response to other long-term treatments in bipolar disorder. Post et al. (1984) suggested that the acute antimanic response to carbamazepine was associated with family history negative for bipolar disorder. In the above-mentioned study by Coryell et al. (2000), a small number of subjects (31) took anticonvulsants carbamazepine or valproate alone for at least 26 weeks. The authors could not find any differences between family histories of those who had high, medium, or low activity of the illness during the treatment. They caution, however, that the probability of type II error was quite high because of the low numbers.

Both theoretically interesting and practically important is the question of specificity of prophylactic treatments. Post et al. (1984) suggested that the long-term treatment response could be specific to an individual patient. For example, subjects who respond to an anticonvulsant may not be lithium responders and vice versa. It is unclear, at present, how far this hypothesis can be extrapolated with respect to family history. Greil et al. (1997) conducted a large prophylactic trial of lithium and carbamazepine in bipolar disorder and found that lithium was more effective in typical patients while carbamazepine had an advantage in subjects with atypical illness. It would be reasonable to predict that these two groups would differ with respect to their family histories. Such a conjecture, however, needs to be tested in a rigorous study. The study by Coryell et al. (2000) included 36 subjects treated with both lithium and anticonvulsants in separate trials. In these patients, it seemed that the morbidity on both treatments was similar. The interpretation of this observation is again obscured by the differences in morbidity before the treatment.

Conclusions

The study of genetic factors in long-term treatment of bipolar disorder has been complicated by methodological difficulties. The results so far are promising, yet not conclusive. New research strategies such as studies of gene expression as well as progress in phenotype definition might provide new insights and lead to results that could have important implications for the management of this severe illness.

Acknowledgements

Parts of this work were supported by grants from the Medical Research Council of Canada and from Ontario Mental Health Foundation. Martin Alda holds an Independent Investigator Award from NARSAD.

REFERENCES

Abou-Saleh M, Coppen A (1986). Who responds to prophylactic lithium? *J Affect Disord* 10, 115–125.

Alda M, Grof P, Grof E, Zvolsky P, Walsh M (1994). Mode of inheritance in families of patients with lithium-responsive affective disorders. *Acta Psychiatr Scand* 90, 304–310.

Alda M, Grof E, Cavazzoni P et al. (1997). Autosomal recessive inheritance of affective disorders in families of responders to lithium prophylaxis? *J Affect Disord* 44, 153–157.

Alda M, Turecki G, Grof P et al. (2000). Association and linkage analyses of CRH and PENK genes in bipolar disorder responsive to lithium: a collaborative IGSLI study. *Am J Med Genet* (*Neuropsychiatr Genet*) 96, 178–181.

Annell AL (1969). Manic-depressive illness in children and effect of treatment with lithium carbonate. *Acta Paedopsychiatr* 36, 292–301.

Berrettini WH, Ferraro TN, Goldin LR et al. (1994). Chromosome 18 DNA markers and manic-depressive illness: evidence for a susceptibility gene. *Proc Natl Acad Sci, USA* 21, 5918–5921.

Cavazzoni P, Alda M, Turecki G et al. (1996). Lithium-responsive affective disorders: no association with the tyrosine hydroxylase gene. *Psychiatry Res* 64, 91–96.

Coryell W, Akiskal H, Leon AC, Turvey C, Solomon D, Endicott J (2000). Family history and symptom levels during treatment for bipolar I affective disorder. *Biol Psychiatry* 47, 1034–1042.

Delong GR (1978). Lithium carbonate treatment of select behavior disorders in children suggesting manic-depressive illness. *J Pediatr* 93, 689–694.

Del Zompo M, Ardau R, Palmas MA, Bocchetta A, Reina A, Piccardi MP (1999). Lithium response: association study with two candidate genes. *Mol Psychiatry* 4, 66–67.

Duffy A, Alda M, Kutcher S, Fusee C, Grof P (1998a). Psychiatric symptoms and syndromes among adolescent children of parents with lithium-responsive or lithium-nonresponsive bipolar disorder. *Am J Psychiatry* 155, 431–433.

Duffy A, Grof P, Grof E, Zvolsky P, Alda M (1998b). Evidence supporting the independent inheritance of primary affective disorders and primary alcoholism in the families of bipolar patients. *J Affect Disord* 50, 91–96.

Duffy A, Grof P, Robertson C, Alda M (2000a). The implications of genetic studies of major mood disorders for clinical practice. *J Clin Psychiatry* 61, 630–637.

Duffy A, Turecki G, Grof P et al. (2000b). Association and linkage studies of candidate genes involved in GABAergic neurotransmission in lithium responsive bipolar disorder. *J Psychiatry Neurosci* 25, 353–358.

Dunner DL, Fleiss JL, Fieve RR (1976). Lithium carbonate prophylaxis failure. *Br J Psychiatry* 129, 40–44.

Engstrom C, Astrom M, Nordqvist-Karlsson B, Adolfsson R, Nylander PO (1997). Relationship between prophylactic effect of lithium therapy and family history of affective disorders. *Biol Psychiatry* 42, 425–433.

Freimer NB, Reus VI, Escamilla MA et al. (1996). Genetic mapping using haplotype, association and linkage methods suggests a locus for severe bipolar disorder (BPI) at 18q22–q23. *Nat Genet* 12, 436–441.

Greil W, Ludwig-Mayerhofer W, Erazo N et al. (1997). Lithium versus carbamazepine in the maintenance treatment of bipolar disorders – a randomised study. *J Affect Disord* 43, 151–161.

Grof P, Alda M (2000). Discrepancies in the efficacy of lithium. *Arch Gen Psychiatry* 57, 191.

Grof P, Alda M, Grof E, Fox D, Cameron P (1993). The challange of predicting response to stabilising lithium treatment. The importance of patient selection. *Br J Psychiatry* 163(Suppl 21), 16–19.

Grof P, Alda M, Grof E, Zvolsky P, Walsh M (1994). Lithium response and genetics of affective disorders. *J Affect Disord* 32, 85–95.

Grof P, Alda M, Ahrens B (1995). Clinical course of affective disorders: were Emil Kraepelin and Jules Angst wrong? *Psychopathology* 28(Suppl 1), 73–80.

Grof P, Duffy A, Cavazzoni P et al. (2000). Is response to prophylactic lithium a familial trait? *Int J Neuropsychopharmacol* 3(Suppl 1), 339–339.

Kim DK, Lim SW, Lee S et al. (2000). Serotonin transporter gene polymorphism and antidepressant response. *Neuroreport* 11, 215–219.

Lipp O, Mahieu B, Souery D et al. (1997). Molecular genetics of bipolar disorders: implication for psychotropic drugs. *Eur Neuropsychopharmacol* 7(Suppl 2), S112–S113.

Lovlie R, Gulbrandsen AK, Molven A, Steen VM (1999). Genomic structure and sequence analysis of a human inositol polyphosphate 1-phosphatase gene (INPP1). *Pharmacogenetics* 9, 517–528.

Maj M, Del Vecchio M, Starace F, Pirozzi R, Kemali D (1984). Prediction of affective psychoses response to lithium prophylaxis: the role of socio-demographic, clinical, psychological and biological variables. *Acta Psychiatr Scand* 69, 37–44.

McKnew DH, Cytryn L, Buchsbaum MS et al. (1981). Lithium in children of lithium-responding parents. *Psychiatry Res* 4, 171–180.

Mendlewicz J (1979). Prediction of treatment outcome: family and twin studies in lithium prophylaxis and the question of lithium red blood cell/plasma ratios. In Cooper TB, Gershon S, Kline NS, Schou M, eds. *Lithium: Controversies and Unresolved Issues.* Amsterdam: Excerpta Medica, pp. 226–240.

Mendlewicz J, Fieve RR, Stallone F (1973). Relationship between the effectiveness of lithium therapy and family history. *Am J Psychiatry* 130, 1011–1013.

Misra PC, Burns BH (1976). "Lithium nonresponders" in a lithium clinic. *Acta Psychiatr Scand* 55, 32–38.

Post RM, Berrettini W, Uhde TW, Kellner C (1984). Selective response to the anticonvulsant carbamazepine in manic-depressive illness: a case study. *J Clin Psychopharmacol* 4, 178–185.

Post RM, Uhde TW, Roy-Byrne PP, Joffe RT (1987). Correlates of antimanic response to carbamazepine. *Psychiatr Res* 21, 71–83.

Prien RF, Caffey EM, Klett CJ (1974). Factors associated with treatment success in lithium carbonate prophylaxis: report of the Veterans Administration and National Institute of Mental Health Collaborative Study Group. *Arch Gen Psychiatry* 31, 189–192.

Schwab SG, Hallmayer J, Lerer B et al. (1998). Support for a chromosome 18p locus conferring susceptibility to functional psychoses in families with schizophrenia, by association and linkage analysis. *Am J Hum Genet* 63, 1139–1152.

Serretti A, Lilli R, Lorenzi C, Franchini L, Smeraldi E (1998). Dopamine receptor D_3 gene and response to lithium prophylaxis in mood disorders. *Int J Neuropsychopharmacol* 1, 125–129.

Serretti A, Lilli R, Lorenzi C, Gasperini M, Smeraldi E (1999a). Tryptophan hydroxylase gene and response to lithium prophylaxis in mood disorders. *J Psychiatr Res* 33, 371–377.

Serretti A, Lilli R, Lorenzi C et al. (1999b). Dopamine receptor D_2 and D_4 genes, GABA(A) alpha-1 subunit genes and response to lithium prophylaxis in mood disorders. *Psychiatry Res* 30, 7–19.

Serretti A, Lorenzi C, Lilli R, Smeraldi E (2000). Serotonin receptor 2A, 2C, 1A genes and response to lithium prophylaxis in mood disorders. *J Psychiatr Res* 34, 89–98.

Shapiro DR, Quitkin FM, Fleiss JL (1989). Response to maintenance therapy in bipolar illness. *Arch Gen Psychiatry* 46, 401–405.

Sjoholt G, Molven A, Lovlie R, Wilcox A, Sikela JM, Steen VM (1997). Genomic structure and chromosomal localization of a human myo-inositol monophosphatase gene (IMPA). *Genomics* 45, 113–122.

Smeraldi E, Petroccione A, Gasperini M, Macciardi F, Orsini A, Kidd KK (1984). Outcomes on lithium treatment as a tool for genetic studies in affective disorders. *J Affect Disord* 6, 139–151.

Smeraldi E, Zanardi R, Benedetti F, Di Bella D, Perez J, Catalano M (1998). Polymorphism within the promoter of the serotonin transporter gene and antidepressant efficacy of fluvoxamine. *Mol Psychiatry* 3, 508–511.

Steen VM, Gulbrandsen AK, Eiken HG, Berle JO (1996). Lack of genetic variation in the coding region of the myo-inositol monophosphatase gene in lithium-treated patients with manic depressive illness. *Pharmacogenetics* 6, 113–116.

Steen VM, Lovlie R, Osher Y, Belmaker RH, Berle JO, Gulbrandsen AK (1998). The polymorphic inositol polyphosphate 1-phosphatase gene as a candidate for pharmacogenetic prediction of lithium-responsive manic-depressive illness. *Pharmacogenetics* 8, 259–268.

Stine OC, Xu J, Koskela R, McMahon FJ et al. (1995). Evidence for linkage of bipolar disorder to chromosome 18 with a parent-of-origin effect. *Am J Hum Genet* 57, 1384–1394.

Strober M, Morrell W, Burroughs J, Lampert C, Danforth H, Freeman R (1988). A family study of bipolar I disorder in adolescence: early onset of symptoms linked to increased familial loading and lithium resistance. *J Affect Disord* 15, 255–268.

Svestka J (1979). Therapy and prophylaxis of manic-depressive psychosis with lithium carbonate, with respect to possibility of prediction of the therapeutic result. *Acta Facult Med Uni Brunensis* 65, 25–102.

Svestka J, Nahunek K (1975). The results of lithium therapy in acute phases of affective psychoses and some other prognosticator factors of lithium prophylaxis. *Activ Nerv Super* (*Praha*) 17, 270–272.

Turecki G, Alda M, Grof P et al. (1996). No association between chromosome-18 markers and lithium responsive affective disorders. *Psychiatry Res* 63, 17–23.

Turecki G, Grof P, Cavazzoni P et al. (1998). Evidence for a role of phospholipase C-gamma1 in the pathogenesis of bipolar disorder. *Mol Psychiatry* 3, 534–538.

Turecki G, Grof P, Cavazzoni P et al. (1999a). MAO-A: association and linkage studies with lithium responsive bipolar disorder. *Psychiatr Genet* 9, 13–16.

Turecki G, Grof P, Cavazzoni P et al. (1999b). Lithium responsive bipolar disorder, unilineality, and chromosome 18: A linkage study. *Am J Med Genet* (*Neuropsychiatr Genet*) 88, 411–415.

Turecki G, Alda M, Grof P et al. (1999c). Expanded polyglutamine tracts: no evidence of a major role in bipolar disorder. *Mol Psychiatry* 4, 220–222.

Turecki G, Alda M, Grof P et al. (2000). Polyglutamine coding genes in bipolar disorder. Lack of association with selected candidate loci. *J Affect Disord* 53, 63–68.

Turecki G, Grof P, Grof E et al. (2001). Mapping susceptibility genes for bipolar disorder: a pharmacogenetic approach based on excellent response to lithium. *Mol Psychiatry* 6, 570–578.

Youngerman J, Canino I (1978). Lithium carbonate use in children and adolescents. A survey of the literature. *Arch Gen Psychiatry* 35, 216–224.

Zanardi R, Benedetti F, Di Bella D, Catalano M, Smeraldi E (2000). Efficacy of paroxetine in depression is influenced by a functional polymorphism within the promoter of the serotonin transporter gene. *J Clin Psychopharmacol* 20, 105–107.

Zvolsky P, Vinarova E, Dostal T, Soucek K (1974). Family history of manic-depressive and endogenous depressive patients and clinical effect of treatment with lithium. *Activ Nerv Super* 16, 194–195.

Zvolsky P, Dvorakova M, Soucek K, Vinarova E, Dostal T (1979). Clinical use of lithium salts from the genetic viewpoint. In Cooper TB, Gershon S, Kline NS, Schou M, eds. *Lithium: Controversies and Unresolved Issues*. Amsterdam: Excerpta Medica, pp. 152–154.

16

Genetic influences on responsiveness to anticonvulsant drugs

Thomas N. Ferraro

Center for Neurobiology and Behavior, Department of Psychiatry, University of Pennsylvania, Philadelphia, USA

OVERVIEW

This chapter addresses pharmacogenetic issues associated with the clinical use of anticonvulsant drugs (ACDs). Individual variability in responsiveness has been documented for nearly all ACDs in common use and current perspectives suggest that genes play a significant causal role. Variation in the DNA sequence of genes that encode drug-metabolizing enzymes is a major factor contributing to differences in drug responsiveness, and several important polymorphisms have been documented to affect the disposition of ACDs, particularly, the influence of *CYP2C9* and *CYP2C19* on metabolism of phenytoin and mephenytoin, respectively. Although the metabolism of other ACDs may also involve polymorphisms producing CYP isoforms, additional studies are needed to determine if these polymorphisms affect pharmacokinetics. A much greater need, however, is for studies that focus on gene variations that encode target proteins against which ACDs act. Studies that relate genetic variation to ACD pharmacodynamics will provide insight into specific gene sequences and protein structures that are most important for drug action. Additionally, this experimental strategy will have the potential of identifying previously unknown drug targets and mechanisms of action. Together, information on genetic contribution to ACD pharmacokinetics and pharmacodynamics will enable more successful and less complicated use of this class of drugs.

Introduction

Clinical experience has documented that patients with epilepsy respond in different ways to standard ACDs. Individuals with similar seizure disorders based on diagnostic criteria exhibit variable responses to the same medication, with some patients deriving significant benefit and others none at all. Additionally, up to one third of patients with epilepsy are refractory to all drug therapies (Porter and Rogawski, 1992; Jallon, 1997; Loscher, 1997). The increasing trend involving use of ACDs for treatment of affective disorders, most notably bipolar disorder (Denicoff, et al., 1997; Mishory et al., 2000; Vasudev et al., 2000), will likely result in similar observations in those patient populations. Thus, understanding individual differences in response to ACDs has many important clinical ramifications.

A consequence of large interindividual differences in responsiveness to ACDs is that it has been difficult to generate standardized treatment regimens even for clinically well-defined epilepsy subtypes. The development of new ACDs is particularly problematic since the least ACD-responsive patients are included in clinical trials. Individual differences in adverse side effects are a major factor influencing the evaluation of new drugs and greatly complicate standardized therapy. Individual variability in response to therapeutic agents has many causes, both genetic and environmental. Until recently, however, attempts to understand failure of drug treatment in epilepsy had been focused almost exclusively on environmental variables such as dosing regimens, drug interactions, and dietary factors. Advances in molecular genetic analysis during the 1990s now provide the means to begin to shift focus to identify genetic factors that influence ACD therapy (Evans and Relling, 1999).

The nature of genetic variation

There are a number of different kinds of natural genetic variation that result in functional protein differences and affect drug responsiveness. The type of variation that is most prevalent in the genome and, arguably, the most relevant to common diseases and complex traits is represented by single nucleotide polymorphisms (SNPs) (Kleyn and Vessell, 1998). SNPs are single base substitutions in a given DNA sequence and are estimated to occur every 500–1000 bases throughout the genome (Johnson and Todd, 2000; McCarthy and Hilfiker, 2000). Protein diversity that extends from SNPs can take the form of single amino acid differences, termed "missense mutations" if the base change occurs within the sequence of a gene exon. Such missense mutations can result in a protein product that exhibits a gain or loss of function. SNPs may also introduce premature stop codons and eliminate functional protein product. Because of the redundancy of the genetic code, many SNPs are masked at the protein level. They are sometimes referred to as "silent mutations." Noncoding sequences help to govern exon splicing, rate of transcription, and mRNA stability (Lewin, 2000). SNPs that occur in noncoding regions can give rise to different amounts of proteins with altered structures and levels of functional activity. While gross mutations such as inversions, translocations, deletions, or insertions can have dramatic functional consequences, careful analysis of SNPs may be the most likely path to advances in pharmacogenomics and a greater understanding of the genetic basis of individual variability in drug responsiveness (Kleyn and Vessell, 1998).

Genetic variability and drug responsiveness

There are many ways in which genetic variability, the differences in the sequence of specific genes, can lead to variability in drug responsiveness and it is likely that each of these mechanisms is involved in determining the effects of ACDs. Up to now, the focus of pharmacogenetic studies has been on "polymorphic drug metabolism" (Lin et al., 1996; Kalow, 1997). This line of research examines variations in the sequence of genes that code for drug-metabolizing enzymes. SNPs have been found to underlie variability in drug-metabolizing capacity and such variability is often documented as differences in drug and metabolite profiles between patients. It is likely that variation in genes coding for proteins involved in other pharmacokinetic processes, including drug absorption, distribution, and excretion, also help to determine individual differences in responsiveness although these mechanisms are not as well studied regarding genetic influences.

Another way in which genetic variation plays a role in drug responses depends upon polymorphisms in genes that code for proteins that are drug targets or that mediate drug action. For example, if the drug target is a neurotransmitter receptor, it can be hypothesized that subtle differences in the amino acid sequence of the proteins that make up the receptor could give rise to important functional differences that affect response. These differences in response apply both to therapeutic effects and adverse effects so that both efficacy and toxicity may be influenced by individual genetic variation. In the future, pharmacogenetic discoveries related to ACDs will make individualization of therapy even more difficult in the sense that the genetic substrate that mediates efficacy may well differ from that which mediates toxicity. As such, two different sets of genes and genotypes will need to be examined in order to match patients with the most appropriate ACD.

In addition to natural variation in the genes that code for primary drug targets or molecules involved in pharmacokinetic processes, another way that genes can affect response to therapy is related to the underlying genetic predisposition to the disease itself. Such is the case in a syndrome called autosomal dominant nocturnal frontal lobe epilepsy, where disease-causing mutations in genes for nicotinic acetylcholine receptor subunits can be demonstrated to yield receptors that are abnormally sensitive to the electrophysiological effects of the drug carbamazepine (Picard et al., 1999). Thus, natural variation in genes that predispose to common forms of epilepsy could also have an influence on the response to ACDs.

Genetic influences on the pharmacology of anticonvulsant drugs

Although it has expanded during the 1990s, the list of drugs used in clinical practice for the treatment of epilepsy is relatively small. This section first presents general comments relevant to the mechanisms of action of conventional classes of ACD and then addresses how these mechanisms are potentially influenced by genetic variation. Subsequently, commonly used drugs are discussed individually in some depth relative to genes that may affect various aspects of their pharmacology, including metabolism.

Among the nonsedating standard ACDs, those most frequently prescribed are phenytoin, carbamazepine, and valproic acid with the depressant drugs phenobarbital and clonazepam also being in common use (McNamara, 1996; Cafiero and Verdone, 1997). Standard ACDs suppress seizure activity in one of three ways: blockade of voltage-dependent sodium channels, blockade of T-type calcium channels, and/or potentiation of α-aminobutyric acid (GABA)-mediated postsynaptic inhibition with increased chloride influx (MacDonald and Kelly, 1993). Frequently, ACDs are shown to have more than one cellular action and there can be uncertainty regarding which actions are most relevant to observed anticonvulsant effects.

It is well documented that barbiturates and benzodiazepines facilitate chloride influx into neurons by virtue of specific allosteric binding sites on GABA-A receptors (MacDonald and Kelly, 1993). GABA-A subunits vary in their ability to bind ACDs such that recombinant receptors comprising only α- and β-subunits respond to barbiturates but not benzodiazepines, which require the presence of a γ-subunit (Mehta and Ticku, 1999; see also Ch. 15). Subtypes of each subunit are encoded by related genes with differing degrees of homology, underscoring the potential influence of genetic variability on overall receptor function since GABA-A receptors comprise multiple subunits (Whiting, 1999). Some of these genes have already been shown to harbor functional SNPs (Cheng et al., 1997; Iwata et al., 2000). Thus, the effect of genetic variability on drug responsiveness is potentially very great. Polymorphisms of α- and β-subunits of GABA-A receptors may alter responsiveness to barbiturates, whereas genetic variation in γ-subunits might be predicted to have the greatest impact upon responsiveness to benzodiazepines.

In general, traditional nonsedating ACDs such as phenytoin, carbamazepine, and valproic acid are thought to produce anticonvulsant effects by virtue of their ability to stabilize the inactive form of sodium channels in a voltage-dependent fashion. This action likely underlies the ability of these drugs to block sodium channels in vitro and to block sustained high-frequency action potential firing in vivo (MacDonald and Kelly, 1993). Sodium channels are multimeric complexes encoded by multiple genes. Again, the large number of polymorphisms already discovered in sodium channel genes (Ludwig et al., 1998; Persu et al., 1999; Xu et al., 1999; Moulard et al., 2000) suggests that these molecules may have a role to play in determining individual differences in response to certain ACDs. Future studies will be aimed at correlating responsiveness in phenytoin- and carbamazepine-treated patients with specific genotypes and haplotypes associated with these candidate genes. The actions of valproic acid may be even more varied than those of phenytoin and carbamazepine, including an ability to block calcium channels (Kelly et al., 1990) and interfere with GABA metabolism (Johanessen, 2000). Therefore the potential sources of genetic variability for responsiveness to this agent are increased in number.

In addition to the conventional ACDs described above, compounds exist with mechanisms of action that either differ from standard drugs or are not yet fully characterized. These compounds and their mechanisms will lead eventually to the investigation of specific, possibly novel, genes in relation to drug responsiveness. Gamma-vinyl-GABA potentiates GABAergic transmission through its ability to inactivate irreversibly the GABA degradative enzyme, GABA transaminase (Jung and Palfreyman, 1995). Therefore, the gene that codes for this enzyme would be a logical candidate for influencing responsiveness to this agent. There are a number of drugs still in the process of gaining wide acceptance and these have been approved mainly for adjunctive therapy of partial and secondary generalized seizures (Bazil and Pedley, 1998) or are still considered investigational. These include compounds such as MK-801, felbamate, gabapentin, lamotrigine, topiramate, tiagabine, retigabine, neurontin, zarontin, and riluzole. Since the mechanisms of action of these drugs have been studied less well (MacDonald and Kelly, 1993; Ikeda et al., 1998), candidate genes that may influence individual responsiveness to them are less well defined. As these drugs gain clinical acceptance and become more widely used, greater interest will be generated in determining genetic influences on patient responsiveness.

Hydantoins

A major polymorphism of oxidative metabolism in humans involves hydroxylation of the anticonvulsant drug mephenytoin. This racemic drug is metabolized in a highly stereospecific manner whereby the (s)-enantiomer undergoes rapid and complete oxidation to a p-hydroxylated derivative and the (R)-enantiomer is subject to a much slower pathway involving N-demethylation to an active metabolite 5-phenyl-5-ethylhydantoin (Guttendorf and Wedlund, 1992). Early pharmacokinetic studies uncovered a familial concurrence of poor hydroxylation capacity, and subsequent population and family studies revealed autosomal recessive inheritance patterns (Kupfer and Preisig, 1984; Wedlund et al., 1984). Lacking the capacity for p-hydroxylation of mephenytoin, poor metabolizers detoxify both enantiomers via N-demethylation, leading to very high 5-phenyl-5-ethylhydantoin levels and exaggerated or toxic responses (Kupfer et al., 1984; Ninomiya et al., 2000). Molecular studies have led to the discovery of CYP2C19 as the P-450 isoform responsible for the stereoselective hydroxylation of mephenytoin (Wrighton et al., 1993; Goldstein et al., 1994; Watanabe et al., 1998) and, further, have uncovered several mutations that lead to the formation of a defective protein and that result in the poor metabolizer phenotype (de Morais et al., 1994; Ferguson et al., 1998; Ibeanu et al., 1998a,b, 1999). There is significant ethnic diversity in the frequency of these polymorphisms, with the poor metabolizer phenotype observed in 2–5% of Caucasian populations from North America and Europe (Kupfer and Preisig, 1984; Wedlund et al., 1984; Goldstein et al., 1997) and in 18–23% of populations from Japan and China (Horai et al., 1989; Goldstein et al., 1997; Xie, 2000). Individuals of other ethnic backgrounds are also characterized by specific *CYP2C19* allele frequencies (Goldstein et al., 1997; Herrlin et al., 1998; Bathum et al., 1999; Xie et al., 1999). Even though substantial progress has been made in identifying the relationship between *CYP2C19* genetics and effects of mephenytoin, the sequence variants discovered so far do not explain all of the individual variability seen clinically, suggesting that other factors exist which influence responsiveness to this drug.

Other drugs that bind to the mephenytoin *p*-hydroxylase isoenzyme include diazepam, flurazepam, and phenytoin, and drugs with metabolism that cosegregates with that of mephenytoin, include mephobarbital, hexobarbital, and diazepam (Inaba et al., 1985). Deficient *p*-hydroxylation of phenytoin has been observed in a small percentage of the population and appears to run in families (Clark, 1985); however, the major P-450 isoform involved in the *p*-hydroxylation of phenytoin is CYP2C9, with CYP2C19 serving a secondary role (Levy, 1995; Hashimoto et al., 1996). The poor metabolizer phenotype is associated with increased phenytoin-induced toxicity, also a familial trait (Gennis et al., 1991), whereas hypermetabolism results in treatment failure (Lebrun and Villeneuve, 1983), indicating that beneficial therapeutic effects as well as adverse effects are significantly influenced by genetic factors. CYP2C9 harbors a conservative Ile359Leu polymorphism, which dramatically alters metabolism of phenytoin (Hashimoto et al., 1996; Takanashi et al., 2000) as well as a more radical but less functionally important Arg144Cys polymorphism (Mamiya et al., 1998). The prevalence of these polymorphisms vary with ethnicity (Bertilsson, 1995) and as a result many studies have focused on identifying polymorphism frequencies in specific populations (Mamiya et al., 1998; Aynacioglu et al., 1999; Bathum et al., 1999) since such data are useful and important for establishing treatment guidelines for individuals of specific ethnic backgrounds. The metabolizing capacity of the CYP2C9 system exhibits a gene dosage effect that distinguishes individuals homozygous for the wild-type allele from those that are heterozygous (Hashimoto et al., 1996). Again, while genetic variation leading to polymorphic metabolism has helped to elucidate the basis of individual differences in response to phenytoin, a significant amount of unexplained response variability still exists.

In order to address residual, nonmetabolic variation in responsiveness to phenytoin, strategies are required that focus on pharmacodynamic aspects of drug action and the potential genetically based variability in cellular targets related to therapeutic effects. Such strategies can be fueled efficiently by studying the sequences of genes with products that are known targets, such as sodium channel genes in the case of phenytoin. The next generation of studies will take advantage of DNA sequence polymorphisms that have already been reported for sodium channel genes (Ludwig et al., 1998; Persu et al., 1999; Xu et al., 1999; Moulard et al., 2000) as well as the many more that will doubtless be identified in the future. Comparison of allele frequencies between carefully matched groups of phenytoin-responsive and phenytoin-unresponsive patients can yield statistical evidence for significant effects of specific genes and specific sequence variants within those genes. This candidate gene approach is useful when the intended drug targets are known; however, a limitation of this strategy is the possibility that the primary endogenous substrate of drug action has not been unequivocally identified. For example, although phenytoin interacts directly with sodium channels (MacDonald and Kelly, 1993), there is evidence that it also interacts with Na^+/K^+-ATPase (Guillaume, 1988). It is possible that other as yet unknown targets for this drug also exist. In such cases, alternative gene identification strategies are required.

Studies using experimental animals offer a means of studying further relevant genes identified in humans and also provide strategies for identifying genes for new or previously unknown drug target molecules. An approach that represents a powerful tool in this regard is called quantitative trait locus (QTL) mapping. One strategy for QTL mapping involves cross-breeding two strains of an organism that have divergent or opposite phenotypes for a given trait and using their second generation progeny to map the location of genes that contribute to the phenotype through phenotype–genotype correlational analysis (Lander and Botstein, 1989), with the ultimate goal being gene identification. QTL studies of pharmacogenetic relevance can be facilitated by exploiting strain differences in responsiveness to specific drugs (Ferraro and Berrettini, 1996). In terms of ACDs, one line of previous work has focused on mapping genes influencing sensitivity or resistance to specific toxic effects, particularly those associated with fetal abnormalities. Strain differences in sensitivity to craniofacial malformation have been reported in mice exposed to phenytoin in utero (Hansen and Hodes, 1983; Brown et al., 1985) and have facilitated mapping genes related to this trait (Karolyi et al., 1990). Although no genes have yet been identified, refined mapping and phenotyping procedures have determined that there may be different genetic influences involved in the craniofacial endophenotypes cleft lip and cleft palate (Diehl and Erickson, 1997).

There is a paucity of published work regarding genetic influences on the pharmacodynamic actions of ACDs relative to their therapeutic effects, although one interesting line of research involves the development of phenytoin-sensitive and phenytoin-resistant strains of rats (Loscher and Rundfeldt, 1991). These experiments were extended to show that rats selectively bred for extreme sensitivity or resistance to phenytoin suppression of amygdala-kindled seizures respond in a correlated fashion to valproate and phenobarbital (Loscher et al., 1993), suggesting that similar genetic influences underlie responsiveness to ACDs with presumably different mechanisms of anticonvulsant action. More recent work has investigated the responsiveness of a variety of inbred strains of rats to phenytoin (Cramer et al., 1998), which will facilitate gene mapping.

Carbamazepine

Apart from the hydantoin-derived ACDs, other commonly prescribed nonsedating drugs are less well studied regarding metabolic polymorphisms. Carbamazepine conversion to its primary metabolite, carbamazepine-10,11-epoxide, has been shown to be mediated primarily by the CYP3A4 isoform (Kerr et al., 1994; Levy, 1995) although some biotransformation has been documented by CYP2C8 as well (Kerr et al., 1994). Idiosyncratic hypersensitivity reactions to carbamazepine are relatively common (McNamara, 1996); however, no data are available for review regarding associations between polymorphisms in P-450 isoforms and ability to metabolize carbamazepine. Nonetheless, several polymorphisms are indeed found in *CYP3A4*. One occurs in the 5′ promoter region (Rebbeck et al., 1998; Westlind et al., 1999) and its frequency exhibits a striking ethnic specificity as it is especially prevalent in individuals of African descent (Ball et al., 1999). This variation does not appear to play a major role in determining constitutive *CYP3A4* expression, however (Ball et al., 1999), and thus it may not significantly influence metabolism of phenytoin. Two other *CYP3A4* alleles have been reported but they are very rare. Both are missense mutations, giving rise to Ser222Pro and Met445Thr (Sata et al., 2000), and thus have the potential to be functionally relevant. It is currently unknown whether these polymorphisms affect carbamazepine metabolism. Genetic influences on clinically relevant adverse effects of carbamazepine are documented in a report of an idiosyncratic hypersensitivity reaction in a pair of identical twins with primary generalized epilepsy (Edwards et al., 1999). Aplastic anemia is a clincally significant adverse effect of carbamazepine therapy, which may be related to the action of myeloperoxidase and formation of the 9-acridine carboxaldehyde metabolite (Uetrecht, 1990). To-date, however, no studies have examined the role of this or other genes that affect carbamazepine metabolism and the ability of this drug to induce aplastic anemia, although some evidence suggests that such an approach might prove useful (Gerson et al., 1983).

The paradigm shift towards identifying genes involved in therapeutic response of ACDs as opposed to polymorphic metabolism is represented by a recent study in which a mutated gene for a nicotinic receptor subunit associated with a rare form of epilepsy (Steinlein et al., 1995) was expressed in *Xenopus* oocytes. It was shown that mutant receptors had acetylcholine-induced responses similar to wild-type cells but that mutants were three times more sensitive to inhibition by carbamazepine (Picard et al., 1999). This study indicates the importance of elucidating underlying genetic basis of disease when focusing on pharmacogenetic aspects of drug action.

Studies relevant to the pharmacogenetics of carbamazepine that involve experimental animals are somewhat scarce. In one study, testing of three different rat strains showed that anticonvulsant effects of carbamazepine were strain dependent and correlated with drug levels (Graumlich et al., 1999). These data suggest that strain-specific pharmacokinetic processes may account for observed differences in response and, as such, they may be less useful regarding application to human research. In another study, ability of carbamazepine to suppress cocaine-induced seizures was tested in three strains of mice; however, all strains exhibited similar responsiveness (Marley et al., 1993), offering no interesting leads for gene mapping.

Valproic acid

Studies related to genetic influences on the effects of valproic acid are not abundant, particularly in humans. As with other ACDs, considerable inconsistencies between dose and serum concentration of valproic acid have been documented (Tisdale et al., 1992) and it is likely that this phenomenon has a genetic component that impacts individual response to treatment and contributes to unexplained response failures and toxicities (McNamara, 1996). Valproic acid metabolism is complex and the bioconversion process results in formation of a number of oxidative metabolites (Prickett and Baille, 1984), one of which, 2-n-propyl-4-pentenoic acid (4-ene-VPA), is associated with significant clinical hepatotoxicity (Rettie et al., 1987). So far, several P-450 isoforms have been implicated in valproic acid biotransformation including CYP2B and CYP4B (Rogiers et al., 1995; Guan et al., 1998), with some evidence to suggest that the CYP2B1 isoform is responsible for forming a metabolite with hepatotoxic properties (Rogiers et al., 1995). Additionally, other CYP isoforms have been implicated in the formation of 4-ene-VPA including CYP2C9 and CYP2A6 (Sadeque et al., 1997). Most of the isoforms involved in valproic acid metabolism are polymorphic, including the *CYP2B* family with nine alleles (Lang et al., 2001), *CYP2A6* with a loss-of-function missense polymorphism (Yamano et al., 1990) and several deletions (Nunoya et al., 1998; Oscarson et al., 1999), and, as described above, *CYP2C9* with four alleles, each resulting in amino acid substitutions and altered enzyme activity (Rettie et al., 1994; Sullivan-Klose et al., 1996; Imai et al., 2000). In spite of the substantial amount of baseline data in the literature on these *CYP* polymorphisms, no studies have yet attempted to correlate relevant *CYP* genotypes in patients receiving valproic acid with drug blood levels or clinical response.

One line of study on pharmacodynamic issues of valproic acid treatment involves genetic models of neural tube defects in mice. These studies address the mechanism of teratogenic effects observed in valproic acid-exposed human fetuses. Support for a genetic component to valproic acid-induced developmental defects in the nervous system is provided by studies of inbred mouse strains that differ significantly in their sensitivity to defects induced by this drug, and further, by evidence that a close correlation exists between sensitivity to valproic acid-induced and spontaneous neural tube defects (Hall et al., 1997). Studies of sensitive and resistant mouse strains have also identified several provocative candidate genes that might be causally related to the development of valproic acid-induced congenital malformations including the gene for 5,10-methylenetetrahydrofolate reductase (Finnell et al., 1997), *Hox* genes (Faiella et al., 2000), the gene for the r1 subunit of ribonucleotide reductase (Craig et al., 2000), and numerous genes for neurotrophic factors (Bennett et al., 2000). So far, however, no studies that examine the role of these genes have been reported in humans.

Benzodiazepines

A wide variety of benzodiazepine compounds are available to treat neurological and psychiatric disorders, with diazepam and clorazepam being the most common ones used for treating patients with epilepsy (McNamara, 1996). While all benzodiazepines are believed to exert their pharmacological effects by facilitating function of GABA-A receptors (MacDonald and Kelly, 1993), some of them have other actions in the brain (Palmada et al., 1999). Additionally, the pharmacokinetic properties of benzodiazepines vary (Baldessarini, 1996). Therefore, genetic variation potentially can affect response to this class of drug in many ways. Most prominently, these include polymorphisms in genes for both cytochrome P-450 drug-metabolizing enzymes and subunits of GABA-A receptors (see Ch. 15).

Although early evidence suggested that pharmacokinetic parameters of diazepam are not under genetic control (Alda et al., 1987), several polymorphic P-450 isoforms that significantly affect the oxidative metabolism of benzodiazepines have been reported more recently. One study in a Chinese population showed that the G681A nucleotide polymorphism of *CYP2C19* segregated with impaired metabolism of both diazepam and desmethyldiazepam (Qin et al., 1999). Another study, in which European-American and African-American men were given midazolam revealed a modest association between systemic clearance of the drug and a polymorphism (A290G) in the 5′ regulatory region of *CYP3A4* (Wandel et al., 2000). The guanine nucleotide, found only in the African-American group, was associated with a 30% reduction in systemic clearance (Wandel et al., 2000). Studies to evaluate the potential significance of CYP2C and CYP3A polymorphisms on functional parameters of benzodiazepine action are needed.

Molecular studies of GABA receptors have begun to define not only the specific subunits required for benzodiazepine sensitivity (Rudolf et al., 1999) but also the specific amino acid residues that mediate GABA and benzodiazepine binding (Benson et al., 1998; Carlson et al., 2000; Hartvig et al., 2000). At the same time, a number of naturally occurring variations of GABA receptor subunit genes are being identified (Cheng et al., 1997; Iwata et al., 2000) and associations with a variety of central nervous system diseases are being investigated (Sander et al., 1996, 1999; Gade-Adavolu et al., 1998; Serretti et al., 1998; Loh et al., 1999, 2000). So far, however, little information regarding the possible association between GABA receptor subunit gene variation and anticonvulsant responses to benzodiazepines is available. One study investigating the influence of a Pro385Ser (C1236T) variation on the sensitivity of oculomotor responses to diazepam showed that the variant serine residue was associated with significantly less diazepam-induced impairment of saccadic velocity (Iwata et al., 1999). Such results provide impetus to examine potential associations between GABA receptor subunit polymorphisms and therapeutic responses to benzodiazepines.

Contributions of animal studies to the pharmacogenetics of benzodiazepines relevant to their behavioral effects have come primarily from comparisons of inbred strains and from studies of other specialized strains such as knockouts and transgenics. Studies of single-gene mutants can evaluate the effects of a defined genetic polymorphism. For example, deletion of the long splice variant of the gene for the γ_2-subunit of the GABA-A receptor yielded a strain of mice that showed enhanced sleep times with both midazolam and zolpidem (Quinlan et al., 2000), demonstrating the importance of the action and processing of this gene in the regulation of benzodiazepine sensitivity. Studies of the effects of benzodiazepines on inbred strains have been much more common. Strain comparisons are useful because they provide a foundation for subsequent studies to identify the genes involved in mediating specific responses with no preconceived notion as to which genes these might be. Behavioral responses to benzodiazepines are complex traits determined by a mix of environmental and genetic influences (Crabbe et al., 1998). If a specific trait or response to drug has a sufficiently large genetic component, mapping studies can be undertaken to determine the genomic location of the major genes involved; however, once genetic mapping is complete, the identification of specific causative genes remains a major task. The correlation of genotype with complex trait phenotype and the resolution of gene mapping is generally insufficient to reduce the chromosomal interval containing the gene of interest to a size small enough to allow positional cloning even for genes that exert very large effects. Consequently, genetic mapping of complex traits in experimental animals must be followed up by other studies that involve systematic reduction of critical intervals and, ultimately, functional analysis of single genes with rigorous quantification of their phenotypic influence.

The use of selectively bred strains of experimental animals has facilitated study of genetic influences on benzodiazepine-associated traits. A particularly useful resource are lines of mice bred specifically for sensitivity and resistance to the ataxic effects of diazepam (Gallagher et al., 1987; Yoong and Wong, 1988). Some of these lines have generated evidence suggesting that common genetic mechanisms are involved in determining responsiveness to benzodiazepines and to volatile anesthetic compounds such as halothane and enflurane (McCrae et al., 1993). The fact that strain differences may be a result of functional differences in neuronal sensitivity (Quinlan et al., 1993) rather than pharmacokinetics (Gallagher et al., 1987) underscores the importance of identifying the genes that mediate these discordant phenotypes. Identification of such genes could significantly advance the therapeutic use of benzodiazepines. Similarly, genes relevant to the anticonvulsant action of benzodiazepines may be amenable to identification using specially bred "ethanol withdrawal seizure prone" and "ethanol withdrawal seizure resistant" mice, since these respective lines differ with regard to the ability of a wide variety of benzodiazepines and barbiturates to increase electrical seizure threshold (Crabbe et al., 1986, 1993). Wistar rat lines selectively bred for high- and low-anxiety-related behavior also differ in their sensitivities to the pharmacological effects of diazepam (Liebsch et al., 1998) and could also be exploited to identify causative genes.

Common, commercially available strains of experimental animals have also provided useful data regarding genetic control of benzodiazepine effects. Inbred strains of mice have been a particular focus and several reported surveys document significant strain differences in behavioral and physiological responses to a variety of benzodiazepines including diazepam (Crabbe et al., 1998; Garrett et al., 1998; Griebel et al., 2000), phenazepam (Seredenin et al., 1990), alprazolam (Weizman et al., 1999), and midazolam (Homanics et al., 1999). Strain differences in benzodiazepine receptor expression may contribute to these opposite behavioral phenotypes (Hode et al., 2000), although the multifactorial nature of drug responsiveness assures that other mechanisms are also involved. Assuming that drug response traits can be shown to be sufficiently heritable, strain survey data can provide a strong foundation to begin to consider strategies for mapping associated genes.

Barbiturates

Like benzodiazepines, the variety of different barbiturate compounds available for clinical use is associated with a complex pharmacokinetic profile for the drug class as a whole. Regarding their use as anticonvulsants, phenobarbital and mephobarbital have found the widest application (Porter et al., 1984; McNamara, 1996). GABA-A receptors are the main target of barbiturates and facilitation of chloride flux through these receptors is believed to be largely responsible for their pharmacological and therapeutic effects (MacDonald and Kelly, 1993; Hobbs et al., 1996).

Therefore, polymorphism in genes that code for GABA-A receptor subunits is a potentially important source of variation in barbiturate treatment response. Nonetheless, other mechanisms and genes may also be relevant (Steinbach et al., 2000).

As is true for other pharmacological classes, large individual differences in response to the clinical effects of barbiturates have been documented previously (Peck et al., 1976; Nightgale, 1988). Studies in monozygotic and dizygotic twin pairs indicate that the rate of metabolism of amobarbital is under genetic control (Endrenyi et al., 1976), and more recent studies have focused on the role of polymorphic cytochrome P-450 isoforms in barbiturate metabolism. Hydroxylation of hexobarbital was shown to be correlated with hydroxylation of mephenytoin (Kato et al., 1992) but not phenobarbital (Schellens et al., 1990), documenting important kinetic differences between compounds closely related pharmacologically and structurally. The CYP2C isoform family has an integral role in barbiturate metabolism since it influences disposition of hexobarbital (Yasumori et al., 1990; Adedoyin et al., 1994) and phenobarbital (Mamiya et al., 2000). Mephobarbital N-demethylation is mediated by CYP2B6 (Kobayashi et al., 1999). The relationships between polymorphisms in CYP isoforms and patient responsiveness to barbiturates remain to be studied.

Studies relevant to genes that influence the action of barbiturates have been carried out with common inbred strains and selectively bred lines of mice. Mice selectively bred for long sleep time and short sleep time in response to ethanol are resistant and sensitive, respectively, to the hypnotic (sleep-inducing) effects of thiopental, phenobarbital, and chlordiazepoxide (McIntyre and Alpern, 1986). These results suggest that a subset of genes with alleles that segregated between the two selectively bred lines mediate responses to a range of central nervous system depressants. The concept that a subset of genes influences response to different types of depressant drug is also supported by studies of withdrawal seizures. Results of experiments involving DBA and C57 mice, inbred strains that are sensitive and resistant to experimental seizures, respectively (Engstrom and Woodbury, 1988; Ferraro et al., 1998, 1999), suggest that similar genes underlie sensitivity to seizures induced by withdrawal from ethanol, pentobarbital, and diazepam (Buck et al., 1999; Metten and Crabbe, 1999). Identification of these genes could provide important information relevant to the therapeutic use of barbiturates and benzodiazepines in so far as understanding genetic susceptibility to adverse effects such as physiological dependence will help to refine treatment regimens for individual patients.

The ability of phenobarbital to induce hepatic microsomal enzyme activity is a well-known factor in studies of drug metabolism and can affect the biodisposition and efficacy of other drugs administered concomitantly (Anderson and Levy,

1995). Great interest exists in defining the properties of genes that have their regulation affected by phenobarbital; recent work indicates the importance of specific 5′ promoter sequences (Ramsden et al., 1999). In vitro studies have examined the effect of phenobarbital on the induction of known genes (Runge et al., 2000; Schilter et al., 2000) whereas newer in vivo approaches enable detection of unknown as well as known genes (Garcia-Allen et al., 2000). Once identified, all of these genes can become candidates to be examined with regard to influences of their variation on barbiturate responsiveness.

Miscellaneous drugs

Among drugs with a longer history of use in the treatment of epilepsy, several studies involving the drug acetazolamide are of interest. These include the successful use of this drug in treating two siblings affected with familial hemiplegic migraine and ataxia resulting from a missense mutation in *CACNA1A*, the gene for the calcium channel (Battistini et al., 1999) and another study in which two strains of mice (one sensitive and one resistant) were used to map genetic loci involved in acetazolamide-induced ectrodactyly (Biddle, 1975). In vitro studies on metabolism of trimethadione suggest that N-demethylation of this compound is mediated primarily by CYP2E1 with some participation by CYP2C8 (Kurata et al., 1998). Functional polymorphisms within *CYP2E1* (Hu et al., 1997) suggest one factor that could influence responsiveness to trimethadione.

Studies of pharmacogenetic relevance to newer ACDs are scarce although a strong foundation for future studies is being developed. For instance, recent work documenting that felbamate blockade of NMDA receptors depends on the presence of the NR2B subunit (Harty and Rogawski, 2000) combined with the recent discovery of a silent mutation in the human gene *NR2B* (Nishiguchi et al., 2000) paves the way for studies to examine the effect of this polymorphism in patients treated with felbamate. Similarly, the ACD gabapentin has been shown to bind an $\alpha_2\delta$-subunit of the calcium channel subunit (Wang et al., 1999), and polymorphisms of genes for related calcium channel subunits, *CACNA1A* (Yue et al., 1997) and *CACNL1A2* (Yamada et al., 1995), have been reported. Genes for specific potassium channels, *KCNQ2* and *KCNQ3*, have been identified as a likely target for the novel ACD retigabine (Main et al., 2000; Wickendon et al., 2000). Since a rare inherited form of epilepsy called benign familial neonatal convulsions has been shown to be caused by missense mutations in these genes (Leppert et al., 1989; Lewis et al., 1993), it is possible that epilepsy patients harboring variants of these or related genes would respond in a unique fashion to drugs such as retigabine. Genes for potassium channel subunits have so far proven to be a rich source of functional polymorphisms (Lai et al., 1994; Sakura et al., 1995; Hansen et al., 1997; Derst et al., 1998; Mylona et al., 1998; Laitinen et al., 2000; Sesti et al., 2000; Vaughn et al.,

2000) and it is likely that drugs designed against potassium channel proteins will be differentially effective in their interaction. MK-801, an investigational compound with anticonvulsant properties, has been the subject of several mouse strain surveys regarding its behavioral effects. Strain-dependent effects of MK-801 for a number of phenotypes have been observed including inhibition of electrical seizure threshold (Deutsch et al., 1998), passive avoidance behavior (Cestari et al., 1999), and "popping" behavior (Deutsch et al., 1997).

Conclusions

Pharmacogenetic studies involving ACDs have focused strongly on polymorphic metabolism, and a number of important associations have been uncovered. Nonetheless, substantial unexplained variability in responsiveness of patients to conventional drug treatments remains and it is probable that additional, as yet undiscovered, genetic factors are involved. Future studies will continue to investigate associations between genes relevant to ACD pharmacokinetics and drug blood levels; however, we need to begin to correlate genotypes with more functional measures of ACD activity. We also need more emphasis on possible associations between variations in genes for drug targets and ACD responsiveness. As genetic polymorphism information on these genes becomes available, it will become feasible to carry out studies involving ACD-treated responsive and unresponsive patients. For those newer drugs with unclear modes of therapeutic action, genetic studies must await further elucidation of drug mechanisms before a candidate gene approach is feasible.

When whole genome scans using dense SNP maps become a reality, there will be less need for candidate gene strategies; however, the current state of the art in complex trait genetics involves association analysis requiring candidate genes. Presently, candidate genes for human association studies derive from a knowledge of drug action and kinetics, or may come from animal models. In either case, identification of specific genetic variation that influences a complex trait requires a combined mathematical and biological approach that starts by determining the relationship between a set of genotypes and phenotypes (Olsen et al., 1999). Several different methods of correlating genotype with complex trait phenotypes that have been developed are used for complex trait analysis in humans (Clayton and Jones, 1999; Page and Amos, 1999; Blangero et al., 2000). Studies in animals can yield important information about complex trait genes and can provide gene candidates for human studies (Ferraro and Berrettini, 1996). On the horizon are new strategies involving experimental animals that promise to enhance further gene mapping and identification in complex trait models (Nadeau and Frankel, 2000; Nadeau et al., 2000; Grupe et al., 2001).

In conclusion, it is clear that the future development of pharmacological strategies to treat disorders of the central nervous system will be most successful when these strategies begin to incorporate knowledge of the effects of genetic variation on individual drug responsiveness. In the case of ACDs, it is likely that patients with seizure disorders will be the primary focus of research; however, it will be crucial to extend these studies to patients with affective disorders, particularly bipolar disorder, since there is a continuing increase in the use of ACDs in this population.

Acknowledgements

Sincere thanks to Russell J. Buono, PhD (Department of Psychiatry, University of Pennsylvania, Philadelphia, PA) and James J. Kocsis, PhD (Department of Biochemistry and Molecular Pharmacology, Thomas Jefferson University, Philadelphia, PA) for suggestions, discussion, and critical reading of this manuscript.

REFERENCES

Adedoyin A, Prakash C, O'Shea D, Blair IA, Wilkinson GR (1994). Stereoselective disposition of hexobarbital and its metabolites: relationship to the *S*-mephenytoin polymorphism in Caucasian and Chinese subjects. *Pharmacogenetics* 4, 27–38.

Alda M, Dvorakova M, Posmurova M, Balikova M, Zvolsky P, Filip V (1987). Pharmacogenetic study with diazepam in twins. *Neuropsychobiology* 17, 4–8.

Anderson GD, Levy RH (1995). Phenobarbital: chemistry and biotransformation. In Levy RH, Mattson RH, Meldrum BS, eds. *Antiepileptic Drugs*, 4th edn. New York: Raven Press, pp. 371–377.

Aynacioglu AS, Brockmoller J, Bauer S et al. (1999). Frequency of cytochrome P-450 CYP2C9 variants in a Turkish population and functional relevance for phenytoin. *Br J Clin Pharmacol* 48, 409–415.

Baldessarini RJ (1996). Drugs and the treatment of psychiatric disorders. In Hardman JG, Limbird LE, eds. *The Pharmacological Basis of Therapeutics*, 9th edn. New York: McGraw-Hill, pp. 461–486.

Ball SE, Scatina J, Kao J et al. (1999). Population distribution and effects on drug metabolism of a genetic variant in the 5′ promoter region of CYP3A4. *Clin Pharmacol Ther* 66, 288–294.

Bathum L, Skjelbo E, Mutabingwa TK, Madsen H, Horder M, Brosen K (1999). Phenotypes and genotypes for CYP2D6 and CYP2C19 in a black Tanzanian population. *Br J Clin Pharmacol* 48, 395–401.

Battistini S, Stenirri S, Piatti M et al. (1999). A new *CACNA1A* gene mutation in acetazolamide-responsive familial hemiplegic migraine and ataxia. *Neurology* 53, 38–43.

Bazil CW, Pedley TA (1998). Advances in the medical treatment of epilepsy. *Annu Rev Med* 49, 135–162.

Bennett GD, Wlodarczyk B, Calvin JA, Craig JC, Finnell RH (2000). Valproic acid-induced alterations in growth and neurotrophic factor gene expression in murine embryos. *Reprod Toxicol* 14, 1–11.

Benson JA, Low K, Keist R, Mohler H, Rudolph U (1998). Pharmacology of recombinant gamma-aminobutyric acid A receptors rendered diazepam-insensitive by point-mutated alpha-subunits. *FEBS Lett* 431, 400–404.

Bertilsson L (1995). Geographical/interracial differences in polymorphic drug oxidation. Current state of knowledge of cytochromes P-450 (CYP) 2D6 and 2C19. *Clin Pharmacokinet* 29, 192–209.

Biddle FG (1975). Teratogenesis of acetazolamide in the CBA/J and SWV strains of mice. II. Genetic control of the teratogenic response. *Teratology* 11, 37–46.

Blangero J, Williams JT, Almasy L (2000). Quantitative trait locus mapping using human pedigrees. *Hum Biol* 72, 35–62.

Brown KS, Evans MI, Harne LC (1985). Genetic variation in spontaneous and diphenylhydantoin-induced craniofacial malformations in mice. *J Craniofacial Genet Dev Biol Suppl* 1, 305–312.

Buck K, Metten P, Belknap J, Crabbe J (1999). Quantitative trait loci affecting risk for pentobarbital withdrawal map near alcohol withdrawal loci on mouse chromosomes 1, 4, and 11. *Mamm Genome* 10, 431–437.

Cafiero C, Verdone J (1997). *Epilepsy: A Guide to Living Well*. Boston, MA: Mosby Consumer Health.

Carlson BX, Engblom AC, Kristiansen U, Schousboe A, Olsen RW (2000). A single glycine residue at the entrance to the first membrane-spanning domain of the gamma-aminobutyric acid type A receptor beta(2) subunit affects allosteric sensitivity to GABA and anesthetics. *Mol Pharmacol* 57, 474–484.

Cestari V, Ciamei A, Castellano C (1999). Strain-dependent effects of MK-801 on passive avoidance behaviour in mice: interactions with morphine and immobilization stress. *Psychopharmacology* 146, 144–152.

Cheng AT, Loh EW, Cheng CY, Wang YC, Hsu YP (1997). Polymorphisms and intron sequences flanking the alternatively spliced 8-amino-acid exon of gamma2 subunit gene for GABAA receptors. *Biochem Biophys Res Commun* 238, 683–685.

Clark DWJ (1985). Genetically determined variability in acetylation and oxidation: therapeutic implications. *Drugs* 29, 32–375.

Clayton D, Jones H (1999). Transmission/disequilibrium tests for extended marker haplotypes. *Am J Hum Genet* 65, 1161–1169.

Crabbe JC, Young ER, Tam B, Kosobud A, Belknap JK, Laursen SE (1986). Genetic differences in anticonvulsant sensitivity in mouse lines selectively bred for ethanol withdrawal severity. *J Pharmacol Exp Ther* 239, 154–159.

Crabbe JC, Merrill CM, Belknap JK (1993). Effect of acute alcohol withdrawal on sensitivity to pro- and anticonvulsant treatments in WSP mice. *Alcohol Clin Exp Res* 17, 1233–1239.

Crabbe JC, Gallaher EJ, Cross SJ, Belknap JK (1998). Genetic determinants of sensitivity to diazepam in inbred mice. *Behav Neurosci* 112, 668–677.

Craig JC, Bennett GD, Miranda RC, Mackler SA, Finnell RH (2000). Ribonucleotide reductase subunit R1: a gene conferring sensitivity to valproic acid-induced neural tube defects in mice. *Teratology* 61, 305–313.

Cramer S, Ebert U, Loscher W (1998). Characterization of phenytoin-resistant kindled rats, a new model of drug-resistant partial epilepsy: comparison of inbred strains. *Epilepsia* 39, 1046–1053.

de Morais SM, Wilkinson GR, Blaisdell J, Nakamura K, Meyer UA, Goldstein JA (1994). The major genetic defect responsible for the polymorphism of *S*-mephenytoin metabolism in humans. *J Biol Chem* 269, 15419–15422.

Denicoff KD, Smith-Jackson EE, Bryan AL, Ali SO, Post RM (1997). Valproate prophylaxis in a prospective clinical trial of refractory bipolar disorder. *J Psychiatry* 154, 1456–1458.

Derst C, Doring F, Preisig-Muller R et al. (1998). Partial gene structure and assignment to chromosome 2q37 of the human inwardly rectifying K^+ channel (Kir7.1) gene (*KCNJ13*). *Genomics* 54, 560–563.

Deutsch SI, Rosse RB, Paul SM, Riggs RL, Mastropaolo J (1997). Inbred mouse strains differ in sensitivity to "popping" behavior elicited by MK-801. *Pharmacol Biochem Behav* 57, 315–317.

Deutsch SI, Mastropaolo J, Powell DG, Rosse RB, Bachus SE (1998). Inbred mouse strains differ in their sensitivity to an antiseizure effect of MK-801. *Clin Neuropharmacol* 21, 255–257.

Diehl SR, Erickson RP (1997). Genome scan for teratogen-induced clefting susceptibility loci in the mouse: evidence of both allelic and locus heterogeneity distinguishing cleft lip and cleft palate. *Proc Natl Acad Sci USA* 94, 5231–5236.

Edwards SG, Hubbard V, Aylett S, Wren D (1999). Concordance of primary generalised epilepsy and carbamazepine hypersensitivity in monozygotic twins. *Postgrad Med J* 75, 680–681.

Endrenyi L, Inaba T, Kalow W (1976). Genetic study of amobarbital elimination based on its kinetics in twins. *Clin Pharmacol Ther* 20, 701–714.

Engstrom F, Woodbury DM (1988). Seizure susceptibility in DBA and C57 mice: the effects of various convulsants. *Epilepsia* 29, 389–395.

Evans WE, Relling MV (1999). Pharmacogenomics: translating functional genomics into rational therapeutics. *Science* 286, 487–491.

Faiella A, Wernig M, Consalez GG et al. (2000). A mouse model for valproate teratogenicity: parental effects, homeotic transformations, and altered *Hox* expression. *Hum Mol Genet* 9, 227–236.

Ferraro TN, Berrettini WH (1996). Quantitative trait loci mapping in mouse models of complex behavior. *Cold Spring Harb Symp Quant Biol* 61, 771–781.

Ferraro TN, Golden GT, Snyder R et al. (1998). Genetic influences on electrical seizure threshold. *Brain Res* 813, 207–210.

Ferraro TN, Golden GT, Smith GG et al. (1999). Mapping loci for pentylenetetrazol seizure susceptibility in mice. *J Neurosci* 19, 6733–6739.

Ferguson RJ, de Morais SM, Benhamou S et al. (1998). A new genetic defect in human *CYP2C19*: mutation of the initiation codon is responsible for poor metabolism of *S*-mephenytoin. *J Pharmacol Exp Ther* 284, 356–361.

Finnell RH, Wlodarczyk BC, Craig JC, Piedrahita JA, Bennett GD (1997). Strain-dependent alterations in the expression of folate pathway genes following teratogenic exposure to valproic acid in a mouse model. *Am J Med Genet* 70, 303–311.

Gade-Andavolu R, MacMurray JP, Blake H, Muhleman D, Tourtellotte W, Comings DE (1998). Association between the gamma-aminobutyric acid A3 receptor gene and multiple sclerosis. *Arch Neurol* 55, 513–516.

Gallagher EJ, Hollister LE, Gionet SE, Crabbe JC (1987). Mouse lines selected for genetic differences in diazepam sensitivity. *Psychopharmacology* 93, 25–30.

Garcia-Allan C, Lord PG, Loughlin JM, Orton TC, Sidaway JE (2000). Identification of phenobarbitone-modulated genes in mouse liver by differential display. *J Biochem Mol Toxicol* 14, 65–72.

Garrett KM, Niekrasz I, Haque D, Parker KM, Seale TW (1998). Genotypic differences between C57BL/6 and A inbred mice in anxiolytic and sedative actions of diazepam. *Behav Genet* 28, 125–136.

Gennis MA, Vemuri R, Burns EA, Hill JV, Miller MA, Spielberg SP (1991). Familial occurrence of hypersensitivity to phenytoin. *Am J Med* 91, 631–634.

Gerson WT, Fine DG, Spielberg SP, Sensenbrenner LL (1983). Anticonvulsant-induced aplastic-anemia: increased susceptibility to toxic drug metabolites in vitro. *Blood* 61, 889–893.

Goldstein JA, Faletto MB, Romkes-Sparkes M et al. (1994). Evidence that CYP2C19 is the major (*S*)-mephenytoin 4′-hydroxylase in humans. *Biochemistry* 33, 1743–1752.

Goldstein JA, Ishizaki T, Chiba K et al. (1997). Frequencies of the defective *CYP2C19* alleles responsible for the mephenytoin poor metabolizer phenotype in various Oriental, Caucasian, Saudi Arabian and American black populations. *Pharmacogenetics* 7, 59–64.

Graumlich JF, McLaughlin RG, Birkhahn D et al. (1999). Carbamazepine pharmacokinetics–pharmacodynamics in genetically epilepsy-prone rats. *Eur J Pharmacol* 369, 305–311.

Greibel G, Belzung C, Perrault G, Sanger DJ (2000). Differences in anxiety-related behaviors and in sensitivity to diazepam in inbred and outbred strains of mice. *Psychopharmacology* (*Berl*) 148, 164–170.

Grupe A, Germer S, Usuka J et al. (2001). In silico mapping of complex disease-related traits in mice. *Science* 292, 1915–1918.

Guan X, Fisher MB, Lang DH, Zheng YM, Koop DR, Rettie AE (1998). Cytochrome P-450-dependent desaturation of lauric acid: isoform selectivity and mechanism of formation of 11-dodecenoic acid. *Chem Biol Interact* 110, 103–121.

Guillaume D (1988). Brain cortical ($Na^+ K^+$)-ATPase in epilepsy. A biochemical study in animals and humans. *Acta Neurol Belg* 88, 257–280.

Guttendorf RJ, Wedlund PJ (1992). Genetic aspects of drug disposition and therapeutics. *J Clin Pharmacol* 32, 107–117.

Hall JL, Harris MJ, Juriloff DM (1997). Effect of multifactorial genetic liability to exencephaly on the teratogenic effect of valproic acid in mice. *Teratology* 55, 306–313.

Hansen DK, Hodes ME (1983). Metabolism of phenytoin in teratogenesis-susceptible and -resistant strains of mice. *Drug Metab Dispos* 11, 21–24.

Hansen L, Echwald SM, Hansen T, Urhammer SA, Clausen JO, Pedersen O (1997). Amino acid polymorphisms in the ATP-regulatable inward rectifier Kir6.2 and their relationships to glucose- and tolbutamide-induced insulin secretion, the insulin sensitivity index, and NIDDM. *Diabetes* 46, 508–512.

Hartvig L, Lukensmejer B, Liljefors T, Dekermendjian K (2000). Two conserved arginines in the extracellular N-terminal domain of the GABA(A) receptor alpha(5) subunit are crucial for receptor function. *J Neurochem* 75, 1746–1753.

Harty TP, Rogawski MA (2000). Felbamate block of recombinant *N*-methyl-D-aspartate receptors: selectivity for the NR2B subunit. *Epilepsy Res* 39, 47–55.

Hashimoto Y, Otsuki Y, Odani A et al. (1996). Effect of CYP2C polymorphisms on the pharmacokinetics of phenytoin in Japanese patients with epilepsy. *Biol Pharm Bull* 19, 1103–1105.

Herrlin K, Massele AY, Jande M et al. (1998). Bantu Tanzanians have a decreased capacity to metabolize omeprazole and mephenytoin in relation to their *CYP2C19* genotype. *Clin Pharmacol Ther* 64, 391–401.

Hobbs WR, Rall TW, Verdoorn TA (1996). Hypnotics and sedatives: ethanol. In Hardman JG, Limbird LE, eds. *The Pharmacological Basis of Therapeutics*, 9th edn. New York: McGraw-Hill, pp. 361–396.

Hode Y, Ratomponirina C, Gobaille S, Maitre M, Kopp C, Misslin R (2000). Hypoexpression of benzodiazepine receptors in the amygdala of neophobic BALB/c mice compared to C57BL/6 mice. *Pharmacol Biochem Behav* 65, 35–38.

Homanics GE, Quinlan JJ, Firestone LL (1999). Pharmacologic and behavioral responses of inbred C57BL/6J and 129/SvJ mouse strains. *Pharmacol Biochem Behav* 63, 21–26.

Horai Y, Nakano M, Ishizaki T et al. (1989). Metoprolol and mephenytoin oxidation polymorphisms in Far Eastern Oriental subjects: Japanese vs mainland Chinese. *Clin Pharmacol Ther* 46, 198–207.

Hu Y, Oscarson M, Johansson I et al. (1997). Genetic polymorphism of human *CYP2E1*: characterization of two variant alleles. *Mol Pharmacol* 51, 370–376.

Ibeanu GC, Goldstein JA, Meyer U et al. (1998a). Identification of new human *CYP2C19* alleles (*CYP2C19*6* and *CYP2C19*2B*) in a Caucasian poor metabolizer of mephenytoin. *J Pharmacol Exp Ther* 286, 1490–1495.

Ibeanu GC, Blaisdell J, Ghanayem BI et al. (1998b). An additional defective allele, *CYP2C19*5*, contributes to the *S*-mephenytoin poor metabolizer phenotype in Caucasians. *Pharmacogenetics* 8, 129–135.

Ibeanu GC, Blaisdell J, Ferguson RJ et al. (1999). A novel transversion in the intron 5 donor splice junction of *CYP2C19* and a sequence polymorphism in exon 3 contribute to the poor metabolizer phenotype for the anticonvulsant drug *S*-mephenytoin. *J Pharmacol Exp Ther* 290, 635–640.

Ikeda A, Hattori H, Odani A, Kimura J, Shibasaki H (1998). Gynaecomastia in association with phenytoin and zonisamide in a patient having a CYP2C subfamily mutation. *J Neurol Neurosurg Psychiatry* 65, 803–804.

Imai J, Ieiri I, Mamiya K et al. (2000). Polymorphism of the cytochrome P-450 (CYP) *2C9* gene in Japanese epileptic patients: genetic analysis of the *CYP2C9* locus. *Pharmacogenetics* 10, 85–89.

Inaba T, Jurima M, Mahon WA, Kalow W (1985). In vitro inhibition studies of two isoenzymes of human liver cytochrome P-450. Mephenytoin *p*-hydroxylase and sparteine monooxygenase. *Drug Metab Dispos* 13, 443–448.

Iwata N, Cowley DS, Radel M, Roy-Byrne PP, Goldman D (1999). Relationship between a GABAA alpha 6 Pro385Ser substitution and benzodiazepine sensitivity. *Am J Psychiatry* 156, 1447–1449.

Iwata N, Virkkunen M, Goldman D (2000). Identification of a naturally occurring Pro385–Ser385 substitution in the GABA(A) receptor alpha6 subunit gene in alcoholics and healthy volunteers. *Mol Psychiatry* 5, 316–319.

Jallon P (1997). The problem of intractability: the continuing need for new medical therapies in epilepsy. *Epilepsia* 38(Suppl 9), S37–S42.

Johannessen CU (2000). Mechanisms of action of valproate: a commentatory. *Neurochem Int* 37, 103–110.

Johnson GC, Todd JA (2000). Strategies in complex disease mapping. *Curr Opin Genet Dev* 10, 330–334.

Jung MJ, Palfreyman MG (1995). Vigabatrin: mechanism of action. In Levy RH, Mattson RH, Meldrum BS, eds. *Antiepileptic Drugs*. New York: Raven Press, pp. 903–913.

Kalow W (1997). Pharmacogenetics in biological perspective. *Pharmacol Rev* 49, 369–379.

Karolyi J, Erickson RP, Liu S, Killewald L (1990). Major effects on teratogen-induced facial cleft-ing in mice determined by a single genetic region. *Genetics* 126, 201–205.

Kato R, Yamazoe Y, Yasumori T (1992). Polymorphism in stereoselective hydroxylations of mephenytoin and hexobarbital by Japanese liver samples in relation to cytochrome P-450 human-2 (IIC9). *Xenobiotica* 22, 1083–1092.

Kelly KM, Gross RA, MacDonald RL (1990). Valproic acid selectively reduces the low threshold (T)-type calcium current in rat nodose neurons. *Neurosci Lett* 116, 233–238.

Kerr BM, Thummel KE, Wurden CJ et al. (1994). Human liver carbamazepine metabolism. Role of CYP3A4 and CYP2C8 in 10, 11-epoxide formation. *Biochem Pharmacol* 47, 1969–1979.

Kleyn PW, Vessell ES (1998). Genetic variation as a guide to drug development. *Science* 281, 1820–1821.

Kobayashi K, Abe S, Nakajima M et al. (1999). Role of human CYP2B6 in *S*-mephobarbital N-demethylation. *Drug Metab Dispos* 27, 1429–1433.

Kupfer A, Preisig R (1984). Pharmacogenetics of mephenytoin: a new drug hydroxylation poly-morphism in man. *Eur J Clin Pharmacol* 26, 753–759.

Kupfer A, Desmond P, Patwardhan R (1984). Mephenytoin hydroxylation deficiency: kinetics after repeated doses. *Clin Pharmacol Ther* 35, 33–39.

Kurata N, Nishimura Y, Iwase M et al. (1998). Trimethadione metabolism by human liver cyto-chrome P-450: evidence for the involvement of CYP2E1. *Xenobiotica* 28, 1041–1047.

Lai LP, Deng CL, Moss AJ, Kass RS, Liang CS (1994). Polymorphism of the gene encoding a human minimal potassium ion channel (*minK*). *Gene* 151, 339–340.

Laitinen P, Fodstad H, Piippo K, et al. (2000). Survey of the coding region of the *HERG* gene in long QT syndrome reveals six novel mutations and an amino acid polymorphism with pos-sible phenotypic effects. *Hum Mutat* 15, 580–581.

Lander ES, Botstein D (1989). Mapping Mendelian factors underlying quantitative traits using RFLP linkage maps. *Genetics* 121, 185–199.

Lang T, Klein K, Fischer J et al. (2001). Extensive genetic polymorphism in the human *CYP2B6* gene with impact on expression and function in human liver. *Pharmacogenetics* 11, 399–415.

Lebrun LH, Villeneuve JP (1983). Hypermetabolism of phenytoin as a cause of treatment failure. *Clin Neuropharmacol* 6, 67–70.

Leppert M, Anderson VE, Quattlebaum T et al. (1989). Benign familial neonatal convulsions linked to genetic markers on chromosome 20. *Nature* 337, 647–648.

Levy RH (1995). Cytochrome P-450 enzymes and antiepileptic drug interactions. *Epilepsia* 36(Suppl 5), S8–S13.

Lewin B (2000). *Genes VII*. New York: Oxford University Press.

Lewis TB, Leach RJ, Ward K, O'Connell P, Ryan SG (1993). Genetic heterogeneity in benign familial neonatal convulsions: identification of a new locus on chromosome 8q. *Am J Hum Genet* 53, 670–675.

Liebsch G, Linthorst AC, Neumann ID, Reul JM, Holsboer F, Landgraf R (1998). Behavioral, physiological, and neuroendocrine stress responses and differential sensitivity to diazepam in two Wistar rat lines selectively bred for high- and low-anxiety-related behavior. *Neuropsychopharmacology* 19, 381–396.

Lin KM, Poland RE, Wan YJ, Smith MW, Lesser IM (1996). The evolving science of pharmacogenetics: clinical and ethnic perspectives. *Psychopharmacol Bull* 32, 205–217.

Loh EW, Smith I, Murray R, McLaughlin M, McNulty S, Ball D (1999). Association between variants at the GABAA beta2, GABAA alpha6 and GABAA gamma2 gene cluster and alcohol dependence in a Scottish population. *Mol Psychiatry* 4, 539–544.

Loh EW, Higuchi S, Matsushita S, Murray R, Chen CK, Ball D (2000). Association analysis of the GABA(A) receptor subunit genes cluster on 5q33–34 and alcohol dependence in a Japanese population. *Mol Psychiatry* 5, 301–307.

Loscher W (1997). Animal models of intractable epilepsy. *Prog Neurobiol* 53, 239–258.

Loscher W, Rundfeldt C (1991). Kindling as a model of drug-resistant partial epilepsy: selection of phenytoin-resistant and nonresistant rats. *J Pharmacol Exp Ther* 258, 483–489.

Loscher W, Rundfeldt C, Honack D (1993). Pharmacological characterization of phenytoin-resistant amygdala-kindled rats, a new model of drug-resistant partial epilepsy. *Epilepsy Res* 15, 207–219.

Ludwig M, Bolkenius U, Wickert L, Bidlingmaier F (1998). Common polymorphisms in genes encoding the human mineralocorticoid receptor and the human amiloride-sensitive sodium channel. *J Steroid Biochem Mol Biol* 64, 227–230.

MacDonald RL, Kelly KM (1993). Antiepileptic drug mechanisms of action. *Epilepsia* 34(Suppl 5), S1–S8.

Main MJ, Cryan JE, Dupere JR, Cox B, Clare JJ, Burbidge SA (2000). Modulation of KCNQ2/3 potassium channels by the novel anticonvulsant retigabine. *Mol Pharmacol* 58, 253–262.

Mamiya K, Ieiri I, Shimamoto J et al. (1998). The effects of genetic polymorphisms of *CYP2C9* and *CYP2C19* on phenytoin metabolism in Japanese adult patients with epilepsy: studies in stereoselective hydroxylation and population pharmacokinetics. *Epilepsia* 39, 1317–1323.

Mamiya K, Hadama A, Yukawa E et al. (2000). *CYP2C19* polymorphism effect on phenobarbitone. Pharmacokinetics in Japanese patients with epilepsy: analysis by population pharmacokinetics. *Eur J Clin Pharmacol* 55, 821–825.

Marley RJ, Shimosato K, Frieman M, Goldberg SR (1993). Genetic differences in the time course for the development and persistence of the anticonvulsant effects of carbamazepine against cocaine seizures. *Brain Res* 600, 193–200.

McCarthy JJ, Hilfiker R (2000). The use of single nucleotide polymorphism maps in pharmacogenomics. *Nat Biotechnol* 18, 505–508.

McCrae AF, Gallagher EJ, Winter PM, Firestone LL (1993). Volatile anesthetic requirements differ in mice selectively bred for sensitivity or resistance to diazepam: implications for the site of anesthesia. *Anesth Analg* 76, 1313–1317.

McIntyre TD, Alpern HP (1986). Thiopental, phenobarbital and chlordiazepoxide induce the same differences in narcotic reaction as ethanol in long-sleep and short-sleep selectively bred mice. *Pharmacol Biochem Behav* 24, 895–898.

McNamara JO (1996). Drugs effective in the therapy of the epilepsies. In Hardman JG, Limbird LE eds. *The Pharmacological Basis of Therapeutics*, 9th edn. New York: McGraw-Hill, pp. 461–486.

Mehta AK, Ticku MK (1999). An update on GABAA receptors. *Brain Res Brain Res Rev* 29, 196–217.

Metten P, Crabbe JC (1999). Genetic determinants of severity of acute withdrawal from diazepam in mice: commonality with ethanol and pentobarbital. *Pharmacol Biochem Behav* 63, 473–479.

Mishory A, Yaroslavsky Y, Bersudsky Y, Belmaker RH (2000). Phenytoin as an antimanic anticonvulsant: a controlled study. *Am J Psychiatry* 157, 463–465.

Moulard B, Buresi C, Malafosse A (2000). Study of the voltage-gated sodium channel beta 1 subunit gene (*SCN1B*) in the benign familial infantile convulsions syndrome (BFIC). *Hum Mutat* 16, 139–142.

Mylona P, Gokhale DA, Taylor GM, Sibley CP, (1998). Detection of a high-frequency silent polymorphism (C→T) in the Kir2.1 (*KCNJ2*) inwardly rectifying potassium channel gene by polymerase chain reaction and single strand conformation polymorphism. *Mole Cell Probes* 12, 331–333.

Nadeau JH, Frankel WN (2000). The roads from phenotypic variation to gene discovery: mutagenesis versus QTLs. *Nat Genet* 25, 381–384.

Nadeau JH, Singer JB, Matin A, Lander ES (2000). Analysing complex genetic traits with chromosome substitution strains. *Nat Genet* 24, 221–215.

Nightgale P (1988). A cause of apparent resistance to thiopentone. *Anesthesia* 43, 68.

Ninomiya H, Mamiya K, Matsuo S, Ieiri I, Higuchi S, Tashiro N (2000). Genetic polymorphism of the *CYP2C* subfamily and excessive serum phenytoin concentration with central nervous system intoxication. *Ther Drug Monit* 22, 230–232.

Nishiguchi N, Shirakawa O, Ono H, Hashimoto T, Maeda K (2000). Novel polymorphism in the gene region encoding the carboxyl-terminal intracellular domain of the NMDA - receptor 2B subunit: analysis of association with schizophrenia. *Am J Psychiatry* 157, 1329–1331.

Nunoya K, Yokoi T, Kimura K et al. (1998). A new deleted allele in the human cytochrome *P-450 2A6* (*CYP2A6*) gene found in individuals showing poor metabolic capacity to coumarin and (+)-*cis*-3,5-dimethyl-2-(3-pyridyl)thiazolidin-4-one hydrochloride (SM-12502). *Pharmacogenetics* 8, 239–249.

Olson JM, Witte JS, Elston RC (1999). Genetic mapping of complex traits. *Stat Med* 18, 2961–2981.

Oscarson M, McLellan RA, Gullsten H et al. (1999). Characterisation and PCR-based detection of a *CYP2A6* gene deletion found at a high frequency in a Chinese population. *FEBS Lett* 448, 105–110.

Page GP, Amos CI (1999). Comparison of linkage-disequilibrium methods for localization of genes influencing quantitative traits in humans. *Am J Hum Genet* 64, 1194–1205.

Palmada M, Bohmer C, Centelles JJ, Kinne RK (1999). Effect of benzodiazepines on the epithelial and neuronal high-affinity glutamate transporter EAAC1. *J Neurochem* 73, 2389–2396.

Peck AW, Adams R, Bye C, Wilkinson RT (1976). Residual effects of hypnotic drugs: evidence for individual differences on vigilance. *Psychopharmacologica* 47, 213–216.

Persu A, Coscoy S, Houot AM, Corvol P, Barbry P, Jeunemaitre X (1999). Polymorphisms of the gamma subunit of the epithelial Na$^+$ channel in essential hypertension. *J Hypertens* 17, 639–645.

Picard F, Bertrand S, Steinlein OK, Bertrand D (1999). Mutated nicotinic receptors responsible for autosomal dominant nocturnal frontal lobe epilepsy are more sensitive to carbamazepine. *Epilepsia* 40, 1198–1209.

Porter RJ, Rogawski MA (1992). New antiepileptic drugs: from serendipity to rational discovery. *Epilepsia* 33(Suppl 1), S1–S6.

Porter RJ, Cereghino JJ, Gladding GD et al. (1984). Antiepileptic drug development program. *Cleve Clin Q* 51, 293–305.

Prickett KS, Baillie TA (1984). Metabolism of valproic acid by hepatic microsomal cytochrome P-450. *Biochem Biophys Res Commun* 122, 1166–1173.

Qin XP, Xie HG, Wang W et al. (1999). Effect of the gene dosage of CgammaP2C19 on diazepam metabolism in Chinese subjects. *Clin Pharmacol Ther* 66, 642–646.

Quinlan JJ, Gallagher EJ, Firestone LL (1993). Halothane's effects on GABA-gated chloride flux in mice selectively bred for sensitivity or resistance to diazepam. *Brain Res* 610, 224–228.

Quinlan JJ, Firestone LL, Homanics GE (2000). Mice lacking the long splice variant of the gamma 2 subunit of the GABA(A) receptor are more sensitive to benzodiazepines. *Pharmacol Biochem Behav* 66, 371–374.

Ramsden R, Beck NB, Sommer KM, Omiecinski CJ (1999). Phenobarbital responsiveness conferred by the 5′-flanking region of the rat *CYP2B2* gene in transgenic mice. *Gene* 228, 169–179.

Rebbeck TR, Jaffe JM, Walker AH, Wein AJ, Malkowicz SB (1998). Modification of clinical presentation of prostate tumors by a novel genetic variant in *CYP3A4*. *J Nat Cancer Inst* 90, 1225–1229.

Rettie AE, Rettenmeier AW, Howald WN, Baillie TA (1987). Cytochrome P-450-catalyzed formation of delta 4–VPA, a toxic metabolite of valproic acid. *Science* 235, 890–893.

Rettie AE, Wienkers LC, Gonzalez FJ, Trager WF, Korzekwa KR (1994). Impaired (S)-warfarin metabolism catalysed by the R144C allelic variant of CYP2C9. *Pharmacogenetics* 4, 39–42.

Rettie AE, Haining RL, Bajpai M, Levy RH (1999). A common genetic basis for idiosyncratic toxicity of warfarin and phenytoin. *Epilepsy Res* 35, 253–255.

Rogiers V, Akrawi M, Vercruysse A, Phillips IR, Shephard EA (1995). Effects of the anticonvulsant, valproate, on the expression of components of the cytochrome-P-450-mediated monooxygenase system and glutathione *S*-transferases. *Eur J Biochem* 231, 337–343.

Rudolph U, Crestani F, Benke D et al. (1999). Benzodiazepine actions mediated by specific gamma-aminobutyric acid(A) receptor subtypes. *Nature* 401, 796–800.

Runge D, Kohler C, Kostrubsky VE et al. (2000). Induction of cytochrome P-450 (CYP)1A1, CYP1A2, and CYP3A4 but not of CYP2C9, CYP2C19, multidrug resistance (MDR-1) and multidrug resistance associated protein (MRP-1) by prototypical inducers in human hepatocytes. *Biochem Biophys Res Commun* 273, 333–341.

Sadeque AJM, Fisher MB, Korzekwa KR, Gonzalez FJ, Rettie AE (1997). Human CYP2C9 and CYP2A6 mediate formation of the hepatotoxin 4-ene-valproic acid. *J Pharmacol Exp Ther* 283, 698–703.

Sakura H, Bond C, Warren-Perry M et al. (1995). Characterization and variation of a human inwardly-rectifying-K-channel gene (*KCNJ6*): a putative ATP-sensitive K-channel subunit. *FEBS Lett* 367, 193–197.

Sander T, Hildmann T, Janz D et al. (1996). Exclusion of linkage between idiopathic generalized epilepsies and the GABAA receptor alpha 1 and gamma 2 subunit gene cluster on chromosome 5. *Epilepsy Res* 23, 235–244.

Sander T, Ball D, Murray R et al. (1999). Association analysis of sequence variants of GABA(A) alpha6, beta2, and gamma2 gene cluster and alcohol dependence. *Alcohol Clin Exp Res* 23, 427–431.

Sata F, Sapone A, Elizondo G et al. (2000). *CYP3A4* allelic variants with amino acid substitutions in exons 7 and 12: evidence for an allelic variant with altered catalytic activity. *Clin Pharmacol Ther* 67, 48–56.

Schellens JH, van der Wart JH, Breimer DD (1990). Relationship between mephenytoin oxidation polymorphism and phenytoin, methylphenytoin and phenobarbitone hydroxylation assessed in a phenotyped panel of healthy subjects. *Br J Clin Pharmacol* 29, 665–671.

Schilter B, Andersen MR, Acharya C, Omiecinski CJ (2000). Activation of cytochrome P-450 gene expression in the rat brain by phenobarbital-like inducers. *J Pharmacol Exp Ther* 294, 916–922.

Seredenin SB, Blednov YuA, Badyshtov BA, Gordey ML, Nagovitsina YA (1990). Pharmacogenetic analysis of mechanisms of emotional stress: effects of benzodiazepines. *Ann Ist Super Sanita* 26, 81–87.

Serretti A, Macciardi F, Cusin C et al. (1998). GABAA alpha-1 subunit gene not associated with depressive symptomatology in mood disorders. *Psychiatr Genet* 8, 251–254.

Sesti F, Abbott GW, Wei J et al. (2000). A common polymorphism associated with antibiotic-induced cardiac arrhythmia. *Proc Natl Acad Sci USA* 97, 10613–10618.

Steinbach JH, Bracamontes J, Yu L, Zhang P, Covey DF (2000). Subunit-specific action of an anti-convulsant thiobutyrolactone on recombinant glycine receptors involves a residue in the M2 membrane-spanning region. *Mol Pharmacol* 58, 11–17.

Steinlein OK, Mulley JC, Propping P et al. (1995). A missense mutation in the neuronal nicotinic acetylcholine receptor alpha 4 subunit is associated with autosomal dominant nocturnal frontal lobe epilepsy. *Nat Genet* 11, 201–203.

Sullivan-Klose TH, Ghanayem BI, Bell DA et al. (1996). The role of the CYP2C9 Leu359 allelic variant in the tolbutamide polymorphism. *Pharmacogenetics* 6, 341–349.

Takanashi K, Tainaka H, Kobayashi K, Yasumori T, Hosakawa M, Chiba K (2000). CYP2C9 Ile359 and Leu359 variants: enzyme kinetic study with seven substrates. *Pharmacogenetics* 10, 95–104.

Tisdale JE, Tsuyuki RT, Oles KS, Penry JK (1992). Relationship between serum concentration and dose of valproic acid during monotherapy in adult outpatients. *Ther Drug Monit* 14, 416–423.

Uetrecht J (1990). Drug metabolism by leukocytes and its role in drug-induced lupus and other idiosyncratic drug reactions. *Crit Rev Toxicol* 20, 213–235.

Vasudev K, Goswami U, Kohli K (2000). Carbamazepine and valproate monotherapy: feasibility, relative safety and efficacy, and therapeutic drug monitoring in manic disorder. *Psychopharmacology* 150, 15–23.

Vaughn J, Wolford JK, Prochazka M, Permana PA (2000). Genomic structure and expression of human KCNJ9 (Kir3.3/GIRK3). *Biochem Biophys Res Commun* 274, 302–309.

Wandel C, Witte JS, Hall JM, Stein CM, Wood AJ, Wilkinson GR (2000). CYP3A activity in African American and European American men: population differences and functional effect of the *CYP3A4*1B5'*-promoter region polymorphism. *Clin Pharmacol Ther* 68, 82–91.

Wang M, Offord J, Oxender DL, Su TZ (1999). Structural requirement of the calcium-channel subunit alpha2delta for gabapentin binding. *Biochem J* 342, 313–320.

Watanabe M, Iwahashi K, Kugoh T, Suwaki H (1998). The relationship between phenytoin pharmacokinetics and the *CYP2C19* genotype in Japanese epileptic patients. *Clin Neuropharmacol* 21, 122–126.

Wedlund PJ, Aslanian WS, McAllister CB, Wilkinson GR, Branch RA (1984). Mephenytoin hydroxylation deficiency in Caucasians: frequency of a new oxidative drug metabolism polymorphism. *Clin Pharmacol Ther* 36, 773–780.

Weizman R, Paz L, Backer MM, Amiri Z, Modai I, Pick CG (1999). Mouse strains differ in their sensitivity to alprazolam in the staircase test. *Brain Res* 839, 58–65.

Westlind A, Lofberg L, Tindberg N, Andersson TB, Ingelman-Sundberg M (1999). Interindividual differences in hepatic expression of CYP3A4: relationship to genetic polymorphism in the 5'-upstream regulatory region. *Biochem Biophys Res Commun* 259, 201–205.

Whiting PJ (1999). The GABA-A receptor gene family: new targets for therapeutic intervention. *Neurochem Int* 34, 387–390.

Wickenden AD, Yu W, Zou A, Jegla T, Wagoner PK (2000). Retigabine, a novel anti-convulsant, enhances activation of KCNQ2/Q3 potassium channels. *Mol Pharmacol* 58, 591–600.

Wrighton SA, Stevens JC, Becker GW, van den Branden M (1993). Isolation and characterization of human liver cytochrome P-450 2C19: correlation between 2C19 and *S*-mephenytoin 4'-hydroxylation. *Arch Biochem Biophys* 306, 240–245.

Xie HG (2000). Genetic variations of S-mephenytoin 4′-hydroxylase (CYP2C19) in the Chinese population. *Life Sci* 66, PL175–PL181.

Xie HG, Kim RB, Stein CM, Wilkinson GR, Wood AJ (1999). Genetic polymorphism of (S)-mephenytoin 4′-hydroxylation in populations of African descent. *Br J Clin Pharmacol* 48, 402–408.

Xu X, Niu T, Chen C, Yang J, Fang Z, Xu X (1999). Identification of a novel intron and 4 polymorphisms in the gene encoding the gamma subunit of the epithelial sodium channel. *Hum Biol* 71, 781–789.

Yamada Y, Masuda K, Li Q et al. (1995). The structures of the human calcium channel alpha 1 subunit (*CACNL1A2*) and beta subunit (*CACNLB3*) genes. *Genomics* 27, 312–319.

Yamano S, Tatsuno J, Gonzalez FJ (1990). The *CYP2A3* gene product catalyzes coumarin 7-hydroxylation in human liver microsomes. *Biochemistry* 29, 1322–1329.

Yasumori T, Murayama N, Yamazoe Y, Kato R (1990). Polymorphism in hydroxylation of mephenytoin and hexobarbital stereoisomers in relation to hepatic P-450 human-2. *Clin Pharmacol Ther* 47, 313–322.

Yoong YL, Wong PT (1988). Selective breeding of mice for differential sensitivity to diazepam. *Behav Genet* 18, 185–191.

Yue Q, Jen JC, Nelson SF, Baloh RW (1997). Progressive ataxia due to a missense mutation in a calcium-channel gene. *Am J Hum Genet* 61, 1078–1087.

17

Apolipoprotein E as a marker in the treatment of Alzheimer's disease

Keith Schappert[1], Pierre Sevigny[1], and Judes Poirier[2]

[1]Mirador DNA Design, Montreal, Canada
[2]McGill Centre for Studies of Aging, Douglas Hospital, Verdun, Canada

OVERVIEW

Recent evidence indicates that apolipoprotein E (ApoE) plays a central role in the brain's response to injury. The coordinated expression of ApoE and its receptors (the so-called low density lipoprotein (LDL) receptor family) appears to regulate the transport and internalization of cholesterol and phospholipids during the early phase of the re-innervation process in the adult brain. During dendritic remodeling and synaptogenesis, neurons progressively repress the synthesis of cholesterol in favor of cholesterol internalization through the apoE/LDL receptor pathway. The discovery, a few years ago, that a polymorphism in the gene for ApoE (the *apoE4* allele), found normally in 15% of the general population, is strongly linked to both sporadic and familial late-onset Alzheimer's disease (AD) raised the possibility that a dysfunction of the lipid transport system, associated with compensatory sprouting and synaptic remodeling, could be central to the AD process. The role of ApoE in the central nervous system (CNS) is particularly important in relation to cholinergic system, which relies to a certain extent on the integrity of phospholipid homeostasis in neurons. Recent evidence indicates that *apoE4* allele has a direct impact on cholinergic system activity in the brain as well as on drug efficacy profile in AD subjects treated with cholinomimetic agents. Furthermore, susceptibility factors such as the gene for butyrylcholinesterase, which acts in a synergistic manner to increase the risk of developing sporadic Alzheimer's disease, were shown to modify treatment outcome significantly in patients with mild-to-moderate AD treated with noncholinergic therapies. These results strongly support the notion that ApoE is not only a major risk factor for AD but also a crucial treatment outcome modifier in subjects with mild-to-moderate AD.

Introduction

Pharmacogenetics, the study of the interplay between drug efficacy and genetics, is not characterized by the nature of the chemical entity nor by the biochemistry of the response but by the fact that a response may lack uniformity and that this lack of uniformity has a genetic basis (Kalow and Grant, 1995). Traditionally, pharmacogenetics focused on the interaction between genetic polymorphisms in drug-metabolizing enzymes, drug-transport enzymes, drug response, and toxicity. However, more recently, the science of pharmacogenetics has begun to focus on genetic polymorphisms in drug targets or genes underlying the disease process and the response to therapy (Farlow et al., 1998; Evans and Relling, 1999; Nebert, 1999; Poirier et al., 1999; McCarthy and Hilfiker, 2000; Rioux, 2000; Roses, 2000). This chapter will focus specifically on the pharmacogenetic role of the risk factor gene *apoE* in Alzheimer's disease (AD) and in the response of patients with AD to treatment.

Pharmacogenetics of Alzheimer's disease

AD is a progressive neurodegenerative disease that has a strong genetic basis (Poirier, 1999). The disease is characterized by the progressive loss of memory, onset of dementia, and finally death. It is estimated that by the 2030s, there will be some 8 million patients with AD in the USA alone. The treatment of this disease represents a large financial burden on the health care system, which has been estimated to be in the 100 billion dollar range. In 1993, it was shown that the frequency of a particular polymorphism in the gene for ApoE, the so-called *apoE4* allele, was increased in both sporadic and some forms of familial AD (Noguchi et al., 1993; Poirier et al., 1993; Strittmatter et al., 1993). The initial observations were rapidly confirmed and it is now an established fact that *apoE4* allele is a risk factor for the development of sporadic AD (Lindsay et al., 1997).

ApoE has been extensively studied in non-nervous tissues as one of several proteins that regulate lipid transport and metabolism. ApoE facilitates cholesterol (and phospholipid) transport between different cell types and different organs. It binds to large lipid–protein particles (called lipoproteins). This binding increases the ability of large lipid complexes to transport cholesterol and phospholipids in the blood and cerebrospinal fluid. The mature form of apoE found in human plasma and in the brain is a single glycosylated 37 kDa polypeptide containing 299 amino acid residues. It was shown to coordinate the mobilization and redistribution of cholesterol in repair, growth, and maintenance of myelin and neuronal membranes during development or after sciatic nerve injury (Beffert et al., 1999). In the brain, apoE coordinates the redistribution of cholesterol and phospholipids during membrane remodeling associated with synaptic plasticity and dendritic remodeling (Poirier, 1994). Deletion of apoE in *apoE* knockout mice causes an age-dependent reduction of synaptic contacts in the cortex and a marked impairment of synaptic plasticity (and re-innervation) in the hippocampus, highlighting the crucial role played by apoE in response to brain damage and neuronal cell loss (Poirier, 1994; Arendt et al., 1997, Beffert et al., 1999).

	E4	E3	E2
ALLELE FREQUENCY ON CHROMOSOME 19 IN EASTERN CANADA	0.152	0.770	0.078

	APO E4	APO E3	APO E2
PROTEIN CODED BY EACH ALLELE (APO E IS 299 AMINO ACID RESIDUES LONG)			
– SITE 112	ARG	CYS	CYS
– SITE 158	ARG	ARG	CYS

PHENOTYPES		RELATIVE CHARGE	%	ISOELECTRIC PROFILE
HOMOZYGOTES	E4/4	+2	3.9	
	E3/3	+1	61.8	
	E2/2	0	2.0	
HETEROZYGOTES	E4/3		20.6	
	E4/2		9.8	
	E3/2		2.0	

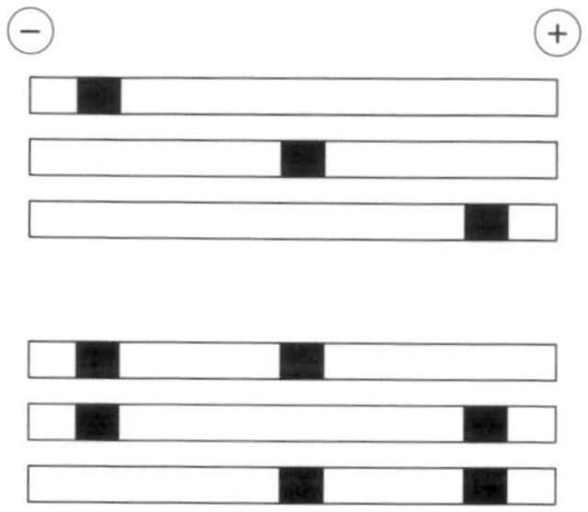

Fig.17.1.   Apolipoprotein E (APO E) polymorphisms, population phenotype distribution, and biochemical properties.

Human ApoE is encoded by a four-exon gene (3.6 kilobases (kb)) on the long arm of chromosome 19 and three major isoforms of ApoE (E4, E3, and E2) differing by a single unit of net charge, which can be easily detected by isoelectrofocusing (Fig. 17.1). These isoforms are expressed from multiple alleles at a single *apoE* genetic locus, giving rise to three common homozygous phenotypes (E4/4, E3/3, and E2/2) and three common heterozygous phenotypes (E4/3, E4/2, and E3/2) (Beffert et al., 1999). Although these different isoforms have been quite well characterized in the periphery, very little is known about the effects of these variants on brain physiology. The strong association between the *apoE4* allele and AD led us to propose that a selective dysfunction of the lipid transport system controlled by ApoE during synaptic remodeling in the CNS could be central to the pathophysiological process that characterizes *apoE4*-carrying subjects with AD (Poirier, 1994). Alternatively, defects in accessory proteins involved in cholesterol homeostasis (such as the ApoE/cholesterol receptors or cholesterol-synthesizing enzymes) could explain some of the key pathophysiological features of subjects with AD who did not carry the *apoE4* allele. The lipid metabolism disturbance theory would also predict that there would be an association between drug response and AD pathology driven by *apoE* genotype. For this chapter, we have divided AD drug therapy into two broad categories, the cholinergic and noncholinergic drugs.

Cholinergic treatments

In 1995, a report was published that retrospectively analyzed the results of an AD clinical trial with the acetylcholinesterase inhibitor tacrine, with respect to each patient's *apoE* genotype (Poirier et al., 1995). Because the majority of a given clinical trial population is not at the extremes of drug response, either extreme or no response, to study this group of patients invites problems in complexity owing to the polygenic nature of a response. Therefore, to reduce the complexity of the genetics of the response and as a means to define an unequivocal phenotype, Poirier and coworkers (1995) chose to analyze the 20 best responders and the 20 worst responders from a group of 202 AD patients that completed a 30-week clinical trial with tacrine. The results indicated that 80% of the non-*apoE4* carriers were responding (demonstrated by a significant improvement in memory tests) to the drug, whereas 50–60% of the *apoE4* carriers were not responding. This study gave the first indication of the possible pharmacogenetic impact of the *apoE* gene in AD treatment and spawned many follow-up studies demonstrating that an individual's *apoE* allele carrier status should be weighted heavily by the physician in treatment.

Farlow and coworkers (1998) published the results of a tacrine trial that involved 528 patients and used an intent-to-treat analysis to examine the effects of tacrine on all the patients as if they had completed the 30-week clinical trial (Fig. 17.2). Overall, the results supported the conclusion of the 1995 Poirier study that showed that the *apoE4* carriers would be less responsive to tacrine treatment than the non-*apoE4* carriers. In addition, Farlow et al. (1998) uncovered a significant gender influence in the response to tacrine. In men, the effect of *apoE* genotype on treatment response was modest, whereas in women the effect was quite strong. Therefore, both *apoE* genotype and gender should be considered when trying to predict a response to tacrine in patients with AD. The influence of apoE on tacrine drug response was yet again confirmed in a study by MacGowan et al. (1998) in which they showed strong indications that apoE genotype affected response to tacrine in the longer term (12 months) as opposed to short term (3 months).

Recently, Farlow and coworkers (1999) published their findings on the influence of *apoE* genotype on the short-term treatment of AD patients with the cholinesterase inhibitor metrifonate. In this study, data from four double-blind placebo-controlled clinical trials were pooled and analyzed retrospectively for the possible interaction between *apoE* genotype and response to metrifonate after 26 weeks for the entire group of 959 patients. The interaction between *apoE* genotype and cognitive performance as measured by the Alzheimer's Disease Assessment Scale–Cognition (ADAS-Cog) score revealed that there was indeed a trend, which did not reach significance for an interaction between *apoE* genotype and treatment effect.

One of the major limitations of studies of the type described in Farlow et al. (1999) is that only a single time point was considered, as often this is the only type

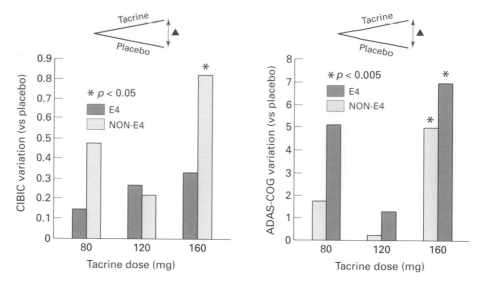

Fig. 17.2. The effect of the apolipoprotein E allele copy number (carrying *apoE4* (E4) or not (NON-E4)) on tacrine drug responsiveness in subjects with Alzheimer's disease. A group of 202 enrolled in a 30 week randomized controlled trial of high-dose tacrine in patients with Alzheimer's disease were selected out of the original 663 cohort. Patients were selected prior to ApoE phenotype determination and blind to genotype. All subjects had completed the study. Phenotypic determination of the *apoE* genotype was performed using frozen serum using the method of Poirier et al. (1993). The graphs represent the group variation using the Clinical Interview-based Impression of Change (CIBIC) score and the Alzheimer's Disease Assessment Scale – Cognition (ADAS-COG) score.

of information that is available for analysis. Very fortunately, we have been able to get access to a 4-year trial of metrifonate and thus have had the rare opportunity of assessing the pharmacogenetic potential of ApoE over an extended period of time. The effects of *apoE* genotype on the response to long-term treatment (240 weeks) was examined in patients with AD and treated with metrifonate, using the Mini-Mental Status Examination (MMSE) as cognitive performance indicator, (Poirier, 1999). In this study, a cohort of AD patients, all under treatment with metrifonate, were retrospectively analyzed for the influence of *apoE* genotype on drug response. The results showed that after 26 weeks of treatment there was no significant difference between the *apoE4* and non-*apE4* carriers. These results are completely consistent with those obtained by Farlow et al. (1999) in their study described above. However, during the longer-term examination of the patients' responses, a difference began to be apparent between the two groups at about 120 weeks, with the difference in response becoming more pronounced as time progressed. After 240 weeks of treatment, there was a clear separation between the two groups and the

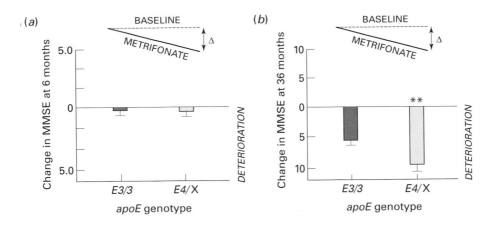

Fig. 17.3.   Variation in Mini Mental State Examination (MMSE) scores in patients with mild-to-moderate Alzheimer's disease treated with metrifonate. Bars represent variations in MMSE scores at 6 (*a*) and 36 (*b*) months compared with baseline values at time zero. Paired t-tests were used to contrast changes over time (** $p < 0.02$). Apolipoprotein E genotype was determined phenotypically by the method of Poirier et al. (1993) and was either E3/3 or E4/X.

non-*apoE4* carriers were the best responders. These results show that *apoE* genotype is affecting the metrifonate response and/or disease progression in a manner that is consistent with reduced disease progression (Fig. 17.3). It also illustrates the limitations in using time periods of less than a year in clinical trials vulnerable to the pharmacogenetic influence of ApoE. However, the long-term study also had limitations, which included the fact that only one cognitive scale (MMSE) was available for the entire duration of the study and that the drop out rate increased over the course of long treatment as an individual patient's condition deteriorated, with the result that only a proportion of the patients were able to reach the 4 year time point.

Riekkinen and coworkers (1998) studied the effects of a single administration of tacrine on electrophysiological parameters associated with memory function in patients with AD. They showed that tacrine responders had a lower frequency of the *apoE4* allele than nonresponders, supporting previous clinical evidence of a role for *apoE* genotype in tacrine drug response. The results suggest that there is a striking difference in the underlying cholinergic pathology between those patients with AD who carry the *apoE4* allele and those who do not.

In contrast to the above mentioned results with tacrine, Oddoze and workers (1998) published the results of a 6-month drug trial with 102 French patients suffering from mild-to-moderate AD disease in which they demonstrate that responders to tacrine, as measured by change in MMSE, were those individuals carrying the *apoE4* allele. The stark contrast between the results of this study and the others conducted with cholinesterase inhibitors is intriguing. However, the consistency of the studies with several cholinesterase inhibitors described above makes it likely that at least one factor, sampling bias, was responsible for the conflicting results described by Oddoze and coworkers. Sampling bias is an important factor that influences genetic studies. It is possible that, by chance, the Oddoze study picked an over-representation of *apoE4* carriers that are responders. There was also an over-representation of female subjects in the study.

Only a few studies reported on the pharmacogenetic impact of *apoE* genotype on the response of AD patients to another type of acetylcholinesterase inhibitor, galantamine (MacGowan et al., 1998). These authors studied the effect of galantamine on cognitive performance (as measured by change in MMSE) in 84 patients with mild-to-moderate AD over the course of 6 months of treatment and found that the best responders belong to the *apoE4* homozygotes subgroup. More recently, Wilcock et al. (2000) examined galantamine efficacy in a large international multicenter randomized trial. They report that, while subjects with and without *apoE4* allele exhibited an improvement on the ADAS-Cog scale, it was the group homozygous for *apoE4* that revealed the most dramatic clinical effect with a mean 6.6 point improvement; whereas subjects lacking *apoE4* exhibited only a 3.8 point improvement over 6 months.

Lastly, Greenberg et al. (2000) published a study from a small clinical trial with the cholinesterase inhibitor donepezil (Aricept), which found that the absence of *apoE4* allele could not predict treatment outcome. However, a careful examination of the results reveals a significant improvement of cognitive parameters in *apoE4* carrier subjects with mild-to-moderate AD. Conversely, a complete absence of efficacy was reported for the subgroup not carrying *apoE4* (see Greenberg et al. (2000), data from Table 4). Several reasons can be invoked to explain the diverging responses that exist between *apoE* genotype and donepezil versus tacrine, galantamine and metrifonate: population biases, sampling error, or, more simply, the biochemistry and pharmacology of donepezil. It is well known that donepesil is a highly selective acetylcholinesterase inhibitor with virtually no butyrylcholinesterase activity. Tacrine, metrifonate, and galantamine, by comparison, have multiple effects on butyrylcholinesterase activity, nicotinic receptor binding, and glutamatergic modulation. It is, therefore, quite possible that target selectivity of each compound is affected differently by the presence of *apoE* polymorphisms in those subjects.

Interestingly, Arai et al. (1996) studied the effect of the topical cholinergic antagonist tropicamide on pupil dilation response in subjects with AD and found that the pupil area was significantly greater in those patients homozygous for *apoE4* compared with subjects not carrying *apoE4*. In a follow-up study, Higuchi and coworkers (1997) studied the effects of tropicamide on cognitively normal individuals and showed that the responders where those individuals carrying at least one *apoE4* allele whereas the nonresponders did not carry *apoE4*. The results of these two studies extend the pharmacogenetic effects of ApoE to non-CNS cholinergic drug response and demonstrate that functional differences exist between the cholinergic neurons of subjects carrying and not carrying *apoE4* in cognitively intact (nondiseased) individuals.

Similarly, the pharmacogenetic profile of xanomeline (Eli Lilly) was assessed in a small phase II drug trial. This compound, which is a muscarinic M_1-specific cholinergic agonist, apparently bypasses the presynaptic cholinergic terminals and directly stimulates the postsynaptic receptor sites in the brain. Since the M_1 sites are particularly insensitive to ApoE4 in postmortem brains of subjects with AD (Poirier et al., 1995), it was postulated that the pharmacogenetic profile of xanomeline would be less dependent on the *apoE4* allele than its acetylcholinesterase inhibitor counterparts. Patients exposed to 75 mg xanomeline daily were monitored over a period of 6 months using the ADAS-Cog as primary outcome variable. Figure 17.4 reveals that, while nearly all treated subjects did show improvement following xanomeline administration, only a small group of subjects homozygous for *apoE4* failed to improve, despite the chronic administration of the M_1 agonist. A second xanomeline phase IIb drug trial was implemented by Eli Lilly in 1997 and the data analysis of more than 180 patients with mild-to-moderate AD revealed a clear pharmacogenomic profile that was virtually identical to the one presented in Figure 17.4 (Alstiel et al., 1998), with *apoE4/apoE4* homozygotes showing no improvement after 6 months of treatment. In addition, the results of both studies suggested that as the number of *apoE4* alleles increased there was a general decline in the odds ratio for a positive therapeutic response.

The drug is currently under investigation in young subjects suffering from schizophrenia.

Noncholinergic drugs

In addition to its impact on drug response to cholinergic drugs, apoE genotype has an effect on noncholinesterase inhibitors used to treat AD. Richard et al. (1997) studied the influence of apoE genotype for the experimental vasopressinergic/noradrenergic drug called S12024. The authors showed that while there was no apparent effect of the drug in the AD group as a whole, the stratification of the AD patients into *apoE4* and non-*apoE4* carriers clearly showed that the former were responding to the drug whereas the latter were not responding (Fig. 17.5).

There are also indications that response to citicoline (cytidine 5'-diphosphocholine) is also pharmacogenetically driven by *apoE* genotype. Citicoline is an endogenous intermediate in the synthesis of membrane lipids and acetylcholine

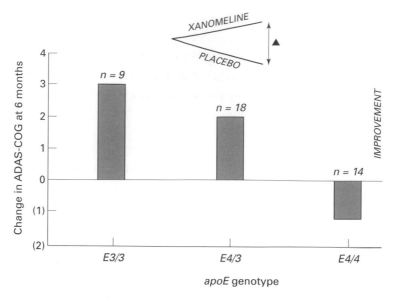

Fig. 17.4.   Xanomeline pharmacogenetic profile in patients with Alzheimer's disease treated for 6 months with a 75 mg dose per day. Genotype is shown for homozygotes for the apolipoprotein E3 (*E3/3*) and E4 (*E4/4*) and for heterozygotes (*E4/3*). Results are expressed as difference between ADAS-COG values (Alzheimer's Disease Assessment Scale–Cognitive score) at the end of the trial minus placebo values (gene dose effect is significant at $p < 0.05$).

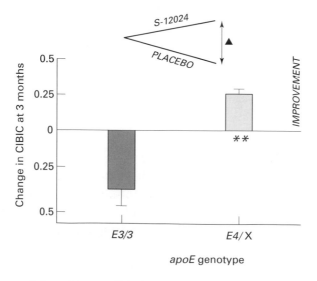

Fig. 17.5.   Variation of mean Clinical Interview Based Impression of Change (CIBIC) scores at entry and after 12 weeks of treatment with S-12024 (Servier, France) in mild-to-moderate Alzheimer's disease. Patients were divided into those carrying the *apoE3* and the *apoE4* allele of the gene for apolipoprotein E. ** $p < 0.015$.

and has been used in the treatment of neurodegenerative disorders like AD. Recently, Alvarez and coworkers (1999) published findings of a double-blind placebo-controlled study with 30 patients with mild-to-moderate AD who were treated with citicoline for 12 weeks. Compared with placebo, citicoline improved cognitive function only in those patients carrying at least one *apoE4* allele.

Conclusions

It appears that not only is the *apoE4* allele an established risk factor for the development of AD, it also has a significant influence on the response of AD patients to treatment with both cholinergic and noncholinergic drugs. These results are intriguing from a mechanistic viewpoint and suggest that the underlying biochemistry and pathology of patients carrying or not carrying *apoE4* are different within the same disease group. Further investigation is needed in order to determine the biochemical reason for the pharmacogenetic effect of the *apoE* alleles. This could lead to the development of a new class of AD drugs that are specifically designed to modify the pharmacogenetic impact of ApoE4, for example, so that those patients would respond to a drug therapy that would ordinarily only be effective in non-*apoE4* carriers.

One of the goals of pharmacogenetics is to deliver the right medicine to the right patient. The retrospective studies described in this chapter show the pharmacogenetic impact of the *apoE* alleles are a step in this direction as there are definitely drugs that work better in non-*apoE4* carriers (for example, tacrine) and those that work better in the *apoE4* carriers (for example, S12024). Prospective clinical trials with *apoE* genotype will need to be carried out in order to verify these findings before they can be applied in drug development and prescription.

Acknowledgements

The research from our laboratory reviewed here was supported by grants from the Alzheimer Society of Canada, the Canadian Institute for Health Research and grants-in-aid from Parke-Davis, Hoechst Marion Roussel, and Nova Molecular Inc. The authors wish to thank Nicole Aumont, Doris Dea, Louise Théroux, Nathalie Gaudreault, and Chantal Arguin for their technical contribution.

REFERENCES

Altstiel LR, Mohs D, Marin L et al. (1998). ApoE genotype and clinical outcome in Alzheimer's disease. *Neurobiol Aging* 19, 140.

Alvarez XA, Mouzo R, Pichel V et al. (1999). Double-blind placebo-controlled study of citicoline in *apoE* genotype Alzheimer's disease patients. *Meth Exp Clin Pharm* 21, 633–644.

Arai H, Terajima M, Nakagawa T, Higuchi S, Mochizuki H, Sasaki H (1996). Pupil dilatation assay by tropicamide is modulated by apolipoprotein E epsilon 4 allele dosage in Alzheimer's disease. *Neuroreport* 22, 918–920.

Arendt T, Schindler C, Bruckner M et al. (1997). Plastic neuronal remodeling is impaired in patients with Alzheimer's disease carrying apolipoprotein $\alpha4$ allele. *J Neurosci* 17, 516–529.

Beffert U, Danik M, Krzykowski P, Ramassamy C, Berrada F, Poirier J (1999). The neurobiology of apolipoproteins and their receptors in the CNS and Alzheimer's disease. *Brain Res Rev* 27, 119–142.

Evans WE, Relling MV (1999). Pharmacogenomics: translating functional genomics into rational therapeutics. *Science* 286, 487–491.

Farlow M, Lahiri DK, Poirier J, Schneider L, Hui SL (1998). Treatment outcome of tacrine therapy depends on apolipoprotein E genotype and gender of the subject with Alzheimer's disease. *Neurology* 50, 669–677.

Farlow MR, Cyrus PA, Nadel A, Labiri DK, Brashear A, Gulanski B (1999). Metrifonate treatment of Alzheimer's disease. *Neurology* 53, 2010–2016.

Greenberg SM, Tennis MK, Brown LB (2000). Donepezil therapy in clinical practice. *Arch Neurol* 57, 94–99.

Higuchi S, Matsushita S, Hasegawa Y, Muramatsu T, Arai H, Hayashida M (1997). Apolipoprotein E epsilon 4 allele and papillary response to tropicamide. *Am J Psychiatry* 154, 694–696.

Kalow W, Grant D (1995). Pharmacogenetics. In Scriver CR, Beaudet AL, Sly WS, eds. *The Metabolic and Molecular Bases of Inherited Disease*. New York: McGraw Hill, pp. 293–326.

Lindsay J and the Apo E and Azlheimer's Disease Meta-analysis Consortium (1997). Effect of age, gender and ethnicity on the association of apolipoprotein E genotype and Alzheimer's disease. *J Am Med Assoc* 278, 1349–1356.

MacGowan SH, Wilcock GK, Scott M (1998). Effect of gender and apolipoprotein E genotype on response to anticholinesterase therapy in Alzheimer's disease. *Int J Geriatr Psychiatry* 13, 625–630.

McCarthy JJ, Hilfiker R (2000). The use of single-nucleotide polymorphism maps in pharmacogenetics. *Nat Biotechnol* 18, 505–508.

Nebert DW (1999). Pharmacogenetics and pharmacogenomics: why is this relevant to the clinical geneticist? *Clin Genet* 56, 247–258.

Noguchi S, Murakami K, Yamada N (1993). Apolipoprotein E and Alzheimer's disease. *Lancet* 342, 737.

Oddoze C, Michel BF, Clavel C, Lucotte G (1998). Apolipoprotein E4 allele predicts a positive response to tacrine in Alzheimer's disease. *Alzheimer's Rep* 1, 13–16.

Poirier J (1994). Apolipoprotein E in animal models of brain injury and in Alzheimer's disease. *Trends Neurosci* 12, 525–530.

Poirier J (1999). Apolipoprotein E: a pharmacogenetic target for the treatment of Alzheimer's disease. *Mol Diag* 4, 335–341.

Poirier J, Aubert I, Quirion R et al. (1995). Apolipoprotein E4 allele as a predictor of cholinergic deficits and treatment outcome in Alzheimer's disease. *Proc Natl Acad Sci USA* 92, 12260–12264.

Poirier J, Davignon J, Bouthillier D, Bertrand P, Gauthier S (1993). Apolipoprotein E and Alzheimer's disease. *Lancet* 342, 697–699.

Richard F, Hetbecque N, Neuman E, Guez E, Levy R, Amouyel P (1997). ApoE genotyping and response to drug treatment in Alzheimer's disease. *Lancet* 349, 539–540.

Riekkinen M, Soininen H, Riekkinen P et al. (1998). Tetrahydroaminoacridine improves the recency effect in Alzheimer's disease. *Neurosci* 83, 471–479.

Roses AD (2000). Pharmacogenetics and future drug development and delivery. *Lancet* 355, 1358–1361.

Rioux PP (2000). Clinical trials in pharmacogenetics and pharmacogenomics: methods and applications. *Am J Health Syst Pharm* 57, 887–898.

Strittmatter WJ, Saunders AM, Schmechel D et al. (1993). Apolipoprotein E: high-avidity binding to beta-amyloid and increased frequency of type 4 allele in late-onset familial Alzheimer disease. *Proc Natl Acad Sci USA* 90, 1977–1981.

Wilcock GK, Lilienfeld S, Gaens E (2000). Efficacy and safety of galantamine in patients with mild to moderate Alzheimer's disease: multicentre randomized controlled trial. *Br Med J* 321, 1–7.

18

Genetic variation and drug dependence risk factors

Joel Gelernter[1] and Henry Kranzler[2]

[1]Yale University School of Medicine and VA CT Healthcare Center, West Haven, USA
[2]University of Connecticut School of Medicine, Farmington, USA

OVERVIEW

This chapter discusses pharmacogenetics in the context of substance abuse and dependence. Owing to the nature of substance-dependence disorders – an exogenous substance is ingested – there is virtually always potential for direct interaction with pharmacogenetic factors, many of which would be expected to be specific to the substance of abuse. Several well-understood examples of such factors are discussed. These issues are placed in the context of identifying and understanding broader genetic risk factors for substance dependence, and of guiding development of pharmacological treatments, both for all patients abusing a given class of substance, and for individual patients based on their specific biochemical make-up as predicted by genetic polymorphism.

Introduction

Genetic factors are important contributors to risk for substance dependence. Some are specific to the substance (e.g., resulting in different euphoric effects by individual), and some are more general (e.g., personality features – novelty seeking, antisocial personality, and so on – which may influence exposure to substances or the transition from substance use to dependence). While the factors that might be mediated by personality and behavior can be conceptualized as analogous to genetic risk factors for other classes of psychiatric disorder, those that are specific to the abused substance could reflect a different set of mechanisms involving genetic variability in receptor–ligand interaction or metabolism of the substance. This can be illustrated by considering two hypothetical limiting cases. In the first limiting case, owing to polymorphic variation, some individuals in the population fail to express a certain receptor, and that receptor is the only one that binds the abused substance. Such individuals would be at decreased risk to become dependent on the substance. In fact, null mutations are known in several important receptors, e.g., the dopamine D_4 receptor encoded by locus *DRD4* (Nöthen et al., 1994). In the second limiting case, imagine that the abused substance is ingested as a prodrug that must be metabolized to a biologically active substance. Suppose further that the enzyme responsible for the bioactivation is defective in some individuals owing to genetic polymorphism. Subjects unable to bioactivate the drug would be at decreased risk of dependence. These cases are simplistic, but similar, less-extreme versions – possibly of the former, and definitely of the latter – are known to exist. Consequently, if the set of all genetically influenced disorders is considered, some forms of substance dependence are uniquely influenced by pharmacogenetic factors. In this chapter, we will explore some of the mechanisms involved, and their implications for diagnosis, treatment, and research.

Genetics of substance dependence: opiates, cocaine, and tobacco

Three drug use disorders constitute the greatest public health problems in the USA: cocaine dependence, opioid dependence, and tobacco, or nicotine, dependence. All of these influence many facets of American society, cutting across geography, race, ethnicity, and status. The population prevalence for a lifetime DSM-III-R (American Psychiatric Association, 1987) diagnosis of cocaine dependence, which was reported (from the National Comorbidity Study) to be 2.7% for individuals between ages 15 and 54 years (Anthony et al., 1994), contrasts with the estimate of 0.2% lifetime prevalence for the broader definition of DSM-III cocaine abuse from the ECA (Epidemiologic Catchment Area) study (Regier et al., 1990). Opioid dependence has a lifetime prevalence of at least 0.4% (reported specifically as heroin dependence: Anthony et al. 1994); dependence or abuse a lifetime prevalence of 0.7% (Regier et al., 1990). At the time of a recent national college survey, prevalence of cigarette use was 28.5% (Rigotti et al., 2000). Elucidating the genetic bases of these disorders would represent major progress towards the goals of improved understanding of etiology, and the development of more effective treatments for such dependences.

Individuals have different vulnerabilities to the development of drug dependence, and the relative contributions of environmental and genetic factors have been examined in a number of studies in animals and humans (Uhl et al., 1995). As Uhl et al. (1995) have pointed out, the mechanisms that underlie interindividual differences in vulnerability to drug dependence are likely to be complex, and, therefore, the genetics will be complex as well. For example, influences that contribute to the initiation of drug use (i.e., experimentation) may differ from those that lead an individual to persist in using the drug (i.e., recreational use), which may also differ from those factors that promote compulsive drug use (i.e., dependence). Genetic factors are likely to play a role in all of these processes, and pharmacogenetic mechanisms are likely to play a prominent role for persistent use and dependence, at least in some individuals.

Heritability of substance dependence

Tsuang et al. (1996) collected data on the Vietnam Era Registry for more than 3000 male twin pairs, among whom drug abuse was defined as at least weekly use of any of a variety of drugs. This study has yielded detailed and comprehensive information regarding heritability of a range of substance-use disorders. Significant pairwise concordance rates showed a familial basis for every one of the drugs considered. The difference in pairwise concordance rates for monozygotic (MZ) and dizygotic (DZ) twins was significant for abuse of or dependence on marijuana, stimulants, cocaine, and for all drugs combined. For opioid dependence, estimated (additive genetic) heritability was 0.43. Despite the large sample, there were relatively few opioid dependence twins; MZ concordance was 13.3% (4/30) and DZ concordance 2.9% (1/34). For stimulant abuse, estimated heritability was 0.44. MZ concordance was 14.1 (21/149) and DZ concordance 5.3 (6/113); the difference between proportions was significant at the $p < 0.05$ level. Tsuang et al. (1998) reported further data from the Vietnam Era Registry focusing on issues relating to comorbidity for different forms of substance-use disorders. They determined that there exist genetic factors both specific to certain individual drugs of abuse, including stimulants, and general to multiple forms of abuse or dependence. Issues of shared genetic factors between substances of abuse are best studied to-date for alcohol and tobacco dependence. Several studies have shown correlation between genetic risk for alcohol and nicotine dependence. True et al. (1999) demonstrated genetic correlation between the disorders of 0.68 in the Vietnam Era Registry. In the same article, the heritability of DSM-III-R nicotine dependence is estimated at 0.60.

Kendler has published twin study data on cocaine dependence demonstrating remarkably high heritability. In a sample of female twins, heritabilities for cocaine abuse and dependence were estimated at 0.79 and 0.65, respectively (Kendler and Prescott, 1998). Data from a sample of male twins showed heritability of liability for cocaine dependence of 0.79 (Kendler et al., 2000). For this study, however, the best-fit model for cocaine *abuse* did not include an additive genetic (a^2) term; Kendler et al. (2000) point out that the power to distinguish between models from this analysis was limited. The twin samples used in these studies were large, but since they were epidemiological samples, the actual numbers of twin pairs from which heritabilities were estimated were considerably smaller. Nonetheless, these data are the best and most specific to-date addressing genetic liability for cocaine abuse and dependence.

Summary: genetic effects and substance dependence

Dependences on cocaine, opioids, and nicotine are both familial and genetically influenced. Some liability factors nonspecifically increase risk for several forms of substance dependence, and others are specific to the substance. Doubtless various combinations of effects (e.g., a particular locus increasing risk for nicotine dependence 10% and cocaine dependence 15%) exist as well. The factors that are specific to substances are the more likely to involve pharmacogenetic mechanisms. Heritability and the increase in risk for first-degree relatives compared with population subjects (λ_1) are such that it should be possible to identify, or at least map, specific risk loci via linkage. However, no such risk loci have been identified unequivocally to-date.

Pharmacogenetics and substance dependence

There is likely to be a large array of genetic influences on each individual's perceptions of the effects of substances of abuse, the time course of those effects, and the occurrence of adverse reactions. Some of these factors will feed back on risk for abusing particular classes of substance, some will be specific to substances within a class (e.g., heroin versus codeine), and others, although they modify the individual's experience, may be orthogonal to risk of dependence. Any of these genetic effects may identify new molecular treatment targets.

Pharmacogenetics is usually discussed in the context of therapeutic agents, but comparable issues pertain for drugs of abuse. That is, genetic factors influence the effects of drugs of abuse, as they do the effects of therapeutic agents, a parallel that holds both for the intended effects of these agents and for their adverse effects. As with therapeutic agents, a distinction can be drawn between genetic effects on risk for substance dependence that are pharmacodynamic in nature and those that are pharmacokinetic.

Pharmacodynamic effects: differing nature of ligand–receptor interaction by individual

Pharmacodynamic effects include, for example, variation in the re-inforcing effects of drugs as a function of genetic differences in receptor–ligand interactions. Genetic variation that could have functional implications has been detected at nearly every neuroreceptor locus where it has been systematically investigated, and in some cases the variation is very extensive (at the D_4 dopamine receptor locus, *DRD4*, for example). Most, if not all, receptors that are known to bind drugs of abuse are already known to show polymorphic variation which at least *could* be functional (serotonin- and dopamine-relevant receptors and transporter are discussed in Chs. 6 and 12 and reviewed in Cravchik and Goldman (2000)). Genetic variation in a receptor that does not affect response to an endogenous ligand could still potentially affect response to an abusable substance if it is physiologically downstream to the interaction, as has been proposed for variation at the D_2 dopamine receptor (*DRD2*) locus (Persico et al., 1996).

Pharmacokinetic effects: differing risk of adverse effects by individual

The best known example of genetic variation affecting risk for substance dependence is the influence of genetic polymorphism at the loci encoding acetaldehyde dehydrogenase and alcohol dehydrogenase on risk of alcohol dependence. The mechanism of this effect is very clear and in some populations it is well established. Ethanol is metabolized to acetaldehyde by alcohol dehydrogenase, for which the most important loci for our purposes are *ADH2* and *ADH3*. Acetaldehyde is metabolized primarily by acetaldehyde dehydrogenase, for which the relevant locus to be considered here is *ALDH2*. Acetaldehyde is toxic and produces a "flushing reaction" characterized by a set of uncomfortable symptoms including flushing, lightheadedness, palpitations, and nausea. Therefore, any deviation from the normal metabolism of ethanol that resulted in increased exposure to acetaldehyde would create an aversive effect of ethanol use, which might decrease risk of alcohol dependence (Goedde et al., 1979). Indeed, a variant that greatly reduces or eliminates acetaldehyde dehydrogenase function (occurring mostly in Asian populations) is protective against alcohol dependence; *ADH* variants that increase function may also be protective (e.g., Thomasson et al. (1991)). These are multiply replicated findings; polymorphic genetic variation is associated with phenotypic variation in a clear and reproducible way. Disulfiram, a medication approved in the 1960s for the treatment of alcohol dependence, is an antagonist of acetaldehyde dehydrogenase. Alcohol consumption by individuals who are pretreated with the medication produces symptoms of acetaldehyde toxicity, which are similar to those associated with variants at *ALDH2*. Although the potential utility of disulfiram for alcoholic relapse prevention was discovered before the variant *ALDH2* alleles were, the use of the medication is congruent to an effort to mimic the protective effects of this genetic polymorphism.

Pharmacogenetics and substance dependence in practice

Specific pharmacogenetic interactions relevant to the understanding of dependence on cocaine, opioids, and nicotine have either been demonstrated or proposed. Below, we discuss examples relevant to each phenotype. There are both pharmacokinetic and pharmacodynamic phenomena relevant to opioid dependence. Pharmacokinetic phenomena relevant to cocaine and nicotine dependence are also discussed.

Opioid dependence: codeine and CYP2D6

Oral opioids such as codeine are metabolized to more active species such as morphine by the P-450 enzyme CYP2D6. The gene that encodes CYP2D6 is polymorphic, with approximately 4% of subjects of European ancestry being poor metabolizers through inheritance of nonfunctional alleles at this locus. Tyndale et al. (1997) found the prevalence of poor metabolizers to be zero among opioid-dependent individuals, 4% among nondependent controls, and 6.5% among individuals dependent on a variety of drugs. They interpreted this as evidence that defective alleles in *CYP2D6* protect against the development of oral opioid dependence. In an effort to mimic this genetic defect, Romach et al. (2000) treated eight long-term opioid users with fluoxetine (an inhibitor of CYP2D6 activity). Opioid use during this 8-week, open-label study declined by 30–100% of baseline, with a parallel decrease in CYP2D6 activity, findings that were interpreted to suggest that fluoxetine may have a role in the treatment of opioid dependence.

Opioid dependence: receptor/ligand interactions

The μ opioid receptor (genetic locus *OPRM1*) plays a central role in mediating the effects of morphine and related opioid agonists (Yu, 1996). Knockout mice unable to produce this protein lack morphine-induced analgesia, morphine place-preference activity, and morphine-induced physical dependence (Matthes et al., 1996; Sora et al., 1997). Genetic variation at loci coding for opiate-system proteins might be expected to affect risk for dependence on drugs and/or alcohol, and possibly other addictive behaviors as well. An approved pharmacological treatment for alcohol dependence, for example, is naltrexone (O'Malley et al., 1992, Volpicelli et al., 1992), a medication that acts as an antagonist of the three opioid receptor types; this medication was first developed for the treatment of opiate dependence, based on its opiate antagonist activity.

A growing body of data supports a role for the endogenous opioid system generally and the opioid μ-receptor specifically in the re-inforcing effects of a variety of drugs that are self-administered by animals and abused by humans, including nicotine, cocaine, amphetamines, alcohol, and cannabinoids. All of these drugs (as well as opioids) have been shown to release dopamine in the nucleus accumbens (Di Chiara and Imperato, 1988; Tanda et al., 1997), which is thought to provide a common pathway for re-inforcement (Koob and LeMoal, 1997). In turn, opioid μ-receptors in the ventral tegmental area are involved in the modulation of nucleus accumbens dopaminergic activity. For example, infusion of a μ-receptor agonist into the ventral tegmental area increases dopamine release in the nucleus accumbens, while infusion of a μ-receptor antagonist decreases dopamine release (Spanagel et al., 1992). Further, alcohol-preferring rats show a significantly higher density of opioid μ-receptors in the ventral tegmental area (and related limbic brain regions), in comparison to alcohol-avoiding rats (de Waele et al. 1995).

Several studies have examined the association between *OPRM1* alleles and alcohol and/or drug dependence. Kranzler et al. (1998) addressed possible association of an single tandem repeat (STR) polymorphism at this locus with substance dependence and Gelernter et al. (1998) described its basic population genetics. They studied this polymorphism in 310 alcohol- and/or drug-dependent subjects (236 European-American and 74 African-American and 118 control subjects 84 European-American and 34 African-American). The primary hypothesis tested was that *OPRM1* alleles would be associated to the presence of a lifetime diagnosis of alcohol, cocaine, or opioid dependence. For this analysis, substance-dependent patients were compared with controls by ethnic origin: 236 substance-dependent European-Americans with 84 controls and 74 African-Americans with 34 ethnically matched controls. Subjects who met criteria for multiple lifetime substance-use disorders were included in more than one specific (secondary) analysis. Among European-Americans, there was a suggestion of association to the presence of alcohol and/or drug dependence (LRT $\chi^2 = 3.52$; $p = 0.03$) (Kranzler et al., 1998); allele frequencies for subjects dependent on any substance differed from those of controls. However, the authors noted that after application of a correction for multiple comparisons, the data failed to support an association of *OPRM1* alleles with substance dependence.

Other authors have looked at single nucleotide polymorphisms (SNPs) at this locus that are more likely to be directly functional. Berrettini et al. (1997) identified two polymorphisms of *OPRM1*, one in a noncoding region, the second producing a nonsynonymous substitution (Ala6Val). They compared the frequency of the variant alleles in a sample of 55 substance-dependent subjects (53% European-American, 47% African-American) with a group of 51 controls (43% European-American, 57% African-American). There was a trend ($p = 0.05$) for the substance-dependent group to have a higher frequency of the Ala6Val variant ($F = 0.22$), compared with controls ($F = 0.10$); however, observations for both ethnic groups were combined. A subsequent report including data from this group did not continue to support this proposed association (Hoehe et al., 2000).

Bergen et al. (1997) directly sequenced 91% of the *OPRM1* coding sequence (1093 base pairs) and 1479 bases of intronic and untranslated sequence. They found four DNA sequence variants, including three nonsynonymous substitutions (Ala6Val, Asn40Asp, and Ser147Cys) and one intronic variant. The variant forms of the exonic polymorphisms were rare in the populations studied. Using *OPRM1* alleles, genotypes, and haplotypes from US Caucasian, Finnish Caucasian, and southwestern American Indian samples, these investigators conducted association and sibling-pair linkage analyses with diagnoses of alcohol dependence and drug dependence. No significant associations were observed. Bond et al. (1998)

described functional variation corresponding to Asn40Asp (A118G); the differing forms vary in their sensitivity to β-endorphin (but not to other possible endogenous and exogenous ligands, including met-enkephalin, dynorphin A, morphine, and methadone, or to naloxone). The observed difference corresponded to about a threefold alteration in affinity. These authors also described a statistically significant association of that variant with opioid dependence, but only in Hispanic subjects; in that population, frequency of the less common allele (Asp or G) was 0.10 in 58 opioid-dependent subjects, but 0.39 in nine nondependent controls.

The reports by Berrettini et al. (1997), Bergen et al. (1997) and Bond et al. (1998) raised important possibilities regarding potential effects of *OPRM1* exon 1 variants on risk for substance dependence and on function of the opioid μ-receptor protein, but these reports are inconsistent, not only in terms of their findings with respect to phenotype but also with respect to allele frequencies observed in similar populations. Gelernter et al. (1999) studied both exon 1 polymorphisms in a total of 891 subjects: control populations of varying geographic origin (European-, African-, and Hispanic-Americans and Ethiopian Jews, Ashkenazi Jews, Japanese, and Bedouins) and varying diagnoses (European-, African-, and Hispanic-American drug-dependent subjects and European-American alcohol-dependent subjects). They reported large differences in allele frequency for both systems by population, a Japanese sample most different from the other populations. They also reported no significant differences in allele frequency for these two exon 1 polymorphisms, within population, by diagnosis. To the extent that the populations overlap, these results were consistent with those of Bergen et al. (1997) and (except for Hispanic controls) Bond et al. (1998).

Hoehe et al. (2000) used multiplex sequence comparison to identify 43 *OPRM1* variants in a sample of 250 individuals (including 51 African-American controls and 158 African-Americans dependent on either cocaine or opioids). These investigators then statistically predicted haplotypes for the sample of African-American controls and affecteds. Using a hierarchical clustering procedure, they proposed to classify the haplotypes into two categories, one of which was reported to be significantly more common among drug-dependent subjects. Based on these findings, these investigators concluded that the pattern of results may reflect either linkage disequilibrium of the region examined with genetic variation that confers risk for drug dependence or the fact that the variation identified through sequence analysis directly accounts for risk for drug dependence. Although in this sample comparable results were obtained following a variety of clustering methods, external validation of the cluster results was not provided. Given that variable findings are often obtained when different samples are analyzed using the same clustering methods, further efforts to replicate this complex statistical approach are required before the validity of the association can be judged. This finding may be interpreted as indicating that many small polymorphisms could be acting similarly in terms of risk for substance dependence, could act together when occurring on a haplotype, or could identify a haplotype containing a truly functional variant. If the first of these is the case, it would be very difficult to validate the finding by designing a study with sufficient power to detect the effect of any one of these polymorphisms; detecting the effect by linkage disequilibrium with a single sufficiently informative polymorphism (as per Kranzler et al., 1998) would provide an alternative strategy. Linkage using affected sibling pairs would also be a strong strategy for validating a finding such as this, owing to the likelihood that affected siblings would be likely to share particular risk alleles (even if they were of small effect populationwise, provided that they incremented risk substantially in a particular individual) identical by descent (IBD). This could be detected first with marker polymorphisms, then examined more closely in those sibling pairs that shared marker alleles IBD. Hoehe et al. (2000) also reported results that were consistent with the observations of Gelernter et al. (1999) regarding allele frequencies for the two exon 1 *OPRM1* polymorphisms, in both case and control African-Americans.

These results regarding a possible relationship of *OPRM1* variation and phenotype are presently equivocal. However, a quantitative trait loci (QTL) linkage mapping study (Berrettini et al., 1994) was consistent with polymorphic variation at the opioid μ-receptor in mouse affecting morphine preference. This result indirectly supports a role for polymorphic variation at this locus affecting opioid intake in rodents, even if not in humans; the support is indirect because QTL mapping studies result in rather broad gene localizations, and the locus cited above, although close to *OPRM1*, is not *necessarily OPRM1*.

Whereas opioidergic medications are used to treat both opioid dependence (agonists such as methadone, L-α-acetylmethadol (LAAM), and buprenorphine are cornerstones in treatment) and alcohol dependence (the antagonist naltrexone is approved by the US Food and Drug Administration, though not widely used, and nalmefene, also an antagonist, is currently in clinical trials), *OPRM1* is a logical candidate for pharmacogenetic investigation in substance dependence. To-date, only Bond et al. (1998) have examined the impact of *OPRM1* polymorphism on ligand binding. There have been no clinical studies addressing response to opioidergic medications in vivo.

Cocaine dependence: cocaine-induced paranoia as a phenotype

Variation in receptor function could, by altering the subjective experience produced by the ingestion of a substance, alter risk for becoming dependent on that substance. Variation in genes with products that participate in metabolic pathways (e.g., CYP2D6 in nicotine metabolism, dopamine β-hydroxylase (DBH) in dopamine metabolism) could also cause differences in risk for substance dependence.

For example, low levels of DBH in the serum or cerebrospinal fluid (CSF) are associated with greater vulnerability to positive psychotic symptoms across several diagnostic groups. The locus encoding DBH is the major quantitative trait locus controlling plasma and CSF DBH levels. Cubells et al. (2000) hypothesized that variants or haplotypes associated with low levels of DBH in the plasma would also associate with greater vulnerability to cocaine-induced paranoia (CIP), possibly by altering synaptic dopamine levels. Gelernter et al. (1994) had previously demonstrated an association of this same trait with another dopamine system gene, *SLC6A3* (dopamine transporter protein), alleles.

These investigators showed that two *DBH* variants are associated with plasma DBH levels, and that among cocaine-dependent European-American subjects evaluated for having ever experienced CIP, a low-DBH-associated haplotype was significantly more frequent in subjects endorsing CIP (29) than in those who reported never having had the experience (16). These investigators concluded that the haplotype associated with low DBH activity is also associated with CIP. Thus, polymorphic variation at the *DBH* locus has been shown to alter sensitivity to at least one adverse effect associated with cocaine abuse.

Tobacco dependence: CYP2A6 and therapeutic agents

Sellers and Tyndale (2000) have outlined a strategy for treating drug dependence based on the pharmacological mimicry of gene defects. These defects are in the genes encoding proteins in the cytochrome P-450 system that catalyze the activation of prodrugs (e.g., codeine to morphine) or the deactivation of biologically active species of drugs (e.g., nicotine to cotinine), thereby modifying the euphoric or aversive effects of the drug. Genetic polymorphisms can thereby modify the risk of dependence on these drugs. Among the polymorphic loci implicated in such effects are *CYP2D6*, discussed above (which encodes CYP2D6, the enzyme that metabolizes codeine, amphetamines, and dextromethorphan), and *CYP2A6* (which encodes CYP2A6, the enzyme that metabolizes nicotine). By mimicking the effects of genetic variants that reduce or abolish enzymatic activity, drugs that inhibit these enzymes may be efficacious treatments for drug dependence.

As noted above, CYP2A6 is responsible for the majority of the metabolic inactivation of nicotine to cotinine. Understanding of the studies discussed below is complicated by the fact that two different polymorphic systems, as well as a deletion, were originally designated by a single set of allele names. Zabetian et al. (2000) normalized allele names for the *CYP2A6* variants, resolving two polymorphisms into "A" and "B" systems (haplotypes introduced in square brackets, below). Consistent with observations that smokers adjust their smoking behavior to maintain constant blood and brain levels of nicotine, Pianezza et al. (1998) found that heterozygotes for the (presumably nonfunctional) variant alleles (*CYP2A6*2*

[*CYP2A6*A2–B1*] and *CYP2A6*3* [*CYP2A6*A1–B2*]) of the gene encoding CYP2A6 smoked fewer cigarettes than homozygotes for the wild-type (*CYP2A6*1* [CYP2A6*A1–B1]) allele, and were less likely to become dependent on nicotine. However, it was subsequently determined that the original genotyping assay for the "B" system (*CYP2A6*3*) was inaccurate, yielding a falsely elevated frequency of that allele. Zabetian et al. (2000) came to a similar conclusion and also presented improved genotyping methods. Rao et al. (2000), using modified genotyping methods, found that individuals with *CYP2A6*A2–B1* or *CYP2A6*4* [CYP2A6*del*] alleles smoked fewer cigarettes per day than wild-type homozygotes. The low allele frequencies for each of the inactive alleles in European populations limit this effect on the population level, in contrast to that predicted by Pianezza et al. (1998), but the finding demonstrates that the principle is nevertheless robust. These investigators also identified a duplicated form of *CYP2A6*. Consistent with this evidence of genetic effects on smoking behavior, Sellers et al. (2000) showed that oral methoxsalen, an inhibitor of CYP2A6, inhibits first-pass metabolism of oral nicotine and the combination reduces smoking in a laboratory setting. Together, these findings provide a promising treatment approach, based on pharmacological manipulation of pharmacokinetic genetic factors that influence substance-use behavior, and demonstrate that even if the effect of a particular polymorphism is small on a population level, it can still provide valuable clues both to disease mechanism and to treatment.

Nicotine metabolism also provides an illustration of the importance of ethnic (population) differences; Pérez-Sable et al. (1998) demonstrated that African-Americans have slower cotinine clearance than European-Americans, a finding that explains, in part, higher levels of cotinine per cigarette consumed, which has been observed in the former population. It is not clear to what extent this effect is genetic in origin; allelic variation at loci involved in metabolism is one possible explanation; Zabetian et al. (2000) did demonstrate a higher frequency of the *CYP2A6*B2* allele in African-Americans than in European-Americans, but this difference is probably not large enough to account for the observations by Pérez-Sable et al. (1998). Even if the effect were purely environmental in origin, it would interact with genetic effects related to nicotine metabolism.

Issues of population genetics and variation by population group

The idea that it is usual for allele frequencies, both at marker loci and for candidate genes, to differ between populations, sometimes greatly (e.g., Gelernter et al., 1998, 1999), is now widely accepted. While this is frequently, and correctly, seen as a potential confounder for case-control genetic association studies, it also sometimes reflects real differences in physiology by population. That is, functional and important variation occurs, not only within but also between populations. This is important, for example, with the alcohol-metabolizing enzymes, discussed above. Variation in allele frequencies by population has profound implications in that the identification of variants important for pharmacogenetics in one population need not generalize to other populations.

Conclusions

Issues relating to pharmacogenetics have a unique role in the investigation of heritable risk factors for drug dependence. The pharmacogenetic research strategy will certainly lead to insight into disease mechanisms but will also yield clinically applicable results relatively quickly (Sellers et al., 2000). Applications will include prediction of risk in unaffected individuals, individualized selection of treatment, and development of new treatments. In a recent review article, Roses (2000) distinguishes the effort to identify genetically based medicine response profiles from the study of disease genetics (which in the case of genetically complex disorders like substance dependence involve susceptibility polymorphisms rather than genetic mutations of large effect). Medicine response profiles involve the specification of a panel of markers, which may be associated to either pharmacokinetic or pharmacodynamic targets, that predict the efficacy, safety, and tolerability of medications in the treatment of specific disorders. Although medicine response profiling and the study of disease genetics overlap and are potentially complementary, the scientific and ethical issues differ substantially.

Medicine response profiling promises to provide an abundance of new targets for medication development. It may also streamline the process of medication development by reducing the universe of potential study participants to those who are more likely to respond favorably, and less likely to experience adverse effects in response, to a particular medication.

Several large-scale gene mapping projects are now underway at different centers with the aim of identifying loci that alter risk for different forms of substance dependence. Upon completion, these are likely to bring with them insights into the relationship of pharmacogenetics and substance dependence by identifying genomic regions that contain risk loci and, ultimately, may lead to the positional cloning of at least some such loci.

Identification of polymorphisms – the currency for identification of pharmacogenetic effects – is still rather labor intensive. There is a large effort presently in progress to identify SNPs throughout the human genome for the purposes of developing a basic understanding of functional variation in the genome, providing markers suitable for linkage or full genome linkage disequilibrium (association) studies, and identifying candidates for influence on phenotype. Undoubtedly, through this project, many polymorphisms important for substance-dependence risk or other modifiers of phenotypes relevant for substance dependence will be discovered. However, it is likely that, for the most part, only common polymorphisms will be discovered. At this point, we have no sure way to predict how many polymorphisms important for substance-dependence pharmacogenetics will be common on a population level. As a general rule, common variants have relatively less effect on phenotype than rare ones. Although some variants we seek will surely have only modest effect, just as surely, others will have dramatic effect and will, therefore, be less common (for example, we can consider the null alleles at the *CYP2D6* and *CYP2A6* loci). Therefore, it is unlikely that this puzzle will be solved through the larger SNP efforts alone; it will be necessary to select subjects who differ in phenotype and carry out mutation detection to find rarer polymorphisms that might have larger effect (e.g., Lappalainen et al., 2002). Ultimately, the Human Genome Project will provide for a major expansion of the scope of substance-dependence pharmacogenetics by expanding our knowledge of the set of genes relevant to addictive processes.

Acknowledgements

This work was supported in part by funds from the US Department of Veterans Affairs (the VA Medical Research Program, and the VA Connecticut–Massachusetts Mental Illness Research, Education and Clinical Center (MIRECC)), NIMH grant K02–MH01387, NIAAA grants R01–AA11330, K02–AA00239, NIDA grants R01–DA12849 and R01–DA12690, and NCRR grant M01–RR06192 (University of Connecticut General Clinical Research Center).

REFERENCES

American Psychiatric Association (1987). *Diagnostic and Statistical Manual of Mental Disorders*, 3rd edn revised. Washington, DC: American Psychiatric Association.

Anthony JC, Warner LA, Kessler RC (1994). Comparative epidemiology of dependence on tobacco, alcohol, controlled substances, and inhalants: basic findings from the National Comorbidity Survey. *Exp Clin Psychopharmacol* 2, 244–268.

Bergen AW, Kokoszka J, Peterson R et al. (1997). μ-Opioid receptor gene variants: lack of association with alcohol dependence. *Mol Psychiatry* 2, 490–494.

Berrettini WH, Ferraro TN, Alexander RC, Buchberg AM, Vogel WH (1994). Quantitative trait loci mapping of three loci controlling morphine preference using inbred mouse strains. *Nat Genet* 7, 54–58.

Berrettini WH, Hoehe MR, Ferraro TN, DeMaria PA, Gottheil E (1997). Human mu opioid receptor gene polymorphisms and vulnerability to substance abuse. *Addict Biol* 2, 303–308.

Bond C, LaForge KS, Tian M et al. (1998). Single-nucleotide polymorphism in the human mu opioid receptor gene alters β-endorphin binding and activity: possible implications for opiate addiction. *Proc Natl Acad Sci USA* 95, 9608–9613.

Cravchik A, Goldman D (2000). Neurochemical individuality: genetic diversity among human dopamine and serotonin receptors and transporters. *Arch Gen Psychiatry* 57, 1105–1114.

Cubells JF, Kranzler HR, McCance-Katz E (2000). A haplotype at the *DBH* locus, associated with low plasma dopamine β-hydroxylase activity, also associates with cocaine-induced paranoia. *Mol Psychiatry* 5, 56–63.

de Waele JP, Kiianmaa K, Gianoulakis C (1995). Distribution of the mu and delta opioid binding sites in the brain of the alcohol-preferring AA and alcohol-avoiding ANA lines of rats. *J Pharmacol Exp Ther* 275, 518–527.

Di Chiara G, Imperato A (1988). Drugs abused by humans preferentially increase synaptic dopamine concentrations in the mesolimbic system of freely moving rats. *Proc Natl Acad Sci USA* 85, 5274–5278.

Gelernter J, Kranzler HR, Satel SL, Rao PA (1994). Genetic association between dopamine transporter protein alleles and cocaine-induced paranoia. *Neuropsychopharmacology* 11, 195–200.

Gelernter J, Kranzler H, Lacobelle J (1998). Population studies of polymorphisms at loci of neuropsychiatric interest (tryptophan hydroxylase (*TPH*), dopamine transporter protein (*SLC6A3*), D3 dopamine receptor (*DRD3*), apolipoprotein E (*apoE*), μ opioid receptor (*OPRM1*), and ciliary neurotrophic factor (*CNTF*)). *Genomics* 52, 289–297.

Gelernter J, Kranzler H, Cubells J (1999). Genetics of two μ opioid receptor gene (OPRM1) exon I polymorphisms: population studies, and allele frequencies in alcohol and drug dependent subjects. *Mol Psychiatry* 4, 476–483.

Goedde HW, Harada S, Agarwal DP (1979). Racial differences in alcohol sensitivity: a new hypothesis. *Hum Genet* 51, 331–334.

Hoehe MR, Kopke K, Wendel B et al. (2000). Sequence variability and candidate gene analysis in complex disease: association of μ opioid receptor gene variation with substance dependence. *Hum Mol Genet* 9, 2895–2908.

Kendler KS, Prescott CA (1998). Cocaine use, abuse and dependence in a population-based sample of female twins. *Br J Psychiatry* 173, 345–350.

Kendler KS, Karkowski LM, Neale MC, Prescott CA (2000). Illicit psychoactive substance use, heavy use, abuse, and dependence in a US population-based sample of male twins. *Arch Gen Psychiatry* 57, 261–269.

Koob GF, LeMoal M (1997). Drug abuse: hedonic homeostatic dysregulation. *Science* 278, 52–58.

Kranzler HA, Gelernter J, O'Malley S, Hernandez-Avila CA, Kaufman D (1998). Association of alcohol or other drug dependence with alleles of the mu opioid receptor gene (*OPRM1*). *Alcohol Clin Exp Res* 22, 1359–1362.

Lappalainen J, Kranzler HR, Malison R et al. (2002). A functional neuropeptide Y Leu7Pro polymorphism is associated with alcohol dependence in a large population sample from the US. *Arch Gen Psychiatry* in press.

Matthes HWD, Maldonado R, Simonin F et al. (1996). Loss of morphine-induced analgesia, reward effect and withdrawal symptoms in mice lacking the μ-opioid-receptor gene. *Nature* 383, 819–823.

Nöthen MM, Cichon S, Hemmer S et al. (1994). Human dopamine D_4 receptor gene: frequent occurrence of a null allele and observation of homozygosity. *Hum Mol Genet* 3, 2207–12.

O'Malley SS, Jaffe AJ, Chang G, Schottenfeld RS, Meyer RE, Rounsaville B (1992). Naltrexone and coping skills therapy for alcohol dependence. A controlled study. *Arch Gen Psychiatry* 49, 881–887.

Pérez-Sable EJ, Herrera B, Jacob III P, Benowitz NL (1998). Nicotine metabolism and intake in black and white smokers. *J Am Med Assoc* 280, 152–156.

Persico AM, Bird G, Gabbay FH, Uhl GR (1996). D_2 dopamine receptor gene *TaqI* A1 and B1 restriction fragment length polymorphisms: enhanced frequencies in psychostimulant-preferring polysubstance abusers. *Biol Psychiatry* 40, 776–784.

Pianezza M, Sellers EM, Tyndale RF (1998). A common genetic defect in nicotine metabolism decreases smoking. *Nature* 393, 750.

Rao Y, Hoffmann E, Zia M et al. (2000). Duplications and defects in the *CYP2A6* gene: identification, genotyping, and in vivo effects on smoking. *Mol Pharmacol* 58, 747–755.

Regier D, Farmer M, Rae D et al. (1990). Comorbidity of mental with alcohol and other drug abuse. Results from the Epidemiologic Catchment Area (ECA) study. *J Am Med Assoc* 264, 2511–2518.

Rigotti NA, Lee JE, Wechsler H (2000). US college students' use of tobacco products: results of a national survey. *J Am Med Assoc* 284, 699–705.

Romach MK, Otton SV, Somer G, Tyndale RF, Sellers EM (2000). Cytochrome P-450 2D6 and treatment of codeine dependence. *J Clin Psychopharmacol* 20, 43–45.

Roses AD (2000). Pharmacogenetics and future drug development and delivery. *Lancet* 355, 1358–1361.

Sellers EM, Tyndale RF (2000). Mimicking gene defects to treat drug dependence. *Ann NY Acad Sci* 909, 233–246.

Sellers EM, Kaplan HL, Tyndale RF (2000). Inhibition of cytochrome P-450 2A6 increases nicotine's oral bioavailability and decreases smoking. *Clin Pharmacol Ther* 68, 35–43.

Sora I, Takahashi N, Funada M et al. (1997). Opiate receptor knockout mice define mu receptor roles in endogenous nociceptive responses and morphine-induced analgesia. *Proc Natl Acad Sci USA* 94, 1544–1549.

Spanagel R, Herz A, Shippenberg TS (1992). Opposing tonically active endogenous opioid systems modulate the mesolimbic dopaminergic pathway. *Proc Natl Acad Sci* USA 89, 2046–2050.

Tanda G, Pontieri FE, Di Chiara G (1997). Cannabinoid and heroin activation of mesolimbic dopamine transmission by a common μ opioid receptor mechanism. *Science* 276, 2048–2050.

Thomasson HR, Edenberg HJ, Crabb DW et al. (1991). Alcohol and aldehyde dehydrogenase genotypes and alcoholism in Chinese men. *Am J Hum Genet* 48, 677–681.

True WR, Xian H, Scherrer JF et al. (1999). Common genetic vulnerability for nicotine and alcohol dependence in men. *Arch Gen Psychiatry* 56, 655–661.

Tsuang MT, Lyons MJ, Eisen SA et al. (1996). Genetic influences on DSM-III-R, drug abuse and dependence: a study of 3372 twin pairs. *Am J Med Genet* (*Neuropsych Genet*) 67, 473–477.

Tsuang MT, Lyons MJ, Meyer JM et al. (1998). Co-occurrence of abuse of different drugs in men; the role of drug-specific and shared vulnerabilities. *Arch Gen Psychiatry* 55, 967–972.

Tyndale RF, Droll KP, Seller EM (1997). Genetically deficient CYP2D6 metabolism provides protection against oral opiate dependence. *Pharmacogenetics* 7, 375–379.

Uhl GR, Elmer GI, LaBuda MC, Pickens RW (1995). Genetic influences in drug abuse. In Bloom FE, Kupfer DJ, eds. *Psychopharmacology: The Fourth Generation of Progress.* New York: Raven Press, pp. 1793–1806.

Volpicelli JR, Alterman AI, Hayashida M, O'Brien CP (1992). Naltrexone in the treatment of alcohol dependence. *Arch Gen Psychiatry* 49, 876–880.

Yu L (1996). The opioid receptor: from molecular cloning to functional studies. *Addict Biol* 1, 19–30.

Zabetian CP, Gelernter J, Cubells JF (2000). Functional variants at CYP2A6: new genotyping methods, population genetics, and relevance to studies of tobacco dependence. *Am J Med Genet* (*Neuropsych Genet*) 96, 638–645.

Part VI

Pharmacogenetics and brain imaging

19

Brain imaging and pharmacogenetics in Alzheimer's disease and schizophrenia

Steven G. Potkin[1], James L. Kennedy[2], and Vincenzo S. Basile[2]

[1] Department of Psychiatry and Human Behavior, University of California, Irvine, USA
[2] Clarke Institute of Psychiatry, University of Toronto, Canada

OVERVIEW

In the future the current trial and error prescribing practices of physicians will be replaced by individualized treatment algorithms based upon each patient's genotype. This advance will be based on the results from large databases relating allelic variation in thousands of genes to medication response including differences in efficacy and side effects. Such databases will produce a series of probabilistic predictions based on the individual's genetic background. As useful as these data-based associations will prove, the basic underlying pathophysiological mechanisms may remain elusive. Brain imaging techniques combined with genetics can contribute to developing an understanding of the pathophysiological mechanism of disease and treatment response. These advances, coupled with developments in gene chip technology and informatics, will lead to surgery/office-based determinations of an individual's genetic background to be used in data-based individualized medication algorithms to optimize treatment.

Introduction

A primary goal of psychiatric genetics is to identify associations between allelic variation in genes and the risk for the development of psychiatric illness. The same association study strategy can be applied to understanding individual patient response to pharmacological treatment, including the occurrence of side effects. Associations between allelic variants and liability to side effects to different pharmacological agents, as well as the hierarchical likelihood of clinical response, can be established. Such associations do not necessarily point the way toward the pathophysiological mechanism of disease and can, in fact, be irrelevant. The association between the apolipoprotein E(ApoE) allele *apoE4* and the onset of Alzheimer's disease and the response to cholinesterase treatment (see Ch. 17) could be examples, in view of the fact that the pathophysiological details have not been established for *apoE* alleles in the disease, although some believe that ApoE plays a key role in amyloid deposition and clearance.

Alzheimer's disease

The *apoE4* allele has been associated with higher risk and/or earlier development of Alzheimer's disease (Roses et al., 1995). Although the genetic association of *apoE4* with the development of Alzheimer's disease is well established, there is now an important need to devise strategies that can fill in the missing links between *apoE* gene variation and the pathophysiological mechanism of Alzheimer's disease. Brain imaging can address and even bridge this gap. Bookheimer et al. (2000) studied 16 neurologically normal subjects who were carriers of the *apoE4* allele and compared them with 14 subjects who were homozygous for the *apoE3* allele. Patterns of brain activation were studied with fMRI (functional magnetic resonance imaging) while subjects memorized and recalled unrelated words. During periods of recall, the *apoE4* carriers had greater average signal increase in the hippocampus and a greater number of active regions throughout the brain than did the *apoE3* homozygotes, suggesting that the *apoE4* carriers needed to activate traditional memory circuits more than the non-*apoE4* carriers as well as to activate additional brain areas in order to perform adequately on the memory task. This study demonstrates that there are different patterns of brain activation during memory tasks that are related to allelic variation. Longitudinal assessment of these subjects provided further evidence for the relevance of the association, as baseline brain activation correlated with the degree of decline in memory revealed longitudinally. Because the subjects were not cognitively impaired at the time of initial imaging, these data suggest that at-risk patients use different memory strategies or require additional brain areas of activation to perform in the normal range. The data from Bookheimer et al. (2000) are very useful in that they also suggest hypotheses regarding how the brain compensates for early pathological changes (Braak and Braak, 1990) that predate clinical symptoms.

The cerebral metabolic rates obtained with positron emission tomography (PET) were able to distinguish carriers of a single copy of the *apoE4* allele from noncarriers (Small et al., 2000). Importantly, these carriers were middle-aged nondemented persons with normal memory performance (Fig. 19.1, color plate). These subjects were followed longitudinally for 2 years and continued to show declines in cortical metabolic rates. In these *apoE4* carriers, who neurocognitively performed normally at baseline, their baseline parietal cortical and posterior cingulate metabolic rates was predictive of memory recall loss two years later. These data suggest that the combination of PET imaging and genetic risk factors can be used for preclinical Alzheimer's detection and have application in monitoring experimental treatments.

This research strategy can also be extended to explaining clinical response to medication, or the development of side effects following specific pharmacological intervention. There is evidence that *apoE4* alleles predict response to cholinesterase treatment (Poirier et al., 1995; also see Ch. 17). The combination of imaging, allelic characterization, and clinical response can synergistically contribute to understanding the role *apoE4* plays in the development of Alzheimer's disease and its response to treatment. This approach was demonstrated by Riekkinen et al. (1997), who investigated the effects of a single challenge dose of tacrine on cortical spectral electroencephalographic activity in patients classified by *apoE4* alleles. The patients with *apoE4*, but not the *apoE3* homozygotes, increased alpha activity and alpha/theta ratio in response to the 50 mg tacrine challenge. The authors interpreted this enhancement of cortical electrical arousal as a reflection of cholinergic therapy enhancing presynaptic nucleus basalis cholinergic neurons. However, these assertions remain speculative, as electroencephalography cannot reveal subcortical structures. PET and fMRI could specifically address this hypothesis.

Schizophrenia

An analogous argument can be made for combining brain imaging with allelic subtyping to understand clinical antipsychotic response in schizophrenia. Although the microscopic neuroanatomy of schizophrenia is not as well developed as it is in Alzheimer's disease, there is accumulating evidence that schizophrenia is a neurodevelopmental disorder (Bunney et al., 1995) that may involve genes which control brain development. Wassink et al. (1999) investigated alleles for brain-derived neurotrophic factor (BDNF) as a candidate gene for schizophrenia. The *BDNF* gene is highly expressed during fetal brain development and continues to be expressed at low levels throughout adulthood. No association was found between the presence or absence of the allele *BDNF1* in proband–parent trios (Wassink et al., 1999). However, subjects who had at least one copy of the *BDNF1* allele had larger parietal lobe volumes by MRI than those that did not. This allelic variation occurs upstream from the transcription initiation site, possibly in the promoter region. As described above, this study could be expanded to incorporate the clinical response dimension. Patients with morphological abnormalities tend to be less responsive to antipsychotic treatment (Jeste et al., 1982).

Side effects and schizophrenia

Following chronic antipsychotic treatment, some individuals develop an oral-facial dyskinesia that may be irreversible. In severe cases, this can involve the trunk and limbs. This disorder is called tardive dyskinesia (TD). Each year approximately 4% of those patients chronically treated with typical antipsychotic drugs develop TD (Kane et al., 1988); however, in most studies, only 20–30% of such treated patients develop TD (Jeste and Caligiuri, 1993). Since not all persons develop TD regard-less of the duration of treatment with antipsychotic medications, there is a variable susceptibility to the development of TD. Why are some patients so resistant to developing TD while others are so sensitive? Genetic variability may account for some of this variability.

Family studies demonstrate that genetic factors contribute to susceptibility to developing TD (Weinhold et al., 1981; Yassa and Ananth, 1981; O'Callaghan et al., 1990). Several genetic studies have examined the putative role of the gene for the dopamine D_3 receptor (*DRD3*) in TD (Steen et al., 1997; Basile et al., 1999; Segman et al., 1999; Rietschel et al., 2000; see also Ch. 11). Polymorphisms at allele *2* (*MscI*) give rise to a serine-to-glycine substitution in the N-terminal domain of D_3 (Ser9Gly). Individuals can be homozygotes for D_{3ser} or D_{3gly} or heterozygotes with $D_{3gly-ser}$. Individuals carrying *DRD3*gly have a higher risk of developing TD.

In 14 subjects who were part of the Basile et al. (1999) study, brain imaging with fluorodeoxyglucose (FDG) was done before and after treatment with haloperidol (Fig. 19.2, color plate). The five patients with *DRD3*gly-gly had significantly higher abnormal involuntary movement scale (AIMS) scores when drug free than the other genotypes, reflecting their increased risk of TD. In patients who were anti-psychotic medication free, there were no differences in basal ganglia metabolism between the *DRD3*gly-gly homozygotes and nonhomozygotes. Following haloper-idol treatment, the patients with *DRD3*gly-gly demonstrated statistically significant increases in caudate and putamen metabolism ($p < 0.01$). In contrast, the other genotypes, who were at lower risk for the development of TD, evidenced no meta-bolic changes following haloperidol treatment. (See Fig. 19.2 (color plate) for the metabolic differences between groups following haloperidol treatment.) Interestingly, D_3 receptor mRNA and protein have been localized to the ventral stri-atum and the ventral putamen in the basal ganglia (motor control) (Joyce and Meador-Woodruff, 1997), the same areas that have increased metabolism in the *DRD3*gly-gly homozygotes on PET. Further, D_3 receptors have been shown to have an inhibitory effect on locomotor activity in rats (Kling-Petersen et al., 1995). In summary, the patients who had increased genetic risk for the development of TD demonstrated increased basal ganglia metabolism after treatment with haloperidol, while those at low genetic risk for TD did not. These studies demonstrate the syn-ergistic effect that brain imaging can have in bridging animal and human studies, and in beginning to understand the pathophysiology of genetic risk factors.

Conclusions

Much has been learned in establishing the efficacy of new pharmacological treat-ments for groups of patients with schizophrenia and Alzheimer's disease.

Comparisons with placebo have clearly defined the side effect profile of these new therapeutic agents. What has remained unclear is why some patients respond to these medications while others do not, and why certain subgroups develop side effects while others are spared. These individual differences are lost in group efficacy analyses but are crucial to developing treatment paradigms. Pharmacogenetics offers the possibility of using differences in genetic background to explain these individual differences in drug response and the development of side effects. The associational link between genetic background and clinical response does not necessarily explain the pathophysiology between genes and treatment response. Brain imaging can play an important role in advancing this understanding. In Alzheimer's disease, *apoE* alleles not only provide information on the risk of developing the disease but can also predict different patterns of brain activation during memory tasks. Changes in patterns of brain activation related to allelic variation can be demonstrated decades before the onset of clinical symptoms. Similarly, in schizophrenia, the risk of TD has been related to *DRD3* alleles. Brain imaging can reveal differences in brain metabolic response to pharmacological treatment that may harbinger the later development of TD. It is noteworthy that the areas of the brain differentially affected by haloperidol treatment are consistent with the distribution of D_3 receptors in the brain. The combined pharmacogenetic and brain imaging approaches that have been used in schizophrenia and Alzheimer's disease can be extended to understand additional treatment side effects, to explain other dimensions of efficacy, and to other neuropsychiatric illnesses.

The ability to extend pharmacogenetics into understanding clinical response and side effects following treatment in neuropsychiatric illness is limited by the database. Large numbers of patients treated under controlled conditions are required to establish associations between genetic variability and these illness-related behaviors. Replication is especially important in establishing the role of such genetic variability. Brain imaging can provide valuable links in understanding the potential importance and clarifying the pathophysiological mechanisms that lie between associations of genetic variability and clinical response. These steps are painstaking and include acquiring large databases with careful clinical evaluation. Replication in additional populations is also necessary to achieve these goals. The use of brain imaging combined with genetics can aid in understanding the pathophysiological mechanism of the disease. Additionally, brain imaging has the ability to bridge between preclinical research and human pharmacological studies.

In the future physicians will be able to obtain DNA from peripheral blood samples and obtain an allelic profile in their surgeries/offices to be used in deciding the optimal treatment algorithm. These treatment decisions will be based on the likelihood of response and development of side effects to a variety of treatments derived from that individual patient's genetic background. Currently, chips the size of a thumbnail containing up to 20 000 genes or SNPs (single nucleotide polymor-phisms) are available that can rapidly determine a person's specific genetic details regarding putative genes that are involved in pharmacogenetic phenotypes (Fig. 19.3, color plate). Technology will not be the limiting factor. Careful clinical assessment of a large number of genotyped individuals will be the limiting step. These advances have the potential to transform clinical prescribing from a trial and error process to a data-driven scientific process of response prediction.

Acknowledgement

This investigation was supported by Public Health Service research grant M01 RR00827 from the National Center for Research Resources.

REFERENCES

Basile VS, Masellis M, Badri F et al. (1999). Association of the *MscI* polymorphism of the dopa-mine D_3 receptor gene with tardive dyskinesia in schizophrenia. Neuropsychopharmacology 21, 17–27.

Bookheimer SY, Strojwas MH, Cohen MS et al. (2000). Patterns of brain activation in people at risk for Alzheimer's disease. *N Engl J Med* 343, 450–456.

Braak H, Braak E (1990). Neurofibrillary changes confined to the entorhinal region and an abun-dance of cortical amyloid in cases of presenile and senile dementia. *Acta Neuropathol* 80, 479–486.

Bunney BG, Potkin SG, Bunney WE Jr. (1995). New morphological and neuropathological find-ings in schizophrenia: a neurodevelopmental perspective. *Clin Neurosci* 3, 81–88.

Jeste DV, Caligiuri MP (1993). Tardive dyskinesia. *Schizophr Bull* 19, 303–315.

Jeste DV, Kleinman JE, Potkin SG, Luchins DJ, Weinberger DR (1982). Ex uno multi: subtyping the schizophrenic syndrome. *Biol Psychiatry* 17, 199–222.

Joyce JN, Meador-Woodruff JH (1997). Linking the family of D_2 receptors to neuronal circuits in human brain: insights into schizophrenia. *Neuropsychopharmacology* 16, 375–384.

Kane JM, Woerner M, Lieberman J (1988). Epidemiological aspects of tardive dyskinesia. *Encephale*, 14, 191–194.

Kling-Petersen T, Ljung E, Svensson K (1995). Effects on locomotor activity after local applica-tion of D_3 preferring compounds in discrete areas of the rat brain. *J Neur Transm Gen Sect* 3, 209–220.

O'Callaghan E, Larkin C, Kinsella A, Waddington JL (1990). Obstetric complications, the puta-tive familial-sporadic distinction, and tardive dyskinesia in schizophrenia. Br J Psychiatry, 157:578–584.

Poirier J, Delisle M-C, Quirion R et al. (1995). Apolipoprotein E4 allele as a predictor of choli-nergic deficits and treatment outcome in Alzheimer disease. *Proc Natl Acad Sci USA* 92, 12260–12264.

Riekkinen P Jr., Soininen H, Partanen J, Paakkonen A, Helisalmi S, Riekkinen P Sr. (1997). The ability of THA treatment to increase corical alpha waves is related to apolipoprotein E genotype of Alzheimer disease patients. *Psychopharmacology* 129, 285–288.

Rietschel M, Krauss H, Müller DJ et al. (2000). Dopamine D$_3$ receptor variant and tardive dyskinesia. *Euro Arch Psychiatr Clin Neurosci* 250, 31–35.

Roses AD, Saunders AM, Corder EH et al. (1995). Influence of the susceptibility genes apolipoprotein E-epsilon 4 and apolipoprotein E-epsilon 2 on the rate of disease expressivity of late-onset Alzheimer's disease. *Arzneimittelforschung*, 45(Suppl 3A), 413–417.

Segman R, Neeman T, Heresco-Levy U et al. (1999). Genotypic association between the dopamine D$_3$ receptor and tardive dyskinesia in chronic schizophrenia. *Mol Psychiatry* 4, 247–253.

Small GW, Ercoli LM, Silverman DHS et al. (2000). Cerebral metabolic and cognitive decline in persons at genetic risk for Alzheimer's disease. *Proc Natl Acad Sci USA* 97, 6037–6042.

Steen VM, Lüvlie R, MacEwan T, McCreadie RG (1997). Dopamine D$_3$-receptor gene variant and susceptibility to tardive dyskinesia in schizophrenic patients. *Mol Psychiatry* 2, 139–145.

Wassink TH, Nelson JJ, Crowe RR, Andreasen NC (1999). Heritability of *BDNF* alleles and their effect on brain morphology in schizophrenia. *Am J Med Genet* 88, 724–728.

Weinhold P, Wegner JT, Kane JM (1981). Familial occurrence of tardive dyskinesia. *J Clin Psychiatry* 42, 165–166.

Yassa R, Ananth J (1981). Familial tardive dyskinesia. *Am J Psychiatry* 138, 1618–1619.

Part VII

Industrial perspectives

20

Pharmacogenetics in psychotropic drug discovery and development

William Z. Potter, AnnCatherine Van Lone, and Larry Altstiel*

Lilly Research Laboratories, Indianapolis, USA
*Present address: Schering-Plough Research Institute, Kenilworth, USA

OVERVIEW

The field of pharmacogenetics impacts all stages of psychotropic drug development. At the level of discovering novel molecular sites of action and screening hundreds of thousands of compounds to find "hits" for these novel targets, the techniques of genomics, proteomics, and molecular biology are now routinely utilized. The vision for the future is that pharmacogenetics will permit matching an individual patient genotype to the specific therapeutic agent that will produce the greatest benefit with the least number of side effects. While industry-sponsored clinical trials present a real opportunity to pursue this vision, ethical and economic hurdles impede progress. The economic hurdles will remain a major barrier until examples of success attract larger investments from the pharmaceutical industry. From the viewpoint of drug development, the only generalizable success to-date has been understanding the genetic basis of variation in drug metabolism. Some convincing instances of predicting susceptibility to side effects has recently emerged. But, putative genetic predictors of *response* in neuropsychiatric disorders have either limited applicability or uncertainty and so they cannot reliably be applied to enrich populations for trials or understand variations in outcome. Given this situation, joint academic–government–industry efforts may provide a means of sharing risks and accelerating research in this promising arena.

Introduction

The 1990s provided a range of new molecular genetic techniques that should ultimately allow identification of the best available pharmacological treatment for each patient. A number of excellent recent reviews make the convincing case that the era of pharmacogenetics has arrived and will provide a new level of drug development and hitherto inaccessible breakthroughs (Rioux, 2000; Roses, 2000). In certain instances such as the treatment of late-stage breast cancer with the recombinant DNA-derived monoclonal antibody trastuzamab, it is now specified in the product labeling that only those 25–30% of patients who overexpress the protein encoded by the *HER*2 gene will benefit from the treatment (Menard et al., 2000). In the field of psychopharmacology, the closest analogous finding is that the small proportion of patients with Alzheimer's disease who are homozygous for the apolipoprotein E allele *apoE4* do not respond to cholinesterase inhibitors (Farlow et al., 1998). When we consider the treatment of psychiatric disorders, we find conflicting reports as to the association of various genotypes with response. Two recent reviews as well as several chapters in this volume provide a thorough overview of the multiple sources of variance that can lead to apparently discordant findings. They also offer tantalizing hints either that certain dopamine or serotonin receptor polymorphisms influence response to neuroleptics (see below) or that serotonin transporter polymorphisms affect response to serotonin uptake inhibitors (Lesch et al., 1996; Smeraldi et al., 1998). It, therefore, seems obvious that in drug development for the central nervous system (CNS) we should place emphasis on whole-genome single nucleotide polymorphism (SNP) disequilibrium mapping of patients in phase II trials followed by a more focused abbreviated SNP linkage disequilibrium mapping in phase III trials, as proposed by Roses (2000).

In what follows, we will discuss why this is not the general case and emphasize the need for "success stories" to allow those involved in leading CNS drug development to obtain the necessary support for a sustainable effort in pharmacogenetics. Average overall costs for any drug from discovery to market, taking into account the more than 90% of compounds selected for development that never make it to registration, is more than US $700 million. In this environment, any addition to a standard protocol that is seen as adding to the cost must be justified in terms of its value. The extraordinary commercial success of multiple selective serotonin uptake inhibitors (SSRI) for depression and the first two relatively nontoxic "atypical" antipsychotics, risperidone and olanzapine, has been built on the same type of protocol used since the 1960s. The only real progress in terms of design has been the inclusion of a broader range of scales that permit some differentiation across treatments, whether it be side effects of antidepressants or therapeutic effects on negative symptoms of schizophrenia. Use of biological measures that might reflect illness and/or genetic predisposition in clinical trials has never extended to large CNS trials despite promising findings in some small studies (Heiligenstein et al., 1994; Berman et al., 1999). Only recently has the US National Institute for Mental Health again funded relatively large-scale studies of pharmacological treatments, but these are not targeted to pharmacogenetic markers. If only by default, the field must depend on industry to apply pharmacogenetics in a clinically meaningful way. Interestingly, the closely related approaches of pharmacogenomics and proteomics have greatly altered the preclinical discovery world within major pharmaceutical companies as well as providing the primary basis for multiple biotechnology companies focused on discovering molecules designed to act on novel targets (Roses, 2000).

Current application of genomics to drug development

In preclinical drug development, genomics is utilized rather than genetics, *per se*. As Roses (2000) summarizes the case:

The difference between the genomic approach and the genetic approach is that the former creates a need to functionally validate the tissue distribution and other aspects of each identified gene and find a relevant disease or clinical indication. In contrast, once the disease-related variants of susceptibility disease genes are identified, a single susceptibility gene is automatically validated in human disease. The major distinction between the genomic and genetic approaches is target selection, with genetically defined genes and variant-specific targets already known to be involved in the disease process. The current vogue of discovery genomics for nonspecific, wholesale gene identification, with each gene in search of a relationship to a disease, creates great opportunities for development of medicines. However, there are also enormous economical costs associated with searching huge lists of genes for "the right disease for the available gene". It is correct to state that target validation is a major challenge to the pharmaceutical industry, but it is also critical to realize that the core problem for drug development is poor target selection. The screening use of unproven technologies to imply disease-related validation, and the huge investment necessary to progress each selected gene to proof of concept in humans, is based on an unproven and cavalier use of the word "validation". Each failure is very expensive in lost time and money.

Nonetheless, industry has come to depend more and more on genomics and its closely related cousin, proteomics, to identify potential drug targets and/or develop methods for the rapid identification of "hits" out of the several hundred thousand compound libraries available to large companies. The stages of drug development and how they utilize the various approaches described below are shown in Figure 20.1.

It is now standard practice to obtain DNA clones, preferably human, for specific known receptors with which cells (such as Chinese Hamster ovary cells) can be transfected for selective expression of DNA to give the coded protein. These cells, in turn, provide a specific receptor preparation, which can be plated on 384-well plates and compounds screened, using robotic processes, to see if they bind to the receptor. With this technique, hundreds of thousands of compounds can be screened within a few weeks. Those compounds that are found to bind at some threshold concentration are then modified by a team of chemists (sometimes a dozen or more), who systematically modify all possible functional groups. The goal is to achieve the best possible balance between potency, selectivity, and physico-chemical properties consistent with brain penetration and lack of susceptibility to extensive metabolism. Our experience with identifying a selective serotonin (5-HT)1f agonist is instructive. From the isolation of the receptor and obtaining its complementary DNA (cDNA) at the end of 1993 through screening (utilizing at that time a 96-well plate) and optimization to a first human dose took less than

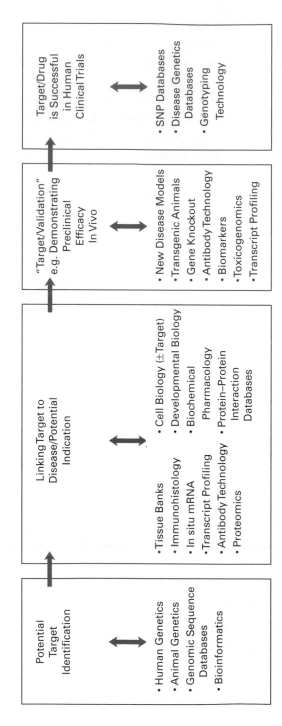

Fig. 20.1.   Stages of drug development and possible relationship to genomics and proteomics. SNP, single nucleotide polymorphism.

2 years. We are now at the point that once a target is identified and its cDNA made available, it is usually possible to identify a selective agonist, antagonist, or potentiator within a year. It can, however, take much longer to find a compound that has the characteristics of a drug: potency, reasonable bioavailability and brain penetration, and a wide enough therapeutic index.

At a more exploratory level, the field uses such techniques as transcriptional profiling to identify novel targets (Bumol and Watanabe, 2001). To-date, we are not aware of any compounds selected for a psychiatric illness that have been developed in this manner. Nonetheless, it is hoped that by studying the effects of available treatments for depression and schizophrenia on mRNAs in various brain regions, novel genes (and/or proteins) that are core to their mechanisms of actions will be found. Compounds targeted to these novel gene products might show greater efficacy and avoid undesirable effects.

The closely related activity of studying protein regulation (proteomics) has been credited with important discoveries relevant to neurological, if not psychiatric, disorders. It can readily be appreciated that there are a multitude of factors distal to basic genetic structure that determine protein regulation; indeed, there are over 200 known possible post-translational modifications of proteins with functional consequences (Banks et al., 2000). These are more and more being detected through improvements in the ability to quantify results from two-dimensional gel electrophoresis, the basic tool of proteomics. Since most drugs exert their effects on proteins, even if a target is identified through genomic techniques, understanding the regulation of the protein should ultimately prove a better way of identifying drugs than the laborious process of evaluating candidates selected primarily on the basis of binding to a particular protein in isolated systems.

Two examples of potential targets for drug development that have emerged from the application of proteomic techniques are discussed in detail elsewhere (Banks et al., 2000). In brief, in the first example, analysis of cerebrospinal fluid from patients with Creutzfeld–Jacob disease and those with the type of dementia associated with the bovine spongiform encephalopathy epidemic identified two relevant proteins. Gel electrophoresis revealed that these were conformational isomers of a normal cellular glycoprotein, isomers which were shown to be variably resistant to proteolytic degradation and associated with different clinical presentations. These insights provide the basis for one current approach to develop a new pharmacological treatment: to select peptides that can reverse the observed conformational changes in the infecting or prion protein (Soto et al., 2000).

The second example relates to Alzheimer's disease. It was the identification of a major protein fragment (beta amyloid) of senile plaques that provided the basis for cloning of the gene for the full-length amyloid precursor protein (APP) (Story and Cappai, 1999). Mutations in APP associated with a high risk of Alzheimer's disease allowed for the isolation of genetic material from humans that was utilized to engineer a mouse strain which deposits excess beta amyloid in the brain. This mouse strain has provided a model in which one can test the ability of compounds to block the deposition of beta amyloid. Certain compounds that have shown efficacy in this model have already entered clinical studies. What is notable here is the interplay of proteomic and genomic approaches to identify a target and to provide a new animal model for the in vivo evaluation of novel agents before they go into human studies. It is hoped that similar models, and other tools such as knockouts of functionally relevant genes, will permit the preclinical assessment of compounds aimed at novel targets, thereby increasing the probability of finding therapeutic effects in humans.

Issues underlying application of genetic polymorphisms to drug development

This brings us back to the other basis of pharmacogenetic and pharmacogenomics research in the field of psychopharmacology: the existence of genetic polymorphism, which is responsible for the observed phenotype described by a particular drug response. However, unlike diseases that are caused solely by the presence of a single gene (e.g., sickle cell anemia, Huntington's disease, etc.), drug response depends upon a large number of factors including drug metabolism, pharmacokinetics, and tolerability, in addition to the susceptibility of the molecular target to pharmacological intervention. Therefore, any attempt to use genetic methods to predict pharmacological response to a particular drug must respect this complexity.

Genetic studies are generally divided into family and association studies. While family-based genetic linkage studies are uncommon in pharmacogenetics and pharmacogenomics, it is important to understand the difference between these two approaches. Genetic linkage refers to the cotransmission of a polymorphic genetic marker and an identifiable trait (phenotype) in families. This phenotype may be a disease, altered drug metabolism, or other observed or quantifiable trait. Genetic linkage between a trait and marker indicates that there is sufficient statistical evidence for cotransmission of the genetic marker and trait. It can be further inferred that the gene(s) responsible for the trait are located on a particular chromosome in the vicinity of the marker. Family-based linkage studies are based on identity by descent (IBD). IBD studies have the advantage that solutions do not depend on prior knowledge of genotype and only presuppose that the trait in question has some sort of genetic basis. IBD linkage studies also allow relatively rapid genomic screening. Genetic markers identified by descent are exact copies of the same founder allele, which is inherited from generation to generation.

The baseline rate of recombination defines the size of IBD regions identified by linkage analysis. With 1 centimorgan representing a 1% recombination rate, it is possible for an IBD region to span several million base pairs. Hence it is likely that any region of this size will contain several genes in which polymorphisms in either coding regions or regulatory elements could be responsible for phenotype. Therefore, genetic linkage is useful for narrowing a region of interest on the chromosome but does not, in most cases, define an exact location of a polymorphism affecting expression of a phenotype. While linkage techniques require relatively few a priori assumptions, these techniques do depend on definitions of phenotype that remain consistent throughout an analysis. These may be disease diagnoses or quantitative trait characteristics such as drug response, which, however, are never assessed through family studies.

IBD methods require the availability of families with affected members. The vast majority of drug studies compare the performance of an experimental therapy with placebo or an established treatment in a large number of unrelated individuals. Consequently, examination of the genetics of drug response in a typical clinical trial is an association or identity by state (IBS) study. Unlike linkage studies that follow the familial association of a founder allele with a phenotype, association studies measure the association of a particular genetic marker with a particular phenotype within a defined population. While IBD regions tend to be large, IBS regions are small. IBS regions may derive from a common ancestral allele from the remote past. However, each of the individuals in an ideal population may be separated by a large number of recombination events. This ensures that regions of identity by state will be smaller than those identified by family study methods. Therefore, IBS association methods have the potential to locate accurately genes responsible for the expression of a particular phenotype.

Association methods have high sensitivity, but the specificity of these studies is susceptible to several forms of artifact. The chief source of error in case-control association studies is population stratification (Malhotra and Goldman, 1999; Risch, 2000). An association study requires, in theory, an ideal population; that is a population of unrelated individuals in which the allelic polymorphism(s) responsible for the expression of a particular phenotype are randomly distributed among the individuals. In such a population, it is possible to ascribe differences in allelic frequency to a particular phenotype. When differences in allelic frequency arise from broadly observable population differences rather than phenotype, it is possible that genetic associations will be either missed or incorrectly assigned. However, some authors have maintained that population stratification issues can be partially overcome with appropriate statistical procedures (Jorm and Easteal, 2000; Lerer et al., 2001). In some cases, age can affect the expression of a particular phenotype. For example, the *apoe4* allele has a strong effect on the age-dependent expression of Alzheimer's disease (Corder et al., 1993); however, these effects can be confounded by other competing causes of mortality influenced by *apoE* genotype (Li et al., 1996).

Despite the potential source of artifact, genetic association studies in the context of drug efficacy trials have significant potential. Large clinical trials generally enroll large numbers of unrelated individuals and, therefore, approximate ideal study populations. Phenotypic determinations, disease diagnosis, therapeutic outcomes, and safety are carefully determined. Consequently, any well-constructed clinical trial offers the potential for a genetic association study.

Determination of the association between genotype and phenotype requires an a priori hypothesis that a particular candidate allele is responsible for expression of the phenotype. Until recently, this involved labor-intensive, serial testing of candidate genes. Early efforts used restriction length fragment polymorphisms, which were supplanted by polymerase chain reaction (PCR) amplification of candidate sequences. However, the discovery and development of SNPs has revolutionized genetic analysis. High-resolution genetic maps of human SNPs now exist and these can be used to place accurately potential loci associated with a particular phenotype (Schorck et al., 2000). A variety of SNP-based technologies exist. Microarrays of DNA probes fixed to solid supports are used to detect genetic polymorphisms. Nonchip SNP-based, solution hybridization technologies are also available. SNP-based techniques are highly parallel. A single SNP chip can simultaneously screen for hundreds of candidate genes. In contrast, previous methods could at best examine a small (<10) number of candidate genes at one time. SNP techniques are also highly automated. Finally, the SNP locations have been determined on chromosomes, thus allowing localization of candidate genes (see Ch. 21).

Industry-based trials remain a promising venue for such genetic research. However, as already suggested, this enthusiasm has been tempered by the significant logistic barriers to industry-sponsored genetic studies. Each patient in a clinical trial is carefully diagnosed and followed closely for both safety and efficacy outcomes. In addition, substantial demographic data are collected. Most industry sponsors have thousands of patients in clinical trials at any given time; therefore, information gathered from these patients in addition to stored DNA allows construction of a central resource for any genetics-based study, a DNA bank. While it seems obvious that a DNA bank could be constructed from patients in clinical trials, rather few such banks exist.

A substantial barrier to DNA bank construction is assurance of individual privacy (Issa, 2000). Considerable concerns have been voiced regarding confidentiality of DNA databases and the potential for genetic discrimination if that confidentiality were violated (Hall and Rich, 2000). Ethical Review Boards have inconsistent policies regarding the collection of patient DNA, and regulatory guidelines vary from country to country (Arledge et al., 2000). It is possible to construct DNA banks that link a DNA sample to a particular individual while stripping all personal identification with that individual. An essential requirement of a DNA bank is rigorous demonstration of confidentiality.

The second barrier is the additional cost of such studies. Database construction, DNA extraction and storage, and facility maintenance are expensive, and the expense has to have tangible justification. Collection of DNA in clinical trials adds additional cost and complexity. In many cases, the present commercial value of pharmacogenetics and pharmacogenomics is largely theoretical. Genetic techniques have the potential to predict adverse events and thereby allow drugs to be given with more assurance of safety. Likewise, there is at least the chance that tests will be discovered that will allow better therapeutic targeting. However it is not a foregone conclusion that these tests will have sufficient predictive value to justify market segmentation based on genotype. Genetic studies can help to identify molecular targets and thereby accelerate drug discovery. However, the future value of these potential discoveries needs to be balanced against present costs.

Despite these concerns about the value of genetic research in the pharmaceutical industry, pharmacogenetics and pharmacogenomics will be a foundation for modern drug development. The major barriers to these efforts are neither scientific nor technical. Indeed, there is at least one area in which the application of pharmacogenetics is recognized as of sufficient value as to be incorporated into current routine drug development: drug metabolism.

Phenotyping/genotyping drug metabolism

It is now known that the major source of the wide interindividual variation in serum concentration per unit dose for many psychotropic drugs is genetic variation in drug-metabolizing enzymes (Weber and Hein, 1995). It is a routine matter to use in vitro systems to assess whether a new compound is metabolized by those mitochondrial P-450 CYP or soluble enzymes such as acetylases, which are known to show functionally relevant genetic variation. By using known inhibitors of these highly polymorphic enzymes, it is possible to estimate the extent to which a new compound depends on a particular enzyme for its metabolism. Compounds shown by these in vitro techniques to depend, for instance, on CYP2D6 or CYP3A4 for their clearance are considered undesirable for clinical development since they can be predicted to show tenfold or greater variation in observed plasma concentrations across subjects given the same dose. Moreover, regulatory agencies such as the US Food and Drug Administration require as part of registration dossiers that it be shown whether or not a new drug has or is likely to have pharmacokinetic interactions with other agents that patients may take. Therefore, if it can be shown – using either human liver microsomal preparations or cell lines transfected with P-450 CYP isozyme-specific DNA – that a new compound is *not* subject to metabolism by highly variable enzymes then expensive and time-consuming clinical drug interaction studies may be avoided. Current submissions to regulatory authorities for marketing approval may include as many as 25–30 separate clinical pharmacological studies, a large proportion of which are directed toward assessing pharmacokinetic drug interactions.

Depending on the preclinical data, regulatory authorities often require direct evidence in humans of the impact of exposing individuals who show a marked deficiency in certain metabolic pathways. Therefore, a business has developed of genotyping healthy subjects to identify, for instance, the 5% of the Caucasian population who have those haplotypes associated with low to absent activity of CYP2D6. These pre-identified subjects are then recruited as paid volunteers for required studies to evaluate whether poor CYP2D6 metabolizers are at greater risk for significant side effects.

Until recently, in actual clinical trials one controlled for pharmacokinetic variance by "phenotyping;" this was measuring plasma concentrations of the actual drug or a test drug such as debrisoquine. A large study of over a thousand subjects in which debrisoquine phenotyping of CYP2D6 activity and genotyping were compared yielded equivalent results in terms of identifying the poor metabolizers (Leathart et al., 1998). In a current drug development program at Lilly Research Laboratories in which children are given tomoxetine, a norepinephrine uptake inhibitor known to be extensively metabolized through CYP2D6, subjects were initially genotyped for the relevant polymorphisms and either excluded or dosed differently if they had the alleles associated with low metabolism. Although there was no known risk to exposing 5% of the children to a ten times higher plasma concentration than the mean of the overall group, it seemed prudent in initial pediatric studies to avoid exposure of a subpopulation to 10-fold higher concentrations than expected to be necessary for efficacy.

In CNS clinical trials in which there is a strong incentive to achieve a target blood concentration, most often in the case of antiepileptic drugs, the process is basically phenotyping drug elimination, which, in turn, is likely to be under genetic control. Lithium, the elimination of which depends primarily on renal function, is an obvious exception. Although knowledge of metabolic genotype should provide a means of controlling pharmacokinetic variance in clinical trials, it is not so clear that this will increase the efficiency of trials in the major psychiatric disorders for which relationships between measured drug concentrations and clinical response are weak at best.

This raises the issue of active metabolites that can potentially contribute to or interfere with efficacy and/or toxicity. The presence of biologically active metabolites of a new drug, metabolites which are unlikely to have been fully studied preclinically, poses an additional burden on the development process. Moreover, active metabolites confound any pharmacokinetic/pharmacodynamic relationship that one is seeking to establish since it cannot be known if effects are caused solely by the parent compound. An ideal drug for testing a hypothesis whether a specific action is associated with a specific effect with minimal interindividual variance is, therefore, a compound with only one known pharmacological action and which is not metabolized by any functionally polymorphic enzymes.

Pharmacogenetics and drug toxicity

Pharmacokinetic variance can also be associated with differential toxicity, another reason to try to avoid this in new compounds. Phenotypic variations in drug metabolism in different ethnic groups, later explored in terms of various genotypes, may be associated with higher or lower rates of drug-associated toxicity. For instance, a higher proportion of Japanese show rapid N-acetylation of several drugs, including isoniazid than do Caucasians, while subjects of Mediterranean origin are predominantly slow acetylators (Weber and Hein, 1985). Similarly, there are ethnic differences in the rate of INH induced hepatotoxicity with slow acetylators at greater risk (Eichelbaum et al., 1982; Peretti et al., 1987). More generally, metabolic variation can be expected to relate to the toxicity of compounds with a relatively narrow therapeutic index. Polymorphisms in *CYP2C9* account for differences in warfarin metabolism and an increased risk of bleeding in poor metabolizers (Aithal et al., 1998). The risk of thiopurine toxicity after a given dose is related to specific thiopurine *S*-methyltransferase alleles, such that genotyping is now being recommended prior to treatment (McLeod et al., 1999; Relling et al., 1999). The likelihood of drug interactions also depends on the major routes of metabolism and their variability. Additionally, susceptibility to experiencing a toxic reaction to a given drug concentration can also vary on a genetic basis. Consequently, complex interactions of pharmacokinetic and pharmacodynamic variability are possible. For instance, inhibition of the CYP3A4 pathway by various added drugs in persons taking terfenadine can produce a range of increases in terfenadine concentrations and an associated risk of fatal arrhythmias, depending on the individual's susceptibility to the QTc syndrome (Saviuc et al., 1993).

Another example of genetically determined variations in side effects observed for a given exposure is provided by tacrine-induced hepatotoxicity. In this instance, a combination of alleles conferring a deficiency of two polymorphically expressed isozymes of glutathione *S*-transferase increase the risk such that 72% of subjects with the double null genotype have markedly elevated alanine aminotransferase levels (Simon et al., 2000). Susceptibility to tardive dyskinesia with neuroleptic drugs may also vary on a genetic basis. It has been reported that functional polymorphisms of *CYP1A2* contribute to such a risk (Basile et al., 2000). Interestingly, there may also be a "small but significant" contribution of polymorphisms in the genes for the $5HT2_c$ and dopamine D_3 receptors to susceptibility to tardive dyskinesia (Segman et al., 2000).

These examples indicate the utility of pharmacogenomics in estimating and possibly controlling the risk of side effects in population studies. With greater knowledge of alleles that confer substantially increased risk to certain side effects, they may ultimately prove to have a prospective application. The alternative approach of genotyping in response to recurrence of an adverse event has been recommended in at least one clinical circumstance: to assess women who experience deep-vein thrombosis while taking oral contraceptives for a susceptibility-conferring genotype at the prothrombin gene locus (Martinelli et al., 1998).

Pharmacogenetic predictors of central nervous system drug response

An even more common problem is variability in clinical, not toxic, responses to a given concentration of a new compound. What is most desirable in drug development, therefore, is prior knowledge as to whether or not there is identifiable genetic variability that can predict the therapeutic response. Although several other chapters in this volume provide detailed examples of promising findings, we will briefly review some of those concerning clozapine response as a basis for some more general points.

To-date, at least two excellent reviews have been compiled of studies on polymorphic variability as a predictor of response to atypical antipsychotics (Brockmoller et al., 1998; Masellis et al., 2000). Table 20.1 builds on these compilations to show the current state of research around genetic predictors of response to clozapine. Several factors mandate caution in relying on the positive association data summarized in Table 20.1. For example, the Lin et al. (1999) and Yu et al. (1999) studies utilized the same patient population, decreasing the external validity (Masellis et al., 2000). In addition, the skewed population in the Yu et al. (1999) trial with a specific six patient subgroup compared with other groups of 52 and 42 subjects could have introduced a type I error. In this report, 52 patients with the 267C/C genotype showed no difference in response from the 42 heterozygotes (267C/T); only the six 267T/T patients responded differently to clozapine. Other studies display similar problems and highlight the need for far more extensive replication, even in the case of clozapine, before one can rely on candidate gene analyses to predict response.

A multipoint haplotype analysis has recently been conducted by Arranz et al. (2000a). Past candidate gene studies were analyzed to determine the most commonly occurring polymorphisms that provided correlation to atypical antipsychotic response. The most common polymorphisms were narrowed by statistical analyses and six were found to have a 76% level of prediction of clozapine response. The authors claim this is the first study to enable individualized neuroleptic treatment based on genetic analysis (Arranz et al., 2000a). Again, replication is needed.

Table 20.1. Studies measuring pharmacogenetic variations and response to clozapine

Receptor	Gene (polymorphism)	Positive associations	Negative associations
Dopamine			
D_2	Promoter region 141Cins/del		Arranz et al., 1998
D_3	Ser9Gly		Shaikh et al., 1996; Malhotra et al., 1998
D_4	*D4.4/D4.7*		Rao et al., 1994; Shaikh et al., 1993, 1995; Kohn et al., 1997
	Val194Gly	Liu et al., 1996	
	Gly11Arg		Rietschel et al., 1996
	12 bp repeat		Rietschel et al., 1996
	13 bp deletion		Rietschel et al., 1996
	48 bp repeats	Hwu et al., 1998	Rietschel et al., 1996
Serotonin			
5-HT_{2A}	102 T/C	Arranz et al., 1995	Nothen et al., 1995; Malhotra et al., 1996a; Jonssen et al., 1996; Lin et al., 1999; Nimgaonkar et al., 1996
	His452Tyr	Arranz et al., 1996	Malhotra et al., 1996a
	Thr25Asp		Masellis et al., 1995
5-HT2C	Cys23Ser	Sodhi et al., 1995	Rietschel et al., 1997; Malhotra et al., 1996b
5-HT6	267T/T	Yu et al., 1999	Masellis et al., 2000
Polymorphism combinations		Arranz et al., 2000b	

Another limitation of the studies summarized in Table 20.1 is the absence of placebo controls. This could be less of a problem if placebo response was negligible or even constant, a situation that does not hold even in the case of antipsychotic trials. Rioux (2000) has recently provided a very clear analysis of the problem with a real life example involving substance P antagonists as possible antidepressants.

Since substance P is extensively metabolized by angiotensin 1-converting enzyme (ACE), variations in ACE amount or activity could affect substance P concentrations and the relative impact of a substance P antagonist. It is known that a functional insertion/deletion polymorphism in the ACE gene has an allele frequency of 34% for the deletion (*D*) and 66% for the insertion (*I*) (Rigat and Alhenc-Gelas, 1990; Todd et al., 1995). Homozygotes for *DD* have higher substance P in the brain than *II* homozygotes, with *ID* heterozygotes having intermediate values. The question then was whether *DD* patients would respond preferentially to a substance P antagonist. In one study, the 11% of subjects observed to be *DD* homozygous had a higher concentration of substance P in the brain and higher likelihood of affective illness than the 43% who were *II* homozygous (Arinami et al., 1996).

Despite a prior positive antidepressant phase II trial of a substance P antagonist (Kramer et al., 1998), a subsequent larger trial failed to show an effect and was essentially uninterpretable given the placebo response rate of 48% (Rioux, 2000). If one reasons, post hoc, that the *DD* homozygous patients with high CNS substance P concentrations were the true patients for this target and that heterozygotes and *II* homozygotes would only respond at the same rate as all patients on placebo, then applying the haplotype frequencies from the literature and equations provided in Rioux's (2000) paper, the 11% of "true" patients would have had to have a 100% response rate.

There is a complex interplay between allele frequency, the percentage treatment–placebo difference in response rates, and the maximum gain in response rate that can be attained by counting only those subjects homozygous for the polymorphism associated with response. In the case of genotype associations with clozapine response (Table 20.1), placebo response has not been taken into account. Nor, to our knowledge, has this been done for any other treatment–genotype association studies for a psychiatric or other CNS disorder. Any degree of placebo response (especially in the subgroup with the genotype that is supposed to predict response) reduces the fraction of the response that can be attributed to drug *and* the maximum possible gain in observing a drug effect through selecting a particular genotype (Rioux, 2000).

This also raises the issue of how one determines "response," which is most often defined as some percentage change on a rating scale or difference in global clinical impression rather than an easily measured quantitative outcome. Ideally, one would have an objective quantitative measure that behaves in a predictable manner across studies and populations rather than the highly variable ones typically employed in studies of CNS disorders. It is usually not feasible to ascertain retrospectively the behavior of outcome measures from standard clinical trials (and impossible in the case of cumulative case series) since the detailed information necessary to do this properly is often not recorded. Only prospective studies can generate data of the type needed to validate the use of genotyping to predict treatment response.

Prospective enrichment of trials through genotyping

The greatest problem for characterizing the increasing number of novel agents targeted to CNS disorders is one of signal detection in clinical trials (Robinson and Rickels, 2000). If we could, for instance, prospectively show a marked difference in categorical antidepressant response between two groups based on genotype in a properly powered study, and this could be replicated, then such enrichment by genotype would become the norm. The reason for emphasizing a prospective design is that equal allocation to treatment and placebo by genotype could be assured, assumptions about relevant variables (e.g. definition of response as final Hamilton Depression Scale 17 score of <7 and nonresponse as $<20\%$ decrease) would be specified, and the study could thereby be properly powered. In the world of clinical trial design, whether or not to use an enrichment strategy depends on performance characteristics of the criteria under just such constraints, since decisions to go forward or not based on results from a proof of concept or phase II study with a new molecule include estimates (or beliefs) about the probability of a type I or II error.

Conclusions

Implementation of prospective studies using genotyping to assess treatment response in a psychiatric disorder will remain a problem for many in the pharmaceutical industry as long as the logistic and ethical issues discussed above are perceived to be significant barriers. Alternatively, it might be possible for academic investigators to initiate such a study with support from multiple sources (including unrestricted grants from industry) and show its feasibility, paying attention to the multiple issues we have raised in this paper. An effort of this type could serve as a major catalyst for fuller engagement of the pharmaceutical industry in capitalizing on the promise of pharmacogenetics for clinical outcome as well as for target identification and preclinical and metabolic studies.

REFERENCES

Aithal GP, Day CP, Kesteven PJ, Daly AK (1999). Association of polymorphisms in the cytochrome P-450 CYP2C9 with warfarin dose requirement and risk of bleeding complications. *Lancet* 353, 717–719.

Arinami T, Li L, Mitsushio H (1996). An insertion/deletion polymorphism in the angiotensin converting enzyme gene is associated with both brain substance P contents and affective disorders. *Biol Psychiatry* 40, 1122–1127.

Arledge T, Freeman A, Arbuckle J, Mosteller M, Mancaso P (2000). Applications of pharmacogenetics to drug development: the Glaxo-Wellcome experience. *Drug Metab Rev*, 32, 387–394.

Arranz M, Collier D, Sodhi M et al. (1995). Association between clozapine response and allelic variation in 5-HT$_{2A}$ receptor gene. *Lancet* 346, 281–282.

Arranz MJ, Lin MW, Powell J, Kerwin R, Collier D (1996). 5HT2A receptor polymorphism and schizophrenia. *Lancet* 347, 1830–1831.

Arranz MJ, Li T, Munro J et al. (1998). Lack of association between a polymorphism in the promoter region of the dopamine-2 receptor gene and clozapine response. *Pharmacogenetics* 8, 481–484.

Arranz MJ, Munro J, Birkett J et al. (2000a). Pharmacogenetic prediction of clozapine response. *Lancet* 355, 1615–1616.

Arranz MJ, Bolonna AA, Munro J, Curtis CJ, Collier DA, Kerwin RW (2000b). The serotonin transporter and clozapine response. *Mol Psychiatry* 5, 124–130.

Banks RE, Dunn MJ, Hochstrasser DF et al. (2000). Proteomics: new perspectives, new biomedical opportunities. *Lancet* 356, 1749–1756.

Basile VS, Ozdemir V, Masellis M et al. (2000). A functional polymorphism of the cytotoxic P450 1A2 (*CYP1A2*) gene: association with tardive dyskinesia in schizophrenia. *Mol Psychiatry* 5, 410–417.

Berman RM, Belanoff JK, Charney DS, Schatzberg AF (1999). Principles of the pharmacotherapy of depression. In *Neurobiology of Mental Illness*. New York: Oxford University Press, pp. 419–432.

Brockmoller J, Kaiser R, Roots I (1998). Receptor polymorphisms and psychotropic drug response. In *Clinical Pharmacology in Psychiatry: Finding the Right Dose of Psychotropic Drugs*, ed. LP Balant, J Benitez, SG Dahl et al., Badajoz, Spain: European Commission, pp. 203–232.

Bumol TF, Watanabe AM (2001). Genetic information, genomic technologies, and the future of drug discovery. *J Am Med Assoc* 285, 551–555.

Collins FS (1999). Shattuck lecture: medical and societal consequences of the human genome project. *N Engl J Med* 341, 28–37.

Corder EH, Saunders AM, Strittmatter WJ et al. (1993). Gene dose of apolipoprotein E type 4 allele and the risk of Alzheimer's disease in late onset families. *Science* 261, 921–923.

Eichelbaum M, Musch E, Castro-Parra M, von Sassen W (1982). Isoniazid hepatotoxicity in relation to acetylator phenotype and isoniazid metabolism. *Br J Clin Pharmacol* 14, 575–576.

Farlow MR, Lahiri DK, Poirier J, Davignon J, Schneider L, Hui SL (1998). Treatment outcome of tacrine therapy depends on apolipoprotein genotype and gender of the subjects with Alzheimer's disease. *Neurology* 50, 669–677.

Hall MA, Rich SS (2000). Genetics privacy laws and patients' fear of discrimination by health insurers: the view from genetics counselors. *J Law Med Ethics* 28, 245–257.

Heiligenstein JH, Faries DE, Rush AJ et al. (1994). Latency to rapid eye movement sleep as a predictor of treatment response to fluoxetine and placebo in nonpsychotic depressed outpatients. *Psychiatr Res* 52, 327–339.

Hwu HG, Hong CJ, Lee YL, Lee PC, Lee S (1998). Dopamine D_4 receptor gene polymorphisms and neuroleptic response in schizophrenia. *Biol Psychiatry* 44, 483–487.

Issa AM (2000). Ethical considerations in pharmacogenomics research. *Trends Pharmacol Sci* 21, 247–249.

Jonssen E, Lannfelt L, Sokoloff P, Schwartz JC, Sedvall G (1996). $5HT_{2A}$ receptor polymorphism and schizophrenia. *Lancet* 347, 1831.

Jorm AF, Easteal S (2000). Assessing candidate genes as risk factors for mental disorders: the value of population-based epidemiological studies. *Soc Psychiatry Psychiatr Epidemiol* 35, 1–4.

Kohn Y, Ebstein RP, Heresco-Levy U et al. (1997). Dopamine D_4 receptor gene polymorphisms: relation to ethnicity, no association with schizophrenia and response to clozapine in Israeli subjects. *Eur Neuropsychopharmacol* 7, 39–43.

Kramer MS, Cutler N, Feighner J et al. (1998). Distinct mechanism of antidepressant activity by blockade of central substance P receptors. *Science* 281, 1640–1645.

Leathart JB, London SJ, Stewart A, Adams JD, Idle JK, Daly AK (1998). CYP2D6 phenotype–genotype relationships in African-Americans and Caucasians in Los Angeles. *Pharmacogenetics* 8, 529–541.

Lerer B, Macciardi F, Segman RH et al. (2001). Variability of $5HT_{2C}$ receptor Cys23Ser polymorphism among European populations and vulnerability to affective disorder. *Mol Psychiatry* in press.

Lesch KP, Bengel D, Heils A et al. (1996). Association of anxiety-related traits with a polymorphism in the serotonin transporter gene regulatory region. *Science* 274, 1527–1531.

Li G, Silverman JM, Altstiel LD et al. (1996). Apolipoprotein E-epsilon 4 allele and familial risk in Alzheimer's disease. *Genet Epidemiol* 13, 285–298.

Lin CH, Tsai SJ, Yu YWY et al. (1999). No evidence for association of serotonin 2A receptor variant (102T/C) with schizophrenia or clozapine response in a Chinese population. *Neuroreport* 10, 57–60.

Liu ISC, Seeman P, Suparna S et al. (1996). Dopamine D_4 receptor variant in Africans, D_4 Valine194Glycine, is insensitive to dopamine and clozapine: report of a homozygous individual. *Am J Med Genet* 61, 277–282.

Malhotra AK, Goldman D (1999). Benefits and pitfalls encountered in psychiatric genetic association studies. *Biol Psychiatry* 45, 544–550.

Malhotra AK, Goldman D, Ozaki N, Breier A, Buchanan R, Pickar D (1996a). Lack of association between polymorphisms in the $5\text{-}HT_{2A}$ receptor gene and the antipsychotic response to clozapine. *Am J Psychiatry* 153, 1092–1094.

Malhotra AK, Goldman D, Ozaki H et al. (1996b). Clozapine response and the $5H_{2C}$ Cys23Ser polymorphism. *Neuroreport* 7, 2100–2102.

Malhotra AK, Goldman D, Buchanan RW et al. (1998). The dopamine D_3 receptor (*DRD3*) Ser9Gly polymorphism and schizophrenia: a haplotype relative risk study and association with clozapine response. *Mol Psychiatry* 3, 72–75.

Martinelli I, Sacchi E, Landi G, Taioli E, Duca F, Mannucci PM (1998). High risk of cerebral vein thrombosis in carriers of a prothrombin-gene mutation and in users of oral contraceptives. *N Eng J Med* 338, 1793–1797.

Masellis M, Paterson AD, Badri F et al. (1995). Genetic variation of the $5\text{-}HT_{2A}$ receptor and response to clozapine. *Lancet* 346, 1108.

Masellis M, Vincenzo SB, Ozdemir V, Meltzer HY, Macciardi FM, Kennedy JL (2000). Pharmacogenomics of antipsychotic treatment: lessons learned from clozapine. *Biol Psychiatry* 47, 252–266.

McLeod HL, Pritchard SC, Githang'a J et al. (1999). Ethnic differences in thiopurine methyltransferase pharmacogenetics: evidence for allele specificity in Caucasian and Kenyan individuals. *Pharmacogenetics* 9, 773–776.

Menard S, Tagliabue E, Campiglio M, Pupa SM (2000). Role of *HER2* gene overexpression in breast carcinoma. *J Cell Physiol* 182, 150–162.

Nimgaonkar VL, Zhang XR, Brar JS, LeLeo M, Ganguli R (1996). 5-HT$_2$ receptor gene locus: association with schizophrenia or treatment response not detected. *Psychiatr Genet* 6, 23–27.

Nothen MM, Reitschel M, Erdmann J et al. (1995). Genetic variation of the 5-HT$_{2A}$ receptor and response to clozapine. *Lancet* 346, 908–909.

Peretti E, Karlaganis G, Lauterburg BH (1987). Increased excretion of toxic hydrazine metabolites of isoniazid by slow acetylators: effect of a slow release preparation of isoniazid. *Eur J Clin Pharmacol* 33, 283–286.

Rao PA, Pickar D, Gejman PV, Ram A, Gershon ES, Gelernter J (1994). Allelic variation of the D$_4$ dopamine receptor (*DRD4*) gene does not predict response to clozapine. *Psychiatry* 51, 912–917.

Relling MV, Hancock ML, Rivera GK et al. (1999). Mercaptopurine therapy intolerance and heterozygosity at the thiopurine *S*-methyltransferase gene locus. *J Nat Cancer Inst* 91, 2001–2008.

Rietschel M, Naber D, Oberlander H et al. (1996). Efficacy and side-effects of clozapine: testing for association with allelic variation in the dopamine D$_4$ receptor gene. *Neuropsychopharmacology* 15, 491–496.

Rietschel M, Naber D, Fimmers R, Moller HJ, Proppine P, Nothen MM (1997). Efficacy and side-effects of clozapine not associated with variation in the 5-HT$_{2C}$ receptor. *Neuroreport* 8, 1999–2003.

Rigat B, Alhenc-Gelas F (1990). An insertion/deletion polymorphism in the angiotensin I-convertin enzyme gene accounting for half the variance of serum enzyme levels. *J Clin Invest* 86, 1343–1346.

Rioux PP (2000). Clinical trials in pharmacogenetics and pharmacogenomics: methods and applications. *Am J Health System Pharm* 57, 887–901.

Risch NJ (2000). Searching for genetic determinants in the new millenium. *Nature* 405, 847–856.

Robinson DS, Rickels K (2000). Concerns about clinical drug trials. *J Clin Psychopharmacol* 20, 593–596.

Roses AD (2000). Pharmacogenetics and the future of drug development and delivery. *Lancet* 355, 1358–1361.

Sato C, Kascsak RJ, Saborio GP et al. (2000). Reversion of prion protein conformational changes by synthetic β-sheet breaker peptides. *Lancet* 355, 192–197.

Saviuc P, Danel V, Dixmerias F (1993). Prolonged QT interval and torsades de pointes following astemizole overdose. *Clin Toxicol* 31, 121.

Schorck NJ, Fallin D, Lanchbury DS (2000). Single nucleotide polymorphisms and the future of genetic epidemiology. *Clin Genet* 58, 250–264.

Segman RH, Heresco-Levy U, Finekl B et al. (2000). Association between the serotonin 2C receptor gene and tardive dyskinesia in chronic schizophrenia: additive contribution of *5-HT2C*ser and *DRD3*gly alleles to susceptibility. *Psychopharmacology* 152, 408–413.

Shaikh S, Collier DA, Kerwin RW et al. (1993). Dopamine D$_4$ receptor subtypes and response to clozapine. *Lancet* 341, 116.

Shaikh S, Collier DA, Sham P et al. (1995). Analysis of clozapine response and polymorphisms of the dopamine D$_4$ receptor gene (*DRD4*) in schizophrenic patients. *Am J Med Genet* 60, 541–545.

Shaikh S, Collier DA, Sham P et al. (1996). Allelic association between a Ser-9-Gly polymorphism in the dopamine D_3 receptor gene and schizophrenia. *Hum Genet* 97, 714–719.

Simon T, Becquemont L, Mary-Krause M et al. (2000). Combined glutathione-*S*-transferase M1 and T1 genetic polymorphism and tacrine hepatotoxicity. *Clin Pharmacol Ther* 67, 432–437.

Smeraldi E, Zanardi R, Benedetti F, DiBella D, Perez J, Catalano M (1998). Polymorphism within the promoter of the serotonin transporter gene and antidepressant efficacy of fluvoxamine. *Mol Psychiatry* 3, 508–511.

Sodhi MS, Arranz MJ, Curtis D et al. (1995). Association between clozapine response and the alleleic variation in the 5-HT_{2C} receptor gene. *Neuroreport* 7, 169–172.

Storey E, Cappai R (1999). The amyloid precursor protein of Alzheimer's disease and the Ab protein. *Neuropathol Appl Neurobiol* 25, 81–97.

Todd GP, Chadwick IG, Higgins KS (1995). Relation between changes in blood pressure and serum ACE activity after a single dose of enalapril and ACE genotype in healthy subjects. *Br J Clin Pharmacol* 39, 131–134.

Weber WW, Hein DW (1985). N-acetylation pharmacogenetics. *Pharmacology* 37, 25–79.

Yu YW, Tsai SJ, Lin CH, Hsu CP, Yang KH, Hong CJ (1999). Serotonin-6 receptor variant (C267T) and clinical response to clozapine. *Neuroreport* 16, 1231–1233.

21

High-throughput single nucleotide polymorphism genotyping

Anne Shalom[1] and Ariel Darvasi[1,2]

[1]The Life Sciences Institute, The Hebrew University of Jerusalem, Israel
[2]IDgene Pharmaceuticals Ltd, Jerusalem, Israel

OVERVIEW

The completion of a draft of the human genome sequence provides unprecedented opportunities for the discovery of important, genetically validated targets in complex, polygenic diseases. The growing catalogs of single nucleotide polymorphisms (SNPs) are becoming the basic tool for use in genetic association studies to identify genes for many medically important conditions. Drug responses is as complex as disease genetics, resulting from underlying genotypic variation at many loci and also from variation in other nongenetic factors. Genomic technologies are increasingly being adopted in the biotechnology and pharmaceutical industries to accelerate identification of disease-validated targets for drug discovery. Improved genotyping methods combined with a large number of defined SNPs will lead to an increasing number of genetically validated targets. In this chapter, the major methodologies that have been developed over the past few years for SNP genotyping are described. Most of these methods have been directed to allowing high-throughput analysis of a large number of SNPs over a large number of samples, at a reduced cost. Using these technologies is likely to provide for a radical change in drug development, prescription and utilization.

Introduction

Complexity of the genetic component of the drug response

Drug response variation among individuals can have important implications and is a major concern for the clinician, as well as for the pharmaceutical industry. In some cases, this variation will affect the daily dosage (which can even vary up to 40-fold) for different individuals. It may even result in total absence of response to a specific drug (such as in schizophrenia, where 30% of the patients do not response to antipsychotic treatment), and in adverse drug reactions. Early studies of the drug response parameter at the population level suggested a Mendelian inheritance pattern. The discipline of pharmacogenetics, therefore, arose from the identification and investigation of the genetic factors underlying clearly observable phenotypes, such as an aberrant clinical response to a given drug (Motulsky, 1957).

Maximizing drug response while minimizing adverse effects for individuals through the study of gene variations is the goal of current pharmacogenomics. Although the two terms pharmacogenetics and pharmacogenomics are often used interchangeably, the latter represents an integrative approach to the genetic basis of drug response. Overall drug response, rather than being a simple Mendelian trait, will in most cases result from the complex interaction of multiple gene products, including those involved in drug absorption, transport pharmacodynamics (drug targets), biotransformation, and excretion (Evans and Relling, 1999). Therefore, an integrative strategy is required to analyze the complex, and often subtle, multigenetically determined phenotypes of a drug response. This strategy involves the genome-wide study of the genetic basis underlying the differences among individuals' responses to drugs.

Until recently, the ability to analyze genetically such complex traits in a comprehensive fashion has been hindered by technical limitations and by a lack of knowledge regarding the identities of the various gene products involved in the intricate network of events that result in patient's response to a given drug. Pharmacogenetics, over its almost 40-year history, has not resulted in major changes in how drugs are discovered or used. The new pharmacogenomics, however, sets out to bring a revolutionary approach to drug development and administration. The rapid expansion of genomics, allowing the systematic examination of variations in the entire human genome, provides the necessary jumping board for this new approach. Such knowledge is now rapidly refining our understanding of the molecular pathways responsible for genetic disease and how they differ from individual to individual, resulting in varying responses to drug treatment.

As the DNA sequence of the human genome is being completely elucidated, large-scale DNA analysis will play a crucial role in determining the relationship between genotype (DNA sequence) and phenotype (disease and health, or drug response) (Cooper and Clayton, 1988). Currently, pharmacogenomics may employ genetic association studies, which have been found to show increased statistical power (Risch and Merikangas, 1996). These studies use powerful experimental and data-handling techniques in DNA analysis to determine the genomic region(s) responsible for the observed phenotypic variation in drug response. Polymorphic, easily detectable molecular markers identify the defined regions. Once established, these markers may allow an efficient and low-cost determination of the complex genetic profiles involved in the drug response. Defining the genetic factors involved in drug response may, in turn, permit prediction of new or existing therapeutic agents for use with maximal efficiency and minimal toxicity.

Properties of single nucleotide polymorphisms

The most common type of human genetic variation is the SNP, a position at which two alternative bases occur at appreciable frequency ($>1\%$) in the human population (Collins et al., 1997). Based on data collected to-date, it has been estimated that humans vary from one another approximately once in every 300 to 1000 nucleotides, which means that there might be about three to ten million sites of significant nucleotide variation in the three billion base human genome. Organizations such as the National Human Genome Research Institute (*http://www.nhgri.nih.gov/*) and the SNP Consortium (*http://snp.cshl.org* – Marshall, 1999) are creating public databases cataloging several hundreds of thousands of these markers. There has been growing recognition that large collections of mapped SNPs would provide a powerful tool for human genetic studies (Risch and Merikangas, 1996; Kruglyak, 1999). SNPs present several advantages over other widely exploited DNA markers, such as microsatellites: SNPs are much more frequent than microsatellites, they are less prone to germline mutations (which makes them easier to follow through the generations), and they can occur within coding or regulatory regions or genes (implying that they may be directly responsible for the traits studied). SNPs found in the coding regions of genes have been termed cSNPs (Cargill et al., 1999). Finally, SNPs are mostly biallelic and relatively easy to score under automation (Wang et al., 1998; Brookes, 1999).

The place of SNPs in pharmacogenomics research

There are three major phases to SNP pharmacogenomics. The first step is SNP discovery and mapping, which consists of the identification and cataloging of SNPs as they appear on the human genome map. The second step, SNP scoring, intends to establish a correlation between specific SNPs and relevant phenotypic variation, such as clinically documented disparities in drug response. The third step, SNP diagnostics, will be the development of SNP-based diagnostic tests to determine the genetic profile of patients, from which a desired/adverse response to a particular drug can be predicted.

Among these, the scoring step holds the greatest potential for uncovering medically important information. Converting raw SNP map data into useful information will lead to the identification of SNP profiles of patients who will benefit from specific drugs. This step necessitates applying high-throughput SNP genotyping methods in the context of well-designed clinical pharmacogenetics correlation studies.

SNP genotyping technologies

Two central elements are essential for realizing the tremendous potential of SNPs in correlation studies (and later in diagnostic tests). The first is access to well-characterized patient and control populations and the second is access to technologies permitting rapid and accurate genotyping of multiple individuals with numerous markers. For example, a genotyping experiment on 5000 individuals using 100 000 SNPs would generate 500 million genotypes. Processing or scoring of large numbers of SNPs in large numbers of patients, with superior accuracy and at the lowest possible cost, is necessary for large-scale correlation studies to be practically feasible (McCarthy and Hilfiker, 2000).

A number of technologies have, therefore, been developed for SNP genotyping, aiming at a high-throughput experimentation profile. Detailed technical reviews of these methods can be found elsewhere (Landegren et al., 1998; Whitcombe et al., 1998; Ravine, 1999; Gray et al., 2000). In this chapter, we shall present the basic principle of the methods employed for SNP allele discrimination and detection. Table 21.1 summarizes the various methods, integrated with a number of specific genotyping technologies appearing in the literature.

Basic methods

Identification of single base substitutions in the DNA can be achieved by a few different ways. Most methods currently adopted require a preliminary amplification, by the polymerase chain reaction (PCR), of a small DNA fragment (usually a few hundred bases long) around the SNP to be analyzed. The next step consists in resolving the allelic state of the fragment at the polymorphism point (usually a two-base alternative); this requires first establishing an assessable discrimination between the alleles. The allelic state is later identified, using an accordingly suitable detection method.

Allele discrimination

There are six major PCR-based strategies for SNP allele discrimination:

Allele-specific amplification

For differential amplification of the SNP alleles, a PCR primer is designed, where the 3′ base corresponds to the polymorphic site. Consequently, only one of the two alleles will allow perfect matching and be amplified. In this case, the SNP detection is concomitant to the amplification step. This strategy has been termed ARMS or allele refractory mutation system (Newton et al., 1989). In realtime PCR, the allele-specific primers are designed to differ significantly in their melting temperature (T_m), by addition of a GC-tail to one of the primers. Allele detection can be achieved by T_m shift measurement (Germer and Higuchi, 1999).

Restriction endonuclease digestion

When a nucleotide substitution creates or eliminates a restriction site, the alleles can be identified by appropriate restriction, followed by electrophoresis for resolution of the digestion products (Middle et al., 2000).

Table 21.1. Summary of single nucleotide polymorphism genotyping technologies[a]

Allele discrimination	Detection method/particularity[b]	Specific name (company)	Application reference[c]
Allele specific amplification	Fluorescence/one allele primer has GC tail, resulting in T_m shift between alleles	T_m shift	Germer and Higuchi, 1999
	Fluorescence polarization	ARMS	Gibson et al., 1997
Restriction digestion	MADGE; MALDI-TOF		Wu et al., 2000; Srinivasan et al., 1998
Primer extension and minisequencing	Fluorescence, electrophoresis		Pastinen et al., 1996
	Pyrophosphate detection	(Pyrosequencing)	Alderborn et al., 2000
	DHPLC		Hoogendoorn et al., 1999
	Fluorescence/flow cytometry on microsphere arrays	GAMMArrays	Cai et al., 2000
	Fluorescence	SBE-Tags	Hirschhorn et al., 2000
	MALDI-TOF/allele-specific elongation	COSBE (Sequenom)	
	MALDI-TOF MS	PROBE	Braun et al., 1997
		PINPOINT	Haff and Smirnov, 1997; Ross et al., 1998
		VSET	Sun et al., 2000
		GOOD	Sauer et al., 2000
	FRET/5' exonuclease assay	TaqMan	Livak et al., 1995
	FRET; fluorescence polarization	TDI	Chen and Kwok, 1997; Chen et al., 1999
	Fluorescence/kinetic PCR	(Roche; Applied Biosystems)	Germer et al., 2000
Allele-specific hybridization	Fluorescence/microarrays	VDA (Affymetrix)	Wang et al., 1998
	Fluorescence/T_m	DASH (Hybaid)	Howell et al., 1999
	FRET/real-time PCR		Nauck et al., 1999
	FRET; MALDI-TOF	Invader (Third Wave Technologies)	Lyamichev et al., 1999; Griffin et al., 1999
	MALDI-TOF	PNA	Ross et al., 1997

Heteroduplex formation	Capillary-CSGE		Rozycka et al., 2000
	Endonuclease cleavage; fluorescence		Del Tito et al., 1998; Babon et al., 1999
	Endonuclease cleavage/microchip electrophoresis	EMD (Variagenics)	Schmalzing et al., 2000
	DHPLC	(Transgenomic)	Giordano et al., 1999
Allele-specific ligation	FRET	DOL	
	FRET	Molecular beacons	
	FRET/rolling circle replication	Padlock probes	
	MALDI-TOF; HPLC	LCR	Jurinke et al., 1996

Notes:

[a] The methods are classified according to allele discrimination strategies and detection methods; when a few variants exist for a given method, the references are presented respective to the variants.

[b] Particularity: refers to a specialized discrimination or detection technique, within a more general category.

[c] The literature cited in the table refers, when possible, to applications of the relevant method, rather than its description.

See the text for explanation of the techniques indicated by abbreviations.

Primer-extension and minisequencing

After amplification of a fragment of the SNP-containing DNA, an oligonucleotide primer is annealed immediately upstream to the polymorphism. In the presence of the appropriate nucleotides, the primer is extended by one or more bases (Fig. 21.1). The alleles can then be distinguished on the basis of size or mass of the extended product either by mass spectrometry or DHPLC (denaturing high performance liquid chromatography), according to specific fluorescence of the incorporated nucleotide (see template directed dye incorporation (TDI) below), by regular electrophoresis-based sequencing techniques, or through hybridization on a high density oligonucleotide array (Yershov et al., 1996). The Pyrosequencing™ strategy (Ahmadian et al., 2000) detects pyrophosphate molecules as they are released during incorporation of the nucleotides in the minisequencing reaction. In the competitive oligonucleotide single base extension (COSBE) assay (Higgins et al., 1997), two primers are simultaneously added to the reaction, corresponding to the alternate alleles; only the perfectly matched primer is extended.

Allele-specific hybridization

The amplified fragments are hybridized over an array of sequence-specific oligonucleotides, using high-stringency hybridization conditions to allow single-base mismatch detection (Saiki et al., 1989; Sapolsky et al., 1999). By using multiplex PCR techniques, many SNPs can be tested simultaneously for each DNA sample (Wang et al., 1998). The dynamic allele specific hybridization (DASH) follows the fluorescence accumulating by a dye binding to double-stranded DNA (e.g., SYBR-green), as the PCR products are hybridized with an allele-specific probe. More specialized hybridization probes have been developed for the purpose of SNP genotyping and are detailed below.

Heteroduplex/homoduplex resolution

If the two allelic forms are present during PCR amplification, heteroduplexes will be formed as a result of annealing between the alternative alleles. Homoduplexes can be distinguished from heteroduplexes either through DHPLC (Giordano et al., 1999) or by enzymatic cleavage of the mismatched molecule (Youil et al., 1995), followed by electrophoretical separation of the digested products. In both methods, artificial heteroduplexes are obtained by addition of wild-type DNA to the tested sample.

Allele-specific ligation

OLA or oligonucleotide ligation assay (Landegren et al., 1988) relies on the high sensitivity of the ligation reaction to mismatches. The amplified fragments are hybridized to allele-specific fluorescent probes. Ligation to a second oligonucleotide will

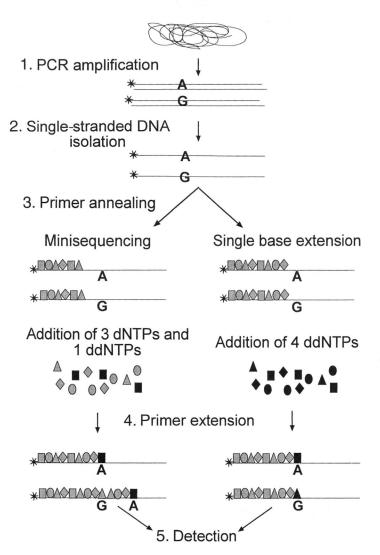

1. PCR amplification

2. Single-stranded DNA isolation

3. Primer annealing

Minisequencing Single base extension

Addition of 3 dNTPs and 1 ddNTPs Addition of 4 ddNTPs

4. Primer extension

5. Detection

Fig. 21.1   Single nucleotide polymorphism (SNP) discrimination by primer extension. Step 1, a SNP-containing DNA fragment is amplified by the polymerase chain reaction (PCR), using one biotinylated (*) primer. Step 2, the single-strand biotinylated, products are purified. Step 3, a new primer is annealed to the single-strand product, upstream to the polymorphic site. Minisequencing primers are typically designated to anneal a few bases away from the SNP, while single-base extension primers anneal immediately adjacent to it. Step 4, primer extension occurs. In minisequencing, the primer extension reaction is carried out in the presence of three deoxynucleotides (dNTP) and one dideoxynucleotide (ddNTP; chain terminator), corresponding to one of the dimorphic nucleotides (for example, ddTTP to complement A on the PCR product). The primer extension proceeds until the chain terminator is incorporated. If the amplified product carries the alternative base, the reaction proceeds through the polymorphic site until it reaches the next nucleotide complementary to the chain terminator. The alleles are resolved according to their size. In single-base extension, the primer extension reaction is carried out in the presence of all four chain terminators, allowing incorporation of a single dideoxynucleotide complementary to the variant nucleotide. Step 5, differential label of the terminators allows identification of the incorporated dideoxynucleotide.

take place only when the probe is perfectly annealed at the polymorphic site. The reaction products are analyzed by enzyme-linked immunosorbant assays (ELISA) (Tobe et al., 1996) or through fluorescence energy resonance transfer (FRET) detection (see below).

Allele detection

Various detection approaches are applicable to the different strategies, based on separation of alternative alleles, or differential detection according to allele-specific labels.

Labeling the amplified product

Labeling is usually necessary and can be achieved either homogeneously or in an allele-specific way. Fluorimetric plus colorimetric detection and phosphorimaging are based on homogeneous internal labeling (fluorescent or radioactive, respectively) of the amplified product or incorporation of a fluorescent dye (e.g. ethidium bromide, or SYBR-green) to the final product. In the minisequencing format, the use of distinct fluorescent labels for the alternative dideoxynucleotides at the SNP site allows direct discrimination between the alleles.

Electrophoresis

Electrophoresis has for long been a choice separation technique for DNA molecular studies. Agarose or acrylamide gel electrophoresis is used for low-throughput analysis of restriction digestion products or sequencing reactions, respectively. These basic methods have been adapted to higher throughput demands, by means of MADGE (microtiter array diagonal electrophoresis; Bolla et al., 1995) or microchip electrophoresis (Schmalzing et al., 2000). Acrylamide gels tend to be replaced by capillary electrophoresis.

Molecular conformation

Under partially denaturing conditions, molecular conformation is sensitive to single base substitutions, which allows allele identification by capillary electrophoresis: single-strand conformation polymorphism (CE-SSCP; Inazuka et al., 1997). Heteroduplexes are identified according to the molecular conformation by CSGE (conformation sensitive gel electrophoresis) recently adapted to higher throughput by capillary CSGE (Rozycka et al., 2000).

Denaturing high performance liquid chromatography

DHPLC has proven an efficient method for heteroduplex identification. Each sample is tested in two separate wells, in one alone and in the other after the wild-type allele is added. Heterozygotes give two peaks and homozygotes give one peak when tested alone. Homozygotes give two peaks after addition of the reference allele only if they possess the alternative allele. DHPLC is also efficient for minisequencing resolution (Hoogendoorn et al., 1999).

MALDI-TOF mass spectrometry

Mass spectrometry (MS) is used to measure the mass-to-charge ratio of ions, from which their molecular weight is inferred. A few MS techniques are applicable to DNA analysis. MALDI (matrix-assisted laser desorption-ionization) allows the production of gas-phase ions from solution and solid phases. In MALDI-TOF, MALDI is coupled to a time-of-flight (TOF) analyzer, in which a detector accurately measures the time required for an ion to traverse the distance between the ion source and detector. SNPs are accurately analyzed by MALDI-TOF in various allele discrimination formats (Griffin and Smith, 2000).

Fluorescence resonance energy transfer

FRET occurs between a fluorescence donor and a fluorescence acceptor in close proximity, if the emission spectrum of the donor overlaps with the excitation spectrum of the acceptor. If the acceptor is nonfluorescent, it acts as a quencher, resulting in a net decrease in photon emission from the donor. If the acceptor is also fluorescent, the decrease in emission from the donor is concomitant with an increase in fluorescence at the emission wavelength of A. The efficiency of energy transfer decreases very rapidly with increasing distance between the donor and acceptor, allowing its use for allele detection in a variety of applications (De Angelis, 1999): TaqMan, realtime PCR, molecular beacons, dye-labeled oligonucleotide ligation (DOL), TDI, Invader (see below).

Fluorescence polarization

Fluorescence polarization takes advantage of the mobility of molecules in solution: fluorescent free nucleotides are more mobile and will, therefore, show no polarization, while nucleotides that have been incorporated in a primer extension reaction to a larger oligonucleotide primer will be detected as polarized molecules, resulting in an amplification of the fluorescence signal.

Methods employing highly specialized probes

Based on the above techniques, specialized probes have been developed that enable a more accurate and/or sensitive assay for genotyping of SNPs.

TaqMan (5′ exonuclease assay)

TaqMan (5′ exonuclease assay; Livak et al., 1995) involves short oligonucleotides probes that undergo FRET in their intact state because they are labeled at each end with a fluorescence donor and acceptor pair. The probe is designed to hybridize to a sequence being amplified in a PCR reaction. If there is a perfect match between the probe and the target, the 5′ exonuclease activity of Taq polymerase will digest the hybridized TaqMan probe during the elongation cycle, separating the donor from the acceptor and resulting in a decrease in FRET.

Molecular beacons

Molecular beacons (Tyagi et al., 1998) are oligonucleotide probes that are chemically modified with a fluorescence donor at their 5′ end and a nonfluorescent quenching acceptor at their 3′ end. In the absence of a perfectly matched target, they assume a stem-and-loop structure in solution. This hairpin conformation positions the donor and the quencher in extremely close proximity, much closer than a pair of fluorophores at opposite ends of a randomly coiled oligonucleotide, resulting in effective fluorescence quenching. In the presence of a perfectly matched sequence, the hairpin loop hybridizes to the target, thus preventing the folding of the probe and separating the donor from the quencher and resulting in a fluorescence increase. The ability of molecular beacons to form hairpin structures significantly enhances their specificity compared with standard oligonucleotide probes of the same size. Scorpion primers (Thelwell et al., 2000) combine the properties of a PCR primer and of a FRET probe similar to the molecular beacons. Sunrise probes (Nazarenko et al., 1997) are hairpin-FRET PCR probes; the FRET is allowed when the hairpin structure serves as a template in the PCR reaction, after a primary round resulting in incorporation of the primers in the template DNA.

Dye-labeled oligonucleotide ligation

DOL (Chen et al., 1998) relies on a ligation assay. The method utilizes two oligonucleotides, one labeled with a fluorescence donor and the other with an acceptor. The probes are designed to hybridize adjacently across the polymorphic site; if both oligonucleotides match perfectly, DNA ligase can join the fragments together, resulting in FRET. A mismatch at the ligation site will result in failure of the ligase to link the labeled oligonucleotides, thus preventing FRET.

Template-directed dye incorporation

TDI (Chen et al., 1997) is a primer-extension strategy based on the FRET detection assay. The primer to be extended is labeled with a fluorescent donor. Incorporation of an acceptor-labeled nucleotide, by the primer extension reaction, brings the fluorophores in close proximity, thus resulting in FRET.

Peptide nucleic acid hybridization probes

Peptide nucleic acid (PNA; Corey, 1997) is a DNA analog containing the four normal nucleotides of DNA attached to a neutrally charged amide backbone. The neutral backbone confers unique characteristics on the hybridization of PNA with DNA, resulting in improved hybridization specificity for complementary DNA sequences. Two similar SNP genotyping approaches using PNA have been independently developed (Griffin et al., 1997; Ross et al., 1997). In both methods, allele-specific PNA probes are hybridized to amplified SNP fragment. The captured PNA are later purified and analyzed by MALDI-TOF MS. Each uniquely mass-labeled PNA probe detected corresponds to a specific SNP allele present in the PCR amplicon.

Non-PCR based strategies and further improvements of general techniques

Ligase chain reaction

In the ligase chain reaction assay (LCR; Barany, 1991), a recurrent ligation reaction is performed on the DNA sample, resulting in an amplified, allele-specific ligation product, which is later detected by usual methods, such as electrophoresis.

Invader™ assay

Invader™ assay involves the sequence-specific hybridization of two oligonucleotides to form a one-base overlapping structure at the polymorphic position (Fig. 21.2). This is followed by enzymatic cleavage of an allele-specific downstream probe, using a "flap" endonuclease. A large excess of the overlapping probe in the reaction results in an amplification of the cleaved product, relative to the original DNA sample. The cleaved product serves as an invader upstream oligonucleotide in a secondary reaction, in which cleavage of the probe results in FRET. A modified version (Griffin et al., 1999) of this assay allows detection by MALDI-TOF MS.

Padlock probes

Padlock probes (Nilsson et al., 1994) are linear oligonucleotides in which the 5′ and 3′ end regions are designed to base-pair next to each other on a target strand. If properly hybridized, then the ends can be joined by enzymatic ligation, converting the probes to circularly closed molecules that are catenated to the target sequences. Because the reaction products remain localized at their target, these probes are suitable for simultaneous analysis of many genes. Many tandem copies of the complement to the circularized molecule can be generated by rolling circle replication (RCR; Baner et al., 1998), resulting in amplification of the detection signals.

Light-up probes

Light-up probes (Isacsson et al., 2000) are PNA probes labeled with a fluorescent dye that has low fluorescence in its unbound state but generates a readily detectable signal when hybridized to its target sequence. This eliminates the need to separate unbound probes from the hybridization complex prior to detection.

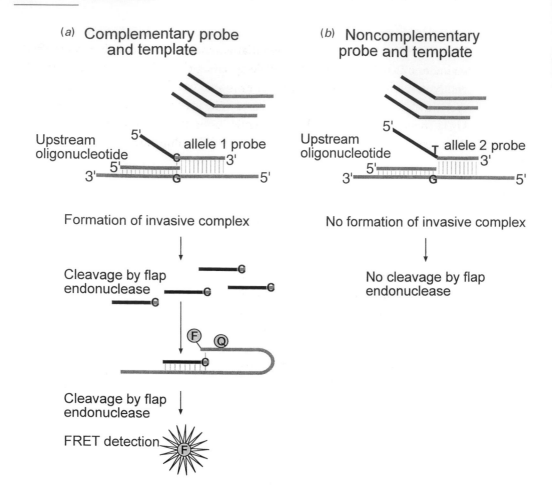

(a) **Complementary probe and template**

(b) **Noncomplementary probe and template**

Fig. 21.2.   Invasive complex cleavage. Two oligonucleotides are simultaneously annealed to the target genomic sequence: A probe and an upstream oligonucleotide are designed to overlap at the single nucleotide polymorphism (SNP). The probe contains an allele-specific region, which forms a duplex with the target, and a noncomplementary 5′ arm region, which serves as a reporter molecule precursor. Cleavage of the downstream probe occurs only when the probe and the upstream oligonucleotide overlap (as in (a) but not in (b)), thus forming at the SNP an invasive complex that is recognized by the flap endonuclease. The cleaved 5′ arm of the probe is used to drive a secondary invasive reaction, resulting in fluorescence energy resonance transfer (FRET) detection.

Realtime polymerase chain reaction

The realtime PCR approach allows simultaneous allele discrimination and detection (Higuchi et al., 1993; Nitsche et al., 1999). A few techniques can be applied in this way, including TaqMan, molecular beacons, allele specific hybridization, and allele-specific amplification. Detection is achieved by FRET, or by fluorescence detection of SYBR-green.

Kinetic polymerase chain reaction

Kinetic PCR is based on the differential amplification of the alternative alleles, owing to mismatch pairing of an allele-specific primer. The mismatched product will be amplified at a lower rate, and thus its realtime detection will occur at a later cycle than the full-match allele. Realtime PCR is conveniently performed on the LightCycler (Roche Molecular Biochemicals) or the ABI PRISM 7700 (Applied Biosystems), which combine a thermocycler with a fluorimeter.

Conclusions

The impressive surge in research in genomics of the last few years has yielded a powerful groundwork for genetic studies, consisting of a high-density SNP genome map, on the one hand, and a wealth of elaborate techniques for high-throughput genotyping, on the other. Even with these tools, the comprehensive dissection of the complex mechanisms of drug response will still be a long drawn-out process, but the impact on medicine will be enormous.

Pharmacogenomics aims at establishing a signature of DNA sequence variants that are characteristic of individual patients in order to assess disease susceptibility and select the optimal drug treatment. As opposed to more generalized genomic studies, pharmacogenomics compares, among affected individuals, the genetic profile of drug responders with that of nonresponders. This approach addresses the complexity of drug response and provides a rational basis for accurately prescribing drugs only to those who will benefit from their use.

Ultimately, as all human genes are discovered, the need for random SNP markers diminishes and gene-based SNP approaches will predominate. This will include not only cSNPs but, most probably, also noncoding SNPs located in the regulatory regions of candidate genes. Common polymorphisms in drug targets dictate that DNA sequence variations are taken into account in the genomic screening processes aimed at new drug development. This will provide new insights for the development of medications that target critical pathways in disease pathogenesis and medications that can be used to prevent diseases in individuals who are genetically predisposed to them. One such approach is exemplified in a recent study showing association between *CYP2D6* variants and Abnormal Involuntary Movement Scale (AIMS) score in schizophrenic patients treated with antipsychotic drugs (Ellingrod et al., 2000).

Implicit in the use of SNP information in both disease-target identification and in preclinical drug development is the consequence that individualized drug prescribing will arise. If a drug is developed with the knowledge that its efficacy or safety is correlated with a specific set of SNPs, then ultimately the use of the drug must be linked to a diagnostic test for that genetic profile. For drugs already on the market, a SNP diagnostic test could be developed to predict the safer and more efficacious use of a compound that may be toxic or not always efficient by allowing the drug prescription only to the patients with a favorable SNP signature.

The application of SNP profiling to the process of drug development and to the rational prescribing of medications developed in this way promises to be one of the most important outgrowths of the Human Genome Project, providing the opportunity for significantly improved health-care delivery in the future.

Acknowledgements

The authors thank Dr Meira Sternfeld for critical reading of the manuscript and for graphic artwork. Ariel Darvasi was supported by the FIRST foundation of the Israel Academy of Sciences.

REFERENCES

Ahmadian A, Gharizadeh B, Gustafsson AC et al. (2000). Single-nucleotide polymorphism analysis by pyrosequencing. *Anal Biochem* 280, 103–110.

Alderborn A, Kristofferson A, Hammerling U (2000). Determination of single-nucleotide polymorphisms by real-time pyrophosphate DNA sequencing. *Genome Res* 10, 1249–1258.

Babon JJ, McKenzie M, Cotton RG (1999). Mutation detection using fluorescent enzyme mismatch cleavage with T4 endonuclease VII. *Electrophoresis* 20, 1162–1170.

Baner J, Nilsson M, Mendel-Hartvig M, Landegren U (1998). Signal amplification of padlock probes by rolling circle replication. *Nucl Acids Res* 26, 5073–5078.

Barany F (1991). Genetic disease detection and DNA amplification using cloned thermostable ligase. *Proc Nat Acad Sci USA* 88, 189–193.

Bolla MK, Haddad L, Humphries SE, Winder AF, Day IN (1995). High-throughput method for determination of apolipoprotein E genotypes with use of restriction digestion analysis by microplate array diagonal gel electrophoresis. *Clin Chem* 41, 1599–1604.

Braun A, Little DP, Koster H (1997). Detecting CFTR gene mutations by using primer oligo base extension and mass spectrometry. *Clin Chem* 43, 1151–1158.

Brookes AJ (1999). The essence of SNPs. *Gene* 234, 177–186.

Cai H, White PS, Torney D et al. (2000). Flow cytometry-based minisequencing: a new platform for high-throughput single-nucleotide polymorphism scoring. *Genomics* 66, 135–143.

Cargill M, Altshuler D, Ireland J et al. (1999). Characterization of single-nucleotide polymorphisms in coding regions of human genes. [Published erratum appears in *Nat Genet* (1999) 23, 373.] *Nat Genet* 22, 231–238.

Chen X, Kwok PY (1997). Template-directed dye-terminator incorporation (TDI) assay: a homogeneous DNA diagnostic method based on fluorescence resonance energy transfer. *Nuc Acids Res* 25, 347–353.

Chen X, Zehbauer B, Gnirke A, Kwok PY (1997). Fluorescence energy transfer detection as a homogeneous DNA diagnostic method. *Proc Nat Acad Sci USA* 94, 10756–10761.

Chen X, Livak KJ, Kwok PY (1998). A homogeneous, ligase-mediated DNA diagnostic test. *Genome Res* 8, 549–556.

Chen X, Levine L, Kwok PY (1999). Fluorescence polarization in homogeneous nucleic acid analysis. *Genome Res* 9, 492–498.

Collins FS, Guyer MS, Charkravarti A (1997). Variations on a theme: cataloging human DNA sequence variation. *Science* 278, 1580–1581.

Cooper DN, Clayton JF (1988). DNA polymorphism and the study of disease associations. *Hum Genet* 78, 299–312.

Corey DR (1997). Peptide nucleic acids: expanding the scope of nucleic acid recognition. *Trends Biotechnol* 15, 224–229.

De Angelis DA (1999). Why FRET over genomics? [In process citation] *Physiol Genomics* 1, 93–99.

Del Tito BJ Jr., Poff HE, III, Novotny MA et al. (1998). Automated fluorescent analysis procedure for enzymatic mutation detection. *Clin Chem* 44, 731–739.

Ellingrod VL, Schultz SK, Arndt S (2000). Association between cytochrome P4502D6 (*CYP2D6*) genotype, antipsychotic exposure, and abnormal involuntary movement scale (AIMS) score. *Psychiatr Genet* 10, 9–11.

Evans WE, Relling MV (1999). Pharmacogenomics: translating functional genomics into rational therapeutics. *Science* 286, 487–491.

Germer S, Higuchi R (1999). Single-tube genotyping without oligonucleotide probes. *Genome Res* 9, 72–78.

Germer S, Holland MJ, Higuchi R (2000). High-throughput SNP allele-frequency determination in pooled DNA samples by kinetic PCR. *Genome Res* 10, 258–266.

Gibson NJ, Gillard HL, Whitcombe D, Ferrie RM, Newton CR, Little S (1997). A homogeneous method for genotyping with fluorescence polarization. *Clin Chem* 43, 1336–1341.

Giordano M, Oefner PJ, Underhill PA, Cavalli Sforza LL, Tosi R, Richiardi PM (1999). Identification by denaturing high-performance liquid chromatography of numerous polymorphisms in a candidate region for multiple sclerosis susceptibility. *Genomics* 56, 247–253.

Gray IC, Campbell DA, Spurr NK (2000). Single nucleotide polymorphisms as tools in human genetics [in process citation]. *Hum Mol Genet* 9, 2403–2408.

Griffin TJ, Smith LM (2000). Single-nucleotide polymorphism analysis by MALDI-TOF mass spectrometry. *Trends Biotechnol* 18, 77–84.

Griffin TJ, Tang W, Smith LM (1997). Genetic analysis by peptide nucleic acid affinity MALDI-TOF mass spectrometry [see comments]. *Nat Biotechnol* 15, 1368–1372.

Griffin TJ, Hall JG, Prudent JR, Smith LM (1999). Direct genetic analysis by matrix-assisted laser desorption/ionization mass spectrometry. *Proc Nat Acad Sci USA* 96, 6301–6306.

Haff LA, Smirnov IP (1997). Single-nucleotide polymorphism identification assays using a thermostable DNA polymerase and delayed extraction MALDI-TOF mass spectrometry. *Genome Res* 7, 378–388.

Higgins GS, Little DP, Koster H (1997). Competitive oligonucleotide single-base extension combined with mass spectrometric detection for mutation screening. *Biotechniques* 23, 710–714.

Higuchi R, Fockler C, Dollinger G, Watson R (1993). Kinetic PCR analysis: real-time monitoring of DNA amplification reactions. *Biotechnology (New York)* 11, 1026–1030.

Hirschhorn JN, Sklar P, Lindblad-Toh K et al. (2000). SBE-TAGS: an array-based method for efficient single-nucleotide polymorphism genotyping. [In Process Citation] *Proc Natl Acad Sci USA* 97, 12164–12169.

Hoogendoorn B, Owen MJ, Oefner PJ, Williams N, Austin J, O'Donovan MC (1999). Genotyping single nucleotide polymorphisms by primer extension and high performance liquid chromatography. *Hum Genet* 104, 89–93.

Howell WM, Jobs M, Gyllensten U, Brookes AJ (1999). Dynamic allele-specific hybridization. A new method for scoring single nucleotide polymorphisms. *Nat Biotechnol* 17, 87–88.

Inazuka M, Wenz HM, Sakabe M, Tahira T, Hayashi K (1997). A streamlined mutation detection system: multicolor post-PCR fluorescence labeling and single-strand conformational polymorphism analysis by capillary electrophoresis. *Genome Res* 7, 1094–1103.

Isacsson J, Cao H, Ohlsson L et al. (2000). Rapid and specific detection of PCR products using light-up probes [in process citation]. *Mol Cell Probes* 14, 321–328.

Jurinke C, van den Boom D, Jacob A, Tang K, Worl R, Koster H (1996). Analysis of ligase chain reaction products via matrix-assisted laser desorption/ionization time-of-flight-mass spectrometry. *Anal Biochem* 237, 174–181.

Kruglyak L (1999). Prospects for whole-genome linkage disequilibrium mapping of common disease genes. *Nat Genet* 22, 139–144.

Landegren U, Kaiser R, Sanders J, Hood L (1988). A ligase-mediated gene detection technique. *Science* 241, 1077–1080.

Landegren U, Nilsson M, Kwok PY (1998). Reading bits of genetic information: methods for single-nucleotide polymorphism analysis. *Genome Res* 8, 769–776.

Livak KJ, Marmaro J, Todd JA (1995). Towards fully automated genome-wide polymorphism screening [letter]. *Nat Genet* 9, 341–342.

Lyamichev V, Mast AL, Hall JG et al. (1999). Polymorphism identification and quantitative detection of genomic DNA by invasive cleavage of oligonucleotide probes. *Nat Biotechnol* 17, 292–296.

Marshall E (1999). Drug firms to create public database of genetic mutations [news; see comments]. *Science* 284, 406–407.

McCarthy JJ, Hilfiker R (2000). The use of single-nucleotide polymorphism maps in pharmacogenomics. *Nat Biotechnol* 18, 505–508.

Middle F, Jones I, McCandless F et al. (2000). Bipolar disorder and variation at a common polymorphism (A1832G) within exon 8 of the *wolfram* gene. *Am J Med Genet* 96, 154–157.

Motulsky A (1957). Drug reactions, enzymes and biochemical genetics. *J Am Med Assoc* 165, 835–837.

Nauck M, Wieland H, Marz W (1999). Rapid, homogeneous genotyping of the 4G/5G polymorphism in the promoter region of the *PAII* gene by fluorescence resonance energy transfer and probe melting curves. *Clin Chem* 45, 1141–1147.

Nazarenko IA, Bhatnagar SK, Hohman RJ (1997). A closed tube format for amplification and detection of DNA based on energy transfer. *Nucl Acids Res* 25, 2516–2521.

Newton CR, Graham A, Heptinstall LE et al. (1989). Analysis of any point mutation in DNA. The amplification refractory mutation system (ARMS). *Nucl Acids Res* 17, 2503–2516.

Nilsson M, Malmgren H, Samiotaki M, Kwiatkowski M, Chowdhary BP, Landegren U (1994). Padlock probes: circularizing oligonucleotides for localized DNA detection. *Science* 265, 2085–2088.

Nitsche A, Steurer N, Schmidt CA, Landt O, Siegert W (1999). Different real-time PCR formats compared for the quantitative detection of human cytomegalovirus DNA. *Clin Chem* 45, 1932–1937.

Pastinen T, Partanen J, Syvanen AC (1996). Multiplex, fluorescent, solid-phase minisequencing for efficient screening of DNA sequence variation. *Clin Chem* 42, 1391–1397.

Ravine D (1999). Automated mutation analysis. *J Inherit Metab Dis* 22, 503–518.

Risch N, Merikangas K (1996). The future of genetic studies of complex human diseases [see comments]. *Science* 273, 1516–1517.

Ross PL, Lee K, Belgrader P (1997). Discrimination of single-nucleotide polymorphisms in human DNA using peptide nucleic acid probes detected by MALDI-TOF mass spectrometry. *Anal Chem* 69, 4197–4202.

Ross PL, Hall L, Smirnov I, Haff L (1998). High level multiplex genotyping by MALDI-TOF mass spectrometry [see comments]. *Nat Biotechnol* 16, 1347–1351.

Rozycka M, Collins N, Stratton MR, Wooster R (2000). Rapid detection of DNA sequence variants by conformation-sensitive capillary electrophoresis. *Genomics* 70, 34–40.

Saiki RK, Walsh PS, Levenson CH, Erlich HA (1989). Genetic analysis of amplified DNA with immobilized sequence-specific oligonucleotide probes. *Proc Nat Acad Sci USA* 86, 6230–6234.

Sapolsky RJ, Hsie L, Berno A, Ghandour G, Mittmann M, Fan JB (1999). High-throughput polymorphism screening and genotyping with high-density oligonucleotide arrays. *Genet Anal* 14, 187–192.

Sauer S, Lechner D, Berlin K et al. (2000). Full flexibility genotyping of single nucleotide polymorphisms by the GOOD assay. *Nucl Acids Res* 28, E100.

Schmalzing D, Belenky A, Novotny MA et al. (2000). Microchip electrophoresis: a method for high-speed SNP detection. *Nucl Acids Res* 28, E43.

Srinivasan JR, Kachman MT, Kileen AA, Akel N, Siemieniak D, Lubman DM (1998). Genotyping of apolipoprotein E by matrix-assisted laser desorption/ionization time-of-flight mass spectrometry. *Rapid Commun Mass Spectrom* 12, 1045–1050.

Sun X, Ding H, Hung K, Guo B (2000). A new MALDI-TOF based mini-sequencing assay for genotyping of SNPS. *Nuc Acids Res* 28, E68.

Thelwell N, Millington S, Solinas A, Booth J, Brown T (2000). Mode of action and application of scorpion primers to mutation detection [in process citation]. *Nucl Acids Res* 28, 3752–3761.

Tobe VO, Taylor SL, Nickerson DA (1996). Single-well genotyping of diallelic sequence variations by a two-color ELISA-based oligonucleotide ligation assay. *Nucl Acids Res* 24, 3728–3732.

Tyagi S, Bratu DP, Kramer FR (1998). Multicolor molecular beacons for allele discrimination. *Nat Biotechnol* 16, 49–53.

Wang DG, Fan JB, Siao CJ et al. (1998). Large-scale identification, mapping, and genotyping of single-nucleotide polymorphisms in the human genome. *Science* 280, 1077–1082.

Whitcombe D, Newton CR, Little S (1998). Advances in approaches to DNA-based diagnostics. *Curr Opin Biotechnol* 9, 602–608.

Wu YY, Delgado R, Costello R, Sunderland T, Dukoff R, Csako G (2000). Quantitative assessment of apolipoprotein E genotypes by image analysis of PCR-RFLP fragments. *Clin Chim Acta* 293, 213–221.

Yershov G, Barsky V, Belgovskiy A et al. (1996). DNA analysis and diagnostics on oligonucleotide microchips. *Proc Nat Acad Sci USA* 93, 4913–4918.

Youil R, Kemper BW, Cotton RG (1995). Screening for mutations by enzyme mismatch cleavage with T4 endonuclease VII. *Proc Nat Acad Sci USA* 92, 87–91.

Index